Medical Management
of the Surgical Patient

Medical Management of the Surgical Patient

3rd edition

Geno J. Merli, MD, FACP

Professor of Medicine
Jefferson Medical College of Thomas Jefferson
    University
Director, Jefferson Center for Vascular Disease
Chief Medical Officer and Senior Vice President
Thomas Jefferson University Hospital
Philadelphia, Pennsylvania

Howard H. Weitz, MD, FACC, FACP

Professor of Medicine
Senior Vice Chair for Academic Affairs
Jefferson Medical College of Thomas Jefferson
    University
Co-Director, Jefferson Heart Institute
Thomas Jefferson University Hospital
Philadelphia, Pennsylvania

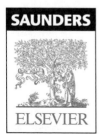

SAUNDERS

ELSEVIER

SAUNDERS
ELSEVIER

1600 John F. Kennedy Boulevard
Suite 1800
Philadelphia, Pennsylvania 19103

MEDICAL MANAGEMENT OF THE SURGICAL PATIENT, 3rd ed.
ISBN: 978-1-4160-2385-2

Notice

Knowledge and best practice in this field are constantly changing. As new research
and experience broaden our knowledge, changes in practice, treatment and drug
therapy may become necessary or appropriate. Readers are advised to check the
most current information provided (i) on procedures featured or (ii) by the manufacturer of each product to be administered, to verify the recommended dose or
formula, the method and duration of administration, and contraindications. It is
the responsibility of practitioners, relying on their own experience and knowledge
of the patient, to make diagnoses, to determine dosages and the best treatment for
each individual patient, and to take all appropriate safety precautions. To the fullest
extent of the law, neither the Publisher nor the editors assume any liability for any
injury and/or damage to persons or property arising out of or related to any use of
the material contained in this book.

Library of Congress Cataloging-in-Publication Data
Medical management of the surgical patient / [edited by] Geno J. Merli, Howard H.
Weitz.—3rd ed.
  p. ; cm.
  Includes bibliographical references and index.
  ISBN 978-1-4160-2385-2
1. Therapeutics, Surgical. I. Merli, Geno J. II. Weitz, Howard H.
  [DNLM: 1. Perioperative CAre. 2. Intraoperative Complications. 3. Postoperative
Complications. 4. Surgical Procedures, Operative. WO 178 M4895 2008]

RD49.M43 2008
617'.9192--dc22   2007041425

Acquisitions Editor: Druanne Martin
Developmental Editor: John Ingram
Publishing Services Manager: Frank Polizzano
Project Manager: Lee Ann Draud
Design Direction: Ellen Zanolle

Printed in the United States of America

Last digit is the print number: 9 8 7 6 5 4 3 2 1

Working together to grow
libraries in developing countries
www.elsevier.com | www.bookaid.org | www.sabre.org

ELSEVIER   BOOK AID   Sabre Foundation

To our wives,
Charlotte
and
Barbara

Contributors

INTEKHAB AHMED, MD
Associate Professor of Clinical Medicine, Jefferson Medical
College of Thomas Jefferson University, Philadelphia,
Pennsylvania
Perioperative Management of Endocrine Disorders

ROBERT F. ATKINS, MD
Anesthesiologist, Department of Anesthesiology, Abington
Memorial Hospital, Abington, Pennsylvania
Selected Medical Challenges of Anesthesia

RODNEY D. BELL, MD
Professor of Neurology and Vice-Chairman for Hospital
Affairs, Department of Neurology, Jefferson Medical College
of Thomas Jefferson University, Philadelphia, Pennsylvania
*Perioperative Assessment and Management of the Surgical Patient
with Neurologic Problems*

BARTOLOME R. CELLI, MD
Professor of Medicine, Tufts University School of Medicine;
Chief, Pulmonary/Critical Care Medicine, St. Elizabeth's
Medical Center, Boston, Massachusetts
*Perioperative Assessment with Management of Patients with
Pulmonary Diseases*

GRETCHEN DIEMER, MD
Clinical Instructor of Medicine, Jefferson Medical College
of Thomas Jefferson University; Assistant Residency
Program Director, Department of Internal Medicine,
Thomas Jefferson University Hospital, Philadelphia,
Pennsylvania
Managing Medication in the Perioperative Period

JOHN A. EVANS, MD
Assistant Professor of Medicine, Duke University School of Medicine, Durham, North Carolina
Gastrointestinal Complications in the Postoperative Period

FREDERICK M. FELLIN, MD
Assistant Professor of Medicine, Jefferson Medical College of Thomas Jefferson University, Philadelphia, Pennsylvania
Perioperative Evaluation of Patients with Hematologic Disorders

JAMES FINK, MD
Instructor of Medicine, Jefferson Medical College of Thomas Jefferson University; Director, Jefferson Hospital Medicine Program, Thomas Jefferson University Hospital, Philadelphia, Pennsylvania
Bariatric Surgery: Preoperative Evaluation and Postoperative Care

DAVID G. FORCIONE, MD
Instructor in Medicine, Harvard Medical School, Boston, Massachusetts
Gastrointestinal Complications in the Postoperative Period

LAWRENCE S. FRIEDMAN, MD
Professor of Medicine, Harvard Medical School, Boston; Professor of Medicine, Tufts University School of Medicine, Boston; Chair, Department of Medicine, Newton-Wellesley Hospital, Newton; Assistant Chief of Medicine, Massachusetts General Hospital, Boston, Massachusetts
Gastrointestinal Complications in the Postoperative Period; Management of the Surgical Patient with Liver Disease

KEVIN FURLONG, DO
Clinical Assistant Professor of Medicine, Jefferson Medical College of Thomas Jefferson University, Philadelphia, Pennsylvania
Perioperative Management of Endocrine Disorders

DEBORAH T. GLASSMAN, MD
Clinical Assistant Professor of Urology, Jefferson Medical
College of Thomas Jefferson University,
Philadelphia, Pennsylvania
Appendix D: Urologic Surgery

MARVIN E. GOZUM, MD
Clinical Assistant Professor of Medicine, Jefferson Medical
College of Thomas Jefferson University; Director of Jefferson
Hospital for the Neurosciences Preoperative Assessment
Center, Division of Internal Medicine, Jefferson Hospital
for the Neurosciences, Philadelphia, Pennsylvania
Perioperative Management of the Ophthalmologic Patient;
Appendix F: Ophthalmologic Surgery

MARK G. GRAHAM, MD
Associate Professor of Medicine, Jefferson Medical College
of Thomas Jefferson University; Director, Jefferson
Hospital Ambulatory Practice, and Associate Director,
Internal Medicine Residency, Thomas Jefferson University
Hospital, Philadelphia, Pennsylvania
Appendix A: Thoracoscopy and Video-Assisted Thorascopic
Surgery; Appendix B: Laparoscopic Surgeries; Appendix E:
Otolaryngologic Surgery

BRENDA HOFFMAN, MD
Associate Professor of Clinical Medicine, University
of Pennsylvania School of Medicine, Philadelphia,
Pennsylvania
Surgery in the Patient with Kidney Disease

DANIEL K. HOLLERAN, MD

Assistant Professor, Jefferson Medical College of Thomas Jefferson University, Philadelphia, Pennsylvania
Perioperative Care of the Patient with Psychiatric Illness

SERGE JABBOUR, MD

Clinical Associate Professor of Medicine, Jefferson Medical College of Thomas Jefferson University, Philadelphia, Pennsylvania
Perioperative Management of Endocrine Disorders

GREGORY C. KANE, MD

Professor of Medicine, and Director, Residency Program, Jefferson Medical College of Thomas Jefferson University, Philadelphia, Pennsylvania
Perioperative Assessment and Management of Patients with Pulmonary Diseases

BARBARA KNIGHT, MD

Instructor, Jefferson Medical College of Thomas Jefferson University, Philadelphia, Pennsylvania
Nonobstetric Surgery in the Pregnant Patient

WALTER K. KRAFT, MD, MS, FACP

Assistant Professor of Pharmacology and Experimental Therapeutics, Jefferson Medical College of Thomas Jefferson University; Medical Director, Clinical Research Unit, Department of Pharmacology and Experimental Therapeutics, Thomas Jefferson University Hospital, Philadelphia, Pennsylvania
Managing Medication in the Perioperative Period

JANINE V. KYRILLOS, MD
Instructor, Division of Internal Medicine, Jefferson Medical College of Thomas Jefferson University; Director, Preventive Health Care Program, Jefferson Internal Medicine Associates, Philadelphia, Pennsylvania
Nonobstetric Surgery in the Pregnant Patient; Appendix E: Otolaryngologic Surgery

KENNETH LIEBMAN, MD
Assistant Professor of Neurosurgery, Jefferson Medical College of Thomas Jefferson University, Philadelphia, Pennsylvania
Appendix H: Neurosurgery

MICHAEL F. LUBIN, MD
Professor of Medicine, Emory University School of Medicine; Director, Preadmission Clinic, Grady Memorial Hospital, Atlanta, Georgia
Perioperative Care of the Elderly Patient

BRIAN F. MANDELL, MD, PHD
Professor and Vice-Chairman of Medicine, Cleveland Clinic Lerner College of Medicine of Case Western Reserve University; Attending Physician, Department of Rheumatic and Immunologic Disease, Cleveland Clinic, Cleveland, Ohio
Perioperative Management of the Patient with Arthritis or Systemic Autoimmune Disease

TRACY McGOWAN, MD
Associate Medical Director, Clinical Affairs, Ortho Biotech, Bridgewater, New Jersey
Surgery in the Patient with Kidney Disease

ROBERT E. MEASLEY, JR., MD
Clinical Assistant Professor of Medicine, Jefferson Medical
College of Thomas Jefferson University; Director of Clinical
Infectious Diseases, Thomas Jefferson University Hospital,
Philadelphia, Pennsylvania
Antimicrobial Prophylaxis: Prevention of Postoperative Infections

L. BERNARDO MENAJOVSKY, MD, MS
Clinical Assistant Professor of Medicine, Jefferson Medical
College of Thomas Jefferson University, Philadelphia,
Pennsylvania
*Prophylaxis for Deep Vein Thrombosis and Pulmonary Embolism
in the Surgical Patient*

GENO J. MERLI, MD, FACP
Professor of Medicine, Jefferson Medical College of Thomas
Jefferson University; Director, Jefferson Center for Vascular
Disease, and Chief Medical Officer and Senior Vice
President, Thomas Jefferson University Hospital,
Philadelphia, Pennsylvania
*The Role and Responsibility of the Medical Consultant;
Prophylaxis for Deep Vein Thrombosis and Pulmonary Embolism
in the Surgical Patient; Perioperative Assessment and
Management of the Surgical Patient with Neurologic Problems;
Appendix G: Orthopedic Surgery; Appendix H: Neurosurgery*

GREGORY MOKRYNSKI, MD
Instructor of Medicine, Jefferson Medical College of Thomas
Jefferson University, Philadelphia, Pennsylvania
Appendix A: Thoracoscopy and Video-Assisted Thorascopic Surgery

JOSEPH M. MONTELLA, MD
Clinical Assistant Professor of Obstetrics and Gynecology,
Jefferson Medical College of Thomas Jefferson University,
Philadelphia, Pennsylvania
Appendix C: Obstetric and Gynecologic Surgery

JACQUELINE G. O'LEARY, MD, MPH
Hepatologist, Baylor University Medical Center, Dallas, Texas
Management of the Surgical Patient with Liver Disease

JAVAD PARVIZI, MD
Associate Professor, Jefferson Medical College of Thomas
Jefferson University, Philadelphia, Pennsylvania
Appendix G: Orthopedic Surgery

JEFFREY M. RIGGIO, MD
Instructor of Medicine and Associate Medical Director of
Informatics, Jefferson Medical College of Thomas Jefferson
University, Philadelphia, Pennsylvania
Appendix B: Laparoscopic Surgeries

ELIZABETH TEPEROV, MD
Clinical Instructor of Medicine, Jefferson Medical College
of Thomas Jefferson University; Director, Hospital Medicine,
Jefferson Hospital for Neurosciences, Philadelphia,
Pennsylvania
The Patient with Substance Abuse Going to Surgery

GEORGE L. TZANIS, MD
Instructor of Medicine, Jefferson Medical College of Thomas
Jefferson University; Associate Director, Jefferson Center for
Vascular Diseases, Philadelphia, Pennsylvania
*Prophylaxis for Deep Vein Thrombosis and Pulmonary Embolism
in the Surgical Patient*

JENNY Y. WANG, MD
Assistant Professor, Jefferson Medical College of Thomas
Jefferson University; Associate Director, Jefferson Hospital
Medicine Program, Thomas Jefferson University Hospital,
Philadelphia, Pennsylvania
Perioperative Care of the Patient with Psychiatric Illness

HOWARD H. WEITZ, MD, FACC, FACP

Professor of Medicine and Senior Vice Chair for Academic Affairs, Jefferson Medical College of Thomas Jefferson University; Co-Director, Jefferson Heart Institute, Thomas Jefferson University Hospital, Philadelphia, Pennsylvania

> *The Role and Responsibility of the Medical Consultant;*
> *Noncardiac Surgery in the Patient with Cardiovascular Disease:*
> *Preoperative Evaluation and Perioperative Care*

SUSAN E. WEST, MD

Assistant Clinical Professor of Medicine, Division of Internal Medicine, Jefferson Medical College of Thomas Jefferson University, Philadelphia, Pennsylvania

> *Appendix C: Obstetric and Gynecologic Surgery; Appendix D:*
> *Urologic Surgery*

BARRY S. ZIRING, MD, MS, FACP

Clinical Assistant Professor, Jefferson Medical College of Thomas Jefferson University; Director, Division of Internal Medicine, Thomas Jefferson University Hospital, Philadelphia, Pennsylvania

> *Preoperative Assessment for the Healthy Patient; Perioperative*
> *Care of the Patient with Psychiatric Illness*

Contents

1 | The Role and Responsibility of the Medical Consultant

GENO J. MERLI, MD
HOWARD H. WEITZ, MD

The role and responsibilities of the medical consultant have changed over the past 30 years. During this time, articles, books, courses, and guidelines by medical societies have defined approaches to assessment, management, and therapeutic interventions to decrease perioperative risk and to provide better care for the surgical patient with medical problems in the perioperative period. This body of information has created an area of expertise and a required knowledge base for all medical consultants. With this ever-expanding database has emerged a defined order of responsibilities that are involved in the process of performing a medical consultation. In this chapter, we review the defined order of this process.

CONDUCT OF THE MEDICAL CONSULTANT

The Ten Commandments for effective consultation were proposed by Goldman and colleagues in 1983 (Box 1-1). These points are the major focus of every medical consultant providing this service in either the hospital or the outpatient setting. We have adapted these Ten Commandments to fit the role and responsibility of the medical consultant in 2007 (Box 1-2):

1. The consultant should know the reason for the consultation and should address only those issues that the requesting physician has indicated. Sometimes the requesting physician has not been clear about the primary reason for the consultation, or the reason for consultation may be listed as "patient known to you." In these

---

Box 1-1 | **TEN COMMANDMENTS OF MEDICAL CONSULTATION**

1. Determine the question.
2. Establish urgency.
3. Look for yourself.
4. Be as brief as appropriate.
5. Be specific.
6. Provide contingency plans.
7. Honor thy turf.
8. Teach with tact.
9. Talk is cheap and effective.
10. Follow up.

From Goldman L, Lee T, Rudd P: Ten commandments for effective consultation. Arch Intern Med 143:1753-1755, 1983.

Box 1-2 | **TEN COMMANDMENTS OF MEDICAL CONSULTATION: 2007**

1. Determine the question and address that question.
2. Perform the consultation in a timely manner.
3. Perform a thorough evaluation.
4. Write as concise a consultation report as appropriate.
5. Make recommendations clear and concise.
6. Provide prompt communication.
7. Do not "clear for OR." Identify risks and attempt to reverse them. Optimize the patient for surgery.
8. Provide appropriate follow-up.
9. Know your role: pure consultant versus co-manager.
10. Provide options and alternative approaches and teach with tact.

---

situations, communication with the requesting physician or the physician's designee is important for defining the focus of evaluation. The consultant's report should always state the reason for the consultation, for example, "Reason for consultation: preoperative evaluation for surgery" or "Asked to evaluate patient for postoperative change in mental status." If another problem unrelated to the reason for consultation is discovered, this should be communicated to the requesting physician.

2. Once a request for a consultation is received by the medical consultant, it should be completed in a timely manner. If the consultation cannot be done because unforeseen circumstances arise, the consultant must notify the requesting physician in ample time for another consultant to complete the task.

3. The evaluation of the patient's history and physical examination should be thorough, with a complete review of old medical records as appropriate and available. The consultant is responsible for obtaining any relevant information for the management of the patient as it pertains to the consultation request. This may include contacting other hospitals or the patient's primary care physician about previous surgical procedures, cardiovascular assessments, and concomitant medical conditions and their management.

4. On completion of this assessment, recommendations should be concise, and therapeutic regimens should be clearly delineated. In our experience, the more extensive and complex management plans are, the greater the likelihood will be that the recommendations will not be implemented.

5. The medical consultant should attempt to provide options or alternative approaches to management. This allows the requesting physician latitude for care should he or she not be comfortable with one form of therapy.

6. Prompt communication, both written and verbal, of the assessment and plan to the requesting physician and medical care team ensures better likelihood that the therapeutic regimens or diagnostic evaluations will be implemented. This also allows any difference of opinion between the consultant and the requesting physician to

be resolved. It is inappropriate to make the medical record the forum for discord between physicians. Conversely, if the consultant and requesting physician cannot agree, the consultant should remove himself or herself from the case and should allow ample time for the requesting physician to obtain another consultant. Documentation in the chart of termination of service should be made, but the reason for disagreement is omitted.

7. We do not use the phrase "Clear for surgery." Although this is a common consultation request, this term is not specific and means different things to different people. "Cleared" may falsely imply that the patient is at no risk or at only minimal risk of surgery, and that is rarely the case. Rather than "clear for surgery," we believe that the roles of the preoperative consultant are to identify and clarify the patient's medical status and risk and to attempt to lower perioperative risk if possible. For many patients, the preoperative consultation may be their most comprehensive medical evaluation. The consultant should convey to the patient appropriate health care issues identified as a result of the preoperative evaluation. The consultant should also be available following surgery to treat any postoperative complications should they occur.

8. Follow-up care should be provided as indicated by the patient's medical problems. This care may include medication adjustment, evaluation of abnormal laboratory test results, or evaluation of new conditions. This sometimes becomes a "gray area" for medical preoperative consultations, because such consultations are often requested only to prepare the patient for surgery. Termination of a consultant's postoperative care should also be documented in the medical record.

9. The consultant must clearly define his or her or role in the care of the patient in the perioperative period. The

consultant may assume one of two roles in the care of patients. He or she may be a pure consultant or may serve as a co-manager with the requesting physician. In the former role, more traditional consultant role recommendations are made and communicated, but care is provided by the requesting physician only. The latter role involves direct care by the consultant in assisting the requesting physician to implement the management plan and to provide follow-up care. This includes order writing, daily notes, and frequent communication. We believe that this co-manager model will continue to evolve, as demonstrated by a study showing that hospitalist management of patients in the perioperative period as part of the surgical team reduced length of stay, utilized fewer special consultants, and reduced the incidence of medical complications.

10. It is the responsibility of the medical consultant to communicate while providing the service of consultation. This should be done in a tactful manner with the patient, nursing staff, and physicians. Embarrassing a requesting physician by exposing his or her lack of knowledge or insight in a case is a grave error. Requesting physicians appreciate consultants who are interested in sharing their insights and experience without condescension. Communication should also include teaching when appropriate.

ASSESSING OPERATIVE RISK

The assessment of operative risk in the preoperative consultation is of significant importance. Various risk factor indices, usually consensus based, are available to help the consultant fulfill that task. One published and validated pulmonary risk assessment matrix accurately predicted postoperative pulmonary complications. The role of the consultant is to estimate the operative risk by identifying the patient's risk factors in combination with the operative procedure and optimizing the patient for surgery.

In 1977, Goldman and co-workers used univariate and multivariate analysis to identify nine risk factors that, if present, were found to increase the risk of cardiac complications in noncardiac surgery. This analysis permitted not only a method for determination of risk but also one for identification of several reversible risk factors that, if alleviated, could result in safer surgery. This work was revised by Detsky and co-workers in 1986, thus allowing a better definition of risk based on the individual's hospital surgical complication rate as well as consideration of some additional risk factors. More recently, the American College of Cardiology and the American Heart Association published practice guidelines for perioperative cardiovascular evaluation of patients undergoing noncardiac surgery. This document is a comprehensive review of the literature with expert consensus; it provides the medical consultant with state-of-the art information.

The perioperative risk for the development of deep venous thrombosis and pulmonary embolism (DVT-PE) has been reported by the American College of Chest Physicians and the International Consensus Statement on Venous Thromboembolism. Patients are categorized into high, moderate, and low risk for the development of DVT-PE on the basis of age, estimated length of surgery, type of procedure, and secondary risk factors (see Table 5-1 in Chapter 5). After risk stratification for the surgical patient, the consultant has the option of applying the most effective prophylaxis recommended by either the American College of Chest Physicians or the International Consensus Statement on Venous Thromboembolism. This risk assessment for DVT-PE is also part of the recommendations by the medical consultant.

More recently, a new area of risk stratification for patients undergoing peripheral revascularization procedures has been developed. These schemes employ the consideration of preexisting risk factors, physical signs and symptoms, laboratory test results, and invasive and noninvasive studies to evaluate underlying cardiovascular disease in this high-risk population, as well as options for managing this patient population. More work in this population will be forthcoming, but for the present the medical consultant must have a working knowledge of these areas. These are but three examples of the new role of the consultant in assessing the patient's risk preoperatively.

PERIOPERATIVE MEDICATIONS

The number of new pharmacologic agents for the treatment of disease continues to grow exponentially. On average, four or more drugs are available to treat a disease process, and each agent has some special action or effect. These differences and the numbers of drugs make it challenging for physicians to maintain a working familiarity with all these agents.

The medical consultant is often faced with preparing patients for surgery for whom he or she has not been the primary physician. In such cases, a variety of medications may be encountered with which the consultant may not be familiar, or the consultant may not agree with their indications. The consultant's responsibility is to decide which of the patient's outpatient medications should be continued in the perioperative period and to develop a strategy for parenteral drug administration for patients who will be unable to resume oral medications immediately following surgery. In some cases, this will be particularly challenging. For patients whose outpatient medication is not available in parenteral form, a substitution will have to be made until oral medications can be resumed. Some medications have specific perioperative recommendations, such as insulin, agents for DVT-PE prophylaxis, and antihypertensive medications. Several medications (e.g., β-blockers) are initiated preoperatively in an effort to decrease the risk of perioperative complications. The medical consultant has the responsibility to know these regimens and to apply them appropriately in the perioperative period. As mentioned earlier, the ever-growing number of medications requires the medical consultant to be up to date on the dosing, administration, and adverse effects of these new agents.

POSTOPERATIVE COMPLICATIONS

As the information base for medical consultation has expanded, the area of postoperative complications has also grown. This focus has been largely on the effects of anesthesia and surgery on the patient.

The role of the consultant is not to select or recommend the anesthetic agent, but rather to understand the effect of the agent on the patient. This is important in patients with concomitant diseases that may be exacerbated by the effects of general, spinal, or local anesthesia. The consultant should also be familiar with the patient's anesthesia record. This document provides important information concerning vital signs, type and amount of fluid administered, and additional intraoperative medications. A postoperative change in mental status, for example, may result from intraoperative hypotension or from a decrease in hemoglobin secondary to the dilutional effect of increased fluid volume.

Our surgical colleagues have long focused on the postoperative complications of procedures. More recently, medical consultation texts have included descriptions of surgical procedures and their complications. It is important that a knowledge of the description, indications, and complications of surgical procedures become part of both the medical consultant's preparation of the patient for surgery and postoperative management. This familiarity with surgical procedures and their postoperative complications allows a better working relationship with the consulting surgeon and frequently a better outcome for the patient.

MEDICAL INSURANCE

Third-party payers were the first to provide definitions, coding, and reimbursement for the responsibilities of the medical consultant. This area will continue to evolve as third-party payers determine compensation for the service provided. The following are descriptions of the responsibilities of the consultant as they pertain to the complexity of the service provided.

A *consultation* includes services rendered by a physician whose opinion or advice is requested by a physician or other appropriate source for the further evaluation or management (or both) of the patient. When the consulting physician assumes responsibility for the continuing care of the patient, any subsequent service rendered by him or her ceases to be a consultation. Five levels of consultation are recognized: limited, intermediate, extended, comprehensive, and complex.

In a *limited consultation,* the physician confines his or her service to the examination or evaluation of a single organ system. This procedure includes documentation of the complaints, evaluation of the present illness, pertinent examination, review of medical data, and establishment of a plan of management relating to the specific problem. An *intermediate consultation* involves examination or evaluation of an organ system, a partial review of the general history, recommendations, and preparation of a report. An *extended consultation* involves the evaluation of problems that do not require a comprehensive evaluation of the patient as a whole. This procedure includes the following: documentation of a history of the chief complaint, past medical history, and pertinent physical examination; review and evaluation of the past medical data; establishment of a plan of investigative or therapeutic management, or both; and the preparation of an appropriate report. A *comprehensive consultation* involves the following: (1) an in-depth evaluation of a patient with a problem requiring the development and documentation of medical data (the chief complaints, present illness, family history, past medical history, personal history, system review, physical examination, and a review of all diagnostic tests and procedures that have previously been performed); (2) the establishment of verification of a plan for further investigative or therapeutic management, or both; and (3) the preparation of a report. The *complex consultation* is an uncommonly performed service that involves an in-depth evaluation of a critical problem that requires unusual knowledge, skill, and judgment on the part of the consulting physician and the preparation of an appropriate report.

MEDICAL-LEGAL LIABILITY

The medical consultant must practice in accordance with the basic principles of medical liability. These principles are quite broad in most jurisdictions. It is our interpretation of the law that a consultant performing a preoperative evaluation must possess and employ the same skill and knowledge possessed by other consultants practicing in this field, giving regard to the state of preoperative evaluation and perioperative care at the time of service. We believe that a consultant will be held liable if his or her actions are inconsistent with the standard of care at the time of the patient encounter if that inconsistency results in injury to the patient. A "poor result" or a "mistake in judgment" alone is not a sufficient basis for liability. Physicians are neither guarantors nor warrantors of the result of a treatment or procedure result. Finally, if more than one diagnostic or treatment plan is recognized as proper, a consultant should not be held responsible if he or she follows one of the recognized plans as opposed to another. We believe that the consultant is responsible for patient care in his or her area of expertise until the problem or question under study has been resolved or the consultant has transferred responsibility to another physician. Finally, if the circumstances surrounding a case raise the issue of medical-legal implications, the hospital's risk management department or the consultant's insurance carrier, or both, should be contacted.

THE CONSULTATION REPORT

The written consultation report should be precise and should include recommended diagnostic tests, dosages and routes of administration of recommended medications, and contingency measures or alternative approaches if the requesting physician is unable to carry out the consultant's primary recommendations. We suggest that the first page of the consultation report contain the following: reason for the consultation, impression of the consultant, and management plan.

CONCLUSION

With the preceding issues in mind, it is obvious that the role and responsibilities of the medical consultant have changed and will continue to evolve as new studies are performed to improve the field. We stress the importance of an orderly and in-depth approach to patient evaluation, accurate documentation, and precise recommendations as well as ongoing communication with the surgical team (Box 1-3). Following these principles will result in effective medical consultation for the surgical patient with medical problems.

Box 1-3	ATTRIBUTES OF EFFECTIVE CONSULTATION

- Timely response
- Precise recommendations
- Follow-up care
- Communication with the requesting physician

Selected Readings

Arozullah AM, Khuri SF, Henderson WG, et al: Development and validation of a multifactorial risk index for predicting postoperative pneumonia after major non-cardiac surgery. Ann Intern Med 135:847-857, 2001.

Boucher C, Brewster D, Darling R, et al: Determination of cardiac risk by dipyridamole-thallium imaging before peripheral vascular surgery. N Engl J Med 312:389-394, 1985.

Detsky A, Abrams H, Forbath N, et al: Cardiac assessment for patients undergoing noncardiac surgery: A multifactorial clinical risk index. Arch Intern Med 146:2131-2134, 1986.

Eagle K, Berger P, Calkins H, et al: ACC/AHA guideline update for perioperative cardiovascular evaluation for non-cardiac surgery: Executive summary. A report of the ACC/AHA Task Force on Practice Guidelines. J Am Coll Cardiol 39:542-553, 2002.

Eagle K, Coley C, Newell J, et al: Combining clinical and thallium data optimizes preoperative assessment of cardiac risk before major vascular surgery. Ann Intern Med 110:859-866, 1989.

Geerts W, Pineo G, Heit J, et al: Prevention of venous thromboembolism. Chest 126(Suppl):338S-400S, 2004.

Goldman D, Brown F, Guarnieri D: Perioperative Medicine: The Medical Care of the Surgical Patient, 2nd ed. New York, McGraw-Hill, 1994.

Goldman L, Caldera D, Nussbaum S, et al: Multifactorial index of cardiac risk in noncardiac surgical procedures. N Engl J Med 297:845-850, 1977.

Goldman L, Lee T, Rudd P: Ten Commandments for effective consultation. Arch Intern Med 143:1753-1755, 1983.

Greenfield L: Complications of Surgery and Trauma, 2nd ed. Philadelphia, JB Lippincott, 1990.

Gross R, Caputo G: Medical Consultation: The Internist on Surgical, Obstetric, and Psychiatric Services, 2nd ed. Baltimore, Williams & Wilkins, 1998.

Hertzer N: Fatal myocardial infarction following lower extremity revascularization. Ann Surg 193:492-498, 1981.

Huddleston J, Long K, Naessens J, et al: A randomized controlled trial of medical and surgical co-management following elective hip and knee arthroplasty. Ann Intern Med 141:28-38, 2004.

Lubin H, Walker H, Smith R: Medical Management of the Surgical Patient, 4th ed. Philadelphia, JB Lippincott, 2006.

Mangano D, Browner W, Hollenberg M, et al: Association of perioperative myocardial ischemia with cardiac morbidity and mortality in men undergoing noncardiac surgery. N Engl J Med 323:1781-1788, 1990.

Mercado D, Betty B: Perioperative medication management. Med Clin North Am 87:41-57, 2003.

Merli G: The hospitalist joins the surgical team. Ann Intern Med 141:67-69, 2004.

Merli G: Prophylaxis for deep vein thrombosis and pulmonary embolism in the surgical patient. *In* Merli G, Weitz H (eds): Medical Management of the Surgical Patient, 3rd ed. Philadelphia, WB Saunders, 2008.

Poldermans D, Boersmae E, Bax J, et al: The effect of bisoprolol on perioperative mortality and myocardial infarction in high risk patients undergoing vascular surgery. N Engl J Med 341:1789-1794, 1997.

Poldermans D, Fioretti P, Forster T, et al: Dobutamine stress echocardiography for assessment of perioperative cardiac risk in patients undergoing major vascular surgery. Circulation 87:1506-1512, 1993.

Prevention and Treatment of Venous Thromboembolism International Consensus Statement: Guidelines according to scientific evidence. Int Angiol 25:101-161, 2006.

Preoperative Assessment for the Healthy Patient

BARRY S. ZIRING, MD

CLINICAL ASSESSMENT OF THE HEALTHY PATIENT

Preoperative evaluation of healthy patients is often done by internists, family physicians, cardiologists, and concurrently by anesthesiologists. The assessment can broadly be divided into defining risks for cardiac complications, complications of anesthesia, and other complications.

Research done over the past 30 years has helped to define who is at risk and which patients need laboratory and other testing to stratify and reduce this risk. This chapter summarizes the data. This research has shown that "healthy patients" require minimal testing. Therefore, the first step in the evaluation should be directed toward defining who is healthy. This is done through conducting a focused history and physical examination.

THE HISTORY

- A complete medication history including nonprescription and herbal medications.
- A review of allergies with particular attention to latex and iodine allergies as well as anesthetic agents.
- A review of surgical history with attention to bleeding complications or coagulation disorders.

Levels of Evidence:

Ⓐ—Randomized controlled trials (RCTs), meta-analyses, well-designed systematic reviews of RCTs. Ⓑ—Case-control or cohort studies, nonrandomized clinical trials, systematic reviews of studies other than RCTs, cross-sectional studies, retrospective studies. Ⓒ—Consensus statements, expert guidelines, usual practice, opinion.

- Social history with careful history of tobacco use and alcohol and drug use and overuse.
- A complete review of systems. This should focus on areas with specific risk to surgery including functional capacity, cardiac symptoms, dyspnea, thyroid disease, prostate disorders, snoring, sleep apnea, and recent infection.
- Family history of perioperative bleeding disorder or anesthetic complication.
- Female patients should be questioned about the possibility of pregnancy and about last menstrual period.

FUNCTIONAL STATUS

Multiple cardiac risk assessment tools have been published. Several of these studies identified poor functional capacity as a clinical predictor of risk. Activity scales such as the Duke Activity Status Index can assess functional capacity (Fig. 2-1). The American College of Cardiology/American Heart Association (ACC/AHA) guidelines for perioperative cardiovascular risk evaluation state that an inability to perform four or more metabolic equivalents (METs) activities, even if the factor limiting the activity is noncardiac (e.g., severe arthritis) is a risk factor for cardiac complications in noncardiac surgery.

BE AWARE OF CARDIAC RISK OF NONCARDIAC PROCEDURES

The ACC/AHA preoperative guidelines divide noncardiac procedures into the following three categories:

High-risk procedures involve cardiac risk greater than 5%. These procedures include emergency major operations, particularly in elderly patients, aortic and major vascular procedures, peripheral vascular surgery, and surgery involving large fluid shifts or blood loss.

Intermediate-risk procedures have a cardiac risk of generally less than 5%. These include carotid endarterectomy, head

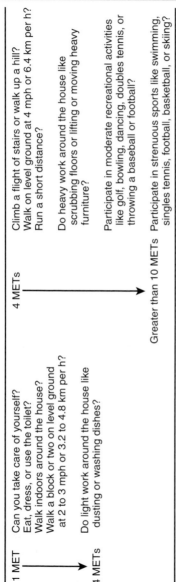

1 MET
Can you take care of yourself?
Eat, dress, or use the toilet?
Walk indoors around the house?
Walk a block or two on level ground at 2 to 3 mph or 3.2 to 4.8 km per h?

Do light work around the house like dusting or washing dishes?

4 METs
Climb a flight of stairs or walk up a hill?
Walk on level ground at 4 mph or 6.4 km per h?
Run a short distance?

Do heavy work around the house like scrubbing floors or lifting or moving heavy furniture?

Participate in moderate recreational activities like golf, bowling, dancing, doubles tennis, or throwing a baseball or football?

Greater than 10 METs
Participate in strenuous sports like swimming, singles tennis, football, basketball, or skiing?

MET indicates metabolic equivalent.

Figure 2-1 • Energy requirement for various activities. (From Hlatky MA, Boineau RE, Higginbotham MB, et al: A brief self-administered questionnaire to determine functional capacity [the Duke Activity Status Index]. Am J Cardiol 64:651-654, 1989; and Eagle KA, Berger PB, Calkins H, et al: ACC/AHA guideline update for perioperative cardiovascular evaluation for noncardiac surgery: a report of the American College of Cardiology/American Heart Association Task Force on Practice Guidelines [Committee to Update the 1996 Guidelines on Perioperative Cardiovascular Evaluation for Noncardiac Surgery]. American College of Cardiology, 2002. Available at http://www.acc.org.)

and neck surgery, intraperitoneal and intrathoracic surgery, orthopedic surgery, and prostate surgery.

Low-risk procedures have a cardiac risk of less than 1%. These include endoscopic procedures, superficial procedures, cataract operations, and breast surgery.

Cataract surgery has been studied and shown to be uniquely safe. A study by Schein and colleagues looked at almost 20,000 patients. Half these patients were randomized to receive a standard battery of medical tests (electrocardiogram [ECG], complete blood count [CBC], and electrolytes) in addition to history and physical examination. Half received only a history and physical examination. The overall rates of events were the same (31.3 events per 1,000 operations). Perioperative death or hospitalization was very rare, and most events were not serious. These authors concluded that **preoperative medical testing before cataract surgery would rarely reduce the risk or severity of an adverse perioperative event** [🅐 *Schein et al, 2000*].

LABORATORY TESTING IN HEALTHY PATIENTS

Preoperative laboratory tests serve to confirm surgical risk factors identified by the history and physical evaluation. Laboratory testing can, when used selectively, identify additional problems as well as establish a basis to allow assessments of abnormalities discovered in the postoperative period. However, when ordered randomly, laboratory tests are more likely to yield false-positive results, which can be confusing and can delay surgery.

Another consideration is medical-legal risk. Physicians have intuitively believed that laboratory tests can protect them from risk. However, many tests that are ordered are neither checked nor acted on preoperatively. Failure to document and address abnormalities that are found by preoperative testing can significantly increase medical-legal risk.

Preoperative Laboratory Testing in the Healthy Elderly Patient

In an evaluation of healthy patients 70 years old or older who underwent elective general surgery (patients whose surgery required local anesthesia or monitored anesthesia care were excluded), the prevalence of abnormal electrolyte values or thrombocytopenia was found to be low (0.5% to 5%). The prevalence of anemia, elevated serum creatinine, or hyperglycemia was higher (10%, 12%, and 7%, respectively). **None of these abnormal preoperative tests was associated with postoperative adverse outcomes** [❸ Dzankic et al, 2001].

Evidence-Based Medicine

More than 100 studies have examined the value of routine preoperative laboratory tests. Two large reviews of the preoperative literature have been published. Results of the study conducted by the American College of Physicians in cooperation with the Blue Cross/Blue Shield Medical Necessity Project were published in 1987. In 1997, Munro and associates published a systematic review of the evidence as part of the Health Technology Assessment program. This project pointed out that there are no controlled trials of the value of preoperative testing. All available evidence has reported the results of case series.

Chest Radiography

The routine chest radiograph is perhaps the most thoroughly studied preoperative test. Proposed reasons for ordering a routine chest radiograph include screening for silent diseases, evaluation of suspected diseases, intrathoracic surgery, establishment of a baseline, and medical-legal consideration (Box 2-1).

The use of the chest radiograph to screen for silent disease may turn out to be the least productive reason for ordering this test because of the low prevalence of occult intrathoracic

Box 2-1	CONSIDERATIONS IN PREOPERATIVE CHEST RADIOGRAPHY

- Findings from routine preoperative chest radiographs are reported as abnormal in 2.5% to 37% of cases.
- These findings lead to a change in management in 0% to 2.1% of patients.
- Limited evidence suggests that a baseline chest radiograph is of value in fewer than 9% of patients.
- No published scientific evidence indicates that routine chest radiographs decrease perioperative risk.

Modified from Munro J, Booth A, Nicholl J: Routine preoperative testing: A systematic review of the evidence. Health Technol Assess 1:i-iv, 1-62, 1997.

disease in an asymptomatic population. For example, the prevalence of tuberculosis is 0.045%, the prevalence of chronic interstitial lung disease is 0.01%, and the prevalence of chronic obstructive lung disease is 1.9%.

Studies that looked at the routine use of chest radiography in an unscreened population showed that the findings on preoperative chest films made almost no difference in the decision to operate. In addition, reviews of all available studies showed that **unexpected chest film abnormalities would lead to an improved outcome in fewer than 2% of patients** [❺ *Tape and Mushlin, 1986*].

A meta-analysis of 21 studies of routine chest radiographs was completed in 1993. In the 21 studies, 14,390 routine chest radiographs were done. There were 1444 abnormal studies, with only 140 abnormalities unexpected. Only 14 (0.1%) resulted in a change in patient management.

The use of preoperative chest radiographs as a baseline for comparison is more controversial. There is no evidence that a baseline radiograph will improve diagnosis in the event of a postoperative complication. However, a study in the United Kingdom showed that pulmonary complications do not always occur in high-risk groups. Therefore, almost all patients would require a baseline film. This practice is unlikely to be justified on a cost-to-benefit basis.

Finally, random ordering of chest radiographic studies in an unselected population will increase the rate of abnormal results. Follow-up of abnormal findings will result in delay of surgery, additional cost, and unnecessary anxiety for the preoperative patient.

Recommendations

1. A chest radiograph is not routinely indicated as part of a preoperative evaluation, before anesthesia, or for baseline assessment.
2. A chest radiograph is not indicated solely because of advanced age.
3. A routine preoperative chest radiograph is generally indicated for patients scheduled for intrathoracic surgical procedures.
4. An admission or preoperative chest radiograph is indicated in patients with signs or symptoms of active chest disease. A history and physical examination will identify most of these patients.
5. Because of the high prevalence of symptoms and signs of chest disease in elderly patients, many older patients require a chest radiograph. Statistically, the yield is higher in this age group, although the physician's judgment is still recommended.

Electrocardiogram

Research on the utility of the preoperative ECG began in the 1970s. Two reasons developed for obtaining a preoperative ECG. First, Goldman and associates identified myocardial infarction (within the preceding 6 months), dysrhythmias, and the presence of congestive heart failure as the factors indicating the highest cardiac risk for surgery. Many patients can be identified on the basis of the history and physical examination. However, certain dysrhythmias and conduction abnormalities (e.g., 2:1 atrioventricular heart block and preexcitation syndrome) can be identified only through an ECG. Second, information from the Framingham study showed that approximately 28% of all myocardial infarctions were not associated with classic symptoms and were discovered only by the appearance of new changes on the ECG.

In the more than 30 years that have followed the publication of the original Goldman cardiac risk index, many studies have reexamined preoperative cardiac risk. The ACC/AHA guidelines recognize previous myocardial infarction or pathologic Q waves as an intermediate clinical predictor of risk. These guidelines recognize an otherwise abnormal ECG (left ventricular hypertrophy, left bundle branch block, ST-T abnormalities) as a minor predictor of cardiac risk (Box 2-2).

As a result of conflicting data regarding the predictive power of a preoperative ECG, there is no consensus regarding the routine use of this test. However, current recommendations have been developed based on the incidence of disease in certain population groups.

Recommendations

1. An ECG is not routinely indicated before noncardiac surgery.
2. Because of the increased prevalence of cardiac disease with increasing age, men 40 to 45 years old or older

---

Box 2-2	**CONSIDERATIONS IN PREOPERATIVE ELECTROCARDIOGRAPHY**

- Findings from routine preoperative electrocardiograms are abnormal in 4.6% to 31.7% of cases and lead to a change in management in 0% to 2.2% of patients.
- The predictive power of electrocardiograms for postoperative cardiac complications in noncardiac surgery is weak.
- No evidence supports the value of recording a preoperative electrocardiogram as a baseline.

Modified from Munro J, Booth A, Nicholl J: Routine preoperative testing: A systematic review of the evidence. Health Technol Assess 1:i-iv, 1-62, 1997.

and women 55 years old or older benefit from a preoperative ECG.

3. Patients with systemic diseases associated with unrecognized cardiac conditions should undergo a preoperative ECG. These systemic diseases include hypertension, peripheral vascular disease, diabetes mellitus, certain malignancies, collagen vascular disease, and certain infectious diseases.

4. Patients who use medications with potential cardiac toxicity, including doxorubicin, phenothiazine, and tricyclic antidepressants, should have a preoperative ECG.

5. Additionally, patients undergoing intrathoracic, intraperitoneal, aortic, or emergency operations should have an ECG.

Complete Blood Count

Several hematologic problems that may be reflected in the CBC can affect operative risk. Anemia most likely increases operative risk, although the hemoglobin value cannot be used as the sole predictor. Traditionally, a hemoglobin value of 9 to 10 g/dL has been used as a minimum for safe surgery, although few data support the use of this particular value. Physical examination may actually give a better estimation of volume status and coincidental surgical risk. Predicted blood loss during surgery may also indicate whether a preoperative CBC will be helpful.

Similarly, a hematocrit greater than 50% may represent a surgical risk because of increased blood viscosity and decreased oxygen transport. The risk of thromboembolism may also be increased at high hemoglobin concentrations. Overall, unexpected hemoglobin abnormalities in routine screening have been found in 0.3% to 30.4% of patients. Isolated unexpected hemoglobin abnormalities rarely affect surgical outcome; therefore, a routine CBC is not recommended (Box 2-3).

Recommendations

1. A CBC is indicated in patients admitted to the hospital for surgery that may involve substantial blood loss.

2. A CBC is not routinely indicated in patients undergoing minor surgery or minor diagnostic procedures.

Box 2-3	CONSIDERATIONS IN PREOPERATIVE HEMOGLOBIN DETERMINATIONS

- Routine preoperative measurement shows that hemoglobin may be lower than 10 to 10.5 g/dL in up to 5% of patients, but it is rarely lower than 9 g/dL.
- The routine test leads to a change in management in 0.1% to 2.7% of patients.

Modified from Munro J, Booth A, Nicholl J: Routine preoperative testing: A systematic review of the evidence. Health Technol Assess 1:i-iv, 1-62, 1997.

3. A CBC is indicated for initial outpatient evaluation (screening). Because many patients do not receive regular medical care, use of the preoperative CBC as a screening test for health maintenance may be indicated in certain patients.
4. A CBC may be useful in subsets of patients with a higher prevalence of anemia, including institutionalized elderly patients ($\geq$75 years old) and recent immigrants from developing countries.
5. A CBC may also be useful in pregnant women in whom iron deficiency anemia or inadequate nutrition is suspected.
6. A CBC is indicated in all patients with a history or physical examination suggestive of anemia or polycythemia.
7. A CBC may be useful for patients with malignancy or chronic renal insufficiency.

Tests of Coagulation and Platelet Count

Tests of coagulation abnormalities have been studied extensively in the setting of preoperative evaluation. Although no absolute consensus exists on the use of the ECG or chest radiograph, there is substantial evidence that coagulation studies are not beneficial when ordered in a low-risk population. A Veterans Administration (VA) study showed only a single patient with potential benefits from random coagulation screening of 750 patients.

Disorders of platelet number and function represent a significant risk because of bleeding complications and thrombosis. Platelet estimation is often included with automated CBCs. However, asymptomatic platelet abnormalities in a patient with no history of bleeding are exceedingly rare. The cost of ordering routine platelet counts in an unselected population is prohibitive. Questioning the patient regarding a history of spontaneous bleeding or bruising, surgical bleeding, or excessive bleeding resulting from dental procedures provides an excellent method of screening (Box 2-4).

Recommendations

1. The activated partial thromboplastin time (aPTT) and prothrombin time (PT) are not indicated in patients without a clinical history or evidence of a bleeding disorder.
2. The PT and aPTT should be evaluated in patients with a clinical finding of liver disease, malabsorption, or malnutrition.

Box 2-4

CONSIDERATIONS IN PREOPERATIVE BLEEDING AND COAGULATION EVALUATIONS

- Abnormalities of bleeding time, prothrombin time, and partial thromboplastin time are found in up to 3.8% to 4.8% and 15.6% of routine preoperative tests, respectively.
- The results of these tests rarely lead to a change in clinical management.
- Routine preoperative platelet counts are low in less than 1.1% of patients, and a low platelet count rarely, if ever, leads to a change in management.

Modified from Munro J, Booth A, Nicholl J: Routine preoperative testing: A systematic review of the evidence. Health Technol Assess 1:i-iv, 1-62, 1997.

3. The PT and aPTT should be determined in patients undergoing insertion of peritoneovenous shunting or extracorporeal circulation or in patients undergoing surgery in which normally minor bleeding complications may produce catastrophic results.
4. The PT, aPTT, and platelet counts should be determined in patients with active bleeding or a history of abnormal bleeding and in patients unable to provide a history.

Electrolytes and Creatinine

Studies have evaluated each of the values reported in a routine seven-factor analysis (SMA-7) (serum sodium, potassium, and chloride concentrations; carbon dioxide content; blood urea nitrogen; glucose; and creatinine concentrations) with respect to the impact on perioperative care. However, in many institutions, ordering the standard automated panel of tests is less expensive than ordering several tests individually. In practical terms, many hospitals provide an SMA-7 at a cost similar to that of a test with one or two values.

The three factors identified by Goldman and associates to correlate with surgical risk are a serum potassium level less than 3, a blood urea nitrogen level higher than 50 mg/dL, and a creatinine level higher than 3 mg/dL. A more recent study showed that a preoperative creatinine level greater than 2.0 mg/dL is a significant independent risk factor for cardiac complications after major noncardiac surgery. This finding is the basis for the ACC/AHA recommendations including renal insufficiency as an intermediate clinical predictor of cardiac complications (Box 2-5).

Screening for any biochemical abnormality in a young, asymptomatic patient has not been demonstrated to result in improved outcome and is not cost effective. In elderly patients and in selected populations, the chance of finding asymptomatic abnormalities increases. Additionally, a serum bicarbonate value less than 20 mmol/L correlates with increased

Box 2-5	CONSIDERATIONS IN PREOPERATIVE SERUM BIOCHEMISTRY EVALUATIONS

- In routine preoperative tests of serum biochemistry, abnormal tests of sodium or potassium are found in up to 1.4% of patients.
- Abnormal creatinine and blood urea nitrogen are found in up to 2.5% of patients.
- Abnormal glucose is found in up to 5.2% of patients.
- The abnormalities rarely result in a change of clinical management.

Modified from Munro J, Booth A, Nicholl J: Routine preoperative testing: A systematic review of the evidence. Health Technol Assess 1:i-iv, 1-62, 1997.

surgical risk. A further use of serum creatinine levels is to adjust drug doses, especially of muscle relaxants and antibiotics, in the perioperative period.

Biochemical Profiles

The 12-test biochemical profile (calcium, alkaline phosphatase, uric acid, lactate dehydrogenase, bilirubin, creatinine, serum glutamic-oxaloacetic acid, cholesterol, phosphorus, protein, albumin, and glucose concentrations) has not been shown to be useful for preoperative evaluation. The yield of true-positive results as opposed to false-positive results in an unselected population is too low to justify general use. Follow-up of false-positive studies has delayed surgery, resulted in longer average length of stay, and increased cost without net benefit.

An exception to this rule is the selected use of biochemical testing of the liver. Although no consensus exists for routine testing to detect subclinical hepatitis, patients with known liver disease, as determined by history and physical examination, should be tested.

Recommendations

1. Biochemical profiles are not routinely indicated before elective admission to the hospital.
2. In selected institutions, biochemical profiles may be less expensive than tests of individual components.

Special Considerations

1. Patients with known liver disease should have at least albumin and bilirubin concentrations determined for assessment using the Child risk classification.
2. Patients with a remote history of hepatitis should have testing of serum aminotransferase, alkaline phosphatase, bilirubin, and albumin levels.
3. Patients with known malignancy may benefit from biochemical testing of the liver as a screen for metastatic disease.

Urinalysis

Multiple studies have shown that abnormalities are commonly found in routine urinalysis. However, abnormalities in protein, ketones, or glucose are also frequently discovered and quantitated in blood chemistry panels. Because blood chemistry panels are more reliable and are ordered in the same population, a urinalysis provides no additional benefit.

A possible exception to this is the finding of asymptomatic bacteriuria. Studies have estimated the frequency of asymptomatic bacteriuria in women at 3.3%. In men, the frequency increases with age. For this reason, urinalysis continues to be used as a preoperative test before the insertion of a prosthetic joint or heart valve. However, at least one study has questioned whether an abnormal preoperative urinalysis predicts wound infection.

Recommendations

1. Urinalysis is not routinely indicated preoperatively.
2. Urinalysis may be useful before any surgical procedure in which urinary tract instrumentation is anticipated,

especially in elderly patients. It may also be useful before joint or valve replacement.

Pregnancy Testing

Because of the risks to the fetus from exposure to anesthetic agents, antibiotics, and radiographs, it may be prudent to test women of childbearing age for pregnancy.

Serum Albumin

Serum albumin has not traditionally been used as a routine preoperative test. There is no evidence for its use in a healthy population. However, the national VA surgical risk study showed that low serum albumin was a better predictor of surgical outcomes than many other preoperative patient characteristics when used in patients with comorbidities. The study showed that a decrease in serum albumin from 46 g/L to less than 21 g/L was associated with an increase in mortality from 1% to 29%. There was an increase in morbidity from 10% to 65%.

SUMMARY

Historically, preoperative tests have been used to find occult disease in low-risk populations. For almost all tests, this approach has been shown to yield a small number of true abnormalities. It also results in many false-positive findings, which can lead to surgical delay and patient anxiety. This approach is not cost effective.

Unfortunately, dissemination of this information sometimes results in minimizing the use of tests when they would be helpful. The current approach is to use the history and physical examination to identify groups at risk for abnormalities and then to order tests to identify and quantitate abnormalities. Based on the likelihood of the disease, the tests shown in Table 2-1 should routinely be ordered for surgery in which low blood loss is anticipated. In addition to

TABLE 2-1	Routine Preoperative Tests for Surgical Procedures Resulting in Low Blood Loss
Patients <40 yr	Hgb for procedures normally involving blood loss exceeding 50 mL
Women	Also consider pregnancy test
Patients 40–59 yr	ECG, Hgb (as above)
Women	Also consider pregnancy test
Patients >60 yr	ECG, Hgb, electrolytes, consider chest radiograph

ECG, electrocardiogram; Hgb, hemoglobin.

the preceding testing, supplemental tests should be ordered in clinical situations in which the likelihood of disease or abnormality is increased (Tables 2-2 to 2-4).

Previous Test Results

Frequently, patients undergoing elective surgery have had recent tests. Several studies looked at the utility and safety of using tests performed within the year before elective surgery.

TABLE 2-2	Supplemental Tests for Patients with Specific Conditions
Diabetes	All diabetic patients should have SMA-7 and ECG regardless of age
Cardiovascular disease	Chest radiograph, ECG, SMA-7
Pulmonary disease	Chest radiograph, ECG
Malignant disease	Chest radiograph, possible liver enzyme tests
Hepatic disease	PT and aPTT, liver enzyme tests
Renal disease	SMA-7, urinalysis
Bleeding disorder	PT and aPTT, platelet determination, possibly bleeding time
Thyroid disorder	ECG, TSH level
Systemic lupus erythematosus	SMA-7, CBC
Dialysis	Chest radiograph, ECG, SMA-7, SMA-12
Oral antibiotics (>2 week's duration) ending within 1 week of surgery	PT and aPTT

aPTT, partial thromboplastin time; CBC, complete blood count; ECG, electrocardiogram; PT, prothrombin time; SMA-7, seven-factor sequential multiple analysis; SMA-12, 12-factor sequential multiple analysis; TSH, thyroid-stimulating hormone.

TABLE 2-3	Supplemental Tests for Surgical Patients Using Specific Medications
Diuretics	SMA-7, ECG
Digoxin	SMA-7, ECG
Steroids	SMA-7
Anticoagulant	PT (warfarin [Coumadin]), aPTT (heparin)
ASA, NSAIDs	Bleeding time (controversial)
Oral antibiotics (>2 week's duration) ending within 1 week of surgery	PT and aPTT

aPTT, partial thromboplastin time; ASA, acetylsalicylic acid; ECG, electrocardiogram; NSAIDs, nonsteroidal anti-inflammatory drugs; PT, prothrombin time; SMA-7, seven-factor sequential multiple analysis.

TABLE 2-4	Special Surgical Cases
Procedure with type and cross	CBC
All gynecologic cases	U/A
Cholecystectomy	Liver enzyme levels, CBC
Urologic case	U/A, culture and sensitivity
Joint replacement or surgery using prosthetic valve	U/A, culture and sensitivity

CBC, complete blood count; U/A, urinalysis.

One study of elderly U.S. veterans examined the following: hemoglobin, white blood cell count, and platelet count; sodium, potassium, and creatinine concentrations; PT and aPTT. Of 3096 previously normal tests, only 13 (0.4%) changed to a value likely to result in changes in patient management. Consequently, **it seems safe to use tests as much as 4 months old if there is no new obvious indication for repeat testing** [❽ MacPherson et al, 1990].

In keeping with the Framingham study and neurologic studies examining the occurrence of silent changes on the ECG, it seems safe to base preoperative evaluation on a normal ECG obtained as much as 4 to 6 months previously. However, any change in the patient's history, physical examination, or performance status should warrant a new preoperative ECG.

Selected Readings

Archer C, Levy EB, Staten M: Value of routine preoperative chest x-rays: A meta-analysis. Can J Anaesth 40:1022-1027, 1993.

Bryson GL, Wyand A, Bragg PR: Preoperative testing is inconsistent with published guidelines and rarely changes management. Can J Anaesth 53:236-241, 2006.

Cebul RD, Beck RJ: Biochemical profiles: Applications in ambulatory screening and preadmission testing of adults. Ann Intern Med 106:403-413, 1987.

Dzankic S, Pastor D, Gonzalez C, Leung J: The prevalence and predictive value of abnormal preoperative laboratory tests in elderly surgical patients. Anesth Analg 93:301-308, 2001. ❸

Eagle KA, Berger PB, Calkins H, et al: ACC/AHA guideline update for perioperative cardiovascular evaluation for noncardiac surgery: A report of the American College of Cardiology/American Heart Association Task Force on Practice Guidelines (Committee to Update the 1996 Guidelines on Perioperative Cardiovascular Evaluation for Noncardiac Surgery). American College of Cardiology, 2002. Available at http://www.acc.org.

Eisenberg J, Goldfarb S: Clinical usefulness of measuring prothrombin time as a routine admission test. Clin Chem 22:1644-1647, 1976.

Gibbs J, Cull W, Henderson W, et al: Preoperative serum albumin level as a predictor of operative mortality and morbidity results from the National VA Surgical Risk Study. Arch Surg 134:36-42, 1999.

Goldberger AL, O'Konski M: Utility of the routine electrocardiogram before surgery and on general hospital admission. Ann Intern Med 105:552-557, 1986.

Goldman L, Caldera DL, Nussbaum SR, et al: Multifactorial index of cardiac risk in noncardiac surgical procedures. N Engl J Med 297:845-850, 1977.

Hlatky MA, Boineau RE, Higginbotham MB, et al: A brief self-administered questionnaire to determine functional capacity (the Duke Activity Status Index). Am J Cardiol 64:651-654, 1989.

Kannel WB, Abbott RD: Incidence and prognosis of unrecognized myocardial infarction: An update on the Framingham study. N Engl J Med 311:1144-1147, 1984.

Kaplan EB, Sheiner LB, Boeckmann AJ, et al: The usefulness of preoperative laboratory screening. JAMA 253:3576-3581, 1985.

Kolwalsyn TJ, Prageer D, Young J: A review of the present status of preoperative hemoglobin requirements. Anesth Analg 51:75, 1972.

Lawrence VA, Kroenke K: The unproven utility of preoperative urinalysis: Clinical use. Arch Intern Med 148:1370-1373, 1988.

Macpherson DS, Snow R, Lofgren RP: Preoperative screening: Value of previous tests. Ann Intern Med 113:969-973,1990. ❸

Munro J, Booth A, Nicholl J: Routine preoperative testing: A systematic review of the evidence. Health Technol Assess 1:i-iv, 1-62, 1997.

Nelson CL, Herndon JE, Mark DB, et al: Relation of clinical and angiographic factors to functional capacity as measured by the Duke Activity Status Index. Am J Cardiol 68:973-975, 1991.

Schein OD, Katz J, Bass EB, et al: The value of routine preoperative medical testing before cataract surgery. N Engl J Med 342:168-175, 2000. **Ⓐ**

Smetana GW, Macpherson DS: The case against routine preoperative laboratory testing. Med Clin North Am 87:7-40, 2003.

Suchman AL, Griner PF: Diagnostic uses of the activated partial thromboplastin time and prothrombin time. Ann Intern Med 104:810-816, 1986.

Tape TG, Mushlin AL: The utility of routine chest radiographs. Ann Intern Med 104:663-670, 1986. **Ⓑ**

3 | Antimicrobial Prophylaxis: Prevention of Postoperative Infections

ROBERT E. MEASLEY, JR., MD

The highly technical and invasive surgical procedures now commonly performed are successful in large part because of perioperative antibiotics. In fact, the greatest impact of antibiotics over the last half-century may ultimately be related to their essential role in supporting surgery.

Although postoperative infection may not be likely, it is still a major component of surgical morbidity and mortality. It accounts for nearly one fourth of all nosocomial infections, second only to urinary tract infections, with an overall incidence of nearly 5%. Surgical site infections (SSIs), as they are now called, account for 60% to 80% of all postoperative infections. Although SSIs usually remain localized, they can spread to adjacent areas and even to the bloodstream, often leading to sepsis and death. The goal of prophylaxis in this setting is to decrease the incidence of infection and its attendant complications.

RISK FACTORS FOR POSTOPERATIVE INFECTIONS

Certain factors have been identified that predispose a patient to the development of a postoperative infection. These include the patient, the surgeon, and the surgical procedure performed (Box 3-1).

Levels of Evidence:

Ⓐ—Randomized controlled trials (RCTs), meta-analyses, well-designed systematic reviews of RCTs. Ⓑ—Case-control or cohort studies, nonrandomized controlled trials, systematic reviews of studies other than RCTs, cross-sectional studies, retrospective studies. Ⓒ—Consensus statements, expert guidelines, usual practice, opinion.

Box 3-1	FACTORS INVOLVED IN THE DEVELOPMENT OF POSTOPERATIVE INFECTIONS

Presence of pathogenic bacteria in sufficient numbers
Local wound environment: blood, tissue fluids, necrotic tissue
Immune status of the host: obesity, age, diabetes mellitus, nutrition
Length of the procedure, surgical skill
Foreign body presence
Type of surgical procedure

The surgical procedure is the factor most often classified and quantitated with regard to postoperative infections. Procedures are grouped according to the risk of contamination of the surgical area with either endogenous or exogenous microorganisms (Table 3-1). In addition to the surgical procedure and type of wound, another important factor influencing the infection rate is the skill of the surgeon. The procedure needs to be performed with adequate débridement, hemostasis, and drainage and as quickly as is safely possible because infection rates double for each hour of surgery.

Surveillance studies have shown the following risk factors for postoperative wound infection:

1. Abdominal surgical procedure
2. Procedure lasting more than 2 hours
3. Contaminated, dirty, or infected procedure by traditional classification (see Table 3-1)
4. Three or more discharge diagnoses that increase the complexity of the patient's condition

PREVENTION OF POSTOPERATIVE INFECTIONS

Many maneuvers other than antimicrobial treatment may decrease the incidence of infection. Several of the risk factors mentioned in Box 3-1 can be influenced only by special

TABLE 3-1	Classification of Surgical Procedures by Degree of Contamination and Risk of Subsequent Infection		
		WOUND INFECTION RATE (%) PREOPERATIVE ANTIBIOTICS ADMINISTERED	
Type of Procedure	Definition	No	Yes
Clean	Atraumatic; no break in technique; gastrointestinal, genitourinary, and respiratory tracts not entered	5.1	0.8
Clean-contaminated	Gastrointestinal or respiratory tract entered but without spillage; oropharynx, sterile genitourinary, or biliary tract entered; minor break in technique	10.1	1.3
Contaminated	Acute inflammation; infected bile or urine; gross spillage from gastrointestinal tract	21.9	10.2
Dirty	Established infection	40	10

preparation of the patient for surgery *before* any perioperative antibiotic use (Box 3-2). Studies suggest that attention to intraoperative temperature control, supplemental oxygen administration, and aggressive fluid resuscitation may also reduce infection rates.

Of the interventions listed in Box 3-2, perhaps the most important for the medical consultant is maximizing of diabetes control. **Considerable evidence indicates that strict perioperative control of blood glucose concentrations with intravenous insulin in patients undergoing cardiac surgery may reduce SSI rates, even in patients without diabetes mellitus [❹ Furnary et al, 1999].** Reversing malnutrition or obesity if time allows, treating remote sites of infection, and, if no active infection exists, avoiding antibiotic use until the time of surgery are other important interventions.

Box 3-2	NONANTIMICROBIAL INTERVENTIONS OF BENEFIT IN DECREASING THE RISK OF SURGICAL WOUND INFECTIONS

PREOPERATIVELY

Minimize preoperative hospitalization.

Treat remote sites of infection.

Avoid shaving or delay it until time of surgery.

Avoid preoperative antibiotic use.

Resolve malnutrition and obesity.

Maximize diabetes control.

INTRAOPERATIVELY/POSTOPERATIVELY

Use careful skin preparation.

Use rigorous aseptic technique.

Use high-flow filtered air or laminar flow.

Minimize dead space.

Minimize the use of catheters and intravenous lines postoperatively.

Maintain adequate hydration, oxygenation, and nutrition postoperatively.

PERIOPERATIVE ANTIBIOTICS

General Principles of Antibiotic Selection and Use

Antibiotic Choice

Cefazolin is the most commonly used antibiotic for prophylaxis. It offers the advantages of a moderately long half-life, activity against most staphylococci and streptococci (in addition to some gram-negative aerobic organisms), and low cost. Cefazolin has had extensive clinical use and has proven effectiveness. For intra-abdominal and pelvic procedures that may involve bowel anaerobes, cefoxitin (Mefoxin) is used instead because of its enhanced activity against these organisms. Recently, ertapenem (Invanz) was also approved for prophylaxis in patients undergoing colorectal surgeries after a trial comparing it with cefotetan showed it to be more effective [Itani et al, 2006]. Ciprofloxacin and levofloxacin are reserved for use in urologic surgery or for gastrointestinal surgery in cases of cephalosporin allergy only. Most authorities still suggest the use of vancomycin in institutions with a high prevalence of methicillin-resistant *Staphylococcus aureus* (MRSA) or methicillin-resistant coagulase-negative staphylococci as postoperative pathogens, but the routine use of vancomycin should be discouraged, to prevent emergence of vancomycin-resistant organisms. Indeed, one study showed that vancomycin did not prevent SSIs any better than cefazolin in a tertiary care institution with just such a high prevalence of MRSA.

In general, newer, broad-spectrum agents, such as third- or fourth-generation cephalosporins, broad-spectrum penicillins, or carbapenems, should be avoided because they are expensive, they are active against organisms rarely encountered in elective surgery, and their use may lead to the emergence of resistant bacterial strains. Antibiotics should be chosen for their activity against the organisms most likely to be involved—it is not necessary to cover all potential pathogens.

Dose Timing and Duration

Adequate tissue antibiotic levels need to be present from the time the incision is made until the procedure is completed. Improper timing of antibiotic administration (either too soon or too late) is responsible for "antibiotic failure" more often than any other factor. **To achieve this objective, the antibiotic chosen should be administered within 60 to 120 minutes before the incision is made** [❶ *Classen et al, 1992*]. Ordering antibiotics to be given "on call" should be avoided because delays in starting surgery may result in inadequate intraoperative tissue levels of antibiotic.

In longer procedures, antibiotics may have to be readministered, especially if the operation is still in progress two half-lives or more after the first dose (e.g., cefazolin, every 2 to 5 hours; cefoxitin, every 2 to 3 hours; clindamycin, every

3 to 6 hours; and vancomycin, every 6 to 12 hours). Prolonged antibiotic use postoperatively (i.e., after wound closure or >24 hours) should be avoided because of the increased risk for developing antimicrobial resistance.

Antimicrobial Prophylaxis for Specific Surgical Procedures

Specific antimicrobial regimens are given in Table 3-2.

Cardiothoracic Surgery

SURGERY INVOLVING MEDIAN STERNOTOMY

Prophylactic antibiotics directed against staphylococci reduce postoperative infections after bypass grafting and valve replacement. If the surgical procedure is lengthy, prophylactic antibiotics may have to be readministered to maintain adequate antibiotic tissue levels and to decrease the risk of SSI. However, continued administration of prophylactic antibiotics until all catheters, wires, and drains have been removed is not appropriate and has been associated with higher rates of resistant organisms when infection occurs.

CARDIAC DEVICE PLACEMENT AND CARDIAC CATHETERIZATION

Although this issue has not been rigorously studied, current consensus favors the use of antimicrobial prophylaxis before placement of pacemakers, defibrillators, ventricular assist devices, ventriculoatrial shunts, and arterial patches. A meta-analysis of seven randomized studies of prophylaxis for permanent pacemaker implantation showed statistically significant reductions in the incidence of SSI, inflammation, and skin erosion. Antibiotic prophylaxis before cardiac catheterization is not currently recommended because of the very low rate of SSIs associated with this procedure.

THORACIC (NONCARDIAC) SURGERY

The use of prophylactic antibiotics in pulmonary resection has been controversial. Evidence in pulmonary resection surgery indicated that prophylactic antibiotics result in a

TABLE 3-2	**Antimicrobial Prophylaxis for Prevention of Specific Surgical Site Infections**		

Nature of Operation	Common Pathogens	Recommended Antimicrobials	Adult Dosage before Surgery[1]
Cardiac	*Staphylococcus aureus, Staphylococcus epidermidis*	Cefazolin or cefuroxime OR vancomycin[3]	1–2 g IV[2] 1.5 g IV[2] 1 g IV
Gastrointestinal			
Esophageal, gastroduodenal	Enteric gram-negative bacilli, gram-positive cocci	*High risk[4] only:* Cefazolin[7]	1–2 g IV
Biliary tract	Enteric gram-negative bacilli, enterococci, clostridia	*High risk[5] only:* Cefazolin[7]	1–2 g IV
Colorectal	Enteric gram-negative bacilli, anaerobes, enterococci	Oral: neomycin plus erythromycin base[6] OR metronidazole[6]	
		Parenteral: cefoxitin OR cefazolin plus metronidazole[7] OR ampicillin/ sulbactam[7]	1–2 g IV 1–2 g IV 0.5 g IV 3 g IV
Appendectomy nonperforated[8]	Enteric gram-negative bacilli, anaerobes, enterococci	cefoxitin[7] OR cefazolin plus metronidazole[7] OR ampicillin/ sulbactam[7]	1–2 g IV 1–2 g IV 0.5 g IV 3 g IV
Genitourinary	Enteric gram-negative bacilli, enterococci	*High risk[9] only:* Ciprofloxacin	500 mg PO or 400 mg IV
Gynecologic and Obstetric			
Vaginal, abdominal, or laparoscopic hysterectomy	Enteric gram-negative bacilli, anaerobes, group B streptococci, enterococci	Cefoxitin[7] or cefazolin[7] OR ampicillin/ sulbactam[7]	1–2 g IV 3 g IV

Table continued on following page

TABLE 3-2	Antimicrobial Prophylaxis for Prevention of Specific Surgical Site Infections (Continued)		

Nature of Operation	Common Pathogens	Recommended Antimicrobials	Adult Dosage before Surgery[1]
Cesarean section	Same as for hysterectomy	Cefazolin[7]	1–2 g IV after cord clamp
Abortion	Same as for hysterectomy	*First trimester, high risk* [10]:	
		Aqueous penicillin G OR doxycycline	2 million units IV 300 mg PO[11]
		Second trimester: Cefazolin[7]	1–2 g IV
Head and Neck Surgery			
Incisions through oral or pharyngeal mucosa	Anaerobes, enteric gram-negative bacilli, S. aureus	Clindamycin plus gentamicin OR cefazolin	600–900 mg IV 1.5 mg/kg IV 1–2 g IV
Neurosurgery	S. aureus, S. epidermidis	Cefazolin OR vancomycin[3]	1–2 g IV 1 g IV
Ophthalmic	S. epidermidis, S. aureus, streptococci, enteric gram-negative bacilli, Pseudomonas spp.	Gentamicin, tobramycin, ciprofloxacin, gatifloxacin, levofloxacin, moxifloxacin, olofloxacin, or neomycin-gramicidin-polymyxin B	Multiple drops topically over 2–24 hr
		Cefazolin	100 mg subconjunctivally
Orthopedic	S. aureus, S. epidermidis	Cefazolin[12] or cefuroxime[12] OR vancomycin[3,12]	1–2 g IV 1.5 g IV 1 g IV
Thoracic (noncardiac)	S. aureus, S. epidermidis, streptococci, enteric gram-negative bacilli	Cefazolin or cefuroxime OR vancomycin[3]	1–2 g IV 1.5 g IV 1 g IV
Vascular			
Arterial surgery involving a prosthesis, abdominal aorta, or groin incision	S. aureus, S. epidermidis, enteric gram-negative bacilli	Cefazolin OR vancomycin[3]	1–2 g IV 1 g IV

Nature of Operation	Common Pathogens	Recommended Antimicrobials	Adult Dosage before Surgery[1]
Vascular—cont'd			
Lower extremity amputation for ischemia	S. aureus, S. epidermidis, enteric gram-negative bacilli, clostridia	Cefazolin OR vancomycin[3]	1–2 g IV 1 g IV

[1]Parenteral prophylactic antimicrobials can be given as a single IV dose begun 60 minutes or less before the operation. For prolonged operations (>4 hours), or those with major blood loss, additional intraoperative doses should be given at intervals 1-2 times the half-life of the drug for the duration of the procedure in patients with normal renal function. If vancomycin or a fluoroquinolone is used, the infusion should be started 60-120 minutes before the initial incision in order to minimize the possibility of an infusion reaction close to the time of induction of anesthesia and to have adequate tissue levels at the time of incision.

[2]Some consultants recommend an additional dose when patients are removed from bypass during open-heart surgery.

[3]Vancomycin is used in hospitals in which methicillin-resistant S. aureus (MRSA) and S. epidermidis are a frequent cause of postoperative wound infection, for patients previously colonized with MRSA, or for those who are allergic to penicillins or cephalosporins. Rapid IV administration may cause hypotension, which could be especially dangerous during induction of anesthesia. Even when the drug is given over 60 minutes, hypotension may occur; treatment with diphenhydramine (Benadryl, and others) and further slowing of the infusion rate may be helpful. Some experts would give 15 mg/kg of vancomycin to patients weighing more than 75 kg, up to a maximum of 1.5 g, with a slower infusion rate (90 minutes for 1.5 g). To provide coverage against gram-negative bacteria, most Medical Letter consultants would also include cefazolin or cefuroxime in the prophylaxis regimen for patients not allergic to cephalosporins; ciprofloxacin, levofloxacin, gentamicin, or aztreonam, each one in combination with vancomycin, can be used in patients who cannot tolerate a cephalosporin.

[4]Morbid obesity, esophageal obstruction, decreased gastric acidity or gastrointestinal motility.

[5]Age >70 years, acute cholecystitis, nonfunctioning gall bladder, obstructive jaundice or common duct stones.

[6]After appropriate diet and catharsis, 1 g of neomycin plus 1 g of erythromycin at 1 PM, 2 PM and 11 PM or 2 g of neomycin plus 2 g of metronidazole at 7 PM and 11 PM the day before an 8 AM operation.

[7]For patients allergic to penicillins and cephalosporins, clindamycin with either gentamicin, ciprofloxacin, levofloxacin, or aztreonam is a reasonable alternative.

[8]For a ruptured viscus, therapy is often continued for about 5 days. Ruptured viscus in postoperative setting (dehiscence) requires antibacterials to include coverage of nosocomial pathogens.

[9]Urine culture positive or unavailable, preoperative catheter, transrectal prostatic biopsy, placement of prosthetic material.

[10]Patients with previous pelvic inflammatory disease, previous gonorrhea, or multiple sex partners.

[11]Divided into 100 mg 1 hour before the abortion and 200 mg 30 minutes after.

[12]If a tourniquet is to be used in the procedure, the entire dose of antibiotic must be infused prior to its inflation.

From Treatment guidelines from the Medical Letter: Antimicrobial prophylaxis for surgery. The Medical Letter (52):83-88, 2006. Reproduced with permission of The Medical Letter, Inc.

significant reduction in the incidence of SSIs, but not of pneumonia or empyema. Other trials showed a benefit after closed-tube thoracostomy for chest trauma. However, the current consensus, despite a lack of hard data, supports the use of antibiotic prophylaxis in most cases of noncardiac thoracic surgery.

Gastrointestinal Surgery

ESOPHAGEAL SURGERY

The esophagus is generally a sterile viscus as a result of peristalsis. However, diseases that lead to obstruction, decreased peristalsis, or stasis prompt proliferation of oral aerobes and anaerobes. In turn, the risk of mediastinal infection is increased, and prophylaxis is generally recommended. One prospective, randomized study in endoscopic sclerotherapy of esophageal varices showed no benefit of prophylactic antibiotics in reducing the risk of bacteremias or SSIs.

GASTRODUODENAL SURGERY

The incidence of postoperative infection in gastroduodenal surgery is proportionate to the number of bacteria within the stomach; consequently, the risk of infection is highest when gastric acidity and gastrointestinal motility are diminished by defects in the gastric mucous membrane or by prolonged therapy with histamine (H_2)-blockers or proton pump inhibitors. Cessation of H_2-blockers or proton-pump inhibitors and preoperative use of a cephalosporin can decrease the incidence of postoperative infection in patients with carcinoma, gastric ulcer, bleeding, obstruction, or perforation. Prophylaxis is also recommended in patients who are morbidly obese. Prophylactic antibiotics are not indicated for routine gastroesophageal endoscopy, but they are indicated before placement of percutaneous gastrostomy tubes.

BILIARY PROCEDURES

The biliary tract is normally sterile, and patients less than 70 years of age who are undergoing elective surgery without preoperative infections are generally not at risk for postoperative infectious complications. Thus, prophylactic antibiotics are generally not indicated in routine elective laparoscopic cholecystectomy. However, prophylaxis is recommended before biliary tract surgery in patients who are at increased risk of infection. This group includes patients more than 70 years of age and those with common bile duct stones, bile duct stricture or obstruction, recent acute cholecystitis, or prior biliary surgery. This recommendation also applies to patients who undergo endoscopic retrograde cholangiopancreatography.

COLORECTAL SURGERY

The risk of significant perioperative infections in patients undergoing colorectal operations may be as high as 40% if prophylactic antibiotics are not used. An oral regimen of luminal catharsis and antibiotics can reduce the postoperative infection rate to less than 7% and appears to be as effective as the use of parenteral antimicrobials. Whether a combination of oral and parenteral agents is better than either regimen alone is unclear, but such a combination is widely employed in the United States. The prophylactic regimen should include an oral lavage solution (e.g., polyethylene glycol) and antimicrobials effective against both aerobic gram-negative bacilli and anaerobes—usually neomycin in combination with either erythromycin or metronidazole.

APPENDECTOMY

Prophylactic antibiotics decrease the incidence of infection after appendectomy. If the appendix has perforated, the patient should be treated as though an infection were present. In that instance, antibiotics should be used therapeutically (i.e., for 5 to 7 days). Regimens with activity against both aerobic gram-negative bacilli and anaerobes are recommended.

PENETRATING ABDOMINAL TRAUMA

Escape of endogenous bacteria as a result of hollow lumen visceral damage is a major risk factor for postoperative infection following penetrating abdominal trauma. Before surgical treatment of penetrating abdominal trauma, a single dose of prophylactic antibiotic is indicated. If at exploratory laparotomy gastrointestinal leakage is observed, antibiotics should be continued on a therapeutic basis. Studies have suggested that shorter courses of antibiotics (e.g., 12 to 24 hours) may be just as effective as 5 days of therapy in patients with penetrating abdominal trauma.

Genitourinary Tract Surgery

In general, antimicrobials are not recommended before urologic operations in patients with documented sterile urine. A basic tenet has been that patients with urine cultures positive for bacteria should be treated to sterilize the urine preoperatively, or these patients should receive a single preoperative dose of an appropriate agent at the time of surgery. Ciprofloxacin is the agent of choice. Prophylactic antibiotics for urologic procedures involving the intestinal tract, such as transrectal prostate biopsy, are recommended. Although no prophylaxis is recommended for transurethral prostatectomy, a meta-analysis of more than 4000 patients with sterile preoperative urine who were undergoing transurethral prostatectomy concluded that antimicrobial prophylaxis significantly decreased the incidence of bacteriuria and septicemia. The implantation of prosthetic devices is increasing, and prophylaxis is recommended for these procedures, usually with vancomycin and ciprofloxacin. Common devices include penile implants, artificial sphincters, synthetic pubovaginal slings, and bone anchors for pelvic floor reconstruction.

Gynecologic Surgery

Perioperative antimicrobials can prevent infection after cesarean section in high-risk situations (premature rupture of membranes). In these cases, most obstetricians administer cefazolin after the umbilical cord is clamped because of concern about masking septic manifestations in the newborn. Antimicrobials are not recommended in uncomplicated cases. First trimester abortion in women at high risk for pelvic infection (pelvic inflammatory disease, previous gonorrhea, or multiple sex partners) warrants prophylaxis with penicillin or doxycycline because controlled trials have shown that these particular agents are effective. In second trimester instillation abortion, cefazolin is recommended. Finally, antimicrobial prophylaxis decreases the incidence of infection after vaginal, abdominal, and laparoscopic hysterectomy. Cefoxitin is currently the first-line agent for these procedures.

Neurosurgery

Antistaphylococcal antibiotics used prophylactically may decrease the incidence of infection following craniotomy. **Prophylaxis before cerebrospinal fluid shunt placement has been associated with a 50% risk reduction of perioperative infection [❶ Langley et al, 1993].** Currently, the use of antibiotic-impregnated shunts has generated interest as another strategy for reducing infection rates. **Although current guidelines for spinal surgery associated with short operative time (e.g., conventional discectomy) state that antibiotic prophylaxis is not warranted, a meta-analysis concluded that prophylaxis was beneficial even in these low-risk cases [❶ Barker, 2002].** For spinal surgery associated with longer operative times (e.g., spinal fusion) or surgery with insertion of prosthetic material, the infection rate is higher than in discectomy. Therefore, despite absence of controlled trials, antibiotic prophylaxis has become more common.

Ophthalmologic Surgery

There are no randomized trials defining the efficacy of prophylaxis before ocular surgery. However, most ophthalmologists use antimicrobial eye drops prophylactically, and some perform subconjunctival injection at the end of the procedure. Nonetheless, consensus is lacking to support a particular choice, route, or duration of antimicrobial prophylaxis. In procedures outside of the globe, prophylactic antibiotics are generally not needed.

Orthopedic Surgery

Antistaphylococcal antibiotics have been shown to be effective in preventing infections of prosthetic joints as well as infections complicating fractures treated with internal fixation hardware. If a proximal tourniquet is used, the antibiotic infusion must be completed before tourniquet inflation. Antibiotic prophylaxis is not indicated in arthroscopic surgery. Although in practice it is usually done, no data support the use of prophylactic antibiotics in patients with prosthetic joints or spinal hardware who undergo dental, gastrointestinal, or genitourinary procedures.

Otolaryngologic Surgery

Wound infections following surgery of the oropharynx are common. Prophylaxis with any one of a variety of antimicrobials has decreased this complication. Clindamycin and gentamicin, or cefazolin, are currently recommended. Infection rates in uncontaminated head and neck surgery (i.e., tonsillectomy, adenoidectomy), however, are too low to justify prophylaxis. Although many otolaryngologists use antimicrobial ear drops before tympanostomy tube placement, any decrease in the degree of purulent otorrhea is largely anecdotal.

Peripheral Vascular Surgery

Preoperative administration of a cephalosporin has been shown to decrease the incidence of postoperative wound infection in the following surgical procedures: abdominal aorta resection with graft placement, lower extremity bypass grafting in which groin incisions are made, and lower extremity amputations for ischemia. Many authorities also recommend using prophylaxis for any procedure involving vascular prosthetic material placement (e.g., hemodialysis access grafts). Antibiotic prophylaxis is not indicated for carotid endarterectomy or upper extremity bypass grafts unless prosthetic material is used.

Selected Readings

Andersen BR, Kallegave FL, Andersen HK: Antibiotics versus placebo for prevention of postoperative infection after appendicectomy. Cochrane Database Syst Rev 2:CD001439, 2003.
Barker FG 2nd: Efficacy of prophylactic antibiotic therapy in spinal surgery: A meta-analysis. Neurosurgery 53:243, 2002. **B**

Bratzler DW, Houck PM, for the Surgical Infection Prevention Guideline Writers Workgroup: Antimicrobial prophylaxis for surgery: An advisory statement from the National Surgical Infection Prevention Project. Clin Infect Dis 38:1706-1715, 2004.

Bratzler DW, Houck PM, Richards C, et al: Use of antimicrobial prophylaxis for major surgery: Baseline results from the national surgical infection prevention project. Arch Surg 140:174-182, 2005.

Burke JF: The effective period of preventive antibiotic action in experimental incisions and dermal lesions. Surgery 50:161-168, 1961.

Chong AJ, Dellinger EP: Infectious complications of surgery in morbidly obese patients. Curr Treat Options Infect Dis 5:387, 2003.

Classen DC, Evans RS, Pestotnik SL, et al: The timing of prophylactic administration of antibiotics and the risk of surgical wound infection. N Engl J Med 326:281-286, 1992. **🅑**

Cornwell EE, Dougherty WR, Berne TV, et al: Duration of antibiotic prophylaxis in high-risk patients with penetrating abdominal trauma: A prospective randomized trial. J Gastrointest Surg 3:648-653, 1999.

Dimick JB, Lipsett PA, Kostuik JP: Spine update: Antimicrobial prophylaxis in spine surgery. Basic principles and recent advances. Spine 25: 2544-2548, 2000.

Furnary AP, Zerr KJ, Grunkemeier GL, Starr A: Continuous intravenous insulin infusion reduces the incidence of deep sternal wound infection in diabetic patients after cardiac surgical procedures. Ann Thorac Surg 67:352-360, 1999. **🅐**

Grief R, Akca O, Horn E-P, et al: Supplemental perioperative oxygen to reduce the incidence of surgical wound infection. N Engl J Med 342: 161-167, 2000.

Itani KMF, Wilson SE, Awad SS, et al: Ertapenem versus cefotetan prophylaxis in elective colorectal surgery. N Engl J Med 355:2640-2651, 2006.

Kurz A, Sessler DI, Lenhardt RA: Perioperative normothermia to reduce the incidence of surgical-wound infection and shorten hospitalization. N Engl J Med 334:1209-1215, 1996.

Langley JM, LeBlanc JC, Drake J, Milner R: Efficacy of antimicrobial prophylaxis in placement of cerebrospinal fluid shunts: Meta-analysis. Clin Infect Dis 17:98-103, 1993. **🅑**

Maki DG, Bohn MJ, Stolz SM, et al: Comparative study of cefazolin, cefamandole, and vancomycin for surgical prophylaxis in cardiac and vascular operations: A double-blind randomized trial. J Thorac Cardiovasc Surg 104:1423-1434, 1992.

Sessler DI, Akca O: Nonpharmacologic prevention of surgical wound infections. Clin Infect Dis 35:1397-1404, 2002.

Strom BL, Abrutyn E, Berlin JA, et al: Dental and cardiac risk factors for infective endocarditis: A population-based, case-control study. Ann Intern Med 129:761-769, 1998.

Ulualp K, Condon RE: Antibiotic prophylaxis for scheduled operative procedures. Infect Dis Clin North Am 6:613-625, 1992.

Zerr KJ, Furnary AP, Grunkemeier GL, et al: Glucose control lowers the risk of wound infection in diabetics after open heart operations. Ann Thorac Surg 63:356-361, 1997.

4 Selected Medical Challenges of Anesthesia

ROBERT F. ATKINS, MD

Although it was once considered legitimate to refuse surgery to a patient because he or she was "too sick to undergo anesthesia," in recent years anesthesia has become much safer. For example, epidemiologic studies conducted over a 30-year period through the late 1970s reported anesthesia-related mortality rates in the range of 1 to 2 per 10,000 anesthesia procedures. Since the early 1980s, reported mortality has declined by at least a factor of 10. During this more recent period, the specialty of anesthesiology has devoted itself to improving patient safety and has been in the vanguard of the effort to develop evidence-based practice guidelines.

Many factors have been important in the reduction of anesthetic risk. They include improvements in anesthetic drugs and in monitoring and equipment technologies, as well as more generalized advances in perioperative medical care. The resulting decline in the frequency of devastating anesthetic complications has largely redirected the attention of patients and physicians to less serious, but more common, adverse sequelae of anesthesia.

Clinicians who are not anesthesiologists are often involved in the care of patients who develop perioperative medical problems related to anesthesia. This chapter deals with some of these common perioperative issues and provides suggestions for assessment and management.

Levels of Evidence:

Ⓐ—Randomized controlled trials (RCTs), meta-analyses, well-designed systematic reviews of RCTs. **Ⓑ**—Case-control or cohort studies, nonrandomized controlled trials, systematic reviews of studies other than RCTs, cross-sectional studies, retrospective studies. **Ⓒ**—Consensus statements, expert guidelines, usual practice, opinion.

SPINAL HEADACHE

Spinal anesthesia (SA) is an extremely popular anesthetic technique that, along with its close relative epidural anesthesia, makes up a significant majority of all regional anesthetics given in the United States. A *regional anesthetic,* which anesthetizes a *region* of the body (e.g., one or more extremities, entire lower half of the body), is distinguished from *local anesthesia,* which focuses on the area surrounding the surgical incision, and from *general anesthesia.* In contrast to general anesthesia, deep unconsciousness is not induced during surgery with regional anesthesia, although intravenous sedation, which produces a mild depression of consciousness in conjunction with anxiolysis, is frequently employed simultaneously to improve the subjective experience for the patient.

Although generally well tolerated, SA can have various sequelae, which are not usually serious. Spinal headache, technically known as *postdural puncture headache* (PDPH), is among the concerns about SA most frequently expressed by patients, especially those with no previous experience with SA or those with a history of PDPH. Moreover, patients suffering from PDPH can be severely incapacitated, often unable to perform basic activities of daily living as a result of pain and associated symptoms.

Etiology and Clinical Characteristics

The underlying cause of PDPH involves a loss of cerebrospinal fluid (CSF) through the puncture site in the dura (and subjacent arachnoid) mater that results in reduced intracranial pressure when the patient assumes an upright posture. This change in pressure, in turn, permits the "sagging" of cerebral structures within the cranial vault and places tension on the sensitive meninges and cerebral vessels. Indeed, the fundamental relationship between posture and the onset of symptoms is a hallmark in the clinical diagnosis of PDPH.

PDPH shares various features with vascular headache, a finding that led to the belief that much of the pain syndrome is vascular in origin. Experimental evidence reveals reproducible, and reversible, compensatory cerebral vasodilation in response to a reduction in intracranial pressure.

The location of the pain of PDPH is typically fronto-occipital, frequently with radiation to the neck and shoulders (Table 4-1). The onset is usually delayed; symptoms rarely begin less than 8 to 12 hours after SA and are most commonly

TABLE 4-1	Spinal Headache: Clinical Features
Etiology	
Intracranial hypotension → reflex cerebral vasodilation	
Location	
Fronto-occipital; nuchal radiation	
Onset	
Earliest, 6–12 hr; 90% in 24–72 hr	
Associated Symptoms	
Nausea, tinnitus, diplopia	
Severity	
Mild:	50%
Moderate:	35%
Severe:	15%
Differential Diagnosis	
Common:	Tension headache, migraine
Rare:	Meningitis, intracranial hematoma, postpartum cortical vein thrombosis (1 in 6000 deliveries)
Pathognomonic Sign	
Relationship with posture: Symptoms worse upright, symptoms rapidly improved supine	
Resolution	
Spontaneous	
Duration variable, correlated with severity at onset	
70% resolved within 5 days	
80%–85% resolved within 7 days	
95% resolved within 6 wk	

first seen on postoperative days 1 to 3. Associated symptoms are not common but can include nausea, tinnitus, hypoacusis, and, in the most severe cases, diplopia resulting from tension on the abducens nerve in the cranial vault. Symptoms are self-limited in most cases, but their duration is highly variable.

Not all headaches that follow SA (or diagnostic lumbar puncture) are PDPHs. The differential diagnosis includes any of the more common headache syndromes as well as various rare, and more serious, causes. The diagnosis is confirmed by the absence of signs of central nervous system (CNS) infection or lateralizing sensorimotor deficit and by the pathognomonic postural component (exacerbation while the patient is upright and relief when the patient is recumbent), without which the diagnosis should not be made.

Epidemiology

Given the ubiquitous loss of CSF that follows dural puncture, the incidence of PDPH after SA is surprisingly low, ranging from 1% to 25% in most contemporary studies. It is unknown why, in similar clinical circumstances, one patient acquires PDPH and another does not. Nonetheless, considerable investigation has been done to elucidate the factors that do affect the incidence of PDPH among various patient groups.

Most of the research on PDPH performed over the past several decades has consistently identified the importance of *age*, *gender*, and *needle size*. PDPH is significantly more frequent with decreasing age, female gender (especially when SA is used for obstetric procedures), and increasing needle diameter (Fig. 4-1). The frequency of PDPH following diagnostic lumbar puncture exceeds that following SA, because larger needles are used in lumbar puncture, and CSF is intentionally withdrawn.

Significantly modifying the effect of needle diameter, however, is the position of the needle tip. First, **the direction of the needle bevel with respect to the patient at the time**

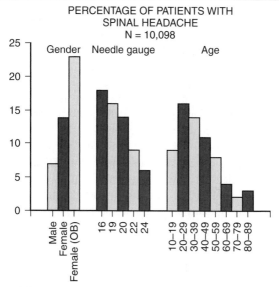

Figure 4-1 • Percentage of patients with spinal headache. OB, obstetric. *(Adapted from Vandam LD, Dripps RD: Long-term follow-up of patients who received 10,098 spinal anesthetics: Syndrome of decreased intracranial pressure [headache and ocular and auditory difficulties]. JAMA 161:586-591, 1956.)*

of dural puncture has a significant influence on the occurrence of PDPH [❶ *Evans et al, 2000*]. Investigators have come to recognize that orienting the bevel of a spinal needle parallel to the longitudinal axis of the vertebral column during insertion (i.e., facing the ceiling or floor with a patient in the lateral decubitus position) produces a significantly lower incidence of PDPH than when the bevel is perpendicular to that axis.

The benefit obtained in parallel bevel orientation has been presumed to be related to the microanatomic arrangement of fibers of connective tissue that form the dura; until recently, these fibers were also thought to be arranged parallel to the long axis of the vertebral column. Thus, a parallel bevel would be expected to produce a less traumatic puncture of the dura and less CSF loss. This explanation has recently been questioned by the results of electron microscopic studies showing that dural fibers are actually arranged randomly, rather than in a precise pattern. Thus, the precise cause of the significant benefit realized with parallel bevel insertion remains unclear.

By far, the most important innovation in spinal needle design has been the replacement of the traditional beveled tip in favor of "pencil point" (e.g., Whitacre, Sprotte) construction (Fig. 4-2). This newer design further reduces dural trauma during lumbar puncture, with an additional reduction in CSF leakage. Numerous clinical and in vitro studies with these needles have yielded overwhelmingly favorable results. Indeed, many anesthesiologists have, with occasional

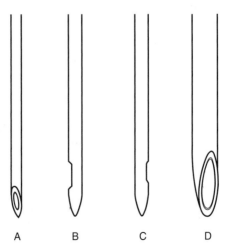

A   B   C   D

Figure 4-2 • Array of needles used for neuraxial anesthesia (A–C are used for spinal anesthesia). **A**, Traditional beveled (Quincke) needle, with orifice within the diagonal cutting tip. **B** and **C**, Newer "pencil point" designs (Sprotte and Whitacre, respectively). These end in a rounded, noncutting tip and have orifices arranged distally on the side. **D**, Standard epidural (Tuohy) needle. This is larger in diameter and has a curved tip containing the orifice oriented perpendicular to its long axis that allows passage of an epidural catheter up the epidural space within the vertebral canal.

exception, abandoned the use of bevel-tipped in favor of pencil point needles.

For unknown reasons, the dominant factor influencing the frequency of PDPH is age. The incidence of PDPH peaks in the young adult population and decreases with increasing age. PDPH is very rare in patients who are more than 70 or less than 10 years old. Anesthesiologists thus have more latitude in the choice of spinal needles in these age groups.

Prognosis and Treatment

The prognosis for PDPH is generally good; 75% of patients have spontaneous resolution of symptoms within 1 week. Unfortunately, in a minority of patients, symptoms can linger for weeks to months. A correlation appears to exist between the severity of pain and the presence of associated symptoms (e.g., diplopia) at onset and the likely duration of symptoms in untreated patients.

Treatment is categorized as conservative or invasive. Conservative treatment is intended to provide symptomatic relief during spontaneous healing of the dural rent. It relies on oral analgesics, especially nonsteroidal anti-inflammatory drugs; narcotics may be appropriate for brief intervals in patients with more severe cases. Other conservative approaches advocated historically and intended to normalize pressure gradients within the neuraxis include forced oral and intravenous fluids, abdominal binders, and bed rest. None of these measures has been shown in clinical studies to offer reproducible benefit.

Although advocating strict bed rest following lumbar puncture as a means of preventing PDPH has remained part of the medical "lore," no evidence indicates that it has any benefit. Patients considering SA often express considerable anxiety about the presumed need to remain in bed following the procedure and deserve reassurance that the practice is not necessary.

The theory that a substantial component of the pain of PDPH is the result of compensatory cerebral vasodilation has led to the use of intravenous caffeine and other methylxanthine derivatives, and more recently sumatriptan, as conservative treatment modalities. Whatever benefit these measures produce tends to be only temporary, and these agents are not without risk.

The "gold standard" in the treatment of PDPH remains the epidural blood patch (EBP) [❽ *Duffy and Crosby, 1999*]. This invasive technique has a 4-decade history of use and has consistently been shown to be highly effective and generally well tolerated. EBP achieves complete and persistent resolution of symptoms in 75% of patients after one treatment and in up to 99% after a second or third procedure. Indeed, many authors maintain that persistent symptoms following two EBPs suggest a misdiagnosis of PDPH.

The technique involves placement of an epidural needle at a level approximating the previous dural puncture site and injecting a 15- to 20-mL sample of the patient's autologous blood, which must be collected aseptically, into the epidural space. The benefit is both immediate, secondary to a tamponade effect that raises intracranial pressure and reduces compensatory cerebral vasodilation, and sustained. The long-term benefit is thought to result from formation of a coagulum in the dural puncture that precludes further loss of CSF; this coagulum also stimulates collagen growth, which presumably promotes healing. Reported recurrences of PDPH 1 to 3 weeks after EBP are presumed to be caused by disruption of the coagulum. For this reason, patients receiving EBP must be instructed to avoid activities that could acutely alter the pressure gradients in the lumbar neuraxis, such as lifting, straining, and possibly airline travel; the use of laxatives and stool softeners should be encouraged.

Side effects of EBP are generally benign and include transient back pain, radicular pain, and fever. Serious sequelae such as persistent radiculopathy, epidural abscess, and spinal cord compression, although theoretically possible, have not been reported. However, because EBP is an invasive procedure, patients must be selected carefully. The complication of inadvertent dural puncture with a (large) epidural needle (incidence, 1% to 3 %) would be highly counterproductive. Patients are usually offered EBP when symptoms have been persistent for several days or are sufficiently severe to interfere with daily activities. A common example of the latter is the postpartum patient whose discharge home is delayed because of PDPH. In this circumstance, the technique has a high acceptance rate.

The understanding that the sustained benefit of EBP is the product of healing and closure of otherwise persistent dural puncture has inspired more recent, innovative treatments. Fibrin glue has been employed as a means of treating disruption in the integrity of various biologic membranes. Case reports have documented the successful use of fibrin glue in the treatment of PDPH. The long-term sequelae of this modality are not yet known, and its role in the approach to PDPH remains to be established.

OBESITY

In 2002, an estimated 30.6% of adults in the United States were obese, more than double the prevalence 20 years earlier. Obesity is thus the most common nutritional-metabolic disorder among patients undergoing surgery. The disorder is both defined and graded by comparison of actual weight with an accepted index of ideal body weight. The currently accepted standard for making this comparison is the calculation of body mass index (Table 4-2). Patients with a body mass index greater than 30 are considered clinically obese; a body mass index greater than 40 defines the state of morbid obesity.

Providing a safe anesthesia experience to a morbidly obese patient undergoing major surgery is among the most difficult tasks anesthesiologists face. The anesthetic challenges that obese patients present, and their perioperative risks, vary in proportion to the severity of the disorder. The anesthetic risks of obesity are caused by technical difficulties imposed

TABLE 4-2	Body Mass Index and Evaluation of Obesity

Calculation of BMI

Standard: weight (kg) ÷ [height (m)]^2
Alternative: {weight (lb) ÷ [height (in)]^2} × 703

Interpretation of BMI

BMI Range	Interpretation
<18.5	Underweight
18.5–24.9	Normal weight
25.0–29.9	Overweight
30.0–39.9	Obese
>40	Morbidly obese

BMI, body mass index.

by the mass of adipose tissue and by the presence of comorbid states (Table 4-3). Of these comorbid conditions, the anesthesiologist is primarily concerned with cardiovascular and airway or pulmonary derangements.

In addition to absolute body mass, the distribution of body fat predicts the extent of comorbidity associated with obesity. Compared with peripheral (gynecoid) obesity, in which adipose distribution is primarily in the hips and lower body, central (android) obesity, involving the waist and upper body, imposes both a greater overall health risk to the patient and a greater technical challenge to the anesthesiologist.

Technical Difficulties

Even mildly obese patients pose challenges to the anesthesiologist. Standard procedures that are often taken for granted in slender patients can be more difficult in mildly to moderately obese patients. These include placement of peripheral intravenous infusion lines, noninvasive blood pressure monitoring, moving and positioning patients on the operating table, laryngoscopy and tracheal intubation, and use of regional anesthetic techniques, all of which can be sufficiently problematic to require advance planning and the use of alternative techniques (e.g., venous cutdown or central venous access, intra-arterial catheters, awake fiberoptic laryngoscopy).

TABLE 4-3	Obesity and Comorbid States

Cardiovascular

Ischemic heart disease
Peripheral vascular disease, deep vein thrombosis
   "Cardiomyopathy of obesity"
   Systemic and pulmonary hypertension
   High cardiac output
   Cardiomegaly, biventricular failure

Pulmonary

Hypoxemia (100% incidence)
   $\downarrow$ FRC, residual volume, expiratory reserve volume $\rightarrow$
   $\downarrow$ Pulmonary compliance (restrictive deficit)
   $\uparrow$ CC; $\downarrow$ (FRC − CC) difference
   $\uparrow$ Oxygen consumption
   Hypoventilation
      Most severe: obesity–hypoventilation (pickwickian) syndrome: 10% incidence
   in morbid obesity
Upper airway obstruction
   Obstructive sleep apnea syndrome: 40%–60% incidence in morbid obesity
   $\uparrow$ Incidence difficult intubation
   $\uparrow$ Incidence regurgitation/pulmonary aspiration

Metabolic

Diabetes mellitus

Gastrointestinal

Delayed gastric emptying
Gastroesophageal reflux
Fatty liver
Biliary disease

Musculoskeletal

Degenerative joint disease
Lumbar disk disease
Osteoporosis

CC, closing capacity; FRC, functional residual capacity.

Unquestionably, such problems become extremely complex in patients with high-moderate and morbid obesity and can add significantly to anesthetic risk. For example, such patients can pose great difficulties with regard to airway management, hypoxemia, traumatic laryngoscopy (e.g., dental, pharyngeal, vocal cord, and tracheal injuries), and pressure-related injuries (ulcers, neuropathy).

Cardiovascular Derangements

Compared with patients of normal weight, obese patients are at increased risk of coronary artery and peripheral vascular disease, and anesthesiologists must be prepared to manage these problems perioperatively. Moreover, chronic obesity produces a characteristic series of hemodynamic abnormalities. Termed the *cardiomyopathy of obesity*, the syndrome includes a high–cardiac output state, systemic and pulmonary hypertension, and cardiac hypertrophy that can lead to biventricular dilation and cardiac failure.

The pathophysiology of this syndrome relates to the presence of the large, metabolically active adipose mass. Although adipose tissue is less vascular on a per weight basis than lean tissue (blood flow, 2 to 3 mL/100 g/minute), a morbidly obese patient weighing 50 kg more than ideal body weight has a cardiac output 1.5 to 2 L/minute greater than normal, with an accompanying increase in total circulating volume (preload). In addition, the metabolic demands cause chronically elevated sympathetic tone (afterload) and increased global oxygen demand. This is often not met by an increase in oxygen supply because of concurrent pulmonary dysfunction, and the chronic hypoxemia that is highly prevalent in obesity increases pulmonary vascular resistance. The ultimate result is biventricular heart failure.

Evidence indicates that the same factors that combine to produce the cardiomyopathy of obesity also predispose obese individuals to a 50% higher risk of new-onset atrial fibrillation, compared with their nonobese counterparts. When this arrhythmia occurs during anesthesia, management of the hemodynamic derangements of obese patients becomes that much more complicated.

Pulmonary Derangements

Abnormalities involving the respiratory system can be severe in obesity and often represent the most difficult aspect of anesthetic care. Four main categories of pulmonary dysfunction that are present in obesity are pertinent to anesthesia (see Table 4-3). An overriding theme is that all these conditions are greatly exaggerated by exposure to anesthetic agents, intravenous sedatives, and frequently the surgical procedure itself. Consequently, pulmonary function, already abnormal preoperatively, is worsened intraoperatively and especially in the immediate postoperative period.

Hypoventilation and Upper Airway Obstruction

As a consequence of the increased volume of subcutaneous tissue involving facial, pharyngeal, and thoracic structures, nearly all obese patients present with some degree of upper airway obstruction; this becomes much more pronounced in recumbency. Moreover, with upper airway obstruction of any cause, airway patency is maintained by an active but subconscious inspiratory muscle tone, which includes pharyngeal structures, aided by gravitational effects in an upright patient. With any depression of consciousness, this tone is reduced or abolished, and upper airway obstruction is exacerbated. In obese patients, this phenomenon is exaggerated, and, especially in that subset of obesity characterized by the *obstructive sleep apnea syndrome*, even nighttime sleep can produce dangerous degrees of upper airway obstruction, hypoventilation, hypoxemia, and microaspiration.

During anesthesia, patients are nearly always in the supine position, and administered medications routinely depress or eliminate consciousness. Further, skeletal muscle relaxant drugs, commonly administered during general anesthesia, abolish any residual inspiratory muscle tone and may worsen upper airway obstruction. In this setting, respiratory gas exchange in obese patients is often severely limited.

Difficulties with Airway Management

Compounding the situation is the finding that because of the mass effect of the adipose tissue, upper airway obstruction is not only more extreme than in nonobese patients but also is much more difficult to overcome manually with standard techniques. Thus, assisted or controlled ventilation by face mask is often impossible, and laryngoscopy and tracheal intubation are considerably more difficult or impossible. Unless anticipated, with appropriate preparations made for the use of alternative techniques (e.g., flexible fiberoptic laryngoscopy), this situation represents a true anesthetic emergency.

Regurgitation and Pulmonary Aspiration

The traditional teaching that obesity correlates with disordered physiology of the upper gastrointestinal tract, including delayed gastric emptying, hypersecretion of gastric juice and acid, and diminished esophageal sphincter tone, suggests that obese patients are predisposed to regurgitation and pulmonary aspiration of gastric contents during general anesthesia, irrespective of the duration of the preoperative fast. However, more recent evidence has called this concept into question. Studies indicate that gastric emptying is actually accelerated in obese individuals, and gastric residual volumes in obese patients undergoing general anesthesia are similar to those of nonobese patients.

However, it is likely premature for anesthesiologists to abandon their historical concern regarding the risk of regurgitation and pulmonary aspiration in obese patients. First, although gastric emptying may not be retarded, obese patients have a higher risk of gastroesophageal reflux, and the extent of symptoms may not correlate with the extent of reflux. Second, studies indicating that the risk of pulmonary aspiration may be no higher in obese than in nonobese patients were performed in patients who were not intubated or in whom intubation was not difficult, and no distinction was made between central and peripheral obesity. Finally, although the consequences of pulmonary aspiration are typically benign, rare but devastating complications can still occur. Because precautions against aspiration (histamine [H_2]-receptor blockers, gastrokinetic agents) are generally well tolerated, many anesthesiologists have not altered their approach to dealing with this risk in the obese population.

Hypoxemia

Chronic hypoxemia is ubiquitous in obesity. As with the other types of pulmonary dysfunction that characterize the syndrome, two features are typical. First, the degree of hypoxemia correlates with the degree of obesity and is significantly worse in patients with obstructive sleep apnea syndrome. Second, the hypoxemia that exists preoperatively as a baseline state in obesity is exaggerated by recumbency, exposure to anesthetics and sedatives, and the effects of surgery.

The pathophysiology of the hypoxemia of obesity can be considered an exaggeration of the "normal pathophysiology" of the respiratory system. This statement is meant to imply that even in physiologically normal individuals, the lungs are imperfect gas exchangers (although they function quite well). During anesthesia and surgery, particularly thoracic or abdominal surgery, these imperfections become magnified and functionally more significant. In obesity, this pattern becomes extreme.

The abnormalities of respiratory gas exchange relate to the fundamental relationship between the functional residual capacity (FRC) of the lungs and their closing capacity (CC) and the way in which this relationship changes during anesthesia and surgery. The FRC is the volume of the lungs at end-expiration, when there is equilibrium of forces favoring expansion and contraction of lung tissue. The CC is that volume, ordinarily less than FRC, at which the forces of contraction gain priority and small airways begin to close. Any circumstances that tend to decrease the difference between FRC and CC favor atelectasis and consequently cause hypoxemia.

In physiologically normal individuals, the FRC is known to be progressively reduced by the following: (1) supine posture, as a result of redistribution of abdominal contents and pressure on the inferior surface of the diaphragm; (2) anesthetic agents and muscle relaxants, which cause a further cephalic displacement of the diaphragm; and (3) surgical retraction (Fig. 4-3). Consequently, during anesthesia even nonobese patients experience sufficient ventilation/perfusion (V/Q) abnormalities that an enriched inspired oxygen concentration is used routinely. In the obese individual, FRC is ordinarily reduced preoperatively because of the enormous increase in intra-abdominal pressure from the adipose mass, which, in conjunction with baseline hypoventilation, accounts for the chronic hypoxemia typically seen. With exposure to anesthesia and surgery, these changes become profound and persist well into the postoperative period.

The anticipated postoperative exacerbation of hypoxemia frequently requires a degree of monitoring and support that is unnecessary in nonobese patients. This ranges from the need for supplemental oxygen guided by pulse oximetry, to reliance on incentive spirometry and chest physical therapy for maintenance of airway patency, to the continuation of tracheal intubation and mechanical ventilation postoperatively. This last approach is particularly likely in the severely obese patient because of the tenuous pulmonary status that precedes surgery,

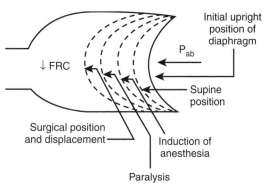

Figure 4-3 • Progressive reduction in functional residual capacity (FRC) resulting from displacement of the diaphragm during anesthesia and surgery. P_{ab}, pressure of abdominal contents. (*From Benumof JL: Respiratory physiology and respiratory function during anesthesia. In Miller RD [ed]: Anesthesia, 3rd ed. New York, Churchill Livingstone, 1990, p 535.*)

and anesthesiologists exercise extreme caution in judging the appropriate timing of extubation in this population.

Regional Anesthesia

Regional anesthetic techniques are often advocated as a means of circumventing the perioperative cardiopulmonary sequelae seen in obesity. Unfortunately, in obese patients regional anesthesia has its own unique problems that can greatly limit its benefit.

First, several inches of subcutaneous tissue may overlie normal landmarks (e.g., spinous processes) and may thus make it completely impossible to perform regional anesthesia, regardless of its apparent advantage. Second, with spinal or epidural anesthesia, the normal dose-response relationships that enable the prediction of a given level of sensory blockade are distorted in obesity, and patients can experience an abnormally high sensory and motor block. The resulting intercostal, and occasionally even diaphragmatic, weakness can profoundly exacerbate the underlying pulmonary dysfunction present in these patients. Third, because the sensory supply of the abdominal and thoracic viscera is through the autonomic nervous system, it is nondiscrete and nonsegmental; this distinctly contrasts with the sensory innervation of the extremities and body wall. An accepted tenet in anesthetic management is that the more rostral the site of surgery within the abdomen, the less adequate will be the sensory block obtained with regional anesthesia. Consequently, the surgical procedure itself may invalidate the use of regional techniques, regardless of the presence of obesity.

Finally, it is extremely difficult for any patient to lie motionless, often in an awkward position, on an operating table for several hours with the knowledge that surgery is ongoing. Added to this is the physical and emotional discomfort of feeling "deafferented" from the waist or chest down, accompanied by pharmacologically induced paraplegia. Thus, the need to provide intravenous sedation to patients during regional anesthesia cannot be overemphasized. Although this approach is generally safe and effective in nonobese patients without concomitant cardiopulmonary dysfunction, the potential hazards of sedative medications in obesity have been discussed and are often paramount in this setting.

Summary

The evaluation and perioperative management of obese patients undergoing surgery can be complex. From the foregoing discussion, certain guidelines are suggested (Table 4-4).

POSTOPERATIVE NEUROLOGIC IMPAIRMENT

General anesthesia entails the creation of a state of coma during surgery from which patients must subsequently be aroused. This is not an all-or-none process but is the result of gradual clearance of drug molecules from active sites in the CNS. Therefore, normal recovery from anesthesia invariably involves some degree of CNS dysfunction.

Anesthesia and recovery room personnel are thoroughly familiar with the range of psychoaffective signs that are typically seen among patients during the immediate postoperative period. Generally brief and clinically unimportant (e.g., somnolence, disorientation, memory impairment), these responses can less commonly become bizarre. Such cases, collectively given the term *emergence delirium,* occasionally require intervention with psychotropic agents during the immediate postoperative period. Nonetheless, even these

TABLE 4-4	Obesity and Anesthesia
Maintain "low thresholds" for the following:	
Expectation of postoperative medical complications	
Especially pulmonary, cardiovascular, diabetic	
Surgical cutdown on peripheral vein/central venous catheter	
Avoiding use of regional techniques, especially if	
Sensory levels required are higher than perineal	
Expected duration of surgery >30 min (increased need for sedation)	
Use of awake fiberoptic intubation and postoperative mechanical ventilation	

more extreme presentations are expected to be transient and without long-term clinical implications.

This benign scenario is not always the case, however, and the challenge for the clinician becomes the need to distinguish normal postoperative neurologic impairment from circumstances that are truly abnormal and worthy of additional evaluation and treatment. Although it is impossible to provide strict distinguishing criteria, it is reasonable to maintain a high index of suspicion in the following circumstances:

1. After a reasonable period of recovery, the patient "just isn't right," exhibits prolonged stupor, excessive disorientation, or extreme agitation after a standard, short-to-moderate duration of general anesthesia in which standard doses of anesthetic agents were used. This is a highly qualitative judgment and thus is the most difficult assessment to make. Such an assessment requires the observation of many patients during postanesthetic recovery to form a basis for comparison.

2. The patient is flaccid and exhibits minimal or absent motor activity during recovery.

3. The patient has new peripheral neurologic deficits postoperatively.

Postoperative Cognitive Dysfunction

Rare among young or middle-aged patients, cognitive impairment after anesthesia is most commonly encountered among elderly patients. When assessed by sensitive neuropsychologic testing, 26% of patients who are more than 60 years old have evidence of *postoperative cognitive dysfunction (POCD)* at 1 week, and 10% at 3 months, after noncardiac surgery. Only rarely does this dysfunction become greatly prolonged. In contrast, POCD is far more common and prolonged after cardiac surgery. The problem of neuropsychiatric impairment following cardiac surgery is complex and is beyond the scope of this discussion.

It is often assumed that extended aftereffects of anesthetic drugs administered to patients during surgery contribute significantly to POCD. This assumption potentially motivates perioperative consultants to advocate the use of regional anesthetic techniques in elderly patients. Evidence that would appear to support this view comes from studies of older anesthetic agents, wherein psychomotor testing has revealed remarkably protracted neurologic impairment after anesthetic exposure.

Current evidence suggests that presumptions about the contributions of general anesthetic agents to the development of POCD may be misguided. First, some of the studies utilizing psychomotor testing in the aftermath of anesthetic exposure involved volunteer subjects rather than patients. Second, disparities between the results of studies using clinical criteria to evaluate postanesthetic patients and the results of trials relying on specialized neuropsychiatric tests suggest that the latter category of evidence may not fully represent actual practice. Third, and most compelling, a substantial body of data indicates that neuropsychiatric outcome in elderly patients, including the incidence of POCD, after general anesthesia does not differ from the outcome observed after regional anesthesia. This is strong evidence that, irrespective of specific anesthetic technique, anesthesia per se is only one among several influences in the perioperative and postoperative periods that may contribute to POCD in elderly patients.

Although the overall long-term clinical significance of POCD is unclear, no doubt exists that its most severe presentation, *postoperative delirium*, can result in significantly increased morbidity and mortality in elderly patients. Postoperative delirium is clinically distinct from the evanescent and benign appearance of emergence delirium, which, as noted previously, is seen during the immediate postoperative recovery period.

Postoperative delirium has attracted considerable study and is the subject of numerous reviews. Although there are accepted criteria for the clinical diagnosis of delirium in the nonsurgical population, it is extremely difficult to apply these criteria in the early postanesthetic period because they are complex, and, for reasons already mentioned, most patients would satisfy them. This realization has prompted efforts to develop algorithms to help predict the emergence of delayed postoperative delirium.

Among the most useful of these algorithms is a clinical prediction rule that employs a specific scoring system based on available preoperative clinical data (Table 4-5) [❽ *Marcantonio et al, 1994*]. The authors of this algorithm arbitrarily omitted from their investigation symptoms of delirium whose onset preceded the second postoperative day, to exclude the influence of residual anesthetic effects and to avoid identifying patients with emergence delirium. Patients who satisfied these risk criteria had more frequent major postoperative complications, longer lengths of stay, and higher rates of discharge to long-term care or rehabilitative facilities.

The importance of identifying patients with the syndrome of (delayed) postoperative delirium emphasizes the need to

TABLE 4-5	Predictors of Delayed Postoperative Delirium
Etiologic Factor	**Point Score**
Age >70 yr	1
History of alcohol abuse	1
TICS <30*	1
SAS class IV†	1
Severe sodium, potassium, glucose abnormalities‡	1
Surgery: abdominal aortic aneurysm repair	2
Surgery: thoracic	1
Total Points	**Delirium Risk (%)**
0	2
1 or 2	11
≥ 3	50

* TICS, Telephone Interview for Cognitive Status (a modification of the Mini-Mental Status Examination).

† SAS, Specific Activity Scale (class IV patients are unable to perform normal daily activities without stopping).

‡ Sodium <130 or >150 mmol/L; potassium <3.0 or >6.0 mmol/L; glucose <60 or >300 mg/dL.

Modified from Marcantonio ER, Goldman L, Mangione CM, et al: A clinical prediction rule for delirium after elective noncardiac surgery. JAMA 271:134–139, 1994.

rule out identifiable causes of short-term mental impairment. Altered mental status resulting from the residual effects of anesthetic, sedative, and analgesic drugs is largely a diagnosis of exclusion. Assuming that other causes have been investigated and ruled out (see later), certain elicited responses can aid in the diagnosis. A traditional rule of thumb holds that one should attempt to reverse whatever residual drug effects are potentially amenable to antidote and observe for transient improvement in mental status. However, only a few anesthetic agents have specific antidotes (Table 4-6). One important caveat: Case reports described the onset of severe acute myocardial ischemia and pulmonary edema in patients who received a standard dose of naloxone (0.4 mg intravenously), an effect that apparently was the result of the stress response caused by acute narcotic reversal in patients with pain. The need to administer small (e.g., 0.04 to 0.08 mg) titrated doses of naloxone cannot be overemphasized.

The differential diagnosis of postoperative delirium includes many of the same preoperative syndromes that may be present in nonsurgical patients presenting with acute delirium (Table 4-7). Among the causes particularly associated with the postoperative period are pain and distention of a hollow viscus, especially the bladder. These are extremely

TABLE 4-6	Reversal of Drug Effects: Anesthetics and Adjunctive Agents
Primary Agent	**"Reversal"**
Neuromuscular blocking agents	Neostigmine, 0.05 mg/kg, PLUS atropine, 0.02 mg/kg
Opioids	Naloxone Caution: Use small doses (e.g., 0.04–0.08-mg increments; 0.16–2.0 mg total)
Benzodiazepines	Flumazenil, 0.2-mg increments q1min (1.0 mg total)
Nonspecific: anticholinergics; inhalation anesthetics; phenothiazines/butyrophenones	Physostigmine, 1–2 mg (variably effective)

TABLE 4-7	Postoperative Delirium: Etiologic Factors

Preoperative

Brain effects:
   Physiologic causes: aging
   Pathologic causes: congenital, traumatic, neoplastic, vascular, idiopathic
Drugs
   Polypharmacy
   Drug intoxication or withdrawal
Endocrine and metabolic
   Hyperthyroidism/hypothyroidism
   Hyponatremia
   Hypoglycemia
Mental status
   Depression
   Dementia
   Anxiety

Intraoperative

Type of surgery: higher incidence with the following:
   Orthopedic, especially repair of femoral neck fracture
   Ophthalmic
   Cardiac
   Urologic (TURP syndrome: hypo-osmolarity, glycine toxicity)
Duration of surgery
Anesthetic drugs used
Complications during surgery
   Hypotension
   Hyperventilation (cerebral ischemia)
   Embolism
   Hypoxemia

Postoperative

Hypoxia
   Respiratory causes
   Perioperative hypoxia
   Residual anesthetics
Hypocarbia
Pain
Distention of hollow viscus (especially bladder)
Sepsis
Sensory deprivation or overload
Electrolyte or metabolic problem

   TURP, transurethral resection of the prostate.
   Modified from Parikh SS, Chung F: Postoperative delirium in the elderly. Anesth Analg 80:1223-1232, 1995.

potent causes of early postanesthetic confusion and agitation, especially in elderly patients, and are often singularly to blame. They should be ruled out in every patient with this presentation.

Postoperative Immobility

Not all patients who exhibit a profound lack of movement during postanesthetic recovery have CNS depression. In the absence of exposure to anesthesia, findings such as no purposeful or reflex movements and absent or significantly diminished spontaneous ventilation raise the likelihood of stupor or coma. By contrast, in the recovery room the possibility exists that a patient with these symptoms may be suffering from profound residual muscle weakness related to unexpectedly prolonged neuromuscular blockade. Resembling myasthenic crisis, the sensorium may be relatively intact.

This assessment is readily made by use of a peripheral nerve stimulator, one of the standard monitoring devices commonly employed during general anesthesia. This device delivers a series of supramaximal stimuli to motor nerves (typically the ulnar nerve at the wrist), and an elicited twitch response is evaluated. Standard patterns of stimulation include the train-of-four, in which four such stimuli are delivered at a frequency of two per second, and a tetanic stimulus at 50 Hz. In both cases, patients should exhibit a normal response that is sustained without loss of amplitude ("fade"). Peripheral nerve stimulators should be readily available in any recovery area, and their use is mandatory in the assessment of such patients.

Postoperative Peripheral Neurologic Deficits

The new onset of a peripheral neurologic deficit postoperatively is often thought to represent an acute CNS event such as a postoperative stroke. Although these findings are alarming, peripheral neurologic deficits can be surprisingly common, and transient, in patients recovering from general anesthesia.

Typically encountered in patients with underlying cerebrovascular disease, they can also be observed in healthy individuals.

In 1981, Rosenberg and colleagues described a high prevalence of neurologic findings such as abnormal corneal and pupillary reflexes, hyperreflexia, and Babinski signs among healthy adults after general anesthesia. Assumed to be unusual manifestations of residual anesthetic effects, all findings resolved spontaneously without sequelae within 40 minutes. More commonly, patients with underlying CNS disease (e.g., tumor, stroke, transient cerebral ischemia) with or without current symptoms, frequently experience either exacerbation of symptoms or unmasking of latent symptoms following exposure to anesthetics and sedatives. This phenomenon has been described as *differential awakening*.

Persistent Neurologic Deficits

Although stroke is a well-described postoperative complication in patients with cerebrovascular disease who are undergoing cardiac and carotid artery surgery, its incidence is surprisingly small (0.2% to 2.9%) in noncardiovascular surgery, even among patients with a history of cerebrovascular disease. When stroke does occur, the onset of symptoms is typically delayed, with peak incidence occurring on the third through fifth postoperative days.

Postoperative dysfunction of a single extremity is typically not related to CNS dysfunction. A much more likely mechanism is postoperative *peripheral sensorimotor neuropathy* (PPSN). In a structured database of more than 6000 closed malpractice claims maintained since 1985 by the American Society of Anesthesiologists (ASA) Committee on Professional Liability, nerve damage was the second most common complication resulting in litigation, and it accounted for 16% of claims. In descending order, the three most common distributions of nerve injury were ulnar, brachial plexus, and lumbosacral nerve root, which together constituted more than half of all nerve damage claims.

Conventional wisdom typically attributes PPSN to the following: (1) direct and indirect nerve injury during use of regional anesthesia; or (2) improper positioning of a patient on the operating table, especially during prolonged surgery, resulting in ischemic compression of peripheral nerves at vulnerable sites. However, PPSN has attracted considerable research attention, and the results have uniformly challenged these assumptions.

For example, in the ASA database, the only categories of neuropathy with a significant association with the use of regional anesthesia were spinal cord damage and lumbosacral nerve damage; ulnar and brachial plexus neuropathies were associated with general anesthesia in most cases (85% and 78%, respectively). However, for all three major distributions of nerve palsy, the mechanism of injury was inapparent in the majority of cases, and the injury was clearly attributable to anesthesias in few cases in which the mechanism was identified.

Among the major categories of PPSN, ulnar neuropathy is the most common and extensively studied. A group of investigators at the Mayo Clinic in Rochester, Minnesota examined this complication both retrospectively (N = 1.13 million) and prospectively (N = 1,502). Their findings revealed that postoperative ulnar neuropathy (PUN) was uncommon (1 in 2729 retrospective data, 0.5% prospective data) and was predominately associated with male gender (relative risk [RR], 4.1), diabetes (RR, 4.3), and duration of hospitalization greater than 14 days (RR, 3.1), and it had the strongest association with obesity (RR, 15.0). There was no significant association with the type of anesthesia or patient position. Moreover, PUN was delayed in onset (peak incidence, postoperative days 2 to 7) and was discernible in the recovery room in only 10% of cases.

Finally, in an independent prospective study employing bilateral nerve conduction evaluation of patients with (unilateral)

PUN, all had slowing of conduction of the contralateral ulnar nerve. This finding suggests that many patients with PUN may have an underlying predisposition to this form of injury and that factors in addition to perioperative body contact play a role in this complication.

PPSN represents a potentially serious adverse postoperative outcome; nearly half of the patients in the Mayo Clinic study had persistent symptoms 1 year after operation. Unfortunately, research into the causes of this complication has thus far failed to identify reliable preventive strategies. Approaches to treatment are nonspecific and are intended primarily to preserve residual extremity function and to minimize contracture deformities. The assistance of physical and occupational therapy services can be invaluable.

Postoperative Visual Loss

An extremely frightening form of postoperative neurologic deficit is *postoperative visual loss (POVL)*; fortunately it is also extremely rare. Although visual disturbances are commonly encountered in the recovery room, they are almost always transient and resolve without long-term sequelae. In contrast, persistent visual loss following nonophthalmologic, noncardiac surgery has been noted to occur in 0.003% to 0.0008% of patients postoperatively.

Despite the rarity of this condition, the emotional impact of POVL on both patient and physician has intensified the focus on this complication. Ischemic optic neuropathy is the most common identifiable cause of POVL (89%); it is most commonly associated with surgery on the spine, with patients in the prone position (67%), and surgery involving cardiopulmonary bypass (14%). Among prone cases, prolonged surgery (>6 hours, mean, 8 hours) and increased blood loss (>1 L, mean, 2.3 L) were independently correlated with POVL; the use of deliberate hypotension is not. However, variances have been shown to be very broad, and at this time, conclusions about cause and prevention are premature.

GENERAL VERSUS REGIONAL ANESTHESIA: WHICH IS SAFER?

In anesthesia and perioperative medicine, there is perhaps no area of greater controversy than the issue whether general or regional anesthesia leads to a better outcome in the high-risk patient. That opinions regarding the relative risks and safety of general and regional anesthesia have been prone to bias is understandable. The study of anesthetic outcome based on rigorous methodology is a comparatively recent undertaking. Historically, clinical teaching and practice were based largely on presumption (e.g., regional anesthesia *appears* to impose less physiologic perturbation than general, so it must be safer). Subsequent efforts at conducting research into anesthetic outcome were often hampered by a variety of methodologic weaknesses, including poorly articulated hypotheses, inadequate sample sizes, conclusions based on intermediate or surrogate endpoints, ambiguous inclusion and exclusion criteria, and poorly standardized treatment protocols. Conclusions based on such questionably designed studies have the potential to reinforce misleading or erroneous presumptions regarding clinical practice.

A 1987 RCT by Yeager and colleagues remains one of the most controversial studies of outcome following general versus regional anesthesia. The investigators concluded that among high-risk patients undergoing major noncardiac surgery, those receiving epidural anesthesia had a substantially lower incidence of major postoperative complications, including mortality, than those receiving general anesthesia. Subsequent analysis of this study resulted in considerable criticism of the authors' conclusions on several levels. Treatment protocols were inadequately standardized, and postoperative analgesic regimens, which may have had a significant independent impact on perioperative outcome, varied substantially between study groups. Moreover, the total number of patients studied was very small (N = 53), thus resulting in an insufficient statistical power to exclude potential sources of bias.

The issue of sample size in RCTs of anesthetic outcome is particularly vexing. That catastrophic anesthetic complications (e.g., mortality) are extremely rare means that to amass data with sufficient statistical power to expose a difference in outcome (if one exists) between two treatment groups would require an enormous number of enrolled patients. Conducting research on this level is generally impractical for a single group of investigators.

Efforts to address the complexity imposed by sample size requirements in RCTs have included such designs as multicenter trials and meta-analyses. Each of these approaches, however, has its own specific statistical drawbacks (e.g., lack of adherence to rigidly standardized protocol among many institutions in multicenter trials, varying quality of study design and statistical techniques among publications included in meta-analyses). Therefore, efforts to reexamine the issue of anesthetic outcome following general versus regional anesthesia have produced variable and often contradictory conclusions and have thus failed to confirm an advantage of regional over general anesthesia.

More recently, Norris and associates published findings of a meticulously conducted RCT examining outcome in patients undergoing abdominal aortic surgery while under general or epidural anesthesia. This study, which adhered to rigorous methodology, found no advantage or disadvantage for either regional or general anesthesia when various outcomes were measured. This finding was echoed by two more recent, large ($N = 915$, $N = 888$) multicenter Australian studies involving high-risk patients undergoing major abdominal surgery while under either epidural anesthesia followed by postoperative epidural analgesia or general anesthesia with conventional postoperative analgesia. Peyton and colleagues concluded that they "were unable to find any significant improvement in major morbidity or mortality after major abdominal surgery from perioperative epidural analgesia."

Thus, the issue whether regional or general anesthesia is safer in the high-risk patient remains largely unresolved [❶ Norris et al, 2001; ❶ Peyton et al, 2003; ❶ Rigg et al, 2002]. Notwithstanding certain specific exceptions that may confer some clinical advantage to the use of regional anesthesia (Table 4-8), one must conclude that the circumstances in which regional techniques provide unequivocal benefit are, at best, rare.

TABLE 4-8	Overview of Traditional Outcome Studies: Does a Consensus Favor Regional Anesthesia?	
Outcome	**Consensus?**	**Comments**
Intraoperative blood loss	Yes	~30% reduction versus general anesthesia; specifically in total hip replacement, radical prostatectomy, lower extremity vascular surgery, total abdominal hysterectomy; ability to extrapolate conclusions from these procedures uncertain
Thromboembolic complications	Yes	Several studies have shown this, but none featured a general anesthesia control group given standard perioperative antithrombotic prophylaxis (e.g., miniheparin, warfarin, compression stockings); thus, applicability to current practice questionable
Lower extremity vascular graft failure	Yes	Two major prospective studies confirmed the value of epidural anesthesia [Christopherson et al, 1993; Tuman et al, 1991]
Postoperative mental status	No	Results highly variable: few studies show benefit, most show no difference, few studies show worse outcome when regional techniques used
Cardiopulmonary complications	No	Most studies reveal insignificant differences, report "trends"; few studies that report statistically significant difference suffer from small sample size (i.e., sampling error)
Perioperative mortality	No	Many studies over several years; favorite patient population: elderly patients undergoing orthopedic procedures on hip joint; samples small but sufficient number of studies for meta-analysis

PREOPERATIVE FASTING: CHANGING CONSENSUS

One of the enduring traditions in anesthesia practice has been the requirement that patients maintain an overnight fast before surgery. The "NPO (nil per os) after midnight" order is familiar to anyone caring for patients perioperatively. The historical imperative regarding this practice results from concern about pulmonary aspiration of gastric contents during anesthesia, one of the earliest described risks of anesthesia and the cause of the first reported anesthetic death.

The dire consequences of pulmonary aspiration of acidic material were first elucidated in the 1940s by Curtis Mendelson, and the acid aspiration syndrome (or Mendelson syndrome) has since been an outcome of general anesthesia greatly feared by patients and physicians alike. However, several more recent insights into the physiology of gastric emptying and the epidemiology of pulmonary aspiration have called into question the validity of the mandatory 8-hour fast. These insights have contributed to a gradual but inexorable reconsideration of this practice.

Declining Incidence of Pulmonary Aspiration

Based on currently available data, the frequency of clinically important pulmonary aspiration during anesthesia is dramatically lower than in decades past. The original study by Mendelson reported 66 cases of clinically significant aspiration pneumonia among 44,016 patients (1 in 667) who were receiving general anesthesia for obstetric procedures between 1932 and 1945. In contrast, large-scale studies since the mid-1980s involving several tens of thousands of adult and pediatric patients receiving general anesthesia have reported frequencies an order of magnitude smaller.

Moreover, the National Health Service of the United Kingdom has maintained an ongoing registry of maternal mortality since the 1950s. Of maternal deaths attributed to anesthesia, 52% to 65% were the result of aspiration in 1952 to 1954, whereas in the 1992 report, there were no defined deaths from that event. Similarly, statistics from the ASA's closed-claim database reveal that sequelae of pulmonary aspiration accounted for only 3.5% of all claims, with no claims related to aspiration reported after 1994.

This decline has several possible explanations. Compared with those used historically, contemporary anesthetic agents and associated medications are safer and are less likely to stimulate regurgitation or active emesis. Epidemiologic studies have been increasingly successful in identifying patients at greater risk for regurgitation and aspiration because of delayed gastric emptying or dysfunction of the gastroesophageal sphincter (Table 4-9). The two most important advances have been the routine use of intravenous agents for induction of general anesthesia and the reliance on endotracheal intubation for a large percentage of surgical procedures performed under general anesthesia. Anesthesia delivered by face mask, a nearly universal technique for more than a century, is currently used only in patients considered at low risk for pulmonary aspiration, in whom the airway is not compromised and controlled mechanical ventilation is not planned. When cases are properly selected, anesthesia by face mask or its more recent popular modification, the laryngeal mask airway, does not increase risk.

Reexamination of Risk

Concomitant with the reduction in the frequency of pulmonary aspiration has been an evolution in an understanding of the relationship between the composition of gastric contents and the risk of acid aspiration syndrome. The rarity of pulmonary aspiration during anesthesia, the large sample size needed to make statistically significant observations, and ethical concerns have hampered research into the risk of anesthesia-related aspiration. Designing a statistically valid study of the various risk factors for this complication

TABLE 4-9	Patients at High Risk for Regurgitation of Gastric Contents

Gastric Distention

Inadequate preoperative fast
Delayed gastric emptying
   Functional
      Pain
      Sepsis
      Obesity
      Pregnancy
      Shock
      Stupor/coma
      Uremia
      Autonomic neuropathy (e.g., diabetes, Shy-Drager syndrome)
      Recent abdominal surgery
   Drug-induced
      Opioids
      Anticholinergics
      Alcohol
      Antiparkinsonian agents
Intestinal obstruction/pseudo-obstruction

Gastroesophageal Reflux

Idiopathic
Obesity-related
Pregnancy-related
Drug-induced
Collagen-vascular (e.g., scleroderma)

Esophageal Disease

Stricture
Webs
Diverticular disease
Neoplasm
Foreign body

is difficult because of the enormous sample sizes required. Moreover, there are serious ethical concerns in studying a complication with potentially devastating consequences. For these reasons, research in this area has been forced to rely on the use of animal experiments or, among human subjects, surrogate end points such as the volume and composition of gastric contents assumed to confer a greater danger.

A long-held belief has been that severe sequelae of pulmo-nary aspiration are more likely when the residual gastric fluid volume exceeds 25 mL (or 0.4 mL/kg in children) and has a pH of less than 2.5. The acceptance of this teaching has pro-moted both strict adherence to the 8-hour fast requirement and an abundance of research into techniques of altering gastric residual volume and acidity preoperatively (e.g., fast-ing, nonparticulate antacids, H_2-receptor blockers, proton pump inhibitors, gastrokinetic agents).

More recent epidemiologic data have revealed that many preoperative patients have gastric contents that qualify as "at risk" by these traditional criteria. Moreover, the prevalence of high-volume, acidic gastric contents is not limited to patients in one of the accepted clinical high-risk categories (see Table 4-9) to whom preoperative prophylactic measures have been primarily directed. These data, in conjunction with the recognition that clinically significant pulmonary aspiration has become rare, have prompted a reexamination of the long-standing acid-volume risk criteria.

Clearance of Gastric Contents

There is no debate that solid, particulate matter and highly acidic material aspirated into the lungs are damaging; at issue is the risk imposed by the residual volume of gastric liquid. The recent scrutiny of its role has taken two directions. No evidence indicates that a complete fast (for solids and liquids) of several hours' duration is mandatory. Further, even with solids, no evidence supports the specific figure of 8 hours as a critical time for gastric emptying in physiologically normal individuals. It is likely that this duration originated as an in-ference drawn from the routine NPO after midnight order, because elective surgery often begins at 8:00 A.M.

Clinical Data

The debate about the validity of an 8-hour preoperative fast is accompanied by the recognition that this duration is fre-quently uncomfortable for patients and frustrating for those interested in the efficient management of an operating suite. Out of concern for the need to maintain a strict period of fasting, patients often omit important oral medications pre-operatively; moreover, patients frequently manifest excessive thirst, nausea, and anxiety. These concerns are especially apparent in children; moreover, in infants a prolonged fast produces a significant risk of dehydration and hypoglycemia. It is therefore not surprising that clinical studies evaluating the composition of gastric contents following various durations of fasting have focused largely on pediatric patients. Since the early 1990s, numerous studies involving children and, more recently, adults have universally found that permitting clear liquids (e.g., water, clear juices, tea, black coffee) up to 2 hours before surgery results in either no difference or, in some cases, a small reduction in gastric residual volumes when compared with prolonged fasting. In addition, no significant differences in gastric pH and no increase in the incidence of regurgitation or aspiration during anesthesia have been reported. Finally, studies in both children and adults have revealed a reduction in preoperative thirst and an improved sense of well-being among patients permitted clear fluids 2 to 3 hours before surgery.

Contemporary Guidelines

In summary, the reappraisal of historical precepts relating to preoperative fasting and the abundance of contemporary clinical data have failed to support the validity of a prolonged, all-inclusive preoperative fast (i.e., for solids and clear liquids). A growing awareness of this fact has inspired a gradual alteration in anesthetic practice nationwide.

In recognition of the need for an evidence-based analysis to address the evolution in clinical practice regarding preoperative fasting, the ASA organized a Task Force on Preoperative Fasting and the Use of Pharmacologic Agents to Reduce the Risk of Pulmonary Aspiration. The task force's guidelines, published in 1999, are summarized in Table 4-10. Although efforts have been made to determine the extent to which the

TABLE 4-10	Current Guidelines for Preoperative Fasting

Ingested Material	Minimum Fasting Period (hr)*
Clear liquids†	2
Breast milk	4
Nonclear liquids, solids‡	6

* These recommendations apply to healthy patients undergoing elective procedures. They are not intended for women in labor.

† Examples of clear liquids include water, fruit juices without pulp, carbonated beverages, clear tea, and black coffee.

‡ This category includes nonhuman milk.

Modified from Practice guidelines for preoperative fasting and the use of pharmacologic agents to reduce the risk of pulmonary aspiration: Application to healthy patients undergoing elective procedures. A report by the American Society of Anesthesiologists Task Force on Preoperative Fasting. Anesthesiology 90:896–905, 1999.

ASA guidelines for preoperative fasting have been embraced on a local level, to date no comprehensive data are available on the adoption of the guidelines nationally. Whereas it can be assumed that growing numbers of institutions have done so, certain aspects of the guidelines require clarification, and, in some cases, exceptions are appropriate.

First, in adults with normal nutritional requirements whose surgery has been electively scheduled, in advance, to occur at a reasonably early hour in the day, it is appropriate to continue employing a routine NPO after midnight order. It would be unwieldy and impractical to individualize the beginning of each patient's period of fasting based on the exact scheduled time of surgery. Moreover, the efficient administration of an operating room schedule requires ongoing flexibility with respect to designated starting times. These are subject to change for a variety of reasons (e.g., change in surgeon availability, cancellation of preceding cases), and they should not depend on the need to complete a preoperative fast tailored to a previously scheduled operating time.

Thus, the liberalization of preoperative fasting requirements through the incorporation of the ASA guidelines is most applicable to patients whose cases are added on to the elective schedule during the day of surgery. This should prove a great benefit by eliminating confusion and disagreement among staff members about when such cases are permitted to begin. Because of the risks to very young children of prolonged fasting, patients younger than 4 years of age should be encouraged to ingest clear liquids 2 to 4 hours preoperatively, even for previously scheduled operations.

Second, when patients present with surgical emergencies, judgment dictates that the risk of delaying surgery outweighs that of not completing a preoperative fast. In such cases, fasting guidelines are abrogated.

Finally, the choice of anesthetic technique is independent of, and unaffected by, the prescribed duration of preoperative fasting. Although local and regional techniques do not entail the intended production of a state of unconsciousness (and the attendant risk of pulmonary aspiration), acute adverse effects requiring the immediate induction of general anesthesia may unexpectedly be encountered during any anesthetic regimen. Thus, SA, for example, is not an acceptable alternative to an insufficient preoperative fast.

Selected Readings

Adams JP, Murphy PG: Obesity in anaesthesia and intensive care. Br J Anaesth 85:91-108, 2000.

American Society of Anesthesiologists Task Force on Preoperative Fasting. Anesthesiology: Practice guidelines for preoperative fasting and the use of pharmacologic agents to reduce the risk of pulmonary aspiration: Application to healthy patients undergoing elective procedures. A report by the American Society of Anesthesiologists Task Force on Preoperative Fasting. Anesthesiology 90:896-905, 1999.

Biring MS, Lewis MI, Liu JT, et al: Pulmonary physiologic changes of morbid obesity. Am J Med Sci 318:293-297, 1999.

Candido KD, Stevens RA: Post-dural puncture headache: Pathophysiology, prevention and treatment. Best Pract Res Clin Anaesthesiol 17:451-469, 2003.

Cheney FW, Domino KB, Caplan RA, et al: Nerve injury associated with anesthesia: A closed claims analysis. Anesthesiology 90:1062-1069, 1999.

Christopherson R, Beattie C, Frank SM, et al: Perioperative morbidity in patients randomized to eqidural or general anesthesia for lower extremity vascular surgery. Perioperative Ischemia Randomized Anesthesia Trial Study Group. Anesthesiology 79:422-434, 1993.

Davignon KR, Dennehy KC: Update on postdural puncture headache. Int Anesthesiol Clin 40:89-102, 2002.

Duffy PJ, Crosby ET: The epidural blood patch: Resolving the controversies. Can J Anaesth 46:878-886, 1999. ❸

Eichenberger A, Proietti S, Wicky S, et al: Morbid obesity and postoperative pulmonary atelectasis: An underestimated problem. Anesth Analg 95:1788-1792, 2002.

Evans RW, Armon C, Frohman EM, et al: Assessment: Prevention of post-lumbar puncture headaches: Report of the therapeutics and technology assessment subcommittee of the American Academy of Neurology. Neurology 55:909-914, 2000. ❹

Johnson T, Monk T, Rasmussen LS, et al: Postoperative cognitive dysfunction in middle-aged patients. Anesthesiology 96:1351-1357, 2002.

Lagasse RS: Anesthesia safety: Model or myth? A review of the published literature and analysis of current original data. Anesthesiology 97:1609-1617, 2002.

Landercasper J, Merz BJ, Cogbill TH, et al: Perioperative stroke risk in 173 consecutive patients with a past history of stroke. Arch Surg 125:986-989, 1990.

Lee LA, Roth S, Posner KL, et al: The American Society of Anesthesiologists Postoperative Visual Loss Registry: Analysis of 93 spine surgery cases with postoperative visual loss. Anesthesiology 105:652-659, 2006.

Liu SS, McDonald SB: Current issues in spinal anesthesia. Anesthesiology 94:888-906, 2001.

Maltby JR, Pytka S, Watson NC, et al: Drinking 300 mL of clear fluid two hours before surgery has no effect on gastric fluid volume and pH in fasting and non-fasting obese patients. Can J Anaesth 51:111-115, 2004.

Marcantonio ER, Goldman L, Mangione CM, et al: A clinical prediction rule for delirium after elective noncardiac surgery. JAMA 271:134-139, 1994. ❸

Moller JT: Cerebral dysfunction after anaesthesia. Acta Anaesthesiol Scand Suppl 110:13-16, 1997.

Norris EJ, Beattie C, Perler BA, et al: Double-masked randomized trial comparing alternate combinations of intraoperative anesthesia and post-operative analgesia in abdominal aortic surgery. Anesthesiology 95:1054-1067, 2001. ❹

O'Brien D: Acute postoperative delirium: Definitions, incidence, recognition, and interventions. J Perianesth Nurs 17:384-392, 2002.

Ogunnaike BO, Jones SB, Jones DB, et al: Anesthetic considerations for bariatric surgery. Anesth Analg 95:1793-1805, 2002.

Parikh SS, Chung F: Postoperative delirium in the elderly. Anesth Analg 80:1223-1232, 1995.

Peyton PJ, Myles PS, Silbert BS, et al: Perioperative epidural analgesia and outcome after major abdominal surgery in high-risk patients. Anesth Analg 96:548-554, 2003. **Ⓐ**

Phillips S, Hutchinson S, Davidson T: Preoperative drinking does not affect gastric contents. Br J Anaesth 70:6-9, 1993.

Rasmussen LS, Johnson T, Kuipers HM, et al: Does anaesthesia cause postoperative cognitive dysfunction? A randomised study of regional versus general anaesthesia in 438 elderly patients. Acta Anaesthesiol Scand 47:260-266, 2003.

Ray CS, Sue DY, Bray G, et al: Effects of obesity on respiratory function. Am Rev Respir Dis 128:501-506, 1983.

Read MS, Vaughan RS: Allowing pre-operative patients to drink: Effects on patients' safety and comfort of unlimited oral water until 2 hours before anaesthesia. Acta Anaesthesiol Scand 35:591-595, 1991.

Rigg JRA, Jamrozik K, Myles PS, et al: Epidural anaesthesia and analgesia and outcome of major surgery: A randomised trial. Lancet 359:1276-1282, 2002. **Ⓐ**

Rosenberg H, Clofine R, Bialik O: Neurologic changes during awakening from anesthesia. Anesthesiology 54:125-130, 1981.

Roth S, Thisted RA, Erickson JP, et al: Eye injuries after nonocular surgery: A study of 60,965 anesthetics from 1988 to 1992. Anesthesiology 85:1020-1027, 1996.

Sarr MG, Felty CL, Hilmer DM, et al: Technical and practical considerations involved in operations on patients weighing more than 270 kg. Arch Surg 130:102-105, 1995.

Tuman KJ, McCarthy RJ, March RJ, et al: Effects of epidural anesthesia and analgesia on coagulation and outcome after major vascular surgery. Anesth Analg 73:696-704, 1991.

Warner MA, Warner DO, Matsumoto JY, et al: Ulnar neuropathy in surgical patients. Anesthesiology 90:54-59, 1999.

Warner MA, Warner ME, Weber JG: Clinical significance of pulmonary aspiration during the perioperative period. Anesthesiology 78:56-62, 1993.

Williams-Russo P, Sharrock NE, Mattis S, et al: Cognitive effects after epidural vs general anesthesia in older adults. A randomized trial. JAMA 274:44-50, 1995.

Yeager MP, Glass DD, Neff RK, et al: Epidural anesthesia and analgesia in high-risk surgical patients. Anesthesiology 66:729-736, 1987.

5 Prophylaxis for Deep Vein Thrombosis and Pulmonary Embolism in the Surgical Patient

GENO J. MERLI, MD
GEORGE L. TZANIS, MD
L. BERNARD MENAJOVSKY, MD, MS

Despite biannual revisions of guidelines by the American College of Chest Physicians (ACCP) for the perioperative prophylaxis of deep vein thrombosis (DVT) and pulmonary embolism (PE), the use of prophylactic regimens is not uniform. The difficulty with complete acceptance of recommended guidelines stems from the following: concern that prophylactic anticoagulation will result in perioperative hemorrhage; willingness to accept some degree of DVT in the calf, with the resultant lower risk of fatal PE, as opposed to the risk of bleeding from more effective prophylaxis that prevents DVT; and in some settings, a lack of familiarity with these guidelines. In an attempt to resolve this issue, surgeons have requested clear-cut guidelines for the identification of a high-risk group of patients in whom prophylaxis of DVT and PE must be more aggressive. The purpose of this chapter is to review the causes, risk factors, methods of prophylaxis, incidence in various procedures, and guidelines for prophylaxis of DVT and PE.

ETIOLOGY

The triad of stasis, intimal injury, and hypercoagulability contributes to thrombosis, DVT, and PE. This section discusses the secondary risk factors that enhance this triad.

The first component of the triad, stasis, results from supine positioning and the effects of anesthesia. Stasis causes venous pooling, which is augmented by the vasodilatory effect of anesthesia and results in increased venous capacitance and decreased venous return from the lower extremities. Venous thrombi composed of platelets, fibrin, and red blood cells develop behind the venous valve cusps or the intramuscular sinuses of the calf secondary to decreased blood flow and stasis.

The second component of the triad is intimal injury, which results from excessive vasodilation caused by vasoactive amines (histamine, serotonin, bradykinin) and anesthesia. Investigators have demonstrated that abrupt venous dilation may cause venous endothelial tears that may serve as the nidus for accumulation of leukocytes, erythrocytes, and platelets. Hypercoagulability is the third risk factor for venous thrombosis in the surgical patient. Stasis and surgery create conditions conducive to clot formation. Impaired venous blood flow results in decreased clearance of activated clotting factors that promotes clot formation in areas of intimal injury and in low-flow areas such as the posterior valve cusp.

RISK FACTOR ASSESSMENT

When the patient's risk for DVT and PE is assessed preoperatively, considerations include the patient's age, the length and type of surgical procedure planned, a history of previous DVT and PE, and additional risk factors. These additional risk factors are increasing age, central venous catheterization, inherited or acquired thrombophilia, cancer therapy (hormonal therapy, chemotherapy, or radiotherapy), prolonged immobilization, paralysis, malignant disease, obesity, varicose veins, estrogen-containing oral contraceptives or hormone replacement therapy, selective estrogen-receptor modulators, nephritic syndrome, heart or respiratory failure, pregnancy or postpartum status, acute medical illness, myeloproliferative disorders, paroxysmal nocturnal hemoglobinuria, smoking, and major or lower extremity trauma (Box 5-1).

Box 5-1	RISK FACTORS FOR VENOUS THROMBOEMBOLISM

1. Surgery
2. Trauma (major or lower extremity)
3. Immobility, paresis
4. Malignant disease
5. Cancer therapy (hormonal therapy, chemotherapy, or radiotherapy)
6. Previous deep vein thrombosis or pulmonary embolism
7. Increasing age
8. Pregnancy and the postpartum period
9. Estrogen-containing oral contraceptives or hormone replacement therapy
10. Selective estrogen-receptor modulators
11. Acute medical illness
12. Heart or respiratory failure
13. Inflammatory bowel disease
14. Nephrotic syndrome
15. Myeloproliferative disorders
16. Paroxysmal nocturnal hemoglobinuria
17. Obesity
18. Smoking
19. Varicose veins
20. Central venous catheters
21. Inherited or acquired thrombophilia

Modified from Geerts WH, Pineo GF, Heit JA, et al: Prevention of venous thromboembolism. Chest 126:338S-400S, 2004. Copyright 2004 by the American College of Chest Physicians. Reproduced with permission of the American College of Chest Physicians in the format Textbook via Copyright Clearance Center.

The patient can be classified as being at low, moderate, high, or very high risk for the development of DVT and PE (Table 5-1). Low-risk patients are less than 40 years old, have no additional risk factors, and are undergoing minor surgery. This group of patients has a 2% risk of calf DVT, a 0.4% risk of proximal vein DVT, and a 0.01% risk of fatal PE if DVT prophylaxis is not used.

TABLE 5-1	Classification of the Risk of Postoperative Deep Venous Thrombosis and Pulmonary Embolism		
Risk Categories	Calf DVT	Proximal DVT	Fatal PE
Very High Risk	40%–80%	10%–20%	0.2%–5%
Age >40 yr			
Multiple additional risk factors*			
Total hip or knee arthroplasty			
Surgery for malignancy			
Hip fracture			
Major trauma			
Spinal cord injury			
High Risk	20%–40%	4%–8%	0.4%–1%
Age >60 or 40–60 yr			
Major surgery			
With additional risk factors*			
Moderate Risk	10%–20%	2%–4%	0.1%–0.4%
Minor surgery			
With additional risk factors*			
Age 40–60 yr			
No additional risk factors			
Low Risk	2%	0.4%	<0.01%
Age <40 yr			
Minor surgery			
No additional risk factors			

*Additional risk factors: increasing age, central venous catheterization, inherited or acquired thrombophilia, cancer therapy (hormonal, chemotherapy, or radiotherapy), prolonged immobilization, paralysis, malignancy, obesity, varicose veins, estrogen-containing oral contraceptives or hormone replacement therapy, selective estrogen-receptor modulators, nephritic syndrome, heart or respiratory failure, pregnancy or postpartum period, acute medical illness, myeloproliferative disorders, paroxysmal nocturnal hemoglobinuria, smoking, trauma (major or lower extremity).

DVT, deep venous thrombosis; PE, pulmonary embolism.

Modified from Geerts WH, Pineo GF, Heit JA, et al: Prevention of venous thromboembolism. Chest 126:338S-400S, 2004. Copyright 2004 by the American College of Chest Physicians. Reproduced with permission of the American College of Chest Physicians in the format Textbook via Copyright Clearance Center.

Moderate-risk patients are those undergoing minor surgery with additional risk factors or those between 40 and 60 years old and who have no additional risk factors. Without prophylaxis, this group has a 10% to 20% risk of the development of calf vein thrombosis, a 2% to 4% risk of a proximal vein clot, and a 0.1% to 0.4% risk of fatal PE.

The high-risk group includes patients having surgery who are more than 60 years old and those between 40 and 60 years old who have additional risk factors. This group has a 20% to 40% risk of calf vein thrombosis, a 4% to 8% risk of proximal vein thrombosis, and a 0.4% to 1% risk of fatal PE if prophylaxis is not used.

Very high-risk patients are more than 40 years old, have multiple additional risk factors, and are undergoing total hip or knee arthroplasty or hip fracture surgery or have major trauma or spinal cord injury. This group has a 40% to 80% risk of calf vein thrombosis, a 10% to 20% risk of proximal vein thrombosis, and a 0.2% to 5% risk of fatal PE with the use of prophylactic regimens.

PROPHYLAXIS MODALITIES

At present, there are seven recognized modalities for DVT and PE prophylaxis. In this section, each modality is reviewed with respect to dose, administration, length of therapy, and adverse reactions.

Heparin (Unfractionated Heparin)

Fixed-Dose Heparin

Heparin is administered subcutaneously at 5000 U 2 hours before surgery. This is followed postoperatively by administration of 5000 U subcutaneously every 8 to 12 hours until the patient is discharged (Box 5-2). In double-blind trials, the incidence of major hemorrhagic events was 1.8% versus 0.8%

Box 5-2	HEPARIN PROPHYLAXIS

1. Administer 5000 U subcutaneously 2 hr before surgery.
2. Administer 5000 U subcutaneously q8h or q12h postoperatively.
3. Maintain the regimen until the patient is discharged.

in the controls. This difference is not statistically significant. The incidence of minor bleeding, such as injection site and wound hematomas, was reported to be significant, with 6.3% in the low-dose heparin group and 4.1% in the controls. Rare complications of low-dose heparin include skin necrosis, thrombocytopenia, and hyperkalemia.

Low-Molecular-Weight Heparin

Low-molecular-weight heparins (LMWHs) are used for the prevention of postoperative DVT in orthopedic and general surgery. This group of heparins was observed to have a more significant inhibitory effect on factor Xa than on factor IIa, as well as a lower bleeding risk than standard heparin. Currently, six LMWH preparations are approved for use in Europe, whereas in the United States only enoxaparin, dalteparin, and fondaparinux are available for orthopedic and general surgery, respectively (Box 5-3). The newest LMWH is fondaparinux. It has a long half-life (17 to 21 hours) and is renally excreted, and its anticoagulant effect is not reversed by protamine. Each of these LMWH s has a different molecular weight, anti-Xa to anti-IIa activity, rates of plasma clearance, and recommended dosage regimens. LMWHs are not bound to plasma proteins

---

Box 5-3	LOW-MOLECULAR-WEIGHT HEPARIN

- Dalteparin: Administer 5000 U subcutaneously q24h (initiated the evening of surgery).
- Fondaparinux: Administer 2.5 mg, subcutaneously beginning 6 hr following surgery and then once daily.
- Enoxaparin: For orthopedic surgery, administer 30 mg subcutaneously q12h (initiated the evening of surgery). For all other surgical procedures, administer 40 mg subcutaneously q24h (initiated the evening of surgery). Patients with a creatinine clearance of less than 30 mL/min should receive 30 mg subcutaneously q24h for both general and orthopedic surgery.

(histidine-rich glycoprotein, platelet factor-4, vitronectin, fibronectin, and von Willebrand factor), endothelial cells, or macrophages, as is standard heparin. This lower affinity contributes to a longer plasma half-life, more complete plasma recovery at all concentrations, and a clearance that is independent of dose and plasma concentration. For DVT prophylaxis, enoxaparin is administered following orthopedic surgery at 30 mg subcutaneously every 12 hours. For all other surgical procedures, enoxaparin is administered at 40 mg subcutaneously once daily. Dalteparin is administered 2 hours before general abdominal surgery at 2500 U subcutaneously and then once daily at 2500 or 5000 U. Fondaparinux has been recently approved for prophylaxis in total hip, knee, and fractured hip surgery at 2.5 mg subcutaneously once daily beginning 6 hours following surgery.

Warfarin

Warfarin prophylaxis can be administered by two methods (Box 5-4). The first protocol is to give warfarin, 10 mg, the night before surgery. This dose is followed by 5 mg the evening of surgery. The daily dose is determined by the prothrombin time (PT) converted to the international normalized ratio (INR). The INR sought is 2 to 3. An alternative approach to warfarin prophylaxis is to give 10 mg of warfarin on the evening of surgery. No warfarin is given on postoperative day 1, and on the second postoperative day, warfarin is given to maintain an INR of 2 to 3. In any of these regimens, patients who are unable to take anything by mouth can receive warfarin intravenously at the same dose as the oral preparation. The preceding therapies are maintained as extended prophylaxis for 4 to 6 weeks at an INR of 2 to 3. The incidence of major postoperative bleeding with warfarin therapy has varied from 5% to 10%. The rare complication of warfarin skin necrosis has not been reported in studies using this agent as prophylaxis for DVT and PE.

Box 5-4	WARFARIN PROPHYLAXIS

METHOD 1
- 10 mg by mouth the evening before surgery
- 5 mg by mouth the evening of surgery
- Adjust dose daily based on an INR of 2 to 3
- Maintain warfarin until discharge

METHOD 2
- 10 mg by mouth the evening of surgery
- No warfarin on postoperative day 1
- On postoperative day 2, begin warfarin to adjust INR to 2 to 3
- Maintain warfarin until discharge

INR, International normalized ratio.

External Pneumatic Compression

External pneumatic compression sleeves are mechanical methods of improving venous return from the lower extremities. They reduce stasis in the gastrocnemius-soleus pump. They are placed on the patient on the morning of surgery and are worn throughout the surgical procedure and continuously for 48 hours afterward. If the patient is ambulatory, the sleeves may be discontinued or replaced by subcutaneous heparin, or both can be used, until hospital discharge. If the patient is nonambulatory, use of the sleeves should be continued until the patient is more active. In this latter group, the sleeves may not be tolerated by the patient because of increased warmth, sweating, or disturbance of sleep. Subcutaneous heparin can be substituted until discharge or when the patient becomes ambulatory. Bed-bound patients wearing the sleeves may have them temporarily removed for skin care, bathing, physical therapy, or bedside commode use. Each manufacturer has specifications regarding the operation and cycle time of the respective device, but no statistically significant difference has been shown in the incidence of DVT related to the brand employed. If a patient has been at bed rest or immobilized for more than 72 hours without any form of prophylaxis, placement of pneumatic sleeves is not recommended because of the possibility of dislodging newly formed clot. In this situation, assessment of the lower extremity by noninvasive testing is recommended to rule out the presence of new DVT. If test results are negative, then venous compression sleeves are used.

A newer mechanical device has come under study for prophylaxis against DVT and PE in the surgical patient. This device operates by compressing the sole of the foot; this compression activates a physiologic pump mechanism and improves venous return in the lower extremity. The arteriovenous impulse system (foot pump) was developed to accomplish this function. Like the external pneumatic compression sleeves, this device is worn during and after the surgical procedure until the patient is ambulatory or the device is replaced by a pharmacologic agent. The foot pump has not been shown to be as effective as the external pneumatic compression sleeves.

Gradient Elastic Stockings

Calf-length gradient elastic stockings are worn during surgery and are maintained until the patient is discharged. The stockings can be removed for skin care and bathing. The use of these stockings has no known complications. This mechanical method of prophylaxis is effective for low-risk procedures.

PROPHYLAXIS FOR SURGERY

Orthopedic Surgery

Prophylaxis for DVT and PE in the orthopedic surgery group has been strongly advocated by the ACCP Consensus Conference on Antithrombotic Therapy and the International

Consensus Statement. Total hip replacement, repair of hip fracture, and total knee replacement constitute the predominant procedures performed in the geriatric patient (Table 5-2). In these types of surgical procedures, DVT may occur as isolated proximal, proximal and distal, or isolated distal thrombosis. This incidence of fatal PE in patients undergoing total joint replacement who have not had DVT prophylaxis has been reported to be as high as 5%. To understand the approach to prophylaxis, the predominant orthopedic procedures are reviewed.

The incidence of DVT in total hip replacement is approximately 45% to 50%. Enoxaparin, dalteparin, fondaparinux, and warfarin are currently the pharmacologic agents of choice for DVT prophylaxis. Warfarin may be administered by any of the methods listed in Table 5-2. Enoxaparin is administered subcutaneously at 30 mg 12 hours postoperatively, then every 12 hours postoperative day 1. Dalteparin is given at 2500 U subcutaneously 4 to 8 hours postoperatively, followed by 5000 IU subcutaneously every 24 hours. Fondaparinux, at 2.5 mg subcutaneously, is given 6 hours postoperatively, then every 24 hours. External pneumatic compression has become a common prophylactic measure in orthopedic surgery. This mechanical prophylaxis does not increase the risk of perioperative bleeding and has been shown to be effective in reducing DVT, but it is recommended as adjuvant therapy for prophylaxis.

Hip fractures have been associated with a DVT incidence of 40% to 45%. By extrapolation of the data from total hip replacement, enoxaparin, dalteparin, fondaparinux, and warfarin should be routinely used as DVT prophylaxis. External pneumatic compression sleeves may be used alone if the bleeding risk is very high or in combination with pharmacologic prophylaxis in this patient group.

The incidence of DVT in total knee replacement has been reported to be 72%. This high rate is attributed to the procedure and to tourniquet application to the limb, which is

TABLE 5-2	Prophylaxis for Orthopedic Surgery

Total Hip Replacement

Incidence: 45%–57% without VTE prophylaxis
Prophylaxis
  LMWH (dalteparin OR enoxaparin OR fondaparinux)
    Dalteparin: 2500 IU, SC, 4–8 hr postop, then 5000 IU, SC, q24h
    Enoxaparin: 30 mg, SC, 12 hr postop, then 30 mg, SC, q12h (creatinine
      clearance <30 mL/min: 30 mg, SC, q24h)
    Fondaparinux: 2.5 mg, SC, 6 hr postop, then 2.5 mg, q24h
  OR
  Warfarin: INR 2–3
Note: ASA, dextran, LDUH, IPC, or VFP should not be used as the only method
  of VTE prophylaxis.

Fractured Hip

Incidence: 36%–60% without VTE prophylaxis
Prophylaxis
  LMWH (fondaparinux OR dalteparin OR enoxaparin)
    Fondaparinux: 2.5 mg, SC, 6 hr postop, then 2.5 mg, q24h
    Dalteparin: 2500 IU, SC, 4–8 hr postop, then 5000 IU, SC, q24h
    Enoxaparin: 30 mg, SC, 12 hr postop, then 30 mg, SC, q12h (creatinine
      clearance <30 mL/min: 30 mg, SC, q24h)
  OR
  Warfarin: INR 2–3
  OR
  UFH: 5000 IU, SC, q8h
Note: Surgery delayed prophylaxis UFH or LMWH should be applied between the
  time of hospital admission and surgery; external pneumatic compression if anti-
  coagulation contraindicated; ASA should not be used as only method of VTE
  prophylaxis.

Total Knee Replacement

Incidence: 40%–84% without VTE prophylaxis
Prophylaxis
  LMWH (enoxaparin OR fondaparinux)
    Enoxaparin: 30 mg, SC, 12 hr postop, then 30 mg, SC, q12h (creatinine
      clearance <30 mL/min: 30 mg, SC, q24h)
    Fondaparinux: 2.5 mg, SC, 6 hr postop, then 2.5 mg, q24h
  OR
  Warfarin: INR 2–3
  OR
  External pneumatic compression
Note: ASA, UFH, VFP should not be used as the only method of VTE prophylaxis.

ASA, acetylsalicylic acid; INR, international normalized ratio; IPC, intermittent
pneumatic compression; LDUH, low-dose unfractionated heparin; LMWH, low-
molecular-weight heparin; postop, postoperatively; SC, subcutaneously; UFH,
unfractionated heparin; VFP, venous foot pump; VTE, venous thromboembolism.

utilized during surgery to decrease bleeding at the surgical site. Enoxaparin, fondaparinux, and warfarin have been recommended as the most effective prophylaxis for DVT prevention. External pneumatic compression sleeves are the most effective nonpharmacologic modality; however, they must be worn continuously to provide the physiologic effect of reducing stasis.

Urologic Surgery

A review of prophylaxis studies in urologic surgery showed that the average male patient was 50 to 70 years old. The incidence of DVT varies in the urologic literature, with an incidence between 31% and 51% in open prostatectomies to 7% to 10% in transurethral resections of the prostate. The patients in these studies had a mixture of benign and malignant diseases. This factor introduces bias into the outcome of these studies. The prophylaxis for DVT has been variable because there are few well-controlled trials. Heparin, external pneumatic compression, and gradient elastic stockings have been advocated as prophylaxis (Table 5-3). The present recommendations are heparin (5000 U subcutaneously beginning 2 hours before surgery, followed by 5000 U subcutaneously every 8 to 12 hours until the patient is discharged or ambulatory) or external pneumatic compression. More trials are necessary in this surgical population.

Neurosurgery

The age group in neurosurgical prophylaxis studies varies from 48 to 60 years. Craniotomies and spinal surgical operations have been the predominant neurosurgical procedures evaluated for prophylaxis. Six major neurosurgical prophylaxis studies have been reported in the literature. Three of the six studies evaluated combined populations of patients undergoing craniotomy and spinal surgery. Two studies evaluated solely craniotomy and aneurysmal resection. In these studies, the incidence of DVT varied between 19% and 43%. Two

TABLE 5-3	Prophylaxis for Urologic Surgery

Incidence of DVT

Open prostatectomy: 31%–51%
TURP: 7%–10%

Prophylaxis: High-Risk Urology Patient

UFH: 5000 U, SC, q8 or 12 h
OR
External pneumatic compression sleeves
OR
Enoxaparin: 40 mg, SC, beginning 12 hours postop, followed by 40 mg, SC, q24h
OR
Dalteparin: 2500 IU, SC, 1–2 hr preop, 2500 IU, SC, 12 hr postop, followed by
    5000 IU, SC, q24h

Prophylaxis: Very High-Risk Urology Patient

External pneumatic compression plus UFH OR LMWH
UFH: 5000 U, SC, q8h
OR
Enoxaparin: 40 mg, SC, beginning 12 hr postop, followed by 40 mg, SC, q24h
OR
Dalteparin: 2500 IU, SC, 1–2 hr preop, 2500 IU, SC, 12 hr postop, followed by
    5000 IU, SC, q24h

Prophylaxis: Low-Risk Urologic Procedure (TURP, cystoscopy)
Early ambulation

DVT, deep venous thrombosis; LMWH, low-molecular-weight heparin; postop, postoperatively; preop, preoperatively; SC, subcutaneously; UFH, unfractionated heparin; TURP, transurethral resection of the prostate; VTE, venous thromboembolism.

significant factors (leg weakness and surgery longer than 4 hours' duration) were identified as risks for the development of DVT. Subcutaneous heparin was shown to be effective. The incidence of DVT was reduced from 34% to 6% with no increased risk of central nervous system bleeding. Studies with external pneumatic compression reported a reduction in DVT from 19% to 1.5%. The current recommendations are to use external pneumatic compression devices as primary prophylaxis for DVT and PE (Table 5-4). In craniotomy, external pneumatic compression sleeves should be worn until the patient is ambulatory. If the patient remains on bed rest for more than 10 days, heparin (5000 U subcutaneously every 12 hours) may be substituted for the compression sleeves. The recommendations given previously should be used for patients

TABLE 5-4	Prophylaxis for Neurosurgery

Incidence of DVT: 19%–34% without VTE prophylaxis

Prophylaxis

External pneumatic compression with or without gradient elastic stockings
OR
Unfractionated heparin: 5000 U, SC, q12h
OR
Enoxaparin: 40 mg, SC, q24h

Very High-Risk Neurosurgery Patients

External pneumatic compression sleeves
AND
Heparin: 5000 U, SC, q12h
OR
Enoxaparin: 40 mg, SC, q24h

DVT, deep venous thrombosis; SC, subcutaneously; VTE, venous thromboembolism.

undergoing spinal surgery. Heparin may be used as prophylaxis if agreed on by the neurosurgeon. Studies using LMWHs are currently in progress.

Gynecologic Surgery

The incidence of DVT in gynecologic surgery varies with respect to the presence of malignant disease and the surgical procedure. In reported studies, patients undergoing abdominal hysterectomy for nonmalignant conditions had an incidence of DVT of 10% to 12%, and those undergoing vaginal hysterectomy had an incidence of 6% to 7%. The incidence of DVT in surgery for malignant disease was reported to be between 12% and 35%. This latter group underwent more extensive surgery for cure or palliation of the malignant condition. The age range in the group undergoing surgery for malignant disease was between 50 and 60 years. Dextran 40 or 70, warfarin, and external pneumatic compression have been evaluated as prophylaxis for DVT in these surgical groups. The current prophylaxis for DVT, in order of preference, is heparin, LMWH, and external pneumatic compression (Table 5-5).

TABLE 5-5	Prophylaxis for Gynecologic Surgery

Incidence of DVT

Surgery for nonmalignant conditions
  Abdominal hysterectomy: 10%–12%
  Vaginal hysterectomy: 6%–7%
Surgery for malignancy: 12%–35%

DVT Prophylaxis

Brief gynecologic procedures for benign disease
  Ambulation
Laparoscopic gynecologic procedures with additional VTE risk factors
  UFH: 5000 U, SC, q12h
  OR
  Enoxaparin: 40 mg, SC, beginning 12 hr postop, followed by 40 mg, SC, q24h
  OR
  Dalteparin: 2500 IU, SC, 1–2 hr preop, 2500 IU, SC, 12 hr postop, followed
    by 5000 IU, SC, q24h
  OR
  External pneumatic compression
Major gynecologic procedure for benign disease without VTE risk factors
  UFH: 5000 U, SC, q12h
  OR
  Enoxaparin: 40 mg, SC, beginning 12 hr postop, followed by 40 mg, SC,
    q24hr
  OR
  Dalteparin: 2500 IU, SC, 1–2 hr preop, 2500 IU, SC, 12 hr postop, fol-
    lowed by 5000 IU, SC, q24h
  OR
  External pneumatic compression
Major gynecologic procedure for malignancy or patients with VTE risk factors
  External pneumatic compression AND either of the following regimens
    (grade 1C)
  UFH: 5000 U, SC, q8h
  OR
  Enoxaparin: 40 mg, SC, beginning 12 hr postop, followed by 40 mg, SC,
    q24h
  OR
  Dalteparin: 2500 IU, SC, 1–2 hr preop, 2500 IU, SC, 12 hr postop, fol-
    lowed by 5000 IU, SC, q24h
Extended prophylaxis for gynecology patients who have undergone surgery for
  malignancy and are >60 yr old or who have had previous VTE (prophylaxis
  should be maintained for 4 wk following hospital discharge)
    Enoxaparin: 40 mg, SC, q24h
    OR
    Dalteparin: 5000 IU, SC, q24h

DVT, deep venous thrombosis; postop, postoperatively; preop, preoperatively;
SC, subcutaneously; UFH, unfractionated heparin; VTE, venous thromboembolism.

General Surgery

The incidence of DVT in general surgery has been documented to be 20% to 30%. These studies evaluated a wide age group of patients undergoing a variety of procedures. The recommended prophylactic agents, in order of preference, are heparin, LMWH, and external pneumatic compression stockings. In high-risk general surgery, low-dose subcutaneous heparin or LMWH should be used. In very high-risk general surgery, low-dose unfractionated or LMWH should be combined with external pneumatic compression sleeves (Table 5-6).

EXTENDED PROPHYLAXIS FOR DEEP VEIN THROMBOSIS AND PULMONARY EMBOLISM

The duration of risk for the development of DVT after release from the hospital following surgery has become an important issue. Despite our most effective DVT and PE prophylaxis regimens, the incidence of DVT has not been reduced to zero. Therefore, the patient's risk of DVT following hospital discharge must be considered, particularly the patient at high risk, such as the patient who has undergone orthopedic surgery or the patient with malignant disease who undergoes surgical treatment.

The ACCP guidelines defined the DVT risk period after discharge following orthopedic surgery to be 28 to 35 days. It has been recommended that prophylaxis with LMWH or warfarin be provided during this period (Table 5-7). For the patient with malignant disease who has undergone surgery for this condition, extended venous thromboembolism (VTE) prophylaxis for 28 to 30 days postoperatively should be considered.

Currently, I recommend that orthopedic surgical patients receive extended prophylaxis with warfarin (an INR 2 to 3) or LMWH (enoxaparin, 40 mg; dalteparin, 5000 IU; or fondaparinux, 2.5 mg every 24 hours) for 28 to 35 days. For

TABLE 5-6	Prophylaxis for General Surgery

Incidence of DVT: 20%–30%

Prophylaxis

Low-risk surgery (minor procedure, age >40 yr, no VTE risk factors)
   Early ambulation
Moderate-risk surgery (nonmajor procedure, age 40–60 yr; VTE risk factors or
   major procedure, age >40 yr, no VTE risk factors)
   Heparin: 5000 U, SC, q12h
      OR
   Enoxaparin: 40 mg, SC, beginning 12 hr postop, followed by 40 mg, SC,
      q24h
      OR
   Dalteparin: 5000 IU, SC, beginning 12 hr postop, followed by 5000 IU, SC,
      q24h
High-risk surgery (nonmajor surgery age >60 yr; VTE risk factors; major surgery,
   age >40 yr, or have VTE risk factors)
   Heparin: 5000 U q8h
      OR
   Enoxaparin: 40 mg, SC, beginning 12 hr postop, followed by 40 mg, SC,
      q24h
      OR
   Dalteparin: 2500 IU, SC, 1–2 hr preop, 2500 IU, SC, 12 hr postop, fol-
      lowed by 5000 IU, SC, q24h
Very high-risk surgery (major surgery, age >40 yr, multiple VTE risk factors)
   External pneumatic compression
      AND
   Heparin: 5000 U, SC, q8h
      OR
   Enoxaparin: 40 mg, SC, beginning 12 hr postop, followed by 40 mg, SC,
      q24h
      OR
   Dalteparin: 5000 IU, SC, beginning 12 hr postop, followed by 5000 IU, SC,
      q24h
   In selected very high-risk general surgery patients, including those who have
      undergone major cancer surgery, extended prophylaxis with LMWH for
      4 wk following discharge
   Enoxaparin: 40 mg, SC, q24h
      OR
   Dalteparin: 5000 IU, SC, q24h

DVT, deep venous thrombosis; LMWH, low-molecular-weight heparin;
postop, postoperatively; preop, preoperatively; SC, subcutaneously; VTE, venous
thromboembolism.

selected very high-risk patients (e.g., history of prior VTE)
who undergo general or gynecologic surgery or for those who
undergo cancer surgery, I recommend that LMWH (enoxaparin, 40 mg every 24 hours) be given for 28 to 30 days
postoperatively (Table 5-8).

TABLE 5-7	Extended Prophylaxis for Orthopedic Surgery

Total Hip Replacement or Hip Fracture Surgery (Patients should receive extended VTE prophylaxis for up to 28 to 30 days following surgery)
LMWH
    Enoxaparin: 40 mg, SC, q24h
    Dalteparin: 5000 IU, SC, q24h
    Fondaparinux: 2.5 mg, SC, q24h
OR
Warfarin: INR 2–3
Total Knee Arthroplasty (Current evidence supports only 14 days extended prophylaxis, but clinical judgment should be exercised especially if risk factors for VTE are present)
LMWH
    Enoxaparin: 40 mg, SC, q24h
    Dalteparin: 5000 IU, SC, q24h
    Fondaparinux: 2.5 mg, SC, q24h
OR
Warfarin: INR 2–3

INR, international normalized ratio; LMWH, low-molecular-weight heparin; SC, subcutaneously; VTE, venous thromboembolism.

TABLE 5-8	Extended Prophylaxis for High-Risk General Surgery and Surgery for Malignant Disease

In selected high-risk general surgical patients, including those who have undergone major cancer surgery or who have had previous venous thromboembolism, extended prophylaxis for 28 to 30 days should be provided
Low-molecular-weight heparin
    Dalteparin: 5000 IU, SC, q24h
    Enoxaparin: 40 mg, SC, q24h

SC, subcutaneously.

SPECIAL ANTICOAGULATION PROBLEMS

Patients receiving long-term oral anticoagulation (warfarin) for various reasons require a tailored management strategy for this agent in the perioperative period. The goals of care are to prevent recurrent thromboembolism during the window when oral anticoagulation is discontinued and to reduce the risk of major bleeding when therapy is reinstituted in the postoperative period. To manage this patient population most effectively, we utilize a "bridge approach" to minimize the total time without therapeutic anticoagulation in selected patient groups (Box 5-5).

Acute Deep Vein Thrombosis or Pulmonary Embolism

The patient with acute DVT or PE before surgery presents a difficult management problem. The approach to this process depends on the urgency of the surgery and the extent of thrombosis. The former point is significant because heparin must be discontinued before the surgical procedure, thereby leaving the patient untreated with an acute DVT or PE. The issue of the extent of thrombosis relates to the risk of PE for an untreated

---

Box 5-5	**BRIDGE APPROACH TO PERIOPERATIVE ANTICOAGULATION**

1. Discontinue warfarin 5 days before surgery.
2. Initiate LMWH (enoxaparin, 1 mg/kg q12h) 24 to 48 hr after discontinuing warfarin.
3. Discontinue LMWH after the morning dose on the day before surgery.
4. At 12 hr postoperatively, initiate prophylaxis with LMWH or UFH, depending on the recommendation made earlier in the chapter. Resume warfarin on postoperative day 1 at the dose the patient was receiving preoperatively. The LMWH or UFH is maintained until the INR has been achieved at 2 to 3 for most indications and at 2.5 to 3.5 for patients with prosthetic cardiac valves.
5. If the patient has a history of developing thromboembolic events following the discontinuation of therapeutic LMWH for the surgical procedure, he or she should be started on a constant infusion of UFH, with appropriate adjustment to achieve a therapeutic aPTT. The choice of UFH is based on the risk of bleeding in the postoperative period that would require immediate discontinuation (shorter half-life than LMWH) and reversal of the medication.

---

aPTT, activated partial thromboplastin time; INR, international normalized ratio; LMWH, low-molecular-weight heparin; UFH, unfractionated heparin.

calf vein thrombosis (15%) or proximal vein thrombosis (50%). The following are the clinical guidelines used for managing patients with a preexisting DVT or PE before surgery.

If the procedure is elective, the patient is treated with heparin and then warfarin, and hospital admission is postponed for 3 to 6 months. On readmission for surgery, prophylaxis for DVT and PE is required because the patient is at very high risk for the development of postoperative thrombosis. The patient whose surgery is an emergency but can be delayed for 7 days, who has either a proximal or distal thrombosis or PE, and whose procedure would allow immediate reinstitution of anticoagulation postoperatively is treated with a constant infusion of heparin. The activated partial thromboplastin time (aPTT) is maintained at 1.5 to 2.5 seconds times the baseline for 7 full days. The heparin infusion is discontinued 6 hours before surgery, and the aPTT, a platelet count, and a complete blood count are evaluated before the procedure. A heparin infusion is reinstituted in 24 to 48 hours from the time of its discontinuation. If the surgical procedure does not allow the resumption of anticoagulation, an inferior vena cava filter should be placed.

The management of the patient undergoing emergency surgery is much more aggressive. Patients with either proximal or distal DVT or PE should have an inferior vena cava filter placed. The filter can be a retrievable or permanent inferior vena caval device. This technique prevents embolization during the risk window of 24 to 72 hours postoperatively for the patient who is unable to resume anticoagulation therapy. Venous imaging may be completed in the postoperative period to evaluate for clot propagation. This recommendation is a clinical judgment.

Antithrombin III Deficiency

Antithrombin-heparin cofactor (AT-III) is one of the α_2-globulins of plasma. AT-III inactivates thrombin, factors XIIa, XIa, IXa, plasmin, and kallikrein. When heparin interacts with AT-III, the combination enhances the inactivation of the preceding serine proteases. Deficiency of AT-III is inherited as an autosomal dominant disorder. Most patients are treated indefinitely with warfarin because of their predisposition to recurrent thrombotic events.

The approach to management in the perioperative period is directed toward the selected prophylaxis for DVT and PE and the planned surgical procedure. If warfarin is not the recommended prophylaxis and therefore not to be administered in the perioperative period, it should be discontinued 3 days before surgery. A functional assay of AT-III is obtained, and the patient is treated with daily AT-III concentrate to raise the level of AT-III to near 100% for surgery. Appropriate VTE prophylaxis should be administered as indicated. If the selected prophylaxis is not warfarin, warfarin should be re-initiated on the third postoperative day, with the aim of attaining an INR of 2 to 3 before nonwarfarin prophylaxis is discontinued.

Protein C and Protein S Deficiency

Protein C deficiency is inherited as an autosomal dominant trait with variable expressivity at the laboratory level and incomplete penetrance at the clinical level. Protein C is a vitamin K–dependent plasma zymogen that is synthesized in the liver. Protein C is activated by thrombin, and this results in inhibition of activated factors V and VIII in addition to an elevation in plasminogen activator levels. Protein S deficiency is inherited as an autosomal dominant trait. It is a vitamin K–dependent plasma protein that acts as a cofactor for the anticoagulant activity of activated protein C. Patients with decreased levels of protein C or S are at high risk for thrombosis when they are in the hypercoagulable state of surgery. Frequently, these patients receive lifelong warfarin therapy. Patients with protein C or S deficiency who are scheduled for surgery should be treated according to the bridge therapy protocol (see Box 5-5).

Factor V Leiden/Activated Protein C Resistance

Activated protein C resistance was first described in 1994, when patients with venous thrombosis were found to be resistant to the normal anticoagulant effects of activated protein C. This protein inhibits coagulation by proteolytically inactivating factors Va and VIIIa. In approximately 90% of these patients, a factor V allele is discovered and results in resistance to protein C. This allele, factor V Leiden, is characterized by a single amino acid change (Arg 506 to Gln) at one of the sites on the factor V molecule when activated protein C cleaves factor Va and inactivates it. Factor V Leiden is present in approximately 5% of healthy people of Northern European ancestry, in 10% of patients presenting with venous thrombosis, and in 30% to 50% of patients investigated for thrombophilia. This entity is rare in patients of African and Asian descent. Factor V Leiden has relatively low risk for thrombosis, but in high-risk situations such as surgery, the risk is increased. These patients must receive appropriate VTE prophylaxis for surgical procedures. Those patients with recurrent thrombotic events and receiving long-term anticoagulation with factor V Leiden should be treated according to the bridge therapy protocol (see Box 5-5).

Prothrombin Gene Mutation (G20210A)

The prothrombin gene mutation (G20210A) was first described in 1996. This mutation was found in the external 3′ untranslated region of the gene and is associated with increased basal levels of functionally normal prothrombin. This mutation is found in 5% to 10% of patients presenting with venous thrombosis and in approximately 15% of patients being investigated for thrombophilia. The risk of venous thrombosis in patients with prothrombin gene mutation is relatively low but is increased in high-risk situations such as surgery. As with factor V Leiden, appropriate VTE prophylaxis must be applied. As described earlier, those patients receiving long-term anticoagulation for this thrombophilia should be treated according to the bridge therapy protocol (see Box 5-5).

Heparin-Induced Thrombocytopenia

Heparin-induced thrombocytopenia is the most frequent and important hematologic drug reaction that occurs secondary to an immunologic mechanism. In 12 prospective studies of more than 1500 patients receiving heparin, pooled data revealed a frequency of thrombocytopenia of 6% and an incidence of thrombocytopenia with arterial thrombosis of less than 1%. This latter form is the most severe clinically. Porcine heparin is associated with a lower incidence of thrombocytopenia than is bovine heparin. The development of thrombocytopenia is independent of the route of administration and occurs between 6 and 12 days after initiation of therapy. In patients with a previously documented episode of thrombocytopenia or thrombocytopenia with arterial thrombosis, reexposure to heparin results in a faster onset of the process.

Because heparin-induced thrombocytopenia and its recurrence cannot be predicted, the surgical patient with a history of this disorder, with or without thrombosis, should have an alternative form of prophylaxis for DVT and PE, as discussed previously for different types of surgical procedures. Although heparin antibodies may be absent 90 days after cessation of heparin, I avoid the repeat use of unfractionated heparin or LMWH in the patient with a prior history of heparin-induced thrombocytopenia. Currently, studies are being conducted with fondaparinux as an agent for VTE prophylaxis in patients with heparin-induced thrombocytopenia because of the low affinity of this agent for binding to platelet factor IV and the theoretically lower risk of precipitating an antibody response.

Antiphospholipid Antibody Syndrome

Antiphospholipid antibodies may be detected by solid-phase anticardiolipin antibody tests and the lupus anticoagulant test. The occurrence of these antibodies has been associated with venous or arterial thrombosis, fetal loss, and possibly thrombocytopenia. These antibodies occur in patients with autoimmune, infectious, drug-induced, malignant, and other disorders. The proposed mechanisms by which antiphospholipid antibodies may mediate thrombosis include the following: inhibition of prostacyclin release from vascular endothelium, a process that results in increased platelet aggregation; inhibition of fibrinolytic activity; inhibition of prekallikrein activity; inhibition of AT-III activity; inhibition of protein C activation; inhibition of thrombomodulin; and binding phospholipid in platelet membranes. The presence of antiphospholipid syndrome may be recognized by the prolongation of aPTT. In two series totaling 23 patients who underwent surgery, only 1 patient experienced bleeding. The prevalence of bleeding is believed to be approximately 0.6%. If the patient has coexisting thrombocytopenia or hypoprothrombinemia, or both, the risk is higher for a hemorrhagic event in the perioperative period. The incidence of thromboembolic complications in patients with lupus anticoagulant is approximately 27%. The literature supports the use of long-term anticoagulation in patients with thromboembolic complications. Corticosteroids, immunosuppressive drugs, or plasmapheresis may be added to the regimen if recurrent thrombosis occurs with adequate anticoagulation.

The approach in the perioperative period to the patient who has a history of antiphospholipid syndrome and no thrombotic complications is to select the appropriate VTE prophylaxis regimen for the surgical procedure. If the patient has a history of recurrent thrombosis and is not receiving long-term anticoagulation therapy, prophylaxis targeted to the high-risk patient should be administered. The patient with antiphospholipid syndrome and recurrent thrombosis who is receiving long-term anticoagulation with warfarin should be treated according to the bridge therapy protocol (see Box 5-5).

Selected Readings

Bergqvist D, Benoni G, Bjorgell O, et al: Low molecular weight heparin (enoxaparin) as prophylaxis against venous thromboembolism after total hip replacement. N Engl J Med 335:696-700, 1996.

Broekman A, Veltkamp J, Bertina R: Congenital protein C and venous thromboembolism. N Engl J Med 308:340-344, 1983.

Caprini J, Scurr J, Hasty J: Role of compression modalities in a prophylactic program for deep vein thrombosis. Semin Thromb Hemost 14:77-87, 1988.

Clagett G, Reisch J: Prevention of venous thromboembolism in general surgical patients: Results of meta-analysis. Ann Surg 208:227-239, 1988.

Cohen AT, Bailey CS, Alikhan R, et al: Extended thromboprophylaxis with low molecular weight heparin reduces symptomatic venous thromboembolism following lower limb arthroplasty: A meta-analysis. Thromb Haemost 85:940-941, 2001.

Douketis JD, Eikelboom JW, Quinlan DJ, et al: Short duration prophylaxis against venous thromboembolism after total hip or knee replacement: A meta-analysis of prospective studies investigating symptomatic outcomes. Arch Intern Med 162:1465-1471, 2002.

Geerts WH, Pineo GF, Heit JA, et al: Prevention of venous thromboembolism. Chest 126:338S-400S, 2004.

Harris E, Asherson R, Hughes G: Antiphospholipid antibodies: Autoantibodies with a difference. Annu Rev Med 39:261-271, 1988.

Hirsh J, Levine M: Low molecular weight heparin. Blood 79:1-17, 1992.

Hull R, Raskob G, McLoughlin D, et al: Effectiveness of intermittent pneumatic leg compression for preventing deep vein thrombosis after total hip replacement. JAMA 263:2313-2317, 1990.

Kelton J, Levine M: Heparin induced thrombocytopenia. Semin Thromb Hemost 12:59-62, 1986.

Merli G: Prophylaxis for deep vein thrombosis and pulmonary embolism in surgery. In Lubin M, Walker H, Smith R (eds): Medical Management of the Surgical Patient, 3rd ed. Philadelphia, JB Lippincott, 2006, pp 221-227.

Much J, Herbst K, Rapaport S: Thrombosis in patients with lupus anticoagulant. Ann Intern Med 92:156, 1980.

Nicolaides A, Fareed J, Kakkar A, et al: Prevention and treatment of venous thromboembolism: International Consensus Statement (guidelines according to scientific evidence). Int Angiol 25:101-161, 2006.

Virchow R: Neuer fall von todlichen: Emboli der Lungenarterie. Arch Pathol Anat 10:225-228, 1856.

Wilson N, Das S, Kakkar V, et al: Thromboembolic prophylaxis in total knee replacement: Evaluation of the A-V impulse system. J Bone Joint Surg Br 74:50-52, 1992.

6 Perioperative Evaluation of Patients with Hematologic Disorders

FREDERICK M. FELLIN, MD

Hematologic abnormalities are fairly common in perioperative patients. Many of these abnormalities are trivial and pose no particular risk to the patient. Some abnormalities, however, can present significant clinical challenges in the perioperative period. This chapter focuses primarily on specific hematologic problems such as anemia, thrombocytosis, and hemostatic abnormalities, with special attention directed to timely diagnosis, risk assessment, and management issues. The paucity of evidence-based guidelines for many of these issues is surprising. Therefore, many of the recommendations are based on standard clinical practice and expert opinion.

ANEMIA

Anemia is the most commonly encountered hematologic problem in the perioperative period. Because the major function of red blood cells is to facilitate oxygen transport to tissues, a sufficient number of red blood cells is crucial to provide adequate oxygenation. Given that additional factors such as cardiac output, pulmonary gas exchange, vessel compliance, blood volume, blood viscosity, and oxygen affinity for hemoglobin contribute to oxygen delivery, the level of hemoglobin itself serves only as a rough guide to the adequacy of oxygenation.

Levels of Evidence:

Ⓐ—Randomized controlled trials (RCTs), meta-analyses, well-designed systematic reviews of RCTs. **Ⓑ**—Case-control or cohort studies, nonrandomized controlled trials, systematic reviews of studies other than RCTs, cross-sectional studies, retrospective studies. **Ⓒ**—Consensus statements, expert guidelines, usual practice, opinion.

The optimal hemoglobin level for the surgical patient has been the subject of much discussion. A value of 10 g/dL had long been accepted as this safe level. However, older anecdotal evidence from patients with hemoglobinopathies or renal failure suggested that even severe degrees of anemia could be tolerated in the perioperative period. More recent reviews of the subject have addressed the issue of transfusion triggers. Few prospective data have been published, but the available information suggests that a hemoglobin value greater than 6 to 8 g/dL is adequate in most circumstances. If patients have coexisting medical issues such as cardiac disease or if significant blood loss is anticipated, higher levels of hemoglobin may be more appropriate. Not all authors agree on these trigger values; some investigators have argued that higher hemoglobin levels (10 to 12 g/dL) may enhance outcomes. Clearly, prospective trials would be helpful to answer these questions definitively. Although, as mentioned, no definitive data are available to quantify risk, information derived from Jehovah's Witnesses who underwent surgical procedures showed that comorbid disease and expected operative blood loss are important covariables in determining morbidity and mortality (Table 6-1). The recommendations given in Table 6-2 are based on this information.

Preoperative Evaluation

A preoperative history should emphasize the personal and family history of anemia or bleeding, ethnic background, medication, alcohol use, toxin exposure, recent illness, and

TABLE 6-1	Postoperative Outcomes
Preoperative Hemoglobin Level	**Mortality**
<6 g/dL	61.5%
6.1–8 g/dL	33%
8.1–10 g/dL	0%
>10 g/dL	7.1%

TABLE 6-2	Transfusion Recommendations
Higher Hemoglobin (>10 g/dL)	**Lower Hemoglobin (7–10 g/dL)**
Coronary artery disease	Younger age
Congestive heart failure	Long life expectancy
Chronic obstructive pulmonary disease	Otherwise good health
Peripheral vascular disease	
Stroke	
Use of β-blockers	
High blood loss	
Older age	
Short life expectancy	

constitutional symptoms (Fig. 6-1). The physical examination should assess jaundice, skin and mucous membrane abnormalities, adenopathy, organomegaly, neurologic dysfunction, and occult blood loss in stool or urine.

The first step in the laboratory evaluation of anemia should be to measure the reticulocyte count. This serves to differentiate anemia caused by inadequate marrow production (low reticulocyte count) from anemia caused by excessive red blood cell loss (high reticulocyte count), related either to acute bleeding or to hemolysis. The absolute reticulocyte count is more helpful because it corrects for the degree of anemia. In the baseline state, there are roughly 5 million red blood cells/µL, and the reticulocyte count is 1% to 2%. Therefore, the baseline reticulocyte number is 50,000 to 100,000 red blood cells/µL. Under stress, the bone marrow can increase red blood cell production approximately eightfold, to 400,000 to 800,000 red blood cells. The following formula is used to determine the absolute reticulocyte count by correcting for the degree of anemia:

$$\text{Absolute reticulocyte count} = \text{Red blood count} \times \text{reticulocyte count}/100$$

During the early stage of acute blood loss, the reticulocyte count may be low for a few days until the bone marrow responds fully.

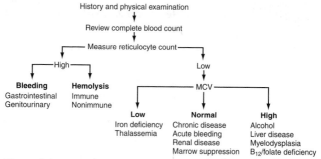

Figure 6-1 • Diagnostic evaluation of anemia. MCV, mean corpuscular volume.

When the reticulocyte count is high, a compensatory phase of acute blood loss or hemolysis is present. The history, physical examination, Coombs test, examination of a peripheral blood smear, and sickle cell preparation or hemoglobin electrophoresis should help the clinician to arrive at a correct diagnosis. If the reticulocyte count is low, the mean corpuscular volume and the peripheral blood smear should be examined to determine whether the patient's anemia is microcytic, normocytic, or macrocytic.

Microcytic anemia is usually the result of iron deficiency or thalassemia. Differentiating iron deficiency from thalassemia minor by examination of a peripheral blood smear may be difficult. Serum iron, iron binding capacity, ferritin, bone marrow evaluation for iron, or determination of hemoglobin A_2 (which is elevated in β-thalassemia) is helpful in establishing a diagnosis. Thalassemia minor rarely causes hemoglobin values lower than 9 g/dL; the more severe forms of thalassemia usually are accompanied by splenomegaly and bizarre red blood cell morphologic features.

Macrocytic anemia is most often the result of alcoholism, liver disease, vitamin B_{12} or folate deficiency, or primary marrow dysfunction (myelodysplasia or "preleukemia"). Ovalomacrocytes and hypersegmented neutrophils are virtually diagnostic of vitamin B_{12} or folate deficiency. Appropriate vitamin levels or bone marrow examination may be necessary to confirm the diagnosis.

Normocytic anemia is most often caused by the following: chronic inflammatory, infectious, or neoplastic disease; uremia; acute blood loss; or bone marrow suppression from drugs or radiation exposure. Additional history and laboratory studies to evaluate these problems usually reveals a cause.

Therapeutic Considerations

The physiologic needs of the patient must be carefully assessed. The clinician must consider all the previous determinants of tissue oxygenation, as well as the consequences of the planned operative procedure, before making a decision to administer red blood cells. When the procedure is elective, it seems prudent to delay surgery, complete the evaluation, and treat the underlying problem (if indicated) to avoid the potential hazards of transfusion. Because reversal of "correctable" anemia (deficiency of vitamin B_{12}, folate, or iron; transient bone marrow suppression; uremia; and immune hemolysis) may take days to weeks, blood transfusion may be the only recourse if surgery is urgently needed. Similarly, "uncorrectable" anemia (myelodysplasia, chronic disease, or thalassemia) requires blood transfusion.

Patients who do need blood transfusion are often concerned about the potential risks associated with blood products. The following list contains recent estimates of the frequency of various transfusion-related complications that indicate the safety of the modern blood supply.

Alloimmunization	1:100
Fever, chill, allergic reactions	1:30 to 1:200
Acute hemolysis	1:12,000 to 1:25,000
Delayed hemolysis	1:5,000 to 1:11,000

Immunosuppression	Unknown
Bacterial infection	1:200,000
Hepatitis B infection	1:137,000
Hepatitis C infection	1:1,000,000
Human immunodeficiency virus infection	1:1,900,000

Management of patients who refuse blood transfusion poses significant issues. Generally, primary blood components are declined, but the use of blood "fractions" such as immune globulin or albumin or the use of intraoperative blood salvage or normovolemic hemodilution may be acceptable to some patients who would otherwise refuse blood transfusion. General guidelines for management of these patients include the following: maintenance of blood volume; limitation of phlebotomy as much as possible; use of folate, iron, and epoetin to enhance erythropoiesis; use of pharmacologic agents to reduce blood loss (antifibrinolytics, recombinant factor VIIa); and consideration of intraoperative blood salvage.

Preoperative donation of autologous blood for elective procedures has become common practice. If more than 1 U of red cells is required, use of epoetin alfa and iron supplements can allow for the collection of as much as 3 to 4 U in a month. Epoetin doses of 50 U/kg to 150 U/kg three times per week have been used.

Management of Specific Disorders

Nutritional Deficiencies and Bone Marrow Suppression

Anemia resulting from major nutritional deficiencies (vitamin B_{12}, folate, or iron) responds to the replacement of the proper nutrient by the appropriate route. A rise in the reticulocyte count, the earliest evidence of successful treatment, takes from 3 days (vitamin B_{12} or folate) to 10 days (iron). Complete correction can take several weeks. Anemia related to bone marrow suppression from radiation therapy or chemotherapy usually begins to be corrected within 2 or 3 weeks of exposure, but, again, full correction may take weeks to occur.

Prolonged bone marrow suppression may result from the use of mitomycin, nitrosoureas, or busulfan. Recombinant erythropoietin is now available to treat chemotherapy-induced anemia in doses of 150 to 300 U/kg three times weekly or 40,000 U once weekly.

Chronic Renal Failure

The anemia of chronic renal failure results from the failure of the diseased kidneys to produce erythropoietin. Erythropoietin replacement has been standard practice for years in patients undergoing dialysis. The use of the hormone in patients with chronic renal failure who are not receiving dialysis is becoming more and more common. The usual dose of erythropoietin in renal failure is 50 U/kg three times per week or 10,000 U weekly. Again, full recovery takes weeks. Iron replacement therapy should be used in all patients.

Thalassemia

Thalassemia is characterized by ineffective production of hemoglobin and intramedullary destruction of red blood cells. Patients with severe thalassemia syndromes often have a history of long-term transfusion therapy and may suffer from multiorgan dysfunction caused by iron overload. A thorough evaluation of cardiac, pulmonary, renal, and hepatic function is indicated in these patients. Patients with less severe thalassemia syndromes usually have mild to moderate anemia and no increased operative risk, except from the anemia itself. Therapy for anemia, in either case, is transfusion.

Sickle Cell Anemia

Sickle cell anemia, the most common hemoglobinopathy, affects approximately 1 in 650 black infants in the United States. It is a structural disorder of hemoglobin that leads to accelerated clearance of red blood cells from the circulation. The pathophysiology consists of repeated polymerization and depolymerization of hemoglobin that produce irreversible red blood cell membrane damage, sludging of blood in capillaries, organ ischemia, and chronic hemolysis. The clinical consequences of these events are recurrent painful crises and dysfunction of the nervous, cardiac, pulmonary, renal, and immune systems. A thorough evaluation is in order in all these patients before any operative procedure is performed. Frequently, folate deficiency and, less commonly, renal insufficiency can exacerbate anemia in these patients.

The use of red blood cell transfusions in the routine preoperative care of patients with sickle cell disease is controversial. Transfusion probably decreases the risk of painful crisis and of acute chest syndrome in surgical patients. However, the intensity of transfusion has ranged from a regimen that raises the hemoglobin level to more than 10 g/dL to exchange transfusion that lowers the hemoglobin S level to less than 30%. A reasonable approach is to avoid transfusion for minor procedures. For most general surgical procedures, a conservative transfusion regimen to raise the hemoglobin level to greater than 10 g/dL is advisable. For high-risk surgical procedures that could result in hypotension, hypoxemia, or acidosis (e.g., major vascular or cardiac surgery), a more aggressive approach to lower hemoglobin S to less than 30% may still be warranted.

Immune Hemolytic Anemia

Immune hemolytic anemias are some of the most difficult problems to manage in the perioperative period. Most immune hemolytic anemias are of the warm antibody type, are mediated by immunoglobulin G, and occur at physiologic temperatures. These are most often idiopathic or associated with autoimmune disorders or lymphoproliferative disorders such as lymphoma or chronic lymphatic leukemia. Less common is the cold antibody type, mediated by immunoglobulin M and most often seen in association with infectious diseases such as *Mycoplasma* infections, mononucleosis, and syphilis.

Two phenomena make this type of anemia difficult to manage. First, the transfused red blood cells are as sensitive to the hemolytic process as are native cells, so their survival is limited. Second, the presence of the autoantibodies can make proper crossmatching difficult if not impossible. An accurate determination of the patient's blood group can be made in spite of the antibody. The real danger is the difficulty of detecting alloantibodies that could lead to a major hemolytic transfusion reaction. Special blood banking procedures are helpful in clarifying these issues.

In general, *warm antibody hemolytic anemia* responds to corticosteroids; a usual starting dose is 1 to 2 mg/kg of prednisone. Improvement typically occurs in several days. If transfusion is necessary, the "least incompatible" units should be used. The blood should be transfused slowly, with careful monitoring for signs and symptoms of hemolytic transfusion reactions, preferably while the patient is awake and able to relate symptoms of a transfusion reaction.

Cold-type immune hemolytic anemia rarely responds to corticosteroids. Management revolves around meticulous maintenance of body temperature and prewarming of all transfused blood products. In addition, washed red blood cells may be safer because infusion of complement components present in plasma may precipitate or aggravate the hemolytic process. In rare circumstances, plasma exchange may be helpful to limit hemolysis.

ERYTHROCYTOSIS

Preoperative Considerations

As with anemia, the major physiologic consequence of erythrocytosis is tissue hypoxemia. The mechanism by which this occurs is through a marked increase in blood viscosity, leading to slowing of capillary blood flow. Although the viscosity of blood is directly proportional to the hematocrit, the rate of rise is slow with a hematocrit less than 50%. With a hematocrit greater than 50%, viscosity increases rapidly, and oxygen transport is progressively diminished. The discovery of erythrocytosis in the perioperative period demands a thorough evaluation because the findings can be a manifestation of a potentially life-threatening disorder.

Erythrocytosis can be divided into two broad categories: relative and absolute. *Relative erythrocytosis* is typically accompanied by a reduced plasma volume. It can be seen in patients with volume contraction resulting from excessive water loss from polyuria or diarrhea, inadequate intake from starvation or vomiting, or excessive third spacing of fluids as in ascites. In addition, relative erythrocytosis can be seen in hypertensive, nonhypoxemic male patients who smoke (so-called stress erythrocytosis). These patients seem to have a chronically contracted plasma volume.

Absolute erythrocytosis can be either primary or secondary. Primary erythrocytosis or polycythemia vera is one of the myeloproliferative disorders. Polycythemia vera is classically associated with increased red blood cell mass, leukocytosis, thrombocytosis, and splenomegaly. Secondary erythrocytosis is always a manifestation of an underlying disorder. This condition can be physiologically appropriate, as in severe pulmonary disease, congenital heart disease with right-to-left shunting, and the unusual cases of hemoglobin variants with high affinity for oxygen. In each of these circumstances, tissue hypoxia stimulates the overproduction of red blood cells as a compensatory mechanism. Unfortunately, this mechanism may, in turn, worsen hypoxemia by increasing blood viscosity. Physiologically inappropriate secondary erythrocytosis is almost always seen in association with renal cysts or with neoplasms of the kidney, liver, uterus, or posterior fossa. These appear to be the result of an inappropriate secretion of erythropoietin.

The physiologically significant consequences of erythrocytosis can be divided into four categories. The first category is related to volume depletion, as seen in patients with relative erythrocytosis and manifested as hypotension, shock, and tissue ischemia. The second category comprises those related to increased blood viscosity, which can manifest as central nervous system symptoms (headache, lethargy, confusion, or delirium), visual disturbances, dyspnea, angina, claudication, or dysesthesias. The third category seems to be unique to polycythemia vera and includes an increased risk of thrombo-hemorrhagic phenomena and postoperative infections. The increase in thrombohemorrhagic events may also be related to the thrombocytosis that often coexists in polycythemia vera. The fourth set of consequences is unrelated to erythrocytosis but consists of manifestations of the underlying disorder, whether it is congenital heart disease, chronic obstructive pulmonary disease, or an occult neoplasm.

Preoperative Evaluation

In the presence of elevated leukocyte and platelet counts and splenomegaly, the diagnosis of polycythemia vera is virtually ensured if the red blood cell mass is increased and the patient has no severe cardiopulmonary disease (Fig. 6-2). If only erythrocytosis is present, the diagnosis centers on the careful evaluation of cardiopulmonary function. In the absence of cardiopulmonary disease or obvious plasma volume deple-tion, determination of red blood cell mass may be helpful but certainly is not necessary to make a diagnosis, particularly if the hematocrit is markedly elevated (>55%). The recent dis-covery of a mutation in the *JAK-2* gene in virtually all patients with polycythemia vera may aid in diagnosis as well.

Therapeutic Considerations

In addition to the indications for phlebotomy given in Box 6-1, considerations in the treatment of erythrocytosis are as follows:

1. In the case of relative erythrocytosis resulting from sig-nificant volume depletion, replacement of plasma volume is all that may be necessary to minimize risk.
2. No intervention is necessary in patients with stress erythrocytosis.

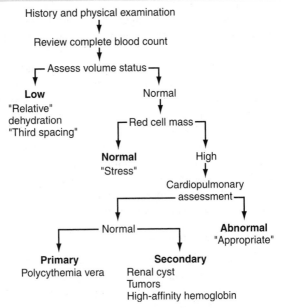

Figure 6-2 • Evaluation of erythrocytosis.

3. Patients with physiologically inappropriate secondary poly-cythemia should undergo phlebotomy (300 to 500 mL) on a daily basis to reduce the hematocrit to less than 45% to 50%, in addition to receiving treatment for the underlying disease. Older patients or those with underlying disease that could be exacerbated by too rapid phlebotomy should have slower phlebotomy (200 to 300 mL) every other day. A more rapid decline in hematocrit can be accomplished by erythrocytopheresis.

4. Patients with physiologically appropriate secondary eryth-rocytosis probably derive some benefit from reduction of the hematocrit to between 55% and 60%. One must balance the decrease in blood viscosity against the potential loss of oxygen-carrying capacity.

Box 6-1	INDICATIONS FOR PHLEBOTOMY IN ERYTHROCYTOSIS

Relative erythrocytosis: Not indicated

Stress erythrocytosis: Not indicated

Appropriate erythrocytosis resulting from cardiopulmonary disease: To hematocrit 50%–60%

Inappropriate primary erythrocytosis (polycythemia vera): To hematocrit <45%

Inappropriate secondary erythrocytosis: To hematocrit <50%

5. Patients with polycythemia vera clearly have an increased risk of thrombohemorrhagic events that can be substantially reduced by maintaining the hematocrit at less than 45% with the use of phlebotomy, with or without cytotoxic chemotherapy. Because it is not certain that an acute reduction in the hematocrit is accompanied by an acute reduction in risk, ideally the hematocrit should be lowered and maintained over a period of weeks to months before an operative procedure. Should surgery be urgently needed, the hematocrit can be safely reduced rapidly by repetitive phlebotomy, accompanied by plasma or colloid infusion to avoid hypotension, or by the use of erythrocytopheresis.

LEUKOPENIA

Preoperative Considerations

Leukopenia is occasionally encountered in patients in the perioperative period. It can occur as a manifestation of a primary hematologic disorder but is more often secondary to nonhematologic causes. The most important consideration is the increased risk of infection in these patients. Neutrophil counts greater than $1000/\mu L$ are rarely associated with a significant increased risk of infection. At lower neutrophil levels, the risk of infection increases significantly as the count falls.

Preoperative Evaluation

The diagnostic evaluation should begin with the identification of the type of leukocyte that is low (Table 6-3). Although most commonly this is the neutrophil, less frequently monocyte or lymphocyte levels can be depressed. The most clinically significant type of leukopenia is related to depressed numbers of neutrophils. Neutropenia has many causes; however, most cases are related to exposure to drugs or radiation. Neutropenia related to radiation or cytotoxic antineoplastic agents is the result of predictable and dose-dependent toxicity to stem cells and granulocytic precursors. Other classes of drugs associated with neutropenia are phenothiazines, anti-inflammatory agents (particularly phenylbutazone), sulfonamides, semisynthetic penicillins, chloramphenicol, and antithyroid drugs. In general, the most common mechanism is idiosyncratic bone marrow suppression. Some drugs may also have an immune component. Other common causes of neutropenia are congenital neutropenia, myelodysplasia, sepsis, viral or rickettsial infection, Felty's syndrome, and systemic lupus erythematosus.

Therapeutic Considerations

If the cytopenia is related to predictable bone marrow suppression from antineoplastic agents or radiation, recovery usually begins 14 to 21 days after exposure. When the cytopenia

TABLE 6-3	Common Causes of Leukopenia	
Neutropenia	**Monocytopenia**	**Lymphopenia**
Chemotherapy	Chemotherapy	Chemotherapy
Other drugs	Aplastic anemia	Corticosteroids
Radiation exposure	Corticosteroids	Severe congestive
Myelodysplasia	Systemic lupus erythematosus	heart failure
Viral infection		Immunodeficiency

is related to an idiosyncratic reaction or to other diseases, recovery may take weeks or months, or the condition may not improve at all. If recovery is expected, it is probably wise to delay surgery until the granulocyte count is increased to greater than 1000/μL. The use of recombinant hematopoietic growth factors such as granulocyte colony-stimulating factor hastens neutrophil recovery in patients with bone marrow suppression related to chemotherapy or radiation. Growth factors can also be useful in many of the other drug-induced types of neutropenia. In the event that recovery is not expected or that surgery is urgently needed while the patient is granulocytopenic, the risk of infection is increased. Whereas empiric antibiotic therapy is not indicated solely because of leukopenia, broad-spectrum antibiotic coverage should be instituted at the first sign of fever or infection. With this aggressive approach to treatment at the first sign of infection, mortality should be reduced substantially. White blood cell transfusions have a limited role in neutropenic patients, although they may offer some utility in the severely neutropenic patient with a documented infection who is not responding to appropriate antibiotic therapy.

LEUKOCYTOSIS

Preoperative Considerations

Leukocytosis is usually an indicator of an underlying inflammatory, infectious, or neoplastic process. Although lymphocytosis is most often associated with chronic lymphatic leukemia, neutrophilia or monocytosis of modest degree is most frequently associated with inflammation or infection. Marked elevation in the neutrophil and monocyte count raises the possibility of chronic leukemia. Moderate leukocytosis, involving mature white cells, carries no significant increase in perioperative risk. In most situations, leukocytosis requires no specific therapy except that of the underlying disorder. If the leukocytosis is related to the effects of leukemia, obviously the underlying illness and its therapy are of paramount importance in determining the perioperative risk.

THROMBOCYTOSIS

Thrombocytosis is present when the platelet count is higher than 500,000/μL. The major complications associated with an elevated platelet count are thrombosis and, to a lesser degree, hemorrhage. The magnitude of the risk varies considerably with the underlying disorder.

Preoperative Considerations

For the purpose of assessing risk, thrombocytosis can be divided into two broad categories (Box 6-2). Primary thrombocytosis is generally regarded as a manifestation of one of the myeloproliferative disorders (polycythemia vera, essential thrombocythemia, chronic myeloid leukemia, or myeloid metaplasia). Within the myeloproliferative disorders, risk varies widely. Thrombocytosis associated with chronic myeloid leukemia carries a low risk of thrombosis or hemorrhage.

Box 6-2	THROMBOHEMORRHAGIC RISK ASSOCIATED WITH THROMBOCYTOSIS

PRIMARY

Polycythemia vera: Thrombosis common, hemorrhage less common

Essential thrombocythemia and myeloid metaplasia: Hemorrhage common, thrombosis less common

Chronic myelogenous leukemia: Bleeding and thrombosis uncommon

SECONDARY

Nonmalignant: No risk

Malignant: Increased risk but not clearly related to platelets

Patients with polycythemia vera, in contrast, are more likely to have thrombosis than are those with essential thrombocythemia or myeloid metaplasia, who more often suffer hemorrhagic events. Individual patients may have both thrombosis and hemorrhage at various times during their illness, and the risk of this combination is higher in older patients and in those who have had prior events. The sites most commonly involved with hemorrhage are the mucosal surfaces, whereas the most common sites for thrombosis are the mesenteric veins, the deep veins of the extremities, and the cerebral, coronary, and peripheral arteries.

Secondary or reactive thrombocytosis can occur in iron deficiency, blood loss, chronic inflammatory states, and neoplastic diseases, as well as in the postoperative period. In general, the risk of thrombosis or hemorrhage is not increased in patients with secondary thrombocytosis. The exception to this rule is the patient with cancer, particularly adenocarcinoma, who often has thromboembolic phenomena related to a hypercoagulable state.

Preoperative Evaluation

The diagnostic evaluation should focus on symptoms and signs of thrombosis, mucosal hemorrhage, acute or chronic bleeding, anemia, infection, and inflammatory disorders or neoplasms. Additional laboratory studies may be helpful in the evaluation. Erythrocytosis and leukocytosis associated with splenomegaly are signs of polycythemia vera. The characteristic leukocytosis with a leftward shift and splenomegaly indicate a probable diagnosis of chronic myeloid leukemia. Iron deficiency should prompt an evaluation for gastrointestinal or genitourinary abnormalities. Appropriate studies to exclude infection are indicated if the situation suggests an infectious cause. If no obvious underlying disorder is found, essential thrombocythemia, which is usually a diagnosis of exclusion, is often the problem, especially in patients who have a history of unexplained thrombosis or hemorrhage.

Therapeutic Considerations

In general, patients with secondary or reactive thrombocytosis require no specific therapy to lower the platelet count. Successful treatment of the underlying disorder often results in normalization of the platelet count. Even if the platelet count remains high, there is no substantial increase in thrombohemorrhagic risk.

Thrombocytosis associated with chronic myeloid leukemia usually does not require specific therapy, although standard therapy with busulfan, hydroxyurea, interferon alfa, or imatinib usually lowers the platelet count. Uncontrolled polycythemia vera is associated with significant perioperative risk. It is not completely clear to what degree this risk depends on the erythrocytosis or the thrombocytosis. Efforts should be made to normalize the platelet count in patients with polycythemia vera who have a hematocrit less than 45%, thrombocytosis, and a history of thrombohemorrhagic events. In addition, older patients or those with significant vascular disease may be more prone to problems and are likely to benefit from lowering the platelet count.

The principles of therapy for essential thrombocythemia include lowering the platelet count in older and sicker patients who have had prior vascular events. The most effective method of lowering the platelet count is with the use of anagrelide or cytotoxic chemotherapy such as hydroxyurea, although it may take days or weeks for a platelet response to occur. If immediate platelet reduction is required, platelet-pheresis, along with the use of cytotoxic agents, is effective in reducing the count to normal levels. Aspirin is rarely indicated in the perioperative therapy of average patients with thrombocytosis because it can lead to an increase in hemorrhagic phenomena. Patients younger than 60 years old, who are nonsmokers, who have no cardiac risk factors, and who have no history of thrombosis typically do not require platelet-lowering therapy before minor surgical procedures if their platelet counts are less than 1,500,000/μL.

Thrombocytosis after splenectomy is a common phenomenon. Platelet counts can occasionally exceed 2,000,000/μL. In the absence of a myeloproliferative disorder, there is no increased risk of thrombosis or hemorrhage, and, therefore, no treatment is indicated. The platelet count should normalize over a period of several weeks to months. Conversely, when splenectomy is performed for a myeloproliferative disorder, the patient may have marked thrombocytosis associated with thrombosis and hemorrhage. In this situation, aggressive preoperative and postoperative cytotoxic treatment is indicated to reduce the preoperative platelet count to the normal range and to maintain this range in the postoperative period.

HEMOSTASIS

Hemostasis is crucial to both the patient and the surgeon during surgical procedures. Without adequate function of the hemostatic system, even the most trivial procedure can quickly result in life-threatening hemorrhage. Because the hemostatic system plays an important role in the ability to perform surgery safely, a basic understanding of the physiology of blood clotting is essential to assess potential abnormalities and to select appropriate therapy.

Preoperative Considerations

Hemostasis is a complex ongoing process involving precise interactions among connective tissue, blood vessels, endothelial cells, platelets and other formed elements of the blood, the soluble coagulation factors, the natural anticoagulant and fibrinolytic substances, and exogenous drugs. Figure 6-3 shows the coagulation scheme with anticoagulant mechanisms. The process of coagulation can be arbitrarily divided into several stages (Box 6-3). The initial stage is damage to the vessel wall. The second stage involves primary vasoconstriction. The third stage involves binding of von Willebrand factor to the subendothelium to facilitate platelet adhesion. Platelet

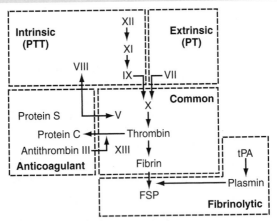

Figure 6-3 • Coagulation scheme with anticoagulant mechanisms. FSP, fibrin split products; PT, prothrombin time; PTT, partial thromboplastin time; tPA, tissue plasminogen activator.

Box 6-3	STEPS IN HEMOSTASIS

1. Injury to vessel wall
2. Primary vasoconstriction
3. Interaction of von Willebrand protein with subendothelium
4. Formation of platelet plug
5. Fibrin formation
6. Clot dissolution and endothelial regeneration

activation follows. At this point, which takes several minutes, hemostasis is maintained by a loose aggregation of platelets called the *platelet plug*. Without stabilization, the plug would break down, and bleeding would recur within minutes to hours. The additional stabilization is provided by the formation of fibrin mesh within and around the platelet plug (see Fig. 6-3). The fibrin is generated by the activation of intrinsic and extrinsic pathways of coagulation. These two pathways converge to activate the common pathway, which leads to the generation of thrombin and the polymerization of fibrin.

Natural anticoagulant pathways involving protein C, protein S, antithrombin, and membrane-bound heparin-like substances tend to limit the coagulative process to the injured area. In addition, the fibrinolytic system is activated simultaneously to limit the coagulation response as well as to prepare for clot dissolution and endothelial regeneration.

Preoperative Evaluation

Abnormalities anywhere in the coagulation pathway can result in abnormal hemostasis. Various laboratory studies help to identify defects in particular stages of the process. The platelet count is a straightforward measure of an important component of the system. The bleeding time is most sensitive to abnormalities in the subendothelial matrix, von Willebrand protein, and qualitative and quantitative disorders of platelets. The partial thromboplastin time (PTT) and the prothrombin time (PT) test the intrinsic and extrinsic pathways, respectively, whereas the thrombin time assesses the clotting ability of fibrinogen. Fibrin split products are an indirect indication of fibrinolytic activation.

The most important component of the evaluation of hemostatic function is a careful history [❹ *Houry et al, 1995*]. Nearly all potential hemostatic problems can be uncovered through careful questioning, although definition of the problem may require extensive laboratory evaluation. Several areas should be stressed in all patients, including unusual bleeding with prior trauma or surgery, episodes of spontaneous bleeding or thrombosis, a family history of bleeding or thrombosis, nutritional habits, drug ingestion, and other medical problems, particularly hepatic or renal disease. Tooth extraction, an "operation" most individuals have undergone, poses the same hemostatic challenge as a major abdominal procedure. Occasionally, unsuspected findings on the physical examination will alert the consultant to the presence of potential bleeding problems. The findings include jaundice, petechiae, ecchymoses, adenopathy, hepatomegaly, and splenomegaly.

Rarely is a previously unsuspected bleeding disorder identified by laboratory screening if the history and physical examination are normal. The most common disorders initially detected by routine laboratory screening are mild to moderate thrombocytopenia or platelet function defects and mild congenital bleeding disorders such as mild hemophilia. Less common are acquired inhibitors of coagulation. The laboratory primarily serves to define the specific bleeding problem and only secondarily screens for problems, because clinically significant bleeding disorders can be associated with relatively normal results on routine screening tests, for example, mild hemophilia or von Willebrand disease.

Although the use of preoperative coagulation testing is commonplace, little evidence supports its widespread use preoperatively. On the contrary, most studies and reviews point to the poor predictive value of preoperative screening tests of coagulation. For example, one review evaluated six studies involving 3786 patients who had preoperative PT measurements. Only 0.3% of patients had an abnormal test result, and surgical management was not changed because of the test, nor was there any predictive value for bleeding complications. Similarly, in a review of seven studies involving almost 6000 patients, 6.5% of patients had an abnormal PTT but no associated bleeding. An extensive review of the bleeding time concluded that this test was a poor predictor of bleeding risk or integrity of the hemostatic system. Therefore, the message is that there is no substitute for a good history in evaluating bleeding risk.

A useful system for risk stratification has been described (Table 6-4). Patients can be classified into three groups based on their histories: those with no suspicion of a bleeding disorder, those with suggestive histories, and those with clearly significant bleeding episodes. Surgical procedures can similarly be divided into those with minimal risk (minor biopsy), those with moderate risk (most general surgical procedures), and those with high hemostatic risk (cardiac, vascular, or emergency procedures). Low-risk patients undergoing

TABLE 6-4	Preoperative Laboratory Coagulation Screen		
	HISTORY		
Hemostatic Challenge	**Negative**	**Suggestive**	**Definite**
Low	None	PLT, BT, PT, PTT	Tests as
Moderate	PLT, PTT	PLT, BT, PT, PTT	necessary to
High	PLT, PTT, BT	As above, plus other tests as needed	make diagnosis

BT, bleeding time; PLT, platelet count; PT, prothrombin time; PTT, partial thromboplastin time.

low-risk procedures probably require no routine coagulation screening. In low-risk patients undergoing moderate-risk surgical procedures, a platelet count and a PTT should be obtained. The bleeding time can be added for high-risk surgical procedures. Patients with suggestive histories should have at least a platelet count, bleeding time, activated PTT, and PT. In this situation, the studies are more helpful in guiding the search for a specific clotting abnormality than in defining one on their own. When no abnormalities are found, the risk is minimal, and additional studies are unlikely to be fruitful. High-risk patients should not undergo surgical procedures until an explanation is given for prior bleeding episodes. In some patients, an extensive laboratory evaluation is necessary to confirm a problem.

Therapeutic Considerations

Thrombocytopenia

Thrombocytopenia is defined as a platelet count less than 150,000/μL. The risk of bleeding varies inversely with the platelet count, assuming that no functional platelet defect is present. A platelet count greater than 100,000/μL should be adequate for all surgical procedures. There should be no significant increase in bleeding for most low- or moderate-risk procedures when the platelet count is between 50,000 and 100,000/μL, but counts higher than 100,000/μL are preferable for high-risk operations (e.g., neurosurgical or spinal surgery). With a platelet count between 25,000 and 50,000/μL, spontaneous bleeding is uncommon, but surgery or trauma can precipitate excessive bleeding. At counts less than 20,000/μL, and particularly less than 10,000/μL, spontaneous bleeding is common, and the operative risk is significant. Should a coexisting platelet function defect be present, bleeding may be a problem at much higher platelet counts. The measurement of bleeding time may be useful in this situation. Although the bleeding time is prolonged in inverse proportion to the platelet count, marked prolongation is uncommon with platelet counts higher than 25,000/μL in the absence of a functional platelet defect.

The three principal mechanisms of thrombocytopenia are decreased production, abnormal sequestration, and increased destruction (Table 6-5). One or all of these mechanisms can be found in most thrombocytopenic patients. Decreased production of platelets is more often related to bone marrow dysfunction resulting from a nutritional deficiency, toxic damage from radiation or chemotherapy or other drugs, or primary bone marrow disease such as leukemia, myelodysplasia, or tumor infiltration. The characteristic feature in most of these disorders is that anemia, leukopenia, or morphologic abnormalities of red or white cells can be demonstrated in almost all circumstances. In addition, a bone marrow examination is nearly always abnormal. If a planned surgical procedure is not urgently required in a patient whose thrombocytopenia is the result of decreased production and is correctable or transient, the procedure should be delayed until the thrombocytopenia resolves. Bone marrow suppression caused by antineoplastic agents, radiation exposure, and most drugs should resolve within 1 to 3 weeks after withdrawal of the offending agent. If thrombocytopenia has an untreatable cause or if surgery is urgent, platelet transfusion is the treatment of choice. Each

TABLE 6-5	Differential Diagnosis of Thrombocytopenia	
Pathophysiology	**Examples**	**Associated Findings**
Decreased production	Aplastic anemia	Anemia, leukopenia, abnormal vitamin B_{12} or smear, abnormal bone marrow Folate deficiency, chemotherapy, or radiation exposure
Sequestration	Hypersplenism	Splenomegaly, anemia, leukopenia, normal smear, hypercellular bone marrow
Increased destruction	Idiopathic thrombocytopenic purpura, drug use, systemic lupus erythematosus, acquired immunodeficiency syndrome	Hematocrit and white blood cell count often normal, normal smear, megakaryocytic hyperplasia

unit of platelets should raise the platelet count by 5,000 to 10,000/μL in a 50-kg person.

Thrombocytopenia resulting from abnormal sequestration is most often seen in the presence of palpable splenomegaly and is frequently associated with leukopenia or anemia. It is uncommon for the platelet count to be less than 40,000 to 50,000/μL unless another problem coexists. The peripheral blood findings are usually minimal, and the bone marrow may show only hyperplasia. Even though therapy is difficult because transfused platelets are rapidly sequestered in the spleen, platelet transfusion remains the mainstay of therapy. On rare occasions, splenectomy may be necessary before a second procedure can be safely performed.

Thrombocytopenia resulting from enhanced destruction is most often immunologically mediated, in idiopathic immune thrombocytopenic purpura (ITP), in drug-induced (from quinine, heparin, or sulfa drugs) or associated underlying immunologic disorders such as lupus erythematosus or acquired immunodeficiency syndrome, or in association with a lymphoproliferative disorder such as chronic lymphatic leukemia or lymphoma. In each situation, the red and white blood cell counts are often normal, and the bone marrow rarely shows anything more than megakaryocytic hyperplasia. The other common causes of enhanced destruction of platelets are infection and disseminated intravascular coagulation (DIC).

The most commonly encountered problem is probably ITP. This disorder is usually acute and transient in children but is most often chronic in adults. It is more common in women than in men, and it usually occurs in the third to fourth decade of life. It usually manifests as mild to moderate thrombocytopenia that generally responds to corticosteroid therapy.

Management of adults with ITP usually involves treatment designed to decrease the immune destruction of platelets. Patients with known ITP who are scheduled for elective surgical procedures should have corticosteroid therapy initiated or adjusted to raise the platelet count to a safe level. This goal can usually be accomplished over 1 to 2 weeks with a dose of 0.5 to 1 mg/kg of prednisone or its equivalent. Corticosteroids should be continued through the perioperative period and tapered over several weeks postoperatively. If surgery is required urgently, higher doses of steroids may be beneficial, but a course of 3 to 5 days of treatment is required to gain a therapeutic response. Infusion of intravenous immune globulin in doses of 0.3 to 0.5 g/kg/day over 3 days may cause a more rapid rise in the platelet count than steroid therapy alone. For Rh-positive patients who have not had splenectomy, infusion of anti-D globulin (50 μg/kg) can accomplish the same result. If at all possible, surgical procedures should be delayed until the thrombocytopenia is controlled. Because platelets in ITP seem to be quite functional, little or no bleeding may occur even at very low counts, and the bleeding time may be relatively normal in spite of marked thrombocytopenia.

Even though the major mechanism of thrombocytopenia in ITP is accelerated destruction of platelets, platelet transfusion can be effective and occasionally lifesaving even in the absence of a demonstrable rise in the platelet count. Platelet life span may be enhanced if transfused platelets are given after intravenous immune globulin. It may occasionally be necessary to perform splenectomy before, or in conjunction with, the planned operative procedure to gain control of disease.

Immune platelet destruction resulting from drugs often does not respond to corticosteroid therapy. Thrombocytopenia associated with other immunologic or lymphoproliferative disorders responds best to control of the underlying disease. If this is not possible, the patient should be managed as in ITP.

Thrombocytopenia can occur as a transient dose-dependent effect of heparin; this is a benign problem. The more serious type of heparin-induced thrombocytopenia results in a thrombotic disorder characterized by antibodies to heparin/platelet factor 4 complex, platelet activation, thrombin generation, and thrombocytopenia, with or without thrombosis (venous or arterial). **The onset of thrombocytopenia and thrombosis is usually 5 to 10 days after the first exposure to heparin and as little as 1 day after repeat challenge with heparin in patients with antibodies who typically had received heparin during the previous 100 days** [◉ *Warkentin, 2003*]. Late-onset thrombosis can occur up to 3 weeks after heparin is stopped. Thrombotic complications may affect any vascular bed. Laboratory testing can be done with either an antibody detection assay (e.g., enzyme-linked immunosorbent assay) or a functional assay (platelet aggregation or serotonin release). The antibody detection assays are very sensitive (>90%) but lack specificity (many patients develop antibodies without thrombocytopenia or thrombosis). The functional assays are very specific but are more difficult to perform. A combination of both types is best for optimal diagnosis. Because neither is available routinely as a "stat" test, one must rely on clinical judgment in the initial evaluation and treatment of the disorder.

If heparin-induced thrombocytopenia is suspected, all heparin products should be stopped promptly, and heparin-coated catheters should be removed. Alternative anticoagulation should be initiated with a direct thrombin inhibitor (either lepirudin or argatroban). Lepirudin is started with a 0.4 mg/kg bolus and is followed with an infusion of 0.15 mg/kg/hour, targeting an activated PTT (aPTT) of 1.5 to 2.5 times control. This agent should be used with dose reduction in patients with renal insufficiency (half dose if serum creatinine is 1 to 2; greater reduction if creatinine is >2). Argatroban is started at 2 μg/kg/minute, targeting an aPTT of 1.5 to 3 times baseline. It should be used with caution in patients with hepatic insufficiency; start with a 75% dose reduction. Warfarin should be started once the thrombosis has responded and the platelet count has improved. The duration of anticoagulant therapy depends on the patient's thrombus burden and whether the patient has sustained a thrombotic event.

Qualitative Platelet Disorders

Qualitative platelet disorders can be congenital or acquired. The acquired disorders are most often caused by drugs (most commonly aspirin and nonsteroidal anti-inflammatory agents, as well as other antiplatelet drugs such as clopidogrel), uremia, or myeloproliferative disorders. The most valuable diagnostic tools are a detailed history and a bleeding time, which is usually prolonged.

No therapy is necessary in most congenital qualitative platelet disorders unless the patient has a significant past history of bleeding or if the morbidity associated with excessive bleeding is great, in which case platelet transfusion is the appropriate therapy. For most other situations, it is sufficient to have platelets available in the event that bleeding occurs.

Drug-induced qualitative platelet dysfunction typically begins to resolve with the discontinuation of the drug (within 24 to 48 hours in the case of nonsteroidal agents and 4 to 7 days for aspirin and possibly longer for other antiplatelet agents). Bleeding time is a poor predictor of bleeding risk [Rodgers and Levin, 1990]. Specifically, a patient with a prolonged bleeding time may not bleed, and a normal bleeding time does not guarantee normal hemostasis. The use of antiplatelet agents is widespread. Although information in the literature seems to indicate increased blood loss during surgery in patients using antiplatelet drugs, transfusion requirements are not usually increased. The impact of antiplatelet therapy on the risks for epidural anesthesia is not well defined. Most patients taking aspirin do not have an increased risk of significant perioperative hemorrhage, but it is reasonable to discontinue aspirin preoperatively because it is not possible to predict who will or will not bleed, particularly in heart surgery, in which an increase in blood loss has been noted. However, there is evidence of an increase in perioperative cardiac events in patients in whom antiplatelet therapy is discontinued, a finding suggesting that the decision to discontinue these agents should be made on an individual basis. For example, patients undergoing most general, vascular, or orthopedic procedures may not have significant issues with a modest increase in surgical blood loss. Conversely, this may be problematic in neurosurgery or in patients requiring epidural or spinal anesthesia. If the agents are stopped, it is recommended that aspirin and clopidogrel be stopped 7 to 10 days preoperatively and short-acting nonsteroidal anti-inflammatory drugs be stopped 1 to 2 days preoperatively. It seems safe to resume antiplatelet agents within the first 24 hours postoperatively. When a surgical procedure is performed in a patient ingesting one of these drugs and bleeding occurs, the appropriate therapy is platelet transfusion. Weaker antiplatelet drugs such as dipyridamole probably pose no substantial hemorrhagic risk for most patients.

Platelet dysfunction resulting from uremia may improve by correcting anemia, if present, and possibly by increasing the intensity of dialysis. The infusion of cryoprecipitate or desmopressin acetate (DDAVP), 0.1 to 0.3 μg/kg over 30 minutes, has also been helpful in patients with uremia.

Abnormalities of Coagulation Tests

The differential diagnostic considerations of abnormal coagulation tests are shown in Box 6-4.

Prolongation of Bleeding Time

Qualitative platelet disorders can prolong the bleeding time. Mild von Willebrand disease may also be associated with a prolonged bleeding time. *Von Willebrand disease* is a congenital disorder characterized by a qualitative or quantitative abnormality of von Willebrand protein. The major clinical abnormalities are easy bruising and mucosal bleeding, but postoperative bleeding can be substantial if the disorder is not recognized. The diagnosis can be confirmed by assay of von Willebrand protein, factor VIII (which is bound to von Willebrand factor in the circulation), and ristocetin cofactor activity (a measure of the ability of the patient's plasma to agglutinate platelets). In the quantitative type (type I), there is an absolute decrease in von Willebrand protein such that von Willebrand protein, factor VIII, and ristocetin cofactor activity are all low. The qualitative type (type II) is characterized by a functional defect in von Willebrand protein.

Box 6-4	DIFFERENTIAL DIAGNOSIS OF ABNORMAL COAGULATION TESTS

Prolonged bleeding time: Thrombocytopenia, platelet function defect, or von Willebrand disease

Prolonged PT: Vitamin K deficiency, liver disease, warfarin use, or factor VII deficiency

Prolonged PTT: Factor XII, XI, IX, or VIII deficiency, heparin use, inhibitors, DIC, or von Willebrand disease

Prolonged PT and PTT: Vitamin K deficiency, warfarin use, or DIC

DIC, disseminated intravascular coagulation; PT, prothrombin time; PTT, partial thromboplastin time.

Von Willebrand protein and factor VIII levels may be normal or only mildly depressed, but ristocetin cofactor activity is low.

Prolongation of Prothrombin Time

Isolated prolongation of the PT is most often related to the following conditions: deficiency of vitamin K, either on a nutritional basis or related to altered absorption from antibiotics or biliary tract obstruction hepatic insufficiency or the use of warfarin-like drugs. Less commonly, the PT can be prolonged because of a deficiency of factor VII or an acquired inhibitor of coagulation. Most of these causes, except factor VII deficiency, should be obvious from the clinical evaluation.

Prolongation of Partial Thromboplastin Time

Obviously, the PTT can be prolonged in patients taking heparin or in patients with type I von Willebrand disease because of low circulating levels of factor VIII. Isolated prolongation of the PTT can be caused by an occult abnormality of the coagulation system. Deficiencies of factor VIII or factor IX in men or factor XI in either sex may result in clinically significant bleeding in the perioperative period. Factor XII deficiency causes a markedly prolonged PTT but no clinical bleeding.

The first step in the evaluation of a prolonged PTT should be to perform the test again with a 1:1 mix of patient plasma and normal plasma. If deficiency of a clotting factor exists, the PTT should correct itself, and specific factor assays can then be performed to establish the particular deficiency. A persistent prolongation of the PTT after the 1:1 mix is an indication of an inhibitor of coagulation, of which two major types are recognized. The first type of inhibitor is usually an antibody with specificity for a particular clotting factor. The most common are antibodies to factors VIII, IX, or X, which can result in excessive, and at times life-threatening, hemorrhage. The second type of inhibitor is the lupus anticoagulant, an antibody with specificity for anionic phospholipids that interfere with the in vitro test. Lupus-like anticoagulants are most often found in patients without systemic lupus erythematosus and are rarely associated with hemorrhage, but they are clinically important because they are often associated with recurrent spontaneous abortions or arterial and venous thrombosis. Special laboratory procedures are necessary to evaluate for these inhibitors.

Simultaneous prolongation of the PT and PTT is usually found in severe liver disease, in severe nutritional deficiency of vitamin K, or with warfarin use. Less commonly, this phenomenon represents underlying DIC.

Treatment of Acquired and Congenital Coagulopathies

Hemophilia A

Hemophilia A is an X-linked recessive disorder characterized by factor VIII deficiency of variable degree. Mild hemophilia characteristically consists of a factor VIII level higher than 6%. This condition is often asymptomatic in the absence of surgery or trauma. Moderate hemophilia with 1% to 5% factor VIII activity may cause occasional spontaneous hemorrhage and massive bleeding with trauma and surgery. Patients with severe hemophilia with factor VIII activity less than 1% suffer a life of recurrent joint and soft tissue hemorrhage. Perioperative management of all patients with hemophilia is complex and usually requires ready access to a laboratory that can perform factor assays quickly and accurately. All patients with hemophilia should be screened preoperatively for factor VIII inhibitors, which occur in approximately 5% to 15% of these patients. Factor VIII inhibitors pose significant problems in management; therefore, surgical procedures in patients with inhibitors should be limited to treatment of life-threatening conditions only and should generally be managed in a center with significant experience in dealing with these problems.

Patients with hemophilia who undergo major surgery should receive factor VIII at a dose of 40 U/kg just before the surgical procedure. Because the half-life of factor VIII is 8 to 12 hours, an infusion of 20 U/kg should be given at 8- to 12-hour intervals postoperatively to maintain a factor VIII level higher than 30% to 50%. The duration of the maintenance therapy depends on the type of operation. Several days may be adequate for a complicated abdominal operation, whereas 4 to 6 weeks may be necessary for major orthopedic surgery. The same procedure can be followed for minor surgery in patients with severe hemophilia, although only 1 to 2 days of maintenance therapy may be necessary. The use of ϵ-aminocaproic acid (Amicar), in doses of 3 g every 4 hours, may be a useful adjunct in the management of patients with hemophilia who undergo oral surgery. Patients with mild hemophilia usually have minimal exposure to blood products except during surgical periods; therefore, cryoprecipitate or preferably recombinant factor VIII should be used. Each unit of cryoprecipitate contains on average 80 to 100 U of factor VIII; therefore, one would use 0.5 U/kg preoperatively and 0.2 U/kg postoperatively every 8 to 12 hours.

Patients with mild hemophilia who are undergoing minor procedures can sometimes be managed simply with an infusion of DDAVP, to increase the release of von Willebrand protein and therefore raise the circulating levels of factor VIII. Patients should have had prior testing with DDAVP to document a response. Those who are responders can then be treated with 0.1 to 0.3 μg/kg of DDAVP as an infusion over 30 minutes about 1 hour before surgery and 8 to 12 hours postoperatively. The response to repeated administrations diminishes rapidly after the second or third dose.

Hemophilia B

The management of hemophilia B, or factor IX deficiency, is similar to the treatment of hemophilia A. Several distinctions are worth noting, however. The volume of distribution of factor IX is greater than that of factor VIII, so twice the number of units will be necessary to achieve the given factor level. Adequate hemostasis can be achieved at a lower factor concentration, however. Because the half-life of factor IX is longer, the usual dosing interval is 24 hours. Thus, the recommended dose of factor IX is 50 U/kg preoperatively and 25 U/kg daily postoperatively. Factor IX concentrates contain small amounts of activated clotting factors and thus are associated with a higher risk of thrombotic events than factor VIII concentrates. Consequently, antifibrinolytic agents such as ϵ-aminocaproic acid should not be used concurrently with factor IX concentrates.

Hemophilia C

Hemophilia C, or factor XI deficiency, variably results in a bleeding diathesis. In patients with a history of prior bleeding, management should be with fresh frozen plasma, 10 to 20 mL/kg preoperatively and 5 to 10 mL/kg every 24 hours postoperatively. A factor XI concentrate is also available. These dosing guidelines are generalizations. The most crucial parameter is the judicious use of factor level assays to guide dosing.

von Willebrand Disease

von Willebrand disease is a congenital abnormality in von Willebrand protein. Because most patients have mild disease, management can usually consist of raising von Willebrand protein levels by the administration of DDAVP. This approach is most effective in type I or quantitative-type disease. As in hemophilia A, patients should be screened for a response well before a surgical procedure is performed. The dose of DDAVP is 0.3 μg/kg over 30 minutes just before the surgical procedure and then every 8 to 12 hours postoperatively. As in hemophilia, the response diminishes after the second dose. Therefore, this approach is useful only for minor procedures. For major procedures or for patients with severe disease, either cryoprecipitate, at a dose of 0.1 to 0.2 U/kg every 12 hours, or intermediate purity factor VIII concentrates, at doses of 40 U/kg/dose every 8 to 12 hours, can be used in the perioperative period. No laboratory test is particularly useful as a guide to dosing, but serial measurements of von Willebrand protein levels may be helpful in determining the frequency of dosing. Although correction of bleeding time is correlated with adequacy of hemostasis, serial bleeding time testing is difficult to perform and uncomfortable for the patient.

Liver Disease

Patients with liver disease have multiple coagulation disorders, including thrombocytopenia, platelet function abnormalities, malabsorption of the fat-soluble vitamin K, and hepatocellular dysfunction leading to abnormal synthesis of clotting factors, decreased clearance of activated clotting factors, and dysfibrinogenemia. Most patients with liver disease should have preoperative screening tests, including PT, PTT, fibrinogen levels, and thrombin time. Although the most common hematologic complication of severe liver disease is bleeding, these patients may be at increased risk for thrombosis or DIC because of abnormal hepatic clearance of activated clotting factors.

Management of these patients is frequently difficult. It is reasonable to administer 10 mg of vitamin K parenterally to any patient with a prolonged PT, although only patients with biliary obstruction or malnutrition are likely to respond. For patients with predominantly hepatocellular disease, the preferred therapy is fresh frozen plasma, which should be given at a dose of 10 to 20 mL/kg to bring the PT to within 2 to 3 seconds of the control value. Because of rapid consumption of clotting factors, it may be necessary to administer additional plasma every few hours, with serial PTs used as a guide.

Platelet transfusion can be useful, particularly in patients with bone marrow suppression. The treatment is somewhat less effective in patients with hypersplenism and may be of some value in patients with prolonged bleeding times.

Postoperative Bleeding

Bleeding in the postoperative period may have numerous causes. Unmasking of a previously unsuspected bleeding disorder such as von Willebrand disease or thrombocytopenia can occur. Drug-related thrombocytopenia, acquired platelet function defects, and abnormal clotting factors resulting from malabsorption or starvation are occasionally noted. Other factors to consider are DIC resulting from sepsis, transfusion reactions, or tissue damage. Dilutional coagulopathies may be caused by inadequate perioperative blood component replacement, particularly in the massively transfused patient. Bleeding may also be related to the use of anticoagulant drugs or inadequate surgical hemostasis in the wound.

A low platelet count is most often seen acutely in association with inadequate replacement during operations in which there is massive blood loss, in DIC resulting from transfusion reaction, or in association with drug toxicity. In a less acute setting, hours to days postoperatively, sepsis and drug-related causes are most common.

Prolonged bleeding time in the postoperative period is most often caused by thrombocytopenia, uremia, or platelet dysfunction after cardiopulmonary bypass. A prolonged PT is typically seen in association with nutritional deficiency of vitamin K, prolonged administration of antibiotics, DIC, or liver disease. A prolonged PTT is usually the result of nutritional deficiency, DIC, or occult von Willebrand disease. Fibrinogen levels are rarely low in any disorder other than severe DIC. Fibrin split products may be elevated postoperatively for various reasons, including DIC, heparin administration, the usual postoperative lysis of hematomas, and significant venous thrombosis.

Postoperative bleeding must be evaluated quickly and efficiently (Box 6-5). A thorough history and physical examination are crucial, with attention paid to all factors described in the preoperative evaluation of hemostatic function. In addition, the clinical characteristic of bleeding may suggest a

Box 6-5	EVALUATION OF A PATIENT WITH POSTOPERATIVE BLEEDING

Obtain history and perform physical examination.

Assess rapidity of bleeding and urgency of intervention.

Order PLT, BT, PT, PTT, fibrinogen, and fibrin split product determinations, and save plasma and serum.

If no urgency, treat based on test results.

If urgency, give fresh frozen plasma and platelets and modify treatment as test results become available.

BT, bleeding time; PLT, platelet count; PT, prothrombin time; PTT, partial thromboplastin time.

specific diagnosis. Immediate bleeding often signifies inadequate surgical hemostasis, inadequate replacement therapy, or severe transfusion reaction with DIC, whereas delayed bleeding is more typical of drug-induced thrombocytopenia, malnutrition, or sepsis with DIC. Brisk bleeding is more likely the result of severe dilutional problems or inadequate surgical hemostasis. Localized bleeding suggests inadequate surgical hemostasis or primary coagulopathy. Generalized bleeding from wounds, venipuncture, urinary catheters, or endotracheal tubes is most often seen in DIC. Laboratory tests should be performed, but frequently therapy must be initiated before results are available. Therefore, a broad array of tests should be requested, including PT, PTT, fibrinogen level, fibrin split products, platelet count, bleeding time, and samples of plasma and serum, which should be saved for additional studies as needed.

MANAGEMENT

Therapeutic intervention depends on the clinical situation as well as on the results of laboratory studies. If bleeding is brisk and no clear cause is determined, it is reasonable to transfuse fresh frozen plasma and platelets as well as red blood cells in anticipation of laboratory studies. It is important to search for the surgical problem to account for bleeding that may require immediate correction. If bleeding is less brisk, management can be tailored to the clinical and laboratory diagnosis, as described for preoperative patients. As previously mentioned, platelet transfusion can be used if bleeding is the result of antiplatelet therapy. Protamine can effectively reverse the anticoagulant effect of heparin and may be of some value in reversing the effect of low-molecular-weight heparins.

Patients who require massive transfusion because of severe bleeding should receive 1 U of fresh frozen plasma and 4 to 6 U of platelets for every 4 U of red blood cells if total blood loss is greater than one blood volume. Treatment of DIC involves correction of the underlying disorder in addition to supportive management with transfusion products. The use of heparin to interrupt the coagulation phase of the syndrome is highly controversial and is reserved for situations in which thrombosis is the significant clinical problem or in which even aggressive replacement therapy fails to curb bleeding. Treatment of the underlying problem is the most important aspect in the therapy of DIC.

Patients who have severe, unexplained blood loss may be candidates to receive recombinant factor VIIa therapy. There is growing interest in the use of this agent to reduce perioperative bleeding, but it should be considered investigational at this point.

Selected Readings

American Society of Anesthesiologists: Practice guidelines for blood component therapy: A report by the American Society of Anesthesiologists Task Force on Blood Component Therapy. Anesthesiology 84:732-747, 1996.

Armas-Loughran B, Kalra R, Carson JL: Evaluation and management of anemia and bleeding disorders in surgical patients. Med Clin North Am 87:229-242, 2003.

Carson JL: Morbidity risk assessment in the surgically anemic patient. Am J Surg 170(Suppl 6A):32S-36S, 1995.

Charache S: Treatment of sickle cell anemia. Annu Rev Med 32:195-206, 1981.

Eschbach JW, Abdulhadi MH, Browne JK, et al: Recombinant human erythropoietin in anemic patients with end stage renal disease: Results of a phase III multicenter clinical trial. Ann Intern Med 111:992-1000, 1989.

Grounds M: Recombinant factor VIIa (rFVIIa) and its use in severe bleeding in surgery and trauma: A review. Blood Rev 17:S11-S21, 2003.

Hardy J, De Moerloose P, Samama M, et al: Massive transfusion and coagulopathy: Pathophysiology and implications for clinical management. Can J Anaesth 51:293-310, 2004.

Houry S, Georgeac C, Hay JM, et al: A prospective multicenter evaluation of preoperative hemostatic screening tests. Am J Surg 170:19-23, 1995. ⓐ

Martlew VJ: Perioperative management of patients with coagulation disorders. Br J Anaesth 84:446-455, 2000.

McKenna R: Abnormal coagulation in the postoperative period contributing to excessive bleeding. Med Clin North Am 85:1277-1310, 2001.

Nash MJ, Cohen H: Management of Jehovah's Witness patients with haematological problems. Blood Rev 18:211-217, 2004.

National Institutes of Health: Consensus conference: Perioperative red blood cell transfusion. JAMA 260:2700-2703, 1988.

Patel T: Surgery in the patient with liver disease. Mayo Clin Proc 74:593-599, 1999.

Rauck R: The anticoagulated patient. Reg Anesth 21(Suppl):51-56, 1996.

Rodgers RP, Levin J: A critical appraisal of the bleeding time. Semin Thromb Hemost 16:1-20, 1990.

Rosse WF: Clinical management of adult ITP prior to splenectomy: A perspective. Blood Rev 16:47-49, 2002.

Samama CM, Bastien O, Forestier F, et al: Antiplatelet agents in the perioperative period: Expert recommendations of the French Society of Anesthesiology and Intensive Care (SFAR) 2001—summary statement. Can J Anaesth 49:S26-S35, 2002.

Smetana GW, Macpherson DS: The case against routine preoperative laboratory testing. Med Clin North Am 87:7-40, 2003.

Spahn D: Perioperative transfusion triggers for red blood cells. Vox Sang 78(Suppl 2):163, 2000.

Spence RK: Surgical red blood cell transfusion practice policies: Blood Management Practice Guidelines Conference. Am J Surg 170(Suppl 6A):3S-15S, 1995.

Tefferi A, Murphy S: Current opinion in essential thrombocythemia: Pathogenesis, diagnosis, and management. Blood Rev 15:121, 2001.

Vichinsky EP, Haberkern CM, Neumayr L, et al: A comparison of conservative and aggressive transfusion regimens in the perioperative management of sickle cell disease: The Preoperative Transfusion in Sickle Cell Disease Study Group. N Engl J Med 333:206-213, 1995.

Warkentin TE, Kelton JG: Delayed-onset heparin-induced thrombocytopenia and thrombosis. Ann Intern Med 135:502-506, 2001.

Warkentin TE: Heparin-induced thrombocytopenia: Pathogenesis and management. Br J Haematol 121:535-555, 2003. ◉

Warkentin TE: Heparin-induced thrombocytopenia: Diagnosis and management. Circulation 110:e454-e458, 2004.

Weaver DW: Differential diagnosis and management of unexplained bleeding. Surg Clin North Am 73:353-361, 1993.

7 Noncardiac Surgery in the Patient with Cardiovascular Disease: Preoperative Evaluation and Perioperative Care

HOWARD H. WEITZ, MD

In 1977, a multifactorial risk factor index was defined by Goldman and associates to identify the high-risk surgical patient preoperatively, as well as to delineate cardiovascular risk factors that could be corrected before surgical procedures, in an effort to decrease cardiovascular morbidity and mortality associated with noncardiac surgery [**Ⓐ** *Goldman et al, 1978*]. Nine clinical or historical features (myocardial infarction [MI] ≤6 months previously; age >70 years; third heart sound [S_3] or jugular venous distention; significant aortic stenosis; rhythm other than sinus on preoperative electrocardiogram [ECG]; more than five ventricular premature contractions per minute at any time before the surgical procedure; poor general medical status; abdominal, thoracic, or aortic surgery; emergency surgery), most of which were reversible, were found to be associated with an increased incidence of perioperative complications. The factors were assigned risk points by multivariate analysis; this approach allowed a preoperative estimate of total cardiac risk and determination of the likelihood of life-threatening complications (e.g., MI, pulmonary edema, ventricular tachycardia,

---

Levels of Evidence:

Ⓐ—Randomized controlled trials (RCTs), meta-analyses, well-designed systematic reviews of RCTs. **Ⓑ**—Case-control or cohort studies, nonrandomized clinical trials, systematic reviews of studies other than RCTs, cross-sectional studies, retrospective studies. **Ⓒ**—Consensus statements, expert guidelines, usual practice, opinion.

and cardiac death). Patients were stratified into four risk classes based on their total accumulated risk points. Risk determined with the original multifactorial cardiac risk index was integrated with the type of surgery to estimate the probability of cardiac complications in noncardiac surgery.

The multifactorial risk index was validated in prospective studies stratifying unselected, consecutive patients who were undergoing noncardiac surgery. The index was less reliable for stratifying risk in selected patient subgroups, particularly those with or at high risk for coronary artery disease and those who were to undergo major vascular surgery. This index and others that were developed contemporaneously were derived from relatively small numbers of patients and predated significant changes in anesthesia and surgery. These measures have therefore not maintained their clinical relevance.

A more recent modification of the multifactorial index has been developed for use with stable patients undergoing major noncardiac surgery and has been shown to perform well as a tool to predict the probability of major cardiac complications. This index uses six readily available clinical factors to place the preoperative patient into one of four risk groups:

- High-risk type of surgery (intraperitoneal, intrathoracic, or suprainguinal vascular)
- History of ischemic heart disease
- History of congestive heart failure (CHF)
- History of cerebrovascular disease
- Diabetes requiring treatment with preoperative insulin
- Renal insufficiency with preoperative serum creatinine concentration higher than 2.0 mg/dL

Rates of major cardiac complications (MI, pulmonary edema, ventricular fibrillation or primary cardiac arrest, and complete heart block) with none, one, two, or three or more of these factors were 0.4%, 0.9%, 7%, and 11%, respectively.

To facilitate preoperative risk assessment of patients with cardiovascular disease, a consensus guideline was developed by a consensus panel of the American College of

Cardiology (ACC) and the American Heart Association (AHA). The panel acknowledged that the number of evidence-based trials pertaining to perioperative cardiovascular evaluation and therapy was limited; therefore, the guidelines are largely based on studies not directly derived from noncardiac surgery and on expert opinion. The guideline initially published in 1996 was revised in 2002 and 2007. It seeks to identify and define those clinical situations in which preoperative testing and intervention may improve patients' perioperative outcome. One of the themes of this guideline is that **cardiac intervention is rarely necessary to lower the risk of surgery** [◉ *Eagle et al, 2002*]. The guideline emphasizes that preoperative tests are recommended only if they have the potential to affect perioperative care, that is, if the information obtained will result in a change in the surgical procedure performed, a change in medical therapy, or lead to the use of perioperative monitoring [◉ *Fleisher et al, 2007*].

These guidelines employ a strategy that requires assessment of active cardiac conditions, clinical predictors, functional status, surgery-specific risk, and history of prior coronary evaluation and/or treatment. The preoperative history and physical examination should focus on identifying the presence of clinical predictors, including the presence of cardiovascular disease and its treatment. A goal of the guideline is the identification of the patient at increased risk who would benefit, in the long term, from medical therapy or coronary artery revascularization. The preoperative evaluation should also aim to identify comorbid conditions that, if present, could increase the risk of perioperative cardiovascular complications. These comorbid conditions include pulmonary disease, renal insufficiency, diabetes mellitus, and anemia.

Active cardiac conditions (Table 7-1), when present, indicate major perioperative cardiac risk. These conditions (referred to as "major clinical risk factors" in the 2002 guideline revision) include unstable coronary syndromes (unstable

TABLE 7-1	Active Cardiac Conditions*

Unstable coronary syndromes (unstable angina, recent MI [MI more than 7 days but less than 1 month before evaluation])
Decompensated heart failure
Significant arrhythmias
Severe valvular disease

*Presence of one or more may result in delay or cancellation of surgery unless surgery is emergent.

MI, myocardial infarction.

From Fleisher LA, Beckman JA, Brown KA, et al: ACC/AHA guidelines on perioperative cardiovascular evaluation and care for noncardiac surgery: A report of the American College of Cardiology/American Heart Association Task Force on Practice Guidelines (Writing Committee to Revise the 2002 Guidelines on Perioperative Cardiovascular Evaluation for Noncardiac Surgery). J Am Coll Cardiol 50: e159-241, 2007.

angina, acute MI [MI within 7 days], or recent MI [MI occurring more than 7 days but less than 1 month before the examination]), decompensated heart failure, significant arrhythmias (supraventricular arrhythmia with uncontrolled ventricular rate, symptomatic arrhythmia in the presence of underlying heart disease, high degree atrioventricular block), and severe valvular disease (critical aortic stenosis). The presence of one or more of these conditions typically leads to cancellation of surgery to allow for treatment and potential resolution of the active cardiac condition. If the surgery is emergent or urgent and cannot be cancelled, the patient typically will require more intensive perioperative monitoring and care.

Clinical risk factors (listed as "intermediate predictors of risk" in the 2002 guideline) (Box 7-1), if present, may also contribute to the risk of perioperative cardiac complication. They have been identified by the Revised Multifactorial Risk Index and include history of ischemic heart disease (e.g., history of prior MI more than 1 month before the examination), compensated or prior CHF, history of cerebrovascular disease, diabetes mellitus, and renal insufficiency (serum Cr

History of ischemic heart disease
History of compensated or prior heart failure
History of cerebrovascular disease
Diabetes mellitus
Renal insufficiency (serum creatinine $\geq$ 2.0)

$\geq$ 2.0 mg/dL). The 2007 guideline revision no longer considers miner predictors of risk (e.g., age > 70 years, abnormal ECG [left ventricular hypertrophy, left bundle branch block, nonspecific ST-T abnormalities], rhythm other than sinus, or uncontrolled systemic hypertension) as determinants of perioperative risk. Although these predictors are markers of cardiovascular disease, they have not been proven to independently result in increased perioperative risk.

Functional capacity (Fig. 7-1) has been shown to be a predictor; poor functional capacity is a marker for subsequent cardiac events. Poor functional capacity, even when not a result of cardiac causes, was empirically postulated in the 1996 initial ACC/AHA preoperative evaluation guideline to be a risk for perioperative cardiac complication. Evidence now supports that postulate. In a series of 600 patients who underwent noncardiac surgery, investigators showed that perioperative myocardial ischemia and cardiovascular events were more common in patients unable to walk four blocks or climb two flights of stairs. Functional capacity may be quantified by evaluating the patient's daily activity. Perioperative cardiac risk is increased in patients unable to reach or exceed an aerobic demand of 4 metabolic equivalents (METs) during normal activity. Energy expenditures of eating, dressing, walking, and other low-level activities range from 1 to 4 METs. More vigorous activity, such as climbing a flight of stairs, brisk walking, or playing golf, is equivalent to 4 to 10 METs. Strenuous activity such as tennis and swimming exceeds 10 METs.

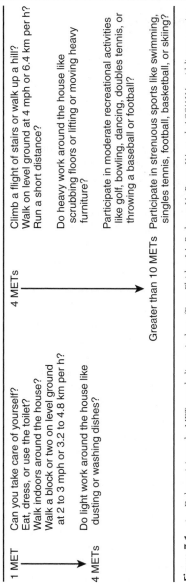

1 MET	Can you take care of yourself? Eat, dress, or use the toilet? Walk indoors around the house? Walk a block or two on level ground at 2 to 3 mph or 3.2 to 4.8 km per h? Do light work around the house like dusting or washing dishes?	4 METs	Climb a flight of stairs or walk up a hill? Walk on level ground at 4 mph or 6.4 km per h? Run a short distance? Do heavy work around the house like scrubbing floors or lifting or moving heavy furniture? Participate in moderate recreational activities like golf, bowling, dancing, doubles tennis, or throwing a baseball or football?
4 METs		Greater than 10 METs	Participate in strenuous sports like swimming, singles tennis, football, basketball, or skiing?

Figure 7-1 • Duke activity scale. MET, metabolic equivalent. *(From Fleisher LA, Beckman JA, Brown KA, et al: ACC/AHA guidelines on perioperative cardiovascular evaluation and care for noncardiac surgery: A report of the American College of Cardiology/American Heart Association Task Force on Practice Guidelines [Writing Committee to Revise the 2002 Guidelines on Perioperative Cardiovascular Evaluation for Noncardiac Surgery]. J Am Coll Cardiol 50:e159-241, 2007.)*

Surgery-specific risk is determined by the type of surgery and its associated hemodynamic stress (Box 7-2). High-risk procedures are those with a reported cardiac risk greater than 5%. They include emergency major operations, particularly in the elderly, aortic and major vascular surgery, peripheral vascular surgery, and anticipated prolonged surgical procedures associated with large fluid shifts or blood

---

Box 7-2	CARDIAC RISK STRATIFICATION FOR NONCARDIAC SURGICAL PROCEDURES

HIGH (REPORTED CARDIAC RISK OFTEN >5%)

Emergency major operations, particularly in elderly patients
Aortic and other major vascular surgery
Peripheral vascular surgery
Anticipated prolonged surgical procedures associated with large fluid shifts or blood loss

INTERMEDIATE (REPORTED CARDIAC RISK <5%)

Carotid endarterectomy
Head and neck surgery
Intraperitoneal and intrathoracic surgery
Orthopedic surgery
Prostate surgery

LOW* (REPORTED CARDIAC RISK <1%)

Endoscopic procedures
Superficial procedures
Cataract surgery
Breast surgery
Ambulatory surgery

---

*Do not generally require further preoperative cardiac testing.

From Fleisher LA, Beckman JA, Brown KA, et al: ACC/AHA 2007 guidelines on perioperative cardiovascular evaluation and care for noncardiac surgery: A report of the American College of Cardiology/American Heart Association Task Force on Practice Guidelines (Writing Committee to Revise the 2002 Guidelines on Perioperative Cardiovascular Evaluation for Noncardiac Surgery). J Am Coll Cardiol 50:e159-241, 2007.

loss. Intermediate-risk procedures are those associated with a risk less than 5% but greater than 1%. They include carotid endarterectomy, head and neck surgery, intraperitoneal and intrathoracic surgery, orthopedic surgery, and prostate surgery. Low-risk procedures are those associated with a cardiac risk lower than 1%. They include endoscopic procedures, superficial procedures, cataract surgery, breast surgery, and ambulatory surgery.

After the patient's active cardiac conditions, clinical risk factors, functional capacity, and surgery-specific risks are identified, the ACC/AHA 2007 Perioperative Guidelines recommend a five-step algorithm to guide decision making regarding further cardiac testing, proceeding to surgery, or both (Fig. 7-2).

1. *Is the surgical procedure an emergency?* If so, the patient should proceed to surgery without delay for further preoperative evaluation. I typically treat patients in this group as though they have coronary artery disease if they have coronary artery disease risk factors or if their functional capacity is poor and coronary disease could be occult (i.e., asymptomatic) as a result of decreased activity. The patient's cardiac risk profile and overall medical state should be assessed in the postoperative period. If the surgical procedure is not an emergency, I then ask the next question:

2. *Does the patient have one or more active cardiac conditions (unstable coronary syndromes, decompensated heart failure, significant arrhythmias, severe valvular disease)?* In this patient group, noncardiac surgery is usually delayed unless it is an emergency. For the patient who has an unstable coronary syndrome, coronary angiography is often performed to define coronary anatomy, and a coronary revascularization procedure is performed, if indicated. For the patient with severe valvular heart disease, evaluation is performed to assess

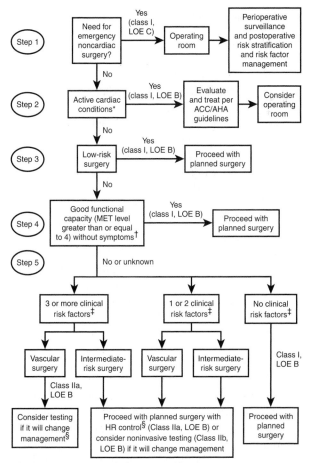

Figure 7-2 • Cardiac evaluation and care algorithm for noncardiac surgery based on active clinical conditions, known cardiovascular disease, or cardiac risk factors for patients 50 years of age or older. *See Table 7-1 for active clinical conditions. †See Figure 7-1 for estimated MET level equivalent. ‡Clinical risk factors include ischemic heart disease, compensated or prior heart failure, diabetes mellitus, renal insufficiency, and cerebrovascular disease. §Consider perioperative beta blockade for populations in which this has been shown to reduce cardiac morbidity/mortality. ACC/AHA, American College of Cardiology/American Heart Association; HR, heart rate; LOE, level of evidence; MET, metabolic equivalent. *(From Fleisher LA, Beckman JA, Brown KA, et al: ACC/AHA guidelines on perioperative cardiovascular evaluation and care for noncardiac surgery: A report of the American College of Cardiology/American Heart Association Task Force on Practice Guidelines [Writing Committee to Revise the 2002 Guidelines on Perioperative Cardiovascular Evaluation for Noncardiac Surgery]. J Am Coll Cardiol 50:e159-241, 2007.)*

whether valve repair or replacement is indicated. For the patient with decompensated congestive heart failure or significant arrhythmias, stabilization of these problems should be undertaken before nonemergency noncardiac surgery is performed.

3. *If the patient does not have one or more active cardiac conditions noted previously, I then ask whether the patient is undergoing low-risk surgery* (see Box 7-2). Because the perioperative cardiac risk (morbidity and mortality <1%) in this patient group is so low, interventions based on cardiac testing typically do not change the outcome. Patients in this category, therefore, usually proceed to surgery.

4. *If the surgery is not low risk, I then ask whether the patient has good functional capacity without provocation of cardiac symptoms.* Functional capacity is quantified by assessing the patient's activities of daily living and expressing that activity in terms of METs. Perioperative cardiac risk has been shown to be increased in patients with poor exercise tolerance (e.g., those who are unable to carry out activity of 4 METs during their daily activities). Cardiac risk is increased even if the inability to perform this degree of activity is the result of a noncardiac cause (e.g., osteoarthritis). As defined by the Duke Activity Status Index, activities that utilize 4 METs include performing light work around the house and climbing a flight of stairs (see Fig. 7-1). If the patient is able to perform 4 or more METs activities without provocation of symptoms, it is unlikely that cardiac stress testing will yield a result that will alter perioperative outcome. If the patient has not had a recent cardiac stress test, I estimate his or her functional capacity by carefully reviewing daily activity level and estimating energy expenditure in METs for the activity.

5. *If the patient has poor functional capacity or a functional capacity that cannot be determined, surgery-specific cardiac*

risk is then determined. This risk is related to the type of surgery and its associated risk as well as to the presence of clinical risk factors, such as history of ischemic heart disease (e.g., mild angina pectoris), prior MI (MI more than 30 days before surgery), compensated or prior congestive heart failure, history of cerebrovascular disease, diabetes mellitus, or renal insufficiency (serum Cr ≥ 2.0). Vascular surgery is associated with the highest degree of cardiac risk because of the hemodynamic stress of the surgery and the fact that many patients who undergo vascular surgery have coexistent coronary artery disease. For the patient who is to undergo vascular surgery or an intermediate-risk procedure and has three or more clinical risk factors, preoperative cardiac stress testing is considered, as the results of testing will alter perioperative management. For the vascular surgery patient or the patient who is to undergo an intermediate-risk surgical procedure and who has one or two clinical risk factors, beta blockers are titrated in the perioperative period to a heart rate less than 65 beats per minute in an effort to decrease perioperative myocardial ischemia. In this patient group, preoperative cardiac stress testing may also be considered if the results will alter perioperative management. A summary of the guideline recommendations for preoperative stress testing is found in Table 7-2. For patients with no clinical risk factors, the guideline suggests that they proceed to surgery.

Although not a component of the formal ACC/AHA preoperative evaluation algorithm at the time of preoperative assessment, I utilize the patient's history of coronary artery revascularization to further assess his or her perioperative risk and management. If the patient has had coronary artery revascularization with coronary artery bypass surgery within the past 5 years or coronary artery angioplasty from 6 months to 5 years previously and has not had symptoms or signs of

TABLE 7-2	Recommendations for Preoperative Noninvasive Stress Testing*

Class IIa recommendation (recommendation in favor of stress testing being useful)

Noninvasive stress testing of patients with three or more clinical risk factors[†] and poor functional capacity (<4 METs) who require vascular surgery is reasonable if it will change management.

Class IIb recommendation (recommendation's usefulness less well established than IIa recommendation)

Noninvasive stress testing may be considered for patients with at least one to two clinical risk factors and poor functional capacity (<4 METs) who require intermediate-risk noncardiac surgery if it will change management.

Noninvasive stress testing may be considered for patients with at least one to two clinical risk factors and good functional capacity (≥4 METs) who are undergoing vascular surgery.

---

*Noninvasive stress testing is not useful for patients who have no clinical risk factors and are undergoing intermediate-risk noncardiac surgery and for patients who are undergoing low-risk noncardiac surgery.

[†]Clinical risk factors: history of ischemic heart disease, history of compensated or prior heart failure, history of cerebrovascular disease, diabetes mellitus, renal insufficiency (serum creatinine ≥2.0).

METs, metabolic equivalents.

From Fleisher LA, Beckman JA, Brown KA, et al: ACC/AHA guidelines on perioperative cardiovascular evaluation and care for noncardiac surgery: A report of the American College of Cardiology/American Heart Association Task Force on Practice Guidelines (Writing Committee to Revise the 2002 Guidelines on Perioperative Cardiovascular Evaluation for Noncardiac Surgery). J Am Coll Cardiol 50: e159-241, 2007.

---

myocardial ischemia, retrospective data suggest that the risk of perioperative MI is low. Data suggest that for this patient group further preoperative cardiac testing is usually unnecessary. I take into consideration the patient's daily activity when answering this question, realizing that for the patient who is sedentary, progression of coronary artery disease may be occult because the physical activity is not strenuous enough to provoke symptoms of ischemia. For the patient who has undergone coronary angioplasty with placement of a non–drug-eluting intracoronary stent, it is recommended that noncardiac surgery be delayed until the patient's mandatory antiplatelet regimen is completed, which is typically 30 to 45 days following stent implantation. This delay is to avoid the risk of major hemorrhage if surgery is performed while the patient is receiving aggressive antiplatelet therapy and to prevent premature termination of antiplatelet therapy, which would increase the stent thrombosis risk dramatically. For the patient who has undergone placement of a drug-eluting stent, the period of dual antiplatelet therapy after stenting (1 year) should similarly be completed before noncardiac surgery is performed.

RISK ASSESSMENT BEFORE ENDOVASCULAR AORTIC ANEURYSM REPAIR

There is evidence that elective endovascular management of aortic and thoracic aneurysms is associated with a lower incidence of perioperative morbidity and mortality than open aneurysm repair. Using current complication rates, I typically classify elective endovascular aortic and thoracic aneurysm repair in the stable patient as an intermediate-risk procedure.

RISK ASSESSMENT BEFORE TRANSPLANT SURGERY

In many instances, transplantation surgery is performed in patients with significant medical comorbidities. The patient who undergoes kidney transplantation is at least at intermediate risk of cardiac complication because of renal insufficiency. Many of these patients also have diabetes mellitus, which contributes to their risk of complication. A retrospective review of 2694 patients who underwent renal transplantation identified age older than 50 years and preexisting heart disease, especially in diabetics, as risk factors that significantly increased the risk of perioperative cardiac complication. In 176 patients who underwent kidney or kidney-pancreas transplant, the occurrence of postoperative cardiac complications correlated with the presence of reversible myocardial perfusion defects on preoperative dipyridamole thallium imaging. For the patient who undergoes liver transplantation, dobutamine stress echocardiography has been shown to have utility in the prediction of postoperative cardiac complications.

Although the guideline algorithm is helpful in assessing preoperative risk and guiding perioperative management, I believe that consideration of the patient's unique history and indications for surgery should be considered when deciding whether specific preoperative cardiac testing is to be used. In some patients, the danger of not performing surgery may be greater than the predicted perioperative risk of cardiac complication, an example being the patient with significant cardiac history who is to undergo a curative surgical procedure for a malignant neoplasm. Another consideration is to weigh the risks that may occur if semiurgent surgery is delayed as a result of stress testing and possible coronary artery revascularization. An example of this scenario is that of the elderly patient with multiple comorbidities who sustains a hip fracture that warrants surgical repair.

ANESTHESIA CONSIDERATIONS

Physiologic Response to Anesthesia and Surgery

Anesthesia and surgery are accompanied by physiologic responses to preserve homeostasis. In the patient with compensated heart disease, these normal responses may precipitate decompensation. Catecholamine production increases in response to the stress of surgery, and it leads to increases in myocardial oxygen demand as well as increased afterload that may provoke myocardial ischemia in the patient with coronary artery disease. In addition, several perioperative factors may lead to decreased myocardial oxygen delivery. Hypoventilation and atelectasis may reduce arterial oxygen saturation. Anemia decreases myocardial oxygen delivery. Volume depletion or perioperative hypotension may result in coronary artery hypoperfusion. Sodium and water retention are increased in response to aldosterone secretion in an effort to maintain intravascular volume. In the patient with impaired ventricular function or "fixed" cardiac output (e.g., critical aortic stenosis, severe left ventricular dysfunction), this process may result in CHF.

Cardiovascular Effects of Anesthetic Agents

Inhalation Agents

Inhalation agents all produce dose-dependent myocardial depression. Nitrous oxide is the least depressant, and because its use is associated with an increase in peripheral vascular resistance, systemic blood pressure is maintained. Halothane, rarely used in adults because of idiosyncratic hepatotoxicity, produces the greatest degree of myocardial depression of all the inhaled agents. All inhalational agents may cause decreases in blood pressure. For halothane and enflurane, blood pressure is decreased by direct myocardial depression in conjunction with decreased cardiac output and stroke volume. For isoflurane, sevoflurane, and desflurane, the associated blood pressure decrease is caused by a reduction in systemic vascular resistance with peripheral vasodilation. This may result in hypotension in the patient who is concurrently receiving vasodilators (nitrates, hydralazine, and nifedipine) or who has intravascular volume depletion. Treatment of hypotension in this setting should be with fluid administration. The depressant effects of inhalational anesthetics may be accentuated in patients with ventricular dysfunction. Desflurane is associated with sympathetic activation and is therefore of limited use in patients with cardiac disease. Sevoflurane appears to be similar to isoflurane and safe in the patient with ischemic heart disease. It has been described as having a more stable effect on heart rate than the other inhaled agents.

Intravenous Anesthetic Agents

Thiopental is the prototypical intravenous barbiturate anesthetic agent. Its cardiac effects during noncardiac surgery can be significant. This drug leads to venous dilation with a reduction in preload as well as myocardial depression. These physiologic responses may result in an increase in heart rate. Thiopental should therefore be used with caution in the patient with decreased preload (e.g., hypovolemia) who is receiving vasodilator medications as well as in the patient in whom increased heart rate would be detrimental (e.g., the patient with ischemia).

Opioids are commonly used in anesthesia to blunt the sympathetic response to intubation and surgical manipulation. Sufentanil and fentanyl are the most frequently used agents of this class. They serve to prevent increases in intraoperative myocardial oxygen demand by maintaining cardiac output and preventing increases in heart rate.

Propofol is commonly used for induction and maintenance of general anesthesia and for sedation during regional anesthesia. It is particularly well suited for use in outpatient surgery because of its short duration of action and antiemetic properties. The use of this drug may be associated with hypotension, especially after bolus administration.

Spinal Anesthesia

Spinal anesthesia is relatively contraindicated in patients with fixed cardiac output (e.g., critical aortic stenosis, severe left ventricular dysfunction) because these patients are unable to augment cardiac output in response to the vasodilation and subsequent hypotension that often accompany this technique.

Regional versus General Anesthesia

Several studies found no difference between the effects of regional and general anesthesia on cardiovascular morbidity or mortality. There are several unique settings in which one modality may be preferable. Regional anesthesia produces less respiratory and cardiac depression than general anesthesia, and the use of regional anesthesia may be advantageous in the patient with left ventricular dysfunction, CHF, or pulmonary disease. Some investigators have suggested that in certain high-risk groups (e.g., those who undergo vascular surgery), epidural analgesia along with general anesthesia is associated with a lower risk of perioperative cardiac complications than general anesthesia alone. In a meta-analysis of 141 randomized trials involving 9559 patients, general anesthesia was compared with neuraxial blockade, such as spinal or epidural anesthesia [◉ Rodgers et al, 2000]. The authors found that neuraxial blockade, with or without general anesthesia, was associated with a 44% decreased incidence of deep vein thrombosis, a 55% decreased incidence of pulmonary embolus, and a 33% decreased incidence of MI. Overall mortality was reduced by approximately 33% in patients receiving neuraxial blockade. The applicability of these data to current care has been questioned. The meta-analysis has been criticized because of the heterogeneity of its component studies, the overestimation of "treatment effect" related to positive publication bias, changes in postoperative management, and the fact that in many of its component studies serum troponin was not used as a marker of MI, with a resulting presumed underdiagnosis of perioperative MI. **Since the publication of this meta-analysis, large, multicenter, retrospective studies have shown no cardiovascular mortality benefit and only minimal morbidity benefit for combined epidural and general anesthesia. The proven benefits of neuraxial anesthesia and analgesia include a reduction in blood loss, superior pain control, decreased postoperative ileus, and fewer pulmonary complications** [◉ Ballantyne et al, 2005].

ISCHEMIC HEART DISEASE

Prevention of Perioperative Myocardial Ischemia and Myocardial Infarction

Perioperative β-blockers have been demonstrated to decrease the risk of perioperative myocardial ischemia and MI in selected patient populations. The ACC/AHA's 2006 "Guideline

Update on Perioperative Cardiovascular Evaluation for Noncardiac Surgery: Focused Update on Perioperative Beta-Blocker Therapy" notes that, for the most part, evidence to support the widespread use of β-blockers to decrease perioperative cardiac risk is lacking. This guideline states that most perioperative β-blocker trials have been inadequately powered, few have been randomized, most have looked only at high-risk populations, and no studies have addressed how, when, and by whom perioperative β-blocker therapy should be implemented and monitored. Many of the patients evaluated in these trials underwent vascular surgery. Despite these concerns, the guideline does recommend that β-**blockers be continued in patients already receiving these agents and should be initiated in patients undergoing vascular surgery who are estimated to be at high cardiac risk as determined by the presence of ischemia on preoperative testing. This guideline states that β-blockers are probably recommended for patients who undergo vascular surgery and who have a history of coronary artery disease or who have multiple coronary artery disease risk factors and for patients with multiple cardiac risk factors who undergo intermediate-risk or high-risk surgical procedures. β-Blockers may be considered for patients who undergo intermediate-risk or high-risk surgical procedures who have a single clinical cardiac risk factor and may also be considered for patients who undergo vascular surgery who have no cardiac risk factors** (Box 7-2)   [● *Fleisher et al, 2006*].

Based on this evidence, I attempt to utilize perioperative β-blockers in all patients who undergo vascular surgery as well as those with known cardiovascular disease or at increased cardiac risk who undergo intermediate-risk or high-risk nonvascular surgery. I attempt to initiate β-blockers at least 1 week preoperatively because I realize that, in many patients, the realities of surgery lead to identification of these patients at time periods considerably less than 1 week preoperatively and

Box 7-2	RECOMMENDATIONS FOR PERIOPERATIVE β-BLOCKER MEDICAL THERAPY

RECOMMENDED

1. Patient already receiving β-blocker therapy
2. Vascular surgery: Myocardial ischemia identified on preoperative testing

PROBABLY RECOMMENDED

1. Vascular surgery: Patient with known coronary artery disease
2. Vascular surgery: Patient with multiple clinical risk factors
3. Intermediate-risk or high-risk surgery: Patient with multiple clinical risk factors

MAY BE CONSIDERED

1. Intermediate-risk or high-risk surgery (including vascular surgery): Single clinical risk factor
2. Vascular surgery: No cardiac risk factors

Adapted from Fleisher LA, Beckman JA, Brown KA, et al: ACC/AHA 2006 guideline update on perioperative cardiovascular evaluation for noncardiac surgery: Focused update on perioperative beta-blocker therapy. A report of the American College of Cardiology/American Heart Association Task Force on Practice Guidelines (Writing Committee to Update the 2002 Guidelines on Perioperative Cardiovascular Evaluation for Noncardiac Surgery). J Am Coll Cardiol 47:2343-2355, 2006.

---

continue for at least 30 days after the surgical procedure. Many patients whom I identify as requiring these agents in the perioperative period have indications for long-term β-blocker use. I attempt to titrate the β-blocker to a heart rate of 60 to 70 beats/minute.

Perioperative α-adrenergic agonists (clonidine, mivazerol) have been demonstrated to decrease perioperative ischemia and mortality following vascular surgery. This approach is not commonly used in the United States.

Emerging evidence suggests that administration of a statin is associated with a reduced incidence of perioperative cardiac complications. Most of this evidence is based on observational studies. Further evidence is needed before statins can be recommended as agents to decrease perioperative cardiovascular risk; however, my approach to patients who are long-term statin recipients is to continue their use in the perioperative period.

No evidence indicates that intraoperative nitrates or calcium channel antagonists are of benefit to prevent intraoperative myocardial ischemia. Prophylactic nitrates may actually be harmful if they lead to excessive preload reduction with subsequent hypotension.

In a study of 300 patients with known coronary artery disease or at high risk for coronary artery disease who underwent abdominal, thoracic, or vascular surgical procedures, maintenance of perioperative normothermia led to a decreased incidence of perioperative morbid events (unstable angina, cardiac arrest, MI: 6.3% morbid events in the hypothermic group versus 1.4% morbid events in the normothermic group), as well as a decrease in episodes of ventricular tachycardia.

Retrospective studies have shown that coronary artery bypass surgery does offer a protective effect for patients whose noncardiac surgical procedure followed coronary artery bypass surgery by up to 6 years. However, when the risk of coronary artery bypass itself is included in overall risk analysis, the protective effect of coronary artery bypass grafting is negated. A prospective randomized trial comparing coronary artery revascularization with intensive medical therapy (β-blockers, aspirin, statins, angiotensin-converting enzyme [ACE] inhibitors) as the preoperative treatment for patients who subsequently underwent vascular surgical procedures showed that **preoperative coronary revascularization did not result in better outcomes than medical therapy in patients with stable coronary artery disease who underwent elective vascular operations** [❹ McFalls et al, 2004].

The ACC/AHA consensus-based guideline for preoperative cardiovascular evaluation before noncardiac surgery recommends that the individual patient's perioperative and long-term risk be considered when deciding whether to perform coronary artery bypass surgery before noncardiac surgical procedures. The guideline advocates that coronary artery bypass surgery be performed before noncardiac surgical procedures in patients who meet established criteria for coronary bypass (i.e., left main coronary stenosis, three-vessel coronary artery disease in conjunction with left ventricular dysfunction, two-vessel coronary disease when one of the vessels is the left anterior descending coronary artery with severe proximal stenosis, and myocardial ischemia despite a maximal medical regimen) [● *Eagle et al, 2004*]. The guideline highlights that coronary artery bypass grafting should be performed in the foregoing patients before high-risk or intermediate-risk noncardiac surgery when long-term outcome would be improved by the coronary procedure.

Investigators have suggested that percutaneous transluminal coronary angioplasty reduces perioperative cardiac morbidity when it is performed to alleviate myocardial ischemia before noncardiac surgery. The few studies that have assessed this technique, however, were nonrandomized and were based on historical controls. In the United States, most patients who undergo coronary artery angioplasty also undergo implantation of an intracoronary stent. For the patient whose stent is drug eluting, it is essential that the antiplatelet regimen (aspirin and clopidogrel) be continued for at least 12 months following placement of a sirolimus-coated or paclitaxel-coated stent. Premature discontinuation of this antiplatelet regimen may result in acute stent thrombosis with subsequent MI. If surgery cannot be performed in the presence of aspirin and clopidogrel, I recommend that the procedure be delayed until the patient's antiplatelet course is completed. If emergency surgery is required and the patient has not completed the post–stent placement antiplatelet regimen, I consider each case on an individual basis. For most patients, I proceed to surgery and utilize platelet transfusions in the event of excessive bleeding. If a patient presents for coronary artery angioplasty and it is known that he or she is to have subsequent noncardiac surgery in less than 12 months, I consider the use of a bare metal stent, which requires only 1 month of antiplatelet therapy (aspirin and clopidogrel). This focused approach serves to reduce the risk of stent thrombosis in those patients whose antiplatelet agents would be prematurely discontinued and to lower the risk of bleeding in those who would undergo surgery while still receiving their antiplatelet regimen.

The Patient with Chronic Coronary Artery Disease

For patients with chronic stable angina, it is important to continue antianginal therapy in the perioperative period. β-Blockers are continued to the time of operation. For prolonged effect, a long-acting preparation (i.e., nadolol or atenolol) may be given on the morning of the surgical procedure. If patients are unable to resume oral intake 24 hours postoperatively, β-blockers may be given intravenously (e.g., propranolol, 0.5 to 2 mg every 1 to 6 hours). Parenteral metoprolol or esmolol may also be used. Oral β-blocker therapy is resumed as soon as possible postoperatively.

Patients who are receiving long-term antianginal treatment with calcium channel antagonists are usually given a long-acting oral preparation on the morning of the surgical procedure. If they are unable to resume oral intake 24 hours postoperatively, I generally add intravenous or topical nitrates to the regimen. The only calcium channel antagonists available for intravenous use are verapamil and diltiazem. Because their effect is primarily antiarrhythmic when they are given intravenously, I do not use these agents as primary anti-ischemic therapy for patients who are unable to take oral medications.

Perioperative Myocardial Infarction

Most perioperative MIs occur during the initial 48 hours after a surgical procedure. Typical characteristics of postoperative MI are that they are of the non–ST-segment elevation

(NSTEMI) type and are typically not accompanied by angina. These MIs are more often accompanied by CHF, arrhythmia, hypotension, confusion, and hyperglycemia in diabetic patients. The presence of any one of these findings in the patient at increased risk for perioperative MI should arouse suspicion that an MI may have occurred. Troponin is the most sensitive and specific biomarker of perioperative MI.

The immediate goals for treatment of perioperative MI are the same as those for treatment of MI in the nonsurgical setting. They include reperfusion of ischemic myocardium supplied by the culprit coronary artery, antithrombotic therapy to prevent rethrombosis of subtotal coronary stenosis, adjunctive measures to decrease ongoing myocardial oxygen demand, and prevention of MI-related left ventricular remodeling.

Thrombolytic therapy is indicated for many patients with acute MI, but it should not be used in the majority of patients who have undergone recent surgery. Although it is not known exactly how soon postoperatively it is safe to use thrombolytic agents, any operation within the previous 2 weeks that could be a source of uncontrollable bleeding with thrombolytic therapy is an absolute contraindication to its use. Recent surgery more than 2 weeks before thrombolytic therapy has also been suggested as a relative contraindication to its use, and the choice must be made on an individual basis. Urgent cardiac catheterization with percutaneous coronary angioplasty should be considered in perioperative patients with evolving acute MIs.

In the absence of contraindications, aspirin (160 to 325 mg) is administered during the acute phase of MI. Aspirin use has been shown to decrease early mortality from MI by as much as 21%. If the patient is unable to tolerate oral medications in the perioperative period, aspirin (325 mg) may be given by rectal suppository. For the patient allergic to aspirin, clopidogrel has been recommended in a consensus guideline of the American College of Chest Physicians.

Heparin has been shown to reduce morbidity and mortality in the peri-MI period for the patient who has not received thrombolytic therapy. Therefore, if there are no contraindications and hemostasis is stable, heparin is utilized in the initial care of the patient with perioperative MI. Evidence indicates that subcutaneous low-molecular-weight heparin (e.g., enoxaparin, 1 mg/kg every 12 hours) is more effective than continuously administered unfractionated heparin, but this determination was made in nonsurgical patients. I believe that, pending study in perioperative patients, either type of heparin preparation would be an acceptable choice.

Although heparin and antiplatelet agents are of benefit after MI, they may increase bleeding following noncardiac surgical procedures. The benefit and risk of these agents must be considered before their use in the perioperative period.

β-Blockers given to patients with acute MIs decrease excessive reflex activation of the sympathetic nervous system, which may increase myocardial ischemia, platelet aggregation, and arrhythmia. These agents reduce post-MI morbidity and mortality. Therefore, in the absence of contraindications, I administer β-blockers to all patients with acute MI. Intravenous β-blockers (propranolol, metoprolol, esmolol) are administered to the patient who is unable to tolerate oral β-blockers. The dose is titrated to decrease the heart rate to less than 70 beats/minute. Contraindications to the use of β-blockers in the perioperative period include significant bradycardia or hypotension, severe left ventricular dysfunction, heart block, and severe bronchospastic lung disease.

Nitroglycerin is effective in decreasing the pain of acute ongoing myocardial ischemia. It is also beneficial when MI is complicated by CHF or pulmonary edema. No evidence indicates that prophylactic nitrates decrease mortality following acute MI. The typical starting dose for nitroglycerin is 5 to 10 μg/minute intravenously for most patients with perioperative MIs. The dose is increased by 5 to 10 μg/minute every 5 to 10 minutes. During titration, continuous monitoring of vital signs is essential. Although titration end points for nitroglycerin vary among individual patients, guidelines suggest the following: (1) control of symptoms or a decrease in mean arterial blood pressure of 10% in patients with normal blood pressure or 30% in patients with hypertension (never a systolic blood pressure <90 mm Hg); (2) a maximum increase in heart rate of more than 10 beats/minute but usually not greater than 110 beats/minute; and (3) a decrease in pulmonary artery end-diastolic pressure of 10% to 30%. For most patients, the final nitrate dose is less than 200 μg/minute.

Evidence indicates that ACE inhibitors given early after MI have increased survival, especially for patients with anterior MIs or those with left ventricular ejection fraction (LVEF) less than 40%.

It is essential that the patient who sustains a perioperative MI be treated following the acute phase in a manner similar to the treatment of MI in the nonsurgical setting. That would include assessment of myocardium at risk with a post-MI stress test in the patient whose MI has been uncomplicated, assessment of cardiac risk factors to include determination of lipid status and initiation of lipid lowering therapy if indicated, smoking cessation counseling, and a plan for cardiac rehabilitation.

HYPERTENSION

Perioperative Hypertension

Despite the extent of preoperative blood pressure control, perioperative hypertension or hypotension each occurs in up to 25% of hypertensive patients who undergo surgery. Two preoperative predictors of perioperative hypertension are previous hypertension, especially a diastolic blood pressure greater than 110 mm Hg, and the type of surgical procedure. Hypertensive events occur most commonly with carotid surgery, abdominal aortic surgery, peripheral vascular procedures, and intraperitoneal or intrathoracic surgery.

Data suggest that diastolic blood pressure of 110 mm Hg or greater is a preoperative marker of perioperative cardiac complications in the patient with chronic hypertension. Therefore, in patients with chronic hypertension, as long as the diastolic blood pressure is less than 110 mm Hg, hypertension in and of itself is not an indication to delay operation.

Data are conflicting regarding the role of preoperative hypertension as a cause of postoperative cardiac complication. In a multivariate analysis of risk factors for perioperative complications in men who underwent noncardiac surgery, the presence of preoperative hypertension increased the odds ratio (OR) for postoperative death to 3.8 times that of normotensive persons. In a case-controlled study of patients who died of a cardiac cause within 30 days of elective surgical procedures, a preoperative history of hypertension was four times more likely than in an equal number of age-matched controls. In contrast, a prospective, randomized, multicenter study of more than 17,000 patients found that although preoperative hypertension was associated with perioperative bradycardia, tachycardia, and hypertension, it was not a predictor of MI or cardiac death.

The importance of systolic hypertension as a risk factor for surgery is unclear. **A meta-analysis showed that there is little evidence for an association between systolic blood pressure of 180 mm Hg or less and perioperative cardiac complications** [● *Howell et al, 2004*].

Perioperative hypertension tends to occur at four distinct time periods: (1) during laryngoscopy and induction of anesthesia, as a result of sympathetic stimulation with adrenergic mediated vasoconstriction; (2) intraoperatively, as a result of acute pain-induced sympathetic stimulation leading to vasoconstriction; (3) in the early postanesthesia period, principally because of pain-induced sympathetic stimulation, hypothermia (which decreases catecholamine reuptake and thereby increases plasma catecholamine levels), hypoxia, or intravascular volume overload from excessive intraoperative fluid therapy; and (4) 24 to 48 hours postoperatively, as fluid is mobilized from the extravascular space. It is also during this period that blood pressure may become elevated in response to discontinuation of chronic antihypertensive medication.

An uncommon cause of perioperative hypertension that has received significant attention is the *clonidine withdrawal syndrome*. This condition has been reported to occur 18 to 24 hours after abruptly stopping clonidine in patients who were almost always taking more than 1.0 mg/day. This syndrome is of particular concern in the perioperative period because there is no rapidly acting, parenteral form of this drug for use in the patient who is unable to take oral medications. Characterized by excessive sympathetic activity with rebound hypertension, the syndrome often resembles the hypertensive crisis of pheochromocytoma. Clonidine withdrawal syndrome may be aggravated by the simultaneous use of propranolol, which blocks peripheral vasodilatory β-receptors and thus leaves vasoconstricting α-receptors unopposed. It may be reversed by reinstitution of clonidine, which can be given intramuscularly, or by treatment with methyldopa or labetalol hydrochloride. Discontinuation syndromes manifested by hypertension may also be provoked by withdrawal of β-blockers, centrally acting antihypertensive agents (e.g., α-methyldopa), and other antihypertensive drugs.

Treatment of Perioperative Hypertension

My initial approach to treatment is prevention. Because many patients who develop postoperative hypertension do so as a result of withdrawal of their long-term antihypertensive regimen, I attempt to minimize this withdrawal in the postoperative period. This approach includes substituting long-acting preparations of the patient's long-term antihypertensive regimen starting, if possible, several days preoperatively, and given in the morning of the day of surgery.

No well-studied indications exist for acute control of hypertension in the perioperative period. I consider the possible causes of the patient's blood pressure elevation and also decide whether the patient's hypertension is a hypertensive emergency or urgency.

Hypertension that occurs in relation to tracheal intubation, surgical incision, and emergence from anesthesia is often the result of increased sympathetic tone. It may be treated with short-acting β-blockers, short-acting narcotics, or, if needed, intravenous nitroprusside.

Hypertensive emergencies are uncommon following noncardiac surgery. They are characterized by severe elevation of blood pressure with associated target organ dysfunction. Examples include the following: hypertensive encephalopathy, intracerebral hemorrhage, subarachnoid hemorrhage, and acute stroke; hypertension-induced acute renal dysfunction; and hypertension associated with unstable angina, acute MI, acute CHF, and acute aortic dissection. Other postoperative situations that may result in a hypertensive emergency include rebound hypertension following withdrawal of antihypertensive medications, hypertension resulting in bleeding from vascular surgical suture lines, hypertension associated with head trauma, and hypertension related to acute catecholamine excess (i.e., pheochromocytoma). My initial approach is to reverse precipitating factors (pain, hypervolemia, hypoxia, hypercarbia, and hypothermia). In the patient with a hypertensive emergency, I usually find it necessary also to administer a parenteral antihypertensive agent. In the acute setting, my treatment goal is to decrease the patient's blood pressure by no more than 25%. This approach decreases the likelihood of too aggressive control, which may result in target organ hypoperfusion. In patients with chronic hypertension, cerebral and renal perfusion autoregulation is shifted to a higher range. The brain and kidneys are particularly prone to hypoperfusion if blood pressure is lowered too rapidly. With the threat of organ injury diminished, I then attempt to control blood pressure to baseline levels over 24 to 48 hours.

My approach to the patient with postoperative hypertension but without evidence of target organ damage is similar to my approach to a patient with a hypertensive urgency. I attempt to reverse precipitating factors (see earlier) and to restore the patient's preoperative antihypertensive medications. For patients who are unable to resume oral intake, I typically administer parenteral alternative antihypertensive agents.

PERIOPERATIVE HYPOTENSION

Perioperative hypotension may result in myocardial ischemia and is a predictor of postoperative cardiac morbidity. A perioperative decrease of mean arterial blood pressure of more than 20 mm Hg has been shown to increase postoperative cardiac complications. The most common causes of perioperative hypotension are intravascular volume depletion and excessive vasodilation. Hypotension may be induced by anesthetic agents. Spinal anesthesia may result in hypotension related to vasodilation. Several of the inhalational anesthetic agents (e.g., isoflurane, desflurane, and sevoflurane) may cause hypotension by peripheral vasodilation as well as by myocardial depression. Other causes of perioperative hypotension include MI, pulmonary embolus, and sepsis. Hypotension caused by volume depletion or vasodilation is best treated by volume expansion. When clinically significant vasodilation-induced hypotension does not respond to this approach, a peripheral vasoconstrictor (phenylephrine) should be considered. Hypotension resulting from direct myocardial depression may be treated with inotropic agents such as dopamine, dobutamine, and milrinone.

VALVULAR HEART DISEASE

Mitral Stenosis

Mitral stenosis in adults is usually a result of rheumatic fever. Rheumatic valvulitis causes scarring of the mitral valve leaflets, with fusion of the commissures as well as subvalvular apparatus. With the reduced incidence of rheumatic fever in developed countries, nonrheumatic causes of mitral valve stenosis should be considered. In elderly patients, idiopathic calcification of the mitral valve annulus with extension to the mitral valve leaflets may result in functional mitral stenosis. Rare causes of mitral stenosis are systemic lupus erythematosus, rheumatoid arthritis, and carcinoid syndrome.

In normal adults, the mitral valve area is 4 to 5 cm^2. Mitral stenosis is critical when the valve area is reduced to 1 cm^2 or less. As mitral valve leaflet fusion progresses, left atrial pressure increases to maintain left ventricular filling, and a diastolic transvalvular pressure gradient exists between the left atrium and the left ventricle. Increased left atrial pressure leads to increased pulmonary vascular pressure. Conditions that decrease diastolic filling time (e.g., tachycardia) as well as those that increase cardiac blood flow across the mitral valve (e.g., physical exercise, fever) further increase left atrial and pulmonary vascular pressure. The pressure gradient across the mitral valve is proportional to the square of the transvalvular flow rate. Therefore, modest increases in transvalvular flow result in significant increases in the pressure gradient. The onset of atrial fibrillation with the loss of the atrial contribution to ventricular filling, as well as decreased diastolic filling time associated with a rapid heart rate, may also lead to increased left atrial pressure. Pulmonary hypertension occurs as mitral stenosis progresses. Although pulmonary venous and arterial hypertension is usually reversible after mechanical correction of mitral stenosis, advanced disease is often associated with mitral regurgitation, hypertrophy of the pulmonary vasculature, and an irreversible component of pulmonary hypertension. Right ventricular pressure overload may occur as a consequence of pulmonary hypertension.

The clinical findings of mitral stenosis result from the inability of the left atrium to empty normally and from pulmonary venous and arterial hypertension. Symptoms such as exertional dyspnea may occur when the mitral valve area decreases to less than 2.5 cm². Rest symptoms such as orthopnea and paroxysmal nocturnal dyspnea are present when the valve area is less than 1.5 cm². Fatigue resulting from decreased cardiac output characterizes late disease. Hoarseness may occur and is caused by compression of the left recurrent laryngeal nerve by the enlarged left atrium and pulmonary artery. Atrial fibrillation commonly accompanies mitral stenosis and is the result of persistently elevated left atrial pressure and left atrial dilation as well as involvement of the left atrium by rheumatic carditis. Atrial fibrillation with rapid ventricular response may lead to pulmonary edema resulting from the decreased diastolic filling time that occurs when heart rate increases. Patients with atrial fibrillation are at high risk for intracardiac thrombus formation with subsequent systemic embolization. The risk of embolization increases with increased size of the left atrium and atrial appendage as well as with decreased cardiac output.

Physical findings of mitral stenosis include an accentuated first heart sound (S_1) that decreases in intensity as stenosis worsens and a high-pitched opening snap heard after the second heart sound (S_2) that is caused by opening of the stenotic but pliable mitral valve. As mitral stenosis progresses, left atrial pressure rises, and the interval between S_2 and the opening snap shortens. When valve mobility is lost, the opening snap disappears. A low-pitched diastolic rumble is heard at the apex, and its duration correlates with the severity of stenosis. Patients in whom sinus rhythm is preserved may have presystolic accentuation of the murmur.

Transthoracic echocardiography is essential in evaluation of these patients. It confirms the diagnosis, identifies the cause (e.g., leaflet fusion of rheumatic mitral valve stenosis, mitral annulus calcification in elderly patients), allows for estimation of valve orifice area, and, with the use of Doppler techniques, facilitates an approximation of the transvalvular pressure gradient. Echocardiography may also facilitate identification of mitral regurgitation, which coexists in as many as 40% of patients with mitral stenosis, as well as other valve lesions. Although it is not indicated in every patient with mitral stenosis, transesophageal echocardiography is an effective tool to determine the presence or absence of left atrial thrombi, the presence of which is a contraindication to restoration of sinus rhythm in the patient with mitral stenosis who is in atrial fibrillation.

Therapy is based on the presence or absence of symptoms and their severity, coexisting pulmonary hypertension resulting from mitral stenosis, and the suitability of the valve to percutaneous balloon mitral valvotomy (i.e., valve with minimal calcification, good leaflet mobility, little involvement of the subvalvular apparatus, and minimal or no valve regurgitation). Asymptomatic patients with moderate or severe mitral stenosis (mitral valve area ≤ 1.5 cm^2) are considered for percutaneous balloon mitral valvotomy if they have suitable valve morphology and pulmonary hypertension (pulmonary artery systolic pressure >50 mm Hg) caused by mitral stenosis. Patients with minimal symptoms often respond to diuretics; those with atrial fibrillation respond to control of the ventricular response with digoxin, β-blockers, or calcium channel antagonists. Survival is decreased when symptoms are more than mild. Therefore, patients with New York Heart Association (NYHA) functional class II symptoms and moderate or severe stenosis (mitral valve area ≤ 1.5 cm^2 or mean gradient ≥ 5 mm Hg) may be considered for mitral balloon valvotomy if they have suitable mitral valve morphology. Balloon mitral valvotomy is contraindicated in patients with left atrial thrombi. The prognosis is poor for patients who have NYHA functional class III or IV symptoms and evidence of severe mitral stenosis if left untreated. These patients should be considered for treatment with either balloon valvotomy or valve replacement. Percutaneous balloon mitral valvuloplasty or mitral valve replacement is indicated before noncardiac surgery only if the patient otherwise meets the indications for interventional treatment of mitral stenosis irrespective of the noncardiac surgical procedure.

Intravascular volume status and heart rate are key factors that require attention in patients undergoing noncardiac surgical procedures. Volume overload must be avoided because further increases in left atrial pressure may result in pulmonary edema. Conversely, excessive volume depletion or preload reduction may decrease left ventricular filling pressure and cardiac output. Perioperative tachycardia may impair left ventricular filling and can be treated with β-blockers, calcium channel antagonists, or digoxin in patients who have atrial fibrillation with rapid ventricular response. Because of the significant hemodynamic alterations that occur with relatively small volume shifts in patients with severe mitral stenosis, invasive hemodynamic monitoring of the pulmonary capillary wedge pressure should be considered if perioperative volume changes are anticipated. Infective endocarditis prophylaxis for indicated procedures is necessary.

Mitral stenosis increases the risk of systemic thromboembolism in the patient with atrial fibrillation. Many of these patients are anticoagulated with warfarin on a long-term basis. For the patient who undergoes a surgical procedure, care should be taken to minimize the perioperative time during which the patient will be not anticoagulated. Strategies include performing the surgical procedure without stopping anticoagulation in the patient in whom perioperative bleeding is unlikely (e.g., cataract surgery) and stopping warfarin 48 to 72 hours preoperatively so the surgical procedure may be performed when the international normalized ratio (INR) is 1.5 or less, with warfarin resumed within 24 hours of surgery. For the patient at significantly increased risk of embolism, such as the patient with mitral stenosis and atrial fibrillation who is elderly, has left ventricular dysfunction, or a history of prior embolism or hypertension, I often stop warfarin several days preoperatively and administer heparin when the INR falls to less than 2.0. Heparin is discontinued 4 to 6 hours preoperatively and is restarted as soon as possible afterward. Warfarin is then reinstituted. Heparin is discontinued when the INR is therapeutic.

An alternative approach, although not studied in prospective randomized trials and not approved by the U.S. Food and Drug Administration for this indication, is to use low-molecular-weight heparin as "bridge" anticoagulation rather than continuous unfractionated heparin. For this purpose, enoxaparin can be given at 1 mg/kg subcutaneously every 12 hours after warfarin is withheld and the INR decreases to less than the therapeutic range. Low-molecular-weight heparin should be stopped 12 hours preoperatively and resumed when hemostasis is stable in the postoperative period. Warfarin is restarted in the postoperative period, and low-molecular-weight heparin is discontinued when the INR is therapeutic.

Mitral Regurgitation

Mitral regurgitation may be caused by one or more abnormalities of the structures that compose the mitral valve apparatus: anterior and posterior valve leaflets, chordae tendineae, papillary muscles, and mitral valve annulus. It may also result from poor alignment of a structurally normal valve apparatus or from mitral annular dilation, both of which are caused by left ventricular dysfunction or dilation. Common causes of mitral apparatus dysfunction are myxomatous degeneration of the mitral valve leaflets or chordae, infective endocarditis that may involve the valve leaflets, coronary artery disease with myocardial ischemia resulting in papillary muscle dysfunction, and rheumatic valve disease. Less common but clinically significant causes of mitral regurgitation include mitral annular calcification (usually limited to elderly persons) and distortion of the mitral valve apparatus as a result of systolic anterior motion of the mitral valve in the setting of hypertrophic cardiomyopathy. Degeneration of the mitral valve may be seen in patients receiving long-term hemodialysis, as well as those with the antiphospholipid antibody syndrome.

The pathophysiology of mitral regurgitation depends on whether the regurgitation is acute or chronic. Acute mitral regurgitation is characterized by sudden increases in left atrial volume and pressure as blood is ejected back into the left atrium during systole. This acute volume overload also results in decreased cardiac output and acute pulmonary edema. The patient with chronic mitral regurgitation develops ventricular dilation slowly, and this helps to accommodate significant increases in blood volume without significant increases in left ventricular end-diastolic pressure. Thus, pulmonary congestion is initially prevented. Although patients may be stable for long periods, chronic left ventricular volume overload eventually leads to left ventricular dysfunction with decreased LVEF, decreased cardiac output, elevated left ventricular filling pressure, and pulmonary congestion.

The total LVEF (forward and regurgitant) is increased in patients with preserved left ventricular function and should be greater than normal (55%). A "normal" LVEF (50% to 55%) in the patient with severe mitral regurgitation gives the appearance that ventricular function is preserved but in reality is evidence of significant left ventricular dysfunction.

In otherwise healthy persons, the sudden onset of fulminant heart failure with the presence of an apical holosystolic murmur strongly suggests acute mitral regurgitation resulting from chordal rupture. CHF in patients with inferior wall MIs indicates the possibility of papillary muscle dysfunction. Sudden respiratory distress after a febrile illness suggests acute mitral regurgitation caused by ruptured chordae or valve leaflet perforation resulting from infective endocarditis.

In the presence of acute mitral regurgitation, patients usually have sinus tachycardia and a nondisplaced hyperdynamic left ventricular apical impulse. An apical systolic murmur begins with S_1 but often ends before S_2 as left atrial and left ventricular pressures equalize and valvular regurgitation ceases. In chronic mitral regurgitation, the left ventricular apical impulse is displaced because of left ventricular dilation. A holosystolic blowing murmur is heard at the apex and radiates to the axilla. S_3 is common and does not necessarily indicate the presence of left ventricular dysfunction. It may occur solely as a result of early diastolic filling. A left parasternal lift and accentuated pulmonic component of S_2 suggest coexistent pulmonary hypertension.

Echocardiography is an essential diagnostic study for evaluation of the patient with mitral regurgitation. It provides a measure of the degree of regurgitation as well as an estimate of left ventricular chamber size and function. This imaging technique usually leads to the identification of the component of the mitral valve apparatus that is responsible for the mitral regurgitation. If tricuspid regurgitation is present, echo-Doppler techniques can be used to measure the pressure gradient between the right ventricle and the right atrium and allow an estimate of pulmonary artery systolic pressure.

When surgical correction of mitral regurgitation is performed, it is desirable to repair rather than replace the valve. Valve repair is associated with lower perioperative mortality and better preservation of left ventricular function and, if sinus rhythm is maintained, freedom from the use of warfarin, as is necessary in the patient with a mechanical valve prosthesis. Patients with mitral valve calcification and scarring as well as those with severe myxomatous degeneration and destruction of the valve and chordae are usually not candidates for valve repair.

Left ventricular function is a major determinant of postoperative survival. Noninvasive measurements of ventricular function, LVEF, and ventricular dimension determined by echocardiography guide the timing of operation. In the patient with severe chronic mitral regurgitation, the normal LVEF should be greater than 60%. An LVEF of 60% or less is indicative of reduced long-term survival. For the patient with severe asymptomatic mitral regurgitation, mitral valve surgery should be performed if there is evidence of left ventricular dysfunction, such as an LVEF of 60% or less. Left ventricular end-systolic dimension should be less than 40 mm in the patient with normal left ventricular function. Therefore, for the patient with asymptomatic severe mitral regurgitation, surgery should be considered when the left ventricular end-systolic dimension exceeds this value. Surgery is considered in the asymptomatic patient with severe mitral regurgitation and preserved left ventricular function if the patient has had a recent onset of episodic or chronic atrial fibrillation or has evidence of pulmonary hypertension (pulmonary artery systolic pressure >50 mm Hg at rest or >60 mm Hg with exercise). In the symptomatic patient with severe mitral regurgitation, surgery should be performed as long as the LVEF is greater than 30% (LVEF <30% in the patient with severe left ventricular dysfunction is indicative of severe left ventricular dysfunction). When the LVEF is less than 30%, operative mortality increases significantly. In this high-risk group, surgery should only be considered if it is highly likely that mitral valve repair will be performed.

The status of left ventricular function is a major determinant of perioperative complications in patients with mitral regurgitation who undergo noncardiac surgery. I believe that patients with chronic severe mitral regurgitation should undergo noninvasive assessment of left ventricular function before noncardiac surgical procedures. If the LVEF is not greater than normal, as would be expected, I am particularly vigilant regarding fluid administration and volume shifts in an effort to avoid the development of CHF. Patients with mitral regurgitation tolerate afterload reduction well in the perioperative period. Agents that increase afterload (e.g., vasopressors) increase the amount of regurgitant blood, and their use should be avoided if possible.

Mitral Valve Prolapse

Mitral valve prolapse (MVP) is a condition in which one or both mitral valve leaflets extend above the mitral annular plane during systole and prolapse into the left atrium. The degree of valve abnormality varies greatly, ranging from relatively normal valves with only intermittent prolapse to markedly abnormal valve structures with valve leaflet thickening, redundancy, and regurgitation. MVP occurs in approximately 3% of the population.

Most persons with MVP are asymptomatic. Some have symptoms that are unrelated to the valve abnormality. These symptoms may be associated with autonomic dysfunction and include chest pain, palpitations, dizziness, and symptoms of panic.

The diagnosis is usually made on hearing the classic midsystolic click and, in patients with mitral regurgitation, a midsystolic to late systolic murmur. Conditions that decrease the size of the left ventricle (i.e., the Valsalva maneuver, dehydration) cause the valve to prolapse earlier, in which case the click is heard closer to S_1, and the intensity and duration of the murmur may be increased. The diagnosis is confirmed by transthoracic echocardiography.

Investigators have suggested that patients with MVP have a slightly higher incidence of cardiac arrhythmias. The cause is unclear, and the risk of serious arrhythmias is low. These arrhythmias often respond to cessation of caffeine or other stimulants and alcohol. β-Adrenergic blockers may be used if these maneuvers are not successful. Patients who have dizziness associated with MVP often have decreased blood volume. The onset of this symptom in the perioperative period should prompt an assessment of volume status and the administration of fluids if indicated.

Aortic Regurgitation

Aortic regurgitation may be caused by processes that affect the aortic valve leaflets (e.g., rheumatic fever, infective endocarditis, congenital bicuspid aortic valve) or the aortic root and valve-supporting structures (aortic dissection, systemic hypertension, cystic medial necrosis, Marfan's syndrome). Eighty percent of cases that come to medical attention are chronic.

Chronic aortic regurgitation is accompanied by left ventricular dilation and a gradual, progressive increase in left ventricular end-diastolic volume with only an initial slight increase in left ventricular end-diastolic pressure. The dilated left ventricle facilitates the rapid return of blood back to the ventricle during diastole, and the result is decreased peripheral arterial diastolic pressure. Left ventricular stroke volume, comprising both forward and regurgitant blood flow, is increased. The heart rate usually remains normal. This compensation often permits patients to remain asymptomatic even with severe aortic regurgitation. This combination of increased stroke volume and decreased diastolic blood pressure explains several of the classic physical findings of chronic aortic regurgitation: wide pulse pressure, water-hammer pulse (brisk pulse upstroke with rapid collapse), de Musset's sign (head bobbing during systole related to increased stroke volume), and Quincke's pulse (visible nail bed capillary pulsations).

Acute aortic regurgitation, in contrast, is characterized by the abrupt regurgitation of blood into a normal left ventricle and leads to a sudden increase in left ventricular volume and marked elevation of left ventricular end-diastolic pressure. Compensatory mechanisms do not occur, as in chronic aortic regurgitation. The heart rate increases, cardiac output decreases, and peripheral vasoconstriction occurs. The wide pulse pressure of chronic aortic regurgitation is not present, and systolic blood pressure may decrease. Acute heart failure and pulmonary edema are common. Because of the absence of chronic compensation, the classic physical findings of chronic aortic regurgitation are not present.

Acute aortic regurgitation may rapidly progress to intractable heart failure. Therefore, it is an indication for urgent aortic valve replacement. In contrast, chronic aortic regurgitation may be associated with minimal or no symptoms for years.

Aortic valve replacement is indicated for patients with acute severe aortic regurgitation. For the patient with chronic severe aortic regurgitation, surgical treatment is indicated if the patient is symptomatic. For the asymptomatic patient with chronic severe aortic regurgitation, surgical treatment is indicated if there is evidence of left ventricular systolic dysfunction (LVEF ≤50% at rest). The risks of surgery increase markedly when the LVEF is less than 25%, but the benefit of surgery often outweighs that risk. For patients with asymptomatic severe aortic regurgitation, aortic valve replacement is indicated in the setting of left ventricular dysfunction (LVEF <50%). Aortic valve replacement is deemed reasonable for patients with severe left ventricular dilatation (left ventricular end-systolic dimension >55 mm) even in the absence of symptoms.

In noncardiac surgery, the operative risk correlates more closely with the status of left ventricular function than with the degree of aortic valve regurgitation. Vasopressors that raise peripheral vascular resistance may increase the degree of regurgitation, and when used, these agents must be administered with caution. Bradycardia is associated with increased diastolic filling time, which raises the magnitude of regurgitant volume by lengthening the period during which regurgitation may occur. In contrast to patients with aortic stenosis, patients with aortic regurgitation typically tolerate vasodilation well, often with an increase in cardiac output. Caution must be exercised to prevent excessive decreases in already lowered diastolic pressure in an effort to preclude reductions in coronary artery perfusion pressure.

Aortic Stenosis

In adults, clinically significant aortic stenosis is usually the result of degenerative calcification of otherwise normal tricuspid aortic valves. When aortic stenosis manifests in adults less than 50 years old, it is usually a result of calcification and fusion of a congenital bicuspid aortic valve. Even when it is severe, aortic stenosis remains clinically silent for many years. The onset of symptoms indicates that patients are at risk for sudden cardiac death. In the patient with untreated symptomatic aortic stenosis, the occurrence of angina or syncope indicates a potential survival of only 2 to 3 years. The onset of CHF is more ominous and suggests the likelihood of death within 1 to 2 years. Sudden death is rare in patients with asymptomatic, hemodynamically severe aortic stenosis (i.e., aortic gradient >50 mm Hg and aortic valve area <1.0 cm^2).

The classic physical findings of significant aortic stenosis are a low-amplitude and slow-rising carotid pulse pressure (pulsus parvus and tardus), a sustained apical impulse, a crescendo-decrescendo harsh systolic murmur heard at the second right intercostal space radiating to the carotids and precordium, an S$_4$, and diminished intensity of the aortic component of S$_2$. As the degree of aortic obstruction increases, the systolic murmur peaks later in systole, and the intensity of the aortic component of S$_2$ decreases and may disappear.

The absence of these classic findings does not rule out the presence of critical aortic stenosis. The intensity of the heart murmur may decrease as the left ventricle fails. The carotid pulse findings may be altered in elderly patients with noncompliant peripheral vasculature. Transthoracic echocardiography is essential to estimate the degree of aortic stenosis more precisely and to quantitate left ventricular function. Echocardiographic correlates of severe aortic stenosis include a maximum velocity across the stenotic aortic valve of more than 4 m/second and a mean aortic valve gradient greater than 40 mm Hg. If the patient has low cardiac output, it may be difficult to distinguish the hemodynamics of severe aortic stenosis from moderate aortic stenosis. In that circumstance, augmentation of cardiac output by exercise or low-dose dobutamine infusion may facilitate hemodynamic assessment.

Adults with critical aortic stenosis (e.g., aortic valve area <1.0 cm^2) should undergo aortic valve replacement once they experience symptoms (e.g., angina, presyncope, syncope, CHF) or manifest evidence of left ventricular dysfunction even without symptoms. Fifty percent of adults with critical aortic stenosis and angina have significant coronary artery disease that may require revascularization at the time of aortic valve replacement. Survival after aortic valve replacement is excellent, and patients with left ventricular dysfunction often experience marked improvement in ventricular function following surgery.

Because the risk of aortic valve replacement exceeds the risk of sudden death in patients with asymptomatic critical aortic stenosis and normal left ventricular function, aortic valve replacement is not performed until the patient develops symptoms of left ventricular dysfunction (i.e., LVEF <50%). An exception is the patient with asymptomatic critical aortic stenosis who requires coronary artery bypass surgery. In this patient, aortic valve replacement at the time of coronary artery bypass surgery is recommended.

Balloon aortic valvuloplasty has been described as a nonsurgical means of decreasing the degree of aortic obstruction in aortic stenosis. The immediate and long-term results of this procedure have been disappointing. Although the aortic valve area following this procedure may be increased up to 60%, many patients with critical aortic stenosis still have significant aortic stenosis after the procedure. Mortality or major morbidity occurs in more than 10% of patients who undergo balloon aortic valvuloplasty, and aortic valve restenosis occurs in 50% of patients within 6 months. This modality has a limited role in patients with aortic stenosis who require noncardiac surgery. It may be considered for those patients with critical aortic stenosis and either CHF or hypotension who require urgent noncardiac surgery. It may also be considered before noncardiac surgical procedures in patients with hemodynamic compromise as a result of critical aortic stenosis who are not candidates for aortic valve replacement.

Aortic stenosis was the only valvular heart disease abnormality found by Goldman and colleagues in their multifactorial cardiac risk index to be associated with an increased risk of perioperative cardiac complications or

death [**A** *Goldman et al, 1978*]. Patients with critical aortic stenosis had a 13% cardiac perioperative mortality, compared with an overall cardiac mortality of 1.9%. Other studies that examined the multifactorial risk index confirmed aortic stenosis to be a risk factor for perioperative cardiac complications. Additional studies found that **aortic stenosis is a risk factor for perioperative cardiac mortality and nonfatal MI, and the severity of aortic stenosis is highly predictive of these complications** [**B** *Kertai et al, 2004*]. One of the hemodynamic consequences of severe aortic stenosis is fixed cardiac output resulting from left ventricular outflow tract obstruction. Patients are unable to increase cardiac output in response to the stress of surgery, and they have decreased left ventricular compliance related to left ventricular hypertrophy. Patients become dependent on adequate preload. Hypovolemia and the vasodilation that may accompany spinal anesthesia or vasodilators are tolerated poorly and may result in profound hypotension. The onset of atrial fibrillation with loss of the atrial contribution to ventricular filling may lead to severe hemodynamic compromise.

I believe that the perioperative approach to patients with aortic stenosis must be individualized and based on the severity of the aortic stenosis, patients' symptoms, left ventricular function, and the anticipated hemodynamic demands of the surgical procedure. All patients with aortic stenosis should receive bacterial endocarditis prophylaxis if indicated. **Most patients with asymptomatic severe aortic stenosis who require urgent noncardiac surgery can do so at relatively low risk with monitoring of anesthesia and attention to fluid balance** [**C** *Bonow et al, 2006*]. Patients with symptomatic severe aortic stenosis or aortic stenosis associated with severe left ventricular dysfunction should undergo aortic valve replacement before noncardiac surgical procedures if possible. If the noncardiac operation cannot be delayed or if patients are not candidates for aortic valve replacement, the risks and benefits of aortic valvuloplasty must be considered. If patients are not candidates for aortic balloon valvuloplasty and surgery is absolutely necessary, the surgical procedure is performed under the guidance of invasive hemodynamic monitoring. The use of vasodilators and anesthetic techniques that may cause vasodilation is avoided if possible.

A unique clinical association that may result in the need for noncardiac surgery in the patient with severe aortic stenosis is bleeding from gastrointestinal dysplasia (Heyde's syndrome). In this syndrome, bleeding often ceases after aortic valve replacement. Although the cause of this relationship is unknown, there have been case reports of deficiency of von Willebrand factor that has normalized after aortic valve replacement.

Treatment of Patients with Prosthetic Heart Valves

The major concerns for the patient with a prosthetic heart valve who undergoes noncardiac surgical procedures are the management of anticoagulation for the patient with a mechanical valve and the need for endocarditis prophylaxis. Few trials describe the rates of prosthetic valve thrombosis in patients who are not receiving anticoagulants. Overall, the risk of valve thrombosis or thromboembolism is higher in patients with valve prostheses in the mitral position. Although data are scant, the incidence of valve thrombosis is probably greater in patients who are not receiving anticoagulants and who have tilting disk valves (e.g., Bjork-Shiley) and lower in patients with leaflet valves (e.g., St. Jude).

Guidelines of the ACC/AHA define the following as risk factors for thrombotic complications in patients with prosthetic heart valves: atrial fibrillation, thromboembolism, left ventricular dysfunction, hypercoagulable conditions, older-generation thrombogenic valves, mechanical tricuspid valves, and the presence of more than one mechanical valve. For patients at low risk of thrombosis (e.g., bileaflet aortic valve with normal left ventricular function), it is recommended that warfarin be stopped 48 to 72 hours preoperatively, so the INR falls to less than 1.5, and restarted within 24 hours after the procedure. For patients at high risk of thrombosis without anticoagulation (e.g., mechanical valve in the mitral position, mechanical aortic valve with one or more of the foregoing risk factors), therapeutic unfractionated heparin should be started when the INR falls to less than 2.0. The heparin should be stopped 4 to 6 hours preoperatively and restarted after the surgical procedure as soon as hemostasis allows. Heparin is continued until the INR becomes therapeutic. The guidelines do support the consideration of low-molecular-weight heparin to prevent valve thrombosis during the period of subtherapeutic INR. For patients at low risk of intraoperative bleeding while they are anticoagulated (e.g., cataract surgery, superficial procedures), my approach has been to reduce the INR briefly to the low or subtherapeutic range preoperatively and to resume the patient's maintenance dose of warfarin after the procedure. Dental extractions can be safely performed on patients at a therapeutic level of anticoagulation.

BACTERIAL ENDOCARDITIS PROPHYLAXIS

In 2007 the AHA issued a major revision of their 1997 guideline for the prevention of infective endocarditis. This guideline revision was based on the following observations: (1) Infective endocarditis is more likely to result from exposure to random bacteremia than from bacteremia caused by a dental, gastrointestinal tract, or genitourinary tract procedure; (2) antibiotic prophylaxis may prevent an exceedingly small number of cases of infective endocarditis that are related to dental, gastrointestinal tract, or genitourinary tract procedures; (3) the risk of antibiotic-associated adverse events exceeds the benefit, if any, from prophylactic antibiotic therapy; (4) maintenance of oral health and hygiene is more important than prophylactic antibiotics in reducing the risk of infective endocarditis; and (5) published data do not demonstrate a benefit from antibiotic prophylaxis.

The revised guidelines recommend that antibiotic prophylaxis be administered only to patients who have cardiac abnormalities associated with the highest risk of adverse outcomes from endocarditis (Box 7-3). This revision, therefore, serves to restrict markedly the number of individuals for whom endocarditis prophylaxis is recommended.

The guideline listing surgical procedures warranting perioperative prophylaxis in this high-risk patient population includes (1) dental procedures that involve manipulation of gingival tissues or periapical regions of teeth or perforation of oral mucosa, (2) invasive procedures of the respiratory tract that involve incision or biopsy of the respiratory mucosa (i.e., tonsillectomy and adenoidectomy), and (3) surgery

---

Box 7-3	CARDIAC CONDITIONS ASSOCIATED WITH THE HIGHEST RISK OF ADVERSE OUTCOME FROM ENDOCARDITIS FOR WHICH PROPHYLAXIS WITH DENTAL PROCEDURES IS RECOMMENDED

Prosthetic cardiac valve

Previous infective endocarditis

Congenital heart disease (CHD)*

Unrepaired cyanotic CHD, including palliative shunts and conduits

Completely repaired congenital heart defect with prosthetic material or device, whether placed by surgery or by catheter intervention, during the first 6 months after the procedure[†]

Repaired CHD with residual defects at the site or adjacent to the site of a prosthetic patch or prosthetic device (which inhibit endothelialization)

---

*Except for the conditions listed above, antibiotic prophylaxis is no longer recommended for any other form of CHD.

[†]Prophylaxis is recommended because endothelialization of prosthetic material occurs within 6 months after the procedure.

From Wilson W, Taubert KA, Gewitz M, et al: Prevention of infective endocarditis. Guidelines from the American Heart Association. Circulation 116:1736-1754, 2007.

involving infected skin, skin structures, or musculoskeletal tissue.

Antibiotic prophylaxis is no longer routinely recommended for genitourinary or gastrointestinal tract procedures. Despite the absence of findings from published studies, it is recommended that patients at high cardiac risk for endocarditis who have an established genitourinary or gastrointestinal tract infection include in their antibiotic regimens an agent active against enterococci, such as penicillin, ampicillin, piperacillin, or vancomycin. For high-risk patients scheduled for an elective cystoscopy or other manipulation of the urinary tract, it is recommended that enterococcal urinary tract infection or colonization be eradicated before the procedure, if possible. Unchanged from the 1997 infective endocarditis antibiotic prophylaxis guideline is the recommendation that antibiotic prophylaxis not be given to the patient who undergoes vaginal delivery and vaginal hysterectomy.

Prophylactic antibiotic regimens should focus on the bacteria at the surgical site most likely to result in bacteremia and endocarditis. For oral and respiratory tract procedures, the relevant bacteria are viridans group streptococci (Table 7-3); for procedures of the gastrointestinal or genitourinary tract, prophylaxis is aimed at enterococci; and for procedures on infected skin, skin structures, or musculoskeletal tissue, the target bacteria are staphylococci and β-hemolytic streptococci.

HYPERTROPHIC CARDIOMYOPATHY

Patients with hypertrophic cardiomyopathy with left ventricular outflow tract obstruction are at risk for worsening of left ventricular outflow tract obstruction in the perioperative period. Factors that may lead to worsening of the left ventricular outflow tract gradient include excessive reductions in preload and afterload, as may occur with volume depletion or vasodilator therapy. Perioperative catecholamine release may directly act on the left ventricular outflow tract to increase myocardial contractility and increase the outflow tract gradient.

TABLE 7-3	Regimens for a Dental Procedure		
Regimen: Single Dose 30-60 Minutes before Procedure			
Situation	**Agent**	**Adults**	**Children**
Oral	Amoxicillin	2 g	50 mg/kg
Unable to take oral medication	Ampicillin OR	2 g IM or IV	50 mg/kd IM or IV
	cefazolin or ceftriaxone	1 g IM or IV	50 mg/kg IM or IV
Allergic to penicillins or ampicillin—oral	Cephalexin*† OR	2 g	50 mg/kg
	clindamycin OR	600 mg	20 mg/kg
	azithromycin or clarithro-mycin	500 mg	15 mg/kg
Allergic to penicillins or ampicillin and unable to take oral medication	Cefazolin or ceftriaxone† OR	1 g IM or IV	50 mg/kg IM or IV
	clindamycin	600 mg IM or IV	20 mg/kg IM or IV

*Or other first- or second-generation oral cephalosporin in equivalent adult or pediatric dosage.

†Cephalosporins should not be used in an individual with a history of anaphylaxis, angioedema, or urticaria with penicillins or ampicillin.

IM, intramuscularly; IV, intravenously.

From Wilson W, Taubert KA, Gewitz M, et al: Prevention of infective endocarditis. Guidelines from the American Heart Association. Circulation 116:1736-1754, 2007.

PREOPERATIVE ARRHYTHMIAS, PERIOPERATIVE ARRHYTHMIAS, CONDUCTION ABNORMALITIES, PACEMAKER MANAGEMENT, AND AUTOMATIC IMPLANTABLE CARDIOVERTER-DEFIBRILLATOR MANAGEMENT

Incidence and Clinical Significance of Perioperative Arrhythmias

Cardiac arrhythmias are common in the perioperative period, and they are usually clinically insignificant. In one study using continuous electrocardiographic monitoring, 84% of patients were documented to have at least transient arrhythmias during their hospitalization for a surgical procedure. Only 5% of these arrhythmias were clinically important. In another study, a 62% incidence of one or more transient arrhythmias in the perioperative period was documented. The dysrhythmias were primarily supraventricular, most commonly wandering atrial pacemaker, isorhythmic AV dissociation, nodal rhythm, and sinus bradycardia. Ventricular premature contractions were common, but paroxysmal ventricular tachycardia was rare. The Multicenter Study of General Anesthesia reported a 70.2% incidence of tachycardia, bradycardia, or dysrhythmia in more than 17,000 patients who underwent a variety of surgical procedures. Adverse outcomes as a result of these dysrhythmias were reported in only 1.6% of the patients.

In a study of men who underwent noncardiac surgical procedures and had known coronary artery disease or significant risk factors for coronary artery disease, frequent or major ventricular arrhythmias (>30 ventricular premature contractions/hour or ventricular tachycardia) occurred in 44% of the patients who were monitored (21% before operation, 16% during operation, and 36% after operation). Preoperative ventricular arrhythmias were associated with the occurrence of intraoperative and postoperative arrhythmias. These arrhythmias were largely benign, and sustained ventricular tachycardia or ventricular fibrillation did not occur.

Multifactorial risk indices identified preoperative ventricular premature contractions and rhythms other than sinus rhythm and markers of risk in noncardiac surgery. I currently believe that ventricular premature contractions and related ventricular ectopy are markers of risk when they occur in the presence of ischemic or structural heart disease. The ACC/AHA practice guideline on perioperative cardiovascular evaluation for noncardiac surgery classifies symptomatic ventricular arrhythmias in the presence of underlying heart disease, supraventricular arrhythmias with uncontrolled ventricular rate, and high-grade AV block in the presence of underlying heart disease as major clinical predictors of increased perioperative cardiovascular risk. This guideline classifies preoperative rhythm other than sinus rhythm (e.g., atrial fibrillation) as a minor risk factor.

I look for evidence of structural or ischemic heart disease, metabolic derangements, and electrolyte abnormalities when arrhythmias or conduction abnormalities are identified preoperatively. I do not consider preoperative ventricular premature contractions or complex ventricular arrhythmias in the absence of heart disease or metabolic or electrolyte abnormality to be significant risk factors. Patients with atrial premature contractions and supraventricular arrhythmias that occur without the development of hemodynamic instability are also not considered to be at increased risk. Although the presence of atrial fibrillation is a minor risk factor for cardiac complication, a challenge in the perioperative period is adjustment of anticoagulation regimens for those patients who are receiving long-term anticoagulant therapy. Patients with chronic atrial fibrillation may be treated with medications to control the ventricular response or with medications to maintain sinus rhythm. Care is required to maintain these medications or appropriate substitutes in the perioperative period.

Risk Factors for and Etiology of Perioperative Arrhythmias and Conduction Abnormalities

In a study of patients who underwent noncardiac surgery and developed supraventricular arrhythmias in the perioperative period, Polanczyk and associates identified the following preoperative correlates for the development of perioperative arrhythmia: male sex (odds ratio [OR], 1.3; 95% confidence interval [CI], 1.0 to 1.7), age 70 years or older (OR, 1.3; CI, 1.0 to 1.7), significant valvular disease (OR, 2.1; CI, 1.2 to 3.6), history of SVA (OR, 3.4; CI, 2.4 to 4.8) or asthma (OR, 2.0; CI, 1.3 to 3.1), CHF (OR, 1.7; CI, 1.1 to 2.7), premature atrial complexes on the preoperative ECG (OR, 2.1; CI, 1.3 to 3.4), American Society of Anesthesiologists class III or IV (OR, 1.4;

CI, 1.1 to 1.9), and type of procedure: abdominal aortic aneurysm (OR, 3.9; CI, 2.4 to 6.3) or abdominal (OR, 2.5; CI, 1.7 to 3.6), vascular (OR, 1.6; CI, 1.1 to 2.4), and intrathoracic (OR, 9.2; CI, 6.7 to 13) procedures. Multiple studies have shown that the only consistent independent risk factor for postoperative atrial fibrillation is age 60 years or older.

Sinus tachycardia is common in the perioperative period and often results from catecholamine release precipitated by stress, pain, or anxiety. Hypovolemia or anemia may cause sinus tachycardia as a compensatory response to increase cardiac output. Less common but ominous causes of sinus tachycardia are perioperative CHF and MI. The anesthetic agent ketamine may induce sinus tachycardia as a result of central sympathetic stimulation. Hypercarbia and hypoxemia resulting from inadequate ventilation may cause sinus tachycardia as well as ventricular tachycardia.

Bradycardia is seen frequently during hospitalization for surgery and has numerous causes. Narcotics, with the exception of meperidine, may cause bradycardia by producing central vagal stimulation. Anticholinesterases administered to antagonize the effect of nondepolarizing neuromuscular blocking agents may result in bradycardia. An imbalance between sympathetic and parasympathetic tone may be produced in patients undergoing spinal or epidural anesthesia if cardiac stimulating sympathetic fibers are anesthetized. This situation can occur if the spinal cord is anesthetized at the level of the sympathetic ganglia (T1 to T4) or if spinal anesthesia is placed two to six segments distant from this region because the anesthetic agent may migrate or ascending preganglionic sympathetic fibers in the paravertebral chain may be blocked. Unopposed parasympathetic (vagal) activity may occur and may lead to peripheral vasodilation and hypotension in addition to bradycardia.

Reflex bradycardia, occasionally associated with heart block and sinus arrest, may occur during surgical procedures (Table 7-4). It is usually caused by a reflex arc whose efferent

TABLE 7-4	Reflex Bradycardia during Surgery
Surgical Procedure	**Afferent Reflex Pathway**
Abdominal manipulation	Celiac plexus
Mesenteric traction	?
Liver biopsy	Hepatic, celiac plexus
Laparoscopy	Parasympathetic stimulation from peritoneal stimulation
Ocular stimulation (oculocardiac reflex)	Parasympathetic fibers in the ciliary nerves and the ophthalmic nerve run to the trigeminal nerve adjacent to the nucleus ambiguus, which is the origin of the vagus
Maxilla or zygoma	Trigeminal nerve stimulation
Neurosurgery (tentorium stimulation)	Ophthalmic nerve innervates tentorium; reflex similar to oculocardiac reflex
Laryngoscopy	Laryngeal stimulation
Blepharoplasty	Same as oculocardiac reflex

limb is the vagus nerve. In addition to bradycardia, this vagally mediated reflex may result in peripheral vasodilation and hypotension. Anesthetic agents such as vecuronium, atracurium, halothane, fentanyl, and succinylcholine may predispose to this reflex. It can be prevented by premedication with an anticholinergic agent such as atropine. If reflex bradycardia does occur, it often can be terminated by discontinuing the procedure or administering anticholinergic agents.

In O'Kelly's study of perioperative ventricular arrhythmias, the presence of preoperative ventricular ectopy was the most significant predictor of intraoperative and postoperative ventricular arrhythmias. Other risk factors were a history of CHF and a history of cigarette smoking. Additional causes of perioperative arrhythmias include hypoxia, hypercarbia, and acute hypokalemia.

Arrhythmias may be precipitated by medications used specifically during ophthalmic surgery as a result of systemic absorption of eye drops. Ophthalmic atropine has been reported to cause supraventricular tachycardia and atrial fibrillation, whereas timolol and pilocarpine eye drops have been reported to cause bradycardia.

Patients with Preoperative Cardiac Arrhythmias

Atrial Fibrillation

If atrial fibrillation is detected during the initial preoperative evaluation, I often delay nonemergency surgical procedures and evaluate the patient as in my approach to patients with newly diagnosed atrial fibrillation who are not undergoing surgical procedures. I attempt to identify precipitating causes. An echocardiogram is performed to evaluate for the presence of structural cardiac abnormalities. Electrolytes as well as thyroid function are assessed. Because the AFFIRM trial found that rhythm control was not superior in terms of mortality to rate control with antithrombotic therapy in patients with persistent or recurrent atrial fibrillation, my approach in patients with newly diagnosed atrial fibrillation is to assess the need for restoration of sinus rhythm versus rate control of atrial fibrillation, to evaluate the need for antithrombotic therapy to prevent stroke, and to control the ventricular response of the atrial fibrillation appropriately. If the patient is unstable (e.g., pulmonary edema, unstable angina), urgent cardioversion may have to be performed. If the patient is stable, my approach is to slow the ventricular rate with AV nodal blocking agents (e.g., diltiazem, verapamil, esmolol, metoprolol, propranolol). Up to two thirds of patients will spontaneously convert to sinus rhythm within 24 hours of the onset of atrial fibrillation. If I am unable to determine the duration of the patient's atrial fibrillation, I initiate warfarin anticoagulation to decrease the likelihood of systemic embolism. For the patient in whom cardioversion is planned, either I perform cardioversion after 3 weeks of therapeutic warfarin therapy or, as an alternate approach, I perform transesophageal echocardiography and attempt cardioversion if there is no evidence of left atrial thrombi. In both approaches, warfarin is continued with maintenance of INR 2.0 to 3.0 for 3 to 4 weeks following conversion. I then schedule the surgical procedure after completion of this warfarin course.

For the patient with chronic atrial fibrillation who receives long-term anticoagulation, the recommendations of the ACC/AHA/European Society of Cardiology 2006 guideline for the management of patients with atrial fibrillation are that for patients with mechanical prosthetic heart valves or those at high risk for systemic thromboembolic phenomena (e.g., prior stroke, transient ischemic attack, systemic embolism), unfractionated or low-molecular-weight heparin should be substituted for warfarin in the perioperative period. My approach to managing the anticoagulants for this high-risk group is to stop warfarin 4 days preoperatively and to begin therapy with full-dose unfractionated heparin, or low-molecular-weight heparin is begun when INR falls to less than the therapeutic level. Unfractionated heparin is discontinued 6 hours preoperatively, whereas if low-molecular-weight heparin is used, it is stopped 12 to 24 hours before the surgical procedure. Heparin (full-dose unfractionated or low-molecular-weight heparin) is restarted along with warfarin as soon as possible following surgery. Heparin is continued until the INR rises to the therapeutic range. **For the patient with atrial fibrillation who does not have a mechanical prosthetic valve or other high-risk markers for thromboembolic phenomena, the guideline suggests that anticoagulation may be interrupted for a period of up to 1 week without substituting heparin for a surgical procedure that carries a risk of bleeding** [● *Fuster et al, 2006*].

Ventricular Arrhythmias

Patients are commonly found to have asymptomatic ventricular ectopy at the time of preoperative evaluation. When significant ventricular ectopy (e.g., frequent ventricular premature contractions, nonsustained ventricular tachycardia) is identified, I search for a metabolic cause such as hypoxia or hypokalemia. If none is identified, I then search for the presence of underlying structural cardiac disease and perform an echocardiogram to evaluate left ventricular function. I frequently perform an exercise stress test or vasodilator myocardial imaging to investigate the possibility that myocardial ischemia is playing a role, although this is controversial in patients without symptoms of ischemic disease. In the patient with normal left ventricular function and no evidence of inducible myocardial ischemia, asymptomatic ventricular ectopy is usually benign. Patients with severe left ventricular dysfunction or inducible myocardial ischemia as a cause of ventricular ectopy are at increased risk of death. These patients are further evaluated in terms of the reversibility of their cardiac dysfunction. For the patient with ischemic left ventricular dysfunction (LVEF ≤30% to 40%) that is optimized on a long-term medical regimen, prophylactic placement of a cardiac defibrillator is considered if the expected survival with good functional capacity exceeds 1 year. The recommendation is similar for the patient with nonischemic cardiomyopathy, although the threshold for defibrillator placement in this group is an LVEF 30% to 35% or lower.

Special consideration must be given to patients who take the antiarrhythmic agent amiodarone. This drug is used to treat serious ventricular arrhythmias and, in low doses, to treat supraventricular tachycardia and atrial fibrillation. One side effect of this drug is chronic pulmonary interstitial disease. Acute life-threatening pulmonary complications such as the acute respiratory distress syndrome have been observed in patients undergoing cardiac, as well as noncardiac, surgical procedures while receiving amiodarone. Respiratory failure has been reported 16 to 72 hours postoperatively, unrelated to the dose of amiodarone. Amiodarone levels persist in the body for weeks after its use has been discontinued, and amiodarone-related postoperative adult respiratory distress syndrome has been observed in patients who stopped taking the drug 6 days preoperatively. The cause of this complication is speculative and may be linked to oxidative lung injury induced by high concentrations of inspired oxygen in the perioperative period. This acute amiodarone pulmonary toxicity should be kept in mind for the patient receiving amiodarone who develops perioperative acute respiratory distress syndrome.

Identification and Treatment of Specific Disorders of Cardiac Rate and Rhythm

The guiding principle in the treatment of perioperative cardiac arrhythmias is that the cause of the arrhythmia should be treated and reversed if possible. In the setting of an unstable or life-threatening tachyarrhythmia, cardioversion is frequently utilized to restore regular rhythm while the cause of the arrhythmia is being identified and treated.

Common causes of perioperative arrhythmias are catecholamine release, alterations in autonomic tone, electrolyte abnormalities (e.g., acute hypokalemia, hyperkalemia), acid-base disturbances (e.g., acidosis, alkalosis), anemia, and acute volume depletion. Less commonly, myocardial ischemia is the cause of serious cardiac arrhythmias or conduction abnormalities. Indications for the treatment of perioperative arrhythmias include hemodynamic instability, myocardial ischemia, and MI or the suspicion that these deleterious consequences may occur if the arrhythmia persists.

Sinus Tachycardia

Sinus tachycardia is the most common perioperative rhythm abnormality and is almost always benign. It is characterized by a heart rate between 100 and 160 beats/minute. The ECG demonstrates a regular rhythm with a normal P wave before each QRS complex. The QRS complex is normal unless patients have myocardial ischemia, aberrant ventricular conduction, or conduction abnormalities. The most common causes of sinus tachycardia are pain, hypovolemia, anemia, hypoxia, fever, and hypercarbia. Treatment is directed at the inciting factor. Patients with coronary artery disease may develop myocardial ischemia as a result of increased heart rate and increased myocardial oxygen demand. β-Adrenergic blockers may be beneficial in this instance to decrease the heart rate and to alleviate myocardial ischemia while the underlying cause of the sinus tachycardia is treated.

Atrial Premature Contractions

Atrial premature contractions are of minor clinical significance, but they may be harbingers of supraventricular tachycardia or atrial fibrillation. They arise in the atria at a site other than the sinus node and therefore are represented on the ECG by a P wave that has a different configuration and occurs earlier in the cardiac cycle than a normal P wave. Atrial premature contractions typically produce a normal QRS complex. If the premature contraction arrives at the ventricular conduction tissue when it is still refractory and has not fully repolarized, it may produce an absent QRS complex or one that is abnormal as a result of aberrant ventricular conduction. The aberrant QRS complex is usually of right bundle branch block morphology because the refractory period of the right bundle is longer than that of the left bundle.

Atrial Flutter and Atrial Fibrillation

No evidence-based guidelines are available for the treatment of atrial fibrillation that occurs following noncardiac surgical procedures. The ACC/AHA/European Society of Cardiology guidelines for the management of patients with atrial fibrillation provide recommendations for treatment of atrial fibrillation that occurs in relation to cardiac surgery. The guidelines do not address atrial flutter or fibrillation that occurs as a result of noncardiac surgery. My recommendations are adapted in large part from my approach to atrial flutter and atrial fibrillation in the nonsurgical setting. I treat perioperative atrial flutter and atrial fibrillation in similar fashion.

Hemodynamic instability and the presence of myocardial ischemia or CHF dictate the treatment that should be employed for postoperative atrial flutter or atrial fibrillation. If atrial fibrillation causes the patient to be unstable, then the immediate goal is to restore sinus rhythm, usually by direct current (DC) cardioversion. If the arrhythmia is well tolerated, the initial plan should be to control the ventricular rate. If patients remain in atrial flutter or fibrillation and are hemodynamically stable, conversion to sinus rhythm may be attempted under elective conditions.

Acute rate control is typically achieved with a continuous intravenous infusion of β-blocker or diltiazem. When patients are switched from continuous intravenous medications to oral medications, I prefer to use β-blockers (if it is possible to do so) because of the long-term beneficial effects of β-blockers in patients with ischemic heart disease.

The postoperative treatment of persistent atrial fibrillation has not been standardized; different centers have different approaches. The basic decision is whether it is best to pursue rhythm control aggressively or whether it is preferable to employ a rate control strategy. Investigators in one study of cardiac surgical patients with postoperative atrial fibrillation who were treated with a rate control strategy noted that 90% of their patients were in sinus rhythm at 4 weeks. I assess the patient's risk of systemic thromboembolism related to atrial fibrillation, and if the risk is moderate or high, I utilize systemic anticoagulation for several weeks postoperatively if the patient has a low risk for bleeding. After that period, the patient's risk for recurrent atrial fibrillation is reassessed, and a decision about long-term therapy can be made.

For patients at high risk for developing bleeding complications and those in whom ventricular rate control is difficult, a rhythm control approach is frequently undertaken. In such patients, I usually restore sinus rhythm with DC electrical countershock. Most antiarrhythmic medications have only moderate efficacy in terminating atrial fibrillation. However, ibutilide, a class III antiarrhythmic medication, is effective in terminating atrial flutter of recent onset. Ibutilide can also be used to lower the atrial defibrillation threshold, an approach that allows a higher success rate for electrical cardioversion. The shorter the duration of the atrial fibrillation, the better the success rate of cardioversion will be. However, new-onset atrial fibrillation has a high spontaneous conversion rate to sinus rhythm.

Because of the known increased risk of acute thromboembolic complication following cardioversion, I do not perform pharmacologic or electrical cardioversion if atrial fibrillation or flutter has persisted for more than 24 to 48 hours. If a rhythm control approach is undertaken, antiarrhythmic medications are usually initiated to prevent the recurrence of atrial fibrillation if the patient reverts to sinus rhythm spontaneously. I prefer to use a class III antiarrhythmic medication, either sotalol or amiodarone, in patients with structural heart disease. I do not use class IC drugs such as propafenone or flecainide in patients with ischemic heart disease; however, I frequently use them in patients without ischemic heart disease.

I prefer to discontinue antiarrhythmic medications 4 to 8 weeks postoperatively unless the patient is at high risk for recurrent atrial fibrillation. No large randomized studies have been performed evaluating the risk-to-benefit ratio of systemic anticoagulation or comparing rhythm control to rate control for the management of postoperative atrial fibrillation. Therefore, an individual approach is required in the management of these conditions.

Of all noncardiac surgical procedures, thoracic operations are probably most often complicated by the onset of postoperative atrial fibrillation. The peak incidence of atrial fibrillation that accompanies thoracic surgery is between postoperative days 2 and 4. The mechanism for thoracic surgery–induced atrial fibrillation is unclear. The pulmonary veins in nonsurgical patients have been found to be a trigger zone for the onset of atrial fibrillation as well as an important factor to sustain atrial fibrillation once it starts. Manipulation of the pulmonary veins may play a role in the occurrence of atrial fibrillation following thoracic surgery. Digoxin is particularly ineffective in the control of ventricular response to atrial fibrillation that follows thoracic surgical procedures.

Paroxysmal Supraventricular Tachycardia

Paroxysmal supraventricular tachycardia (PSVT) is characterized by the sudden onset of a rapid regular rhythm with rates between 150 and 250 beats/minute. The most common mechanism requires two different electrical pathways, one to conduct more rapidly than the other. With *AV nodal reentrant tachycardia* (AVNRT), the most common type of PSVT, a premature atrial complex that is blocked in the fast pathway and is redirected through the slow pathway typically triggers the tachycardia. The electrical impulse, after proceeding down the slow pathway, reenters the fast pathway in retrograde fashion. It then travels back, in antegrade fashion, toward the ventricles and again reenters the fast pathway to travel back to the atria in retrograde fashion. In AVNRT this circuit is found in the AV node. Reentrant PSVT that utilizes an accessory pathway outside the AV node (e.g., Wolff-Parkinson-White syndrome) is called *AV reentrant tachycardia* (AVRT). On occasion, atrial tachycardia or atrial flutter has the 12-lead ECG pattern of PSVT.

The management of PSVT is identical regardless of whether the mechanism is AVNRT or AVRT. If patients are hemodynamically unstable and have angina or CHF because of the tachycardia, immediate synchronized DC cardioversion should be performed. PSVT is usually responsive to DC cardioversion with a synchronized 50-J monophasic shock. If a 50-J monophasic shock does not restore sinus rhythm, then shocks at higher energy levels should be administered (i.e., 100 J, 200 J). If the QRS complex is wide and the rhythm has not been definitely proved to be supraventricular, the arrhythmia should be treated as ventricular tachycardia. If patients are hemodynamically stable during narrow-complex PSVT, vagal maneuvers or medical therapy (e.g., adenosine, calcium channel blockers, β-blockers) may suffice to terminate the arrhythmia. Vagal maneuvers slow conduction through the AV node by increasing parasympathetic tone. These maneuvers terminate the arrhythmia by disrupting the reentrant circuit that is necessary to sustain the tachycardia. The most effective vagal maneuver is the Valsalva maneuver (54% termination rate). However, the Valsalva maneuver may be impossible to perform in the perioperative period, either because of the inability of patients to cooperate or because of the high sympathetic tone. Carotid sinus massage has a success rate of 17% using the right carotid and 5% using the left, and it may be the easiest vagal maneuver to perform in the perioperative period. It must be performed while using electrocardiographic monitoring; intravenous atropine and other antiarrhythmic drugs should be available in the event that advanced heart block or another arrhythmia occurs. Carotid sinus massage should not be used in elderly patients or in those with carotid bruits or known cerebrovascular disease because of the risk of inducing a stroke. If vagal maneuvers are unsuccessful or contraindicated and patients remain hemodynamically stable, intravenous adenosine should be administered. This agent is the initial drug of choice for the conversion of hemodynamically stable PSVT and is successful in more than 90% of cases. Adenosine should be given as a 6-mg rapid infusion over 1 to 3 seconds. If conversion is not achieved after 1 or 2 minutes, an additional 12-mg rapid infusion should be given. If the second dose is unsuccessful and the patient remains hemodynamically stable, then the 2005 guidelines for Advanced Cardiac Life Support (ACLS) suggest that further treatment consist of an attempt at rate control with intravenous diltiazem or β-blocker. If patients become hemodynamically unstable during attempts at conversion to sinus rhythm using medical therapy, DC cardioversion should be performed promptly. In one of the few studies of PSVT in postsurgical patients, adenosine had only a 44% successful conversion rate, and arrhythmia recurrences were common (52% of patients). The high recurrence rate of PSVT suggests that many patients will require suppressive therapy while they are critically ill.

Multifocal Atrial Tachycardia

Multifocal atrial tachycardia (MAT) is an automatic arrhythmia characterized by an atrial rate greater than 100 beats/minute with organized, discrete, nonsinus P waves of at least three different forms in the same lead on the ECG. MAT is usually associated with severe pulmonary disease and often accompanies critical illness. When the onset of MAT occurs in the perioperative period, respiratory failure, pneumonia, and CHF are common causes. Therapy centers on treating the pulmonary, cardiac, or other acute illness that led to the onset of the arrhythmia. When MAT persists despite these maneuvers, additional medical therapy may be indicated if the arrhythmia is hemodynamically significant (i.e., contributing to hypotension, CHF, or myocardial ischemia). Intravenous magnesium may be helpful for patients with hypomagnesemia or hypokalemia. β-Blockers may be effective in decreasing the ventricular rate, but these drugs must be used with extreme caution, if at all, in patients with reversible airway disease or severe acute CHF. For patients with bronchospastic lung disease, verapamil may be used instead of β-blockers. This drug slows the tachycardia rate by decreasing the degree of atrial ectopy. Digitalis preparations are rarely effective in the treatment of MAT. Aminophylline, even at therapeutic levels, may aggravate the tachycardia by increasing the atrial rate and the number of ectopic atrial beats. MAT is usually resistant to DC cardioversion as well as to therapy with quinidine, lidocaine, and procainamide.

Ventricular Premature Contractions and Nonsustained Ventricular Tachycardia

No specific medical therapy is indicated for patients who develop asymptomatic, hemodynamically insignificant ventricular premature contractions or nonsustained ventricular tachycardia in the perioperative period. The cause of these dysrhythmias should be determined and the provoking factors corrected if possible. Common causes of acute ventricular arrhythmias in the perioperative period include acute myocardial ischemia, hypoxia, hypokalemia, and hypomagnesemia. Right-sided heart catheters may cause ventricular irritability and ectopy as a result of trauma to the right ventricular outflow tract in patients who require these devices to aid in hemodynamic monitoring during the perioperative period. This condition should resolve on repositioning or removal of the monitoring catheter.

No well-studied data are available regarding the treatment of symptomatic or hemodynamically significant nonsustained ventricular tachycardia that develops acutely in the perioperative period. My approach is to conduct an immediate search for a reversible cause. I occasionally initiate medical antiarrhythmic therapy with intravenous β-blockers, lidocaine, or procainamide.

Sustained Ventricular Tachycardia and Ventricular Fibrillation

Patients who develop sustained ventricular tachycardia or ventricular fibrillation in the perioperative period should be treated according to the ACLS protocol. Patients who have ventricular fibrillation or hemodynamically unstable ventricular tachycardia should undergo immediate DC cardioversion. For the patient with hemodynamically stable ventricular tachycardia, an alternate approach to cardioversion is the use of intravenous amiodarone or lidocaine. If these agents are ineffective in restoring normal rhythm, DC cardioversion should be performed. Readers are referred to the ACLS guidelines for further information (http://circ.ahajournals.org/cgi/content/full/112/24_suppl/IV-67).

Wide-Complex Tachycardia of Unknown Type

Supraventricular tachycardia may occasionally be accompanied by aberrant ventricular conduction, resulting in a wide QRS complex. Although criteria have been established to aid in the identification of the arrhythmia, a definite diagnosis is often elusive. A 12-lead ECG should be obtained. When AV dissociation is present (e.g., loss of a 1:1 relationship between

P wave and QRS complex), the ECG is highly specific for ventricular tachycardia. I treat the patient with perioperative wide-complex tachycardia of unknown type in the manner recommended by the 2005 ACLS Guidelines. For the hemodynamically stable patient, I utilize intravenous amiodarone (150 mg intravenously run over 10 minutes, maximum total dose 2.2 g in 24 hours). If this is ineffective or if the patient develops hemodynamic instability, synchronized cardioversion should be used.

Perioperative Conduction Abnormalities

In the perioperative period, sinus bradycardia and Mobitz I type of second-degree AV block are common. Mobitz I AV block is a progressive prolongation of the P-R interval until a P wave is not conducted to the ventricles. The P wave that follows is conducted to the ventricles with a P-R interval that is shorter than the P-R interval that was associated with the last conducted P wave. These conduction abnormalities usually result from enhanced vagal tone and, if they are hemodynamically significant, typically respond to 0.5 to 1 mg of intravenous atropine.

Mobitz II second-degree AV block (a fixed P-R interval with P wave conduction to the ventricles blocked on a constant [e.g., 2:1, 3:1, 4:1] or variable basis) is usually caused by diffuse disease of the conduction system distal to the AV node. Many patients with this conduction disturbance are at high risk for progression to complete heart block, and a means of providing temporary-demand cardiac pacing should be quickly available in the event this occurs. New-onset Mobitz II AV block in the perioperative period should initiate a search for myocardial ischemia or MI.

Third-degree AV block occurs when no atrial impulses reach the ventricles. An associated ventricular rate of 40 to 60 beats/minute with normal-appearing QRS complexes suggests that the escape rhythm originates at the level of the AV node. This type of heart block may result from enhanced vagal tone, from medications that depress AV nodal conduction (e.g., β-blockers, digitalis), and less commonly, from AV nodal ischemia. It is often reversible and may respond to the administration of intravenous atropine or the discontinuation of offending pharmacologic agents. When complete heart block is associated with a ventricular escape rate of 20 to 40 beats/minute and the QRS complex is wide, the escape rhythm originates from the ventricles. This finding strongly suggests the presence of extensive conduction system disease and warrants the placement of a cardiac pacemaker.

Chronic bifascicular block (i.e., right bundle branch block, with either left anterior hemiblock or left posterior hemiblock, or left bundle branch block) rarely progresses to advanced hemodynamically significant heart block in the perioperative period. The preoperative insertion of a temporary pacemaker therefore is not generally indicated for this patient group. Possible exceptions are patients with preexisting left bundle branch block who are undergoing perioperative pulmonary artery catheterization. Transient right bundle branch block, which is well tolerated in physiologically normal patients, may occur in as many as 5% of patients who undergo pulmonary artery catheterization. Transient complete heart block has been reported in patients with preexisting left bundle branch block who have developed acute right bundle branch block related to this procedure. Given the potential for this significant complication, a method for pacing the left ventricle should be available in the event complete heart block develops in this clinical setting. A temporary pacemaker should be inserted preoperatively if patients meet the criteria for permanent pacemaker implantation and a permanent pacing device has not yet been implanted (Box 7-4).

Long QT Syndrome

The long QT syndrome is a heterogeneous group of disorders characterized by a prolonged QT interval when corrected for heart rate, malignant ventricular arrhythmias (classically the

Box 7-4	SELECTED INDICATIONS FOR IMPLANTATION OF CARDIAC PACEMAKERS

Third-degree or advanced second-degree AV block associated with
  Symptomatic bradycardia
  Documented asystole >3 seconds or escape rate <40 beats/minute in an awake, symptom-free patient
Second-degree AV block, regardless of site or type, with symptomatic bradycardia
Bifascicular block with intermittent complete heart block with symptomatic bradycardia
Symptomatic bifascicular block with intermittent type II second-degree AV block
Sinus node dysfunction with documented symptomatic bradycardia
Following acute myocardial infarction
  Persistent second-degree AV block in the His-Purkinje system with bilateral bundle branch block or third-degree AV block within or below the His-Purkinje system
  Persistent and symptomatic second- or third-degree AV block

AV, atrioventricular.
Adapted from Gregoratus G, Abrams J, Epstein A, et al: ACC/AHA/NASPE 2002 guideline update for implantation of cardiac pacemakers and antiarrhythmia devices. Available at www.acc.org/clinical/guidelines/pacemaker/pacemaker.pdf.

torsades de pointes form of ventricular tachycardia), and the risk of sudden death. It is most commonly acquired as a result of a drug or metabolic abnormality (Box 7-5). It may also occur as a congenital form inherited as a result of either autosomal dominant or recessive genetic mutations. To date, seven different genetic defects have been identified that encode for abnormal cardiac ion channels and that may result in long QT syndrome.

The approach to patients in the perioperative period depends on whether the long QT syndrome is congenital or

Box 7-5	SELECTED CAUSES OF ACQUIRED LONG QT SYNDROME

ANTIARRHYTHMIC DRUGS

Type IA agents (e.g., quinidine, procainamide, disopyramide)
Type III agents (amiodarone, sotalol)

NONCARDIAC DRUGS

Phenothiazines
Tricyclic antidepressants
Haloperidol
Selective serotonin reuptake inhibitors
Antibiotics (e.g., erythromycin, azithromycin, clarithromycin, ampicillin, trimethoprim-sulfamethoxazole, ketoconazole, itraconazole)

METABOLIC AND ELECTROLYTE DISORDERS

Hypokalemia
Hypomagnesemia
Nutritional disorders (starvation, liquid protein diets)

CENTRAL NERVOUS SYSTEM DISORDERS

Subarachnoid hemorrhage
Intracerebral hemorrhage
Head trauma
Encephalitis

acquired. Congenital long QT syndrome is adrenergic dependent, and ventricular arrhythmias are typically provoked by sympathetic stimulation (i.e., pain, physical exertion). Long-term treatment with β-blockers, permanent pacing, or left cervicothoracic sympathectomy is frequently effective. Implantation of an implantable cardioverter-defibrillator (ICD) is recommended for selected patients who have syncope, sustained ventricular arrhythmias, or aborted sudden cardiac death despite this standard therapy. ICD implantation as primary treatment should be considered in the patient in whom aborted sudden cardiac death is the initial presentation of the long QT syndrome and in those patients with long QT syndrome who have a strong family history of sudden cardiac death.

For patients with congenital long QT syndrome, I provide perioperative β-blockade to blunt the adrenergic response to the surgery. β-Blockers also shift the rate-adjusted QT interval to the normal range, and this feature may contribute to their efficacy. I attempt to avoid anesthetics that may prolong the QT interval (e.g., succinylcholine, propofol, enflurane, or halothane). Although isoflurane has been demonstrated to prolong the QT interval in physiologically normal persons, it shortens the QT interval in patients with long QT syndrome and has been proposed as an acceptable anesthetic agent for this patient group. Thiopental has also been reported to prolong the QT interval in physiologically normal persons but has no effect on the QT duration in patients with long QT syndrome. Finally, I minimize sympathetic stimulation and provide adequate sedation to blunt the adrenergic response to surgery. In patients who have acquired long QT syndrome, I discontinue administration of the offending drug or correct the metabolic or electrolyte abnormality before undertaking surgical procedures.

Despite these measures, malignant ventricular arrhythmias may still occur in the patient with long QT syndrome in the perioperative period. The treatment for ventricular ectopy is the same for idiopathic and acquired long QT syndrome. Intravenous magnesium sulfate, 2 g given over 1 to 2 minutes, with a follow-up dose 15 minutes later if required, is often effective in restoring regular rhythm. Immediate ventricular pacing should be used if magnesium sulfate is ineffective. Pacing at rates of 70 to 80 beats/minute may shorten the QT interval and decrease the dispersion of refractoriness of the cardiac conduction system. Intravenous isoproterenol may be used cautiously to increase the heart rate and to suppress ventricular arrhythmia until temporary ventricular pacing is achieved. If these methods are unsuccessful in restoring the patient's baseline stable rhythm, DC cardioversion should be considered.

Cardiac Conduction Issues in the Patient with a Cardiac Transplant Who Requires Noncardiac Surgery

Cardiac physiology is altered after cardiac transplantation. Because the transplanted heart is denervated, cardiac reflexes mediated by the autonomic nervous system are blunted or absent. As a result, heart rate abnormalities may be seen in the perioperative period. The resting heart rate is higher than normal, but the heart rate response to stress is less than that of an innervated heart. When the heart rate does increase as a result of stress, it does so gradually in response to circulating catecholamines. Reflex tachycardia does not occur in response to vasodilation or volume loss. The effect of certain cardiac drugs on cardiac conduction is altered. Agents that affect the heart indirectly through their action on the autonomic nervous system are generally ineffective. Therefore, the chronotropic effect of atropine is absent, as is the AV nodal inhibitory effect of digoxin. The antiarrhythmic efficacy of β-blockers and calcium channel antagonists (e.g., verapamil, diltiazem) is unchanged. The transplanted heart becomes overly sensitive to adenosine, and reduced doses (i.e., one third to one half lower than those given to patients with intact cardiac innervation) should be used when this drug is administered to control arrhythmias.

Bradyarrhythmias Following Acute Spinal Cord Injury

Acute injury to the cervical spinal cord is frequently accompanied by clinically significant bradyarrhythmias and, in some cases, hypotension. Acute autonomic dysfunction is thought to be the cause. Sympathetic nerves exit the spinal cord in preganglionic fibers at the first through fourth thoracic levels. In patients with a complete cervical spinal cord lesion, sympathetic control from higher centers is interrupted. Parasympathetic control, which is mediated by the vagus nerve, is unaffected by spinal cord interruption. The clinical picture is therefore one of unopposed parasympathetic activity in the setting of markedly reduced sympathetic activity. Sympathetic stimulation with low-dose isoproterenol has been used in several patients for the treatment of clinically significant bradyarrhythmias. These cardiovascular abnormalities have been demonstrated to resolve within 14 to 30 days following acute cervical spinal cord injury. The reason for resolution is not known, but it may be related to adaptive sympathetic disinhibition (i.e., loss of reflex sympathetic inhibitory control from higher centers or increase in the number and function of adrenergic receptors).

Management of Permanent Cardiac Pacemakers

Although most pacemakers are implanted as treatment of bradyarrhythmias or conduction system abnormalities, other indications for pacemakers include treatment of heart failure in the patient with severe left ventricular dysfunction (biventricular pacemaker), neurocardiogenic syncope, long QT syndrome, and selected patients with hypertrophic cardiomyopathy. It is important to know the indication that led to implantation of the patient's pacemaker and whether the patient is pacemaker dependent.

There is no industry-wide standard regarding pacemaker programming or estimation of battery reserve. It is therefore important that the type of pacemaker and the name of its manufacturer be identified preoperatively. If the patient or the patient's physician is unable to provide this information, it may be identified by chest radiography, which reveals radiopaque identification markers on the pacemaker generator. The pacemaker should be tested and its settings recorded.

Although pacemaker problems are uncommon in the perioperative period, one series identified a pacemaker abnormality (e.g., inhibition, acceleration, change in pacing mode) in 13% of patients with pacemakers. The most significant pacemaker problem in the perioperative period is alteration of pacemaker function inhibition resulting from electrocautery-induced electromagnetic interference (EMI). If the pacemaker interprets EMI as the patient's electrical heart activity, the pacemaker may be inhibited. If the patient has a dual-chamber pacemaker and EMI is sensed only by the atrial sensing circuitry, then the ventricular pacing channel may pace at the pacemaker upper rate limit. Some pacemakers respond to the "noise" of EMI by pacing in an asynchronous (fixed-rate) mode. Some older pacemakers may respond to EMI by reprogramming. The pacemaker response to the electrical interference of electrocautery may be obtained from the pacemaker manufacturer. This alteration of pacemaker function may be prevented by avoiding the application of electrocautery directly over the pacemaker pulse generator and by keeping the electrocautery current path, which is from electrode tip to the ground plate, as far away as possible from the pulse generator. The pacemaker should be programmed to the asynchronous (fixed-rate) mode so that it does not inhibit in response to EMI. Many pacemakers operate in an asynchronous mode if a magnet is applied to the skin over the pulse generator. Although that has been a common approach to perioperative pacemaker management, some newer pacemakers have a programmable option that prevents this pacemaker response to magnet application.

Since the early 1990s, many pacemakers have adaptive rate systems devised to facilitate a change in heart rate response to a change in the desired cardiac output. Various biologic parameters have been used to trigger heart rate responses. The most common parameters include sensation of vibration at the pulse generator site as a manifestation of perceived patient physical activity and respiratory rate as determined by a minute ventilation sensor. The adaptive rate system may therefore sense surgically induced vibration or shivering, which commonly occurs on recovery from anesthesia, and may thus pace inappropriately at a high rate. Similarly, intraoperative hyperventilation may also lead the pacemaker to generate a faster heart rate than actually desired if the pacemaker adaptive rate sensor is linked to the patient's minute ventilation. For these reasons, the rate responsive feature should be deactivated during surgical procedures.

For patients who require placement of central venous catheters or right-sided heart pulmonary artery catheters, care should be taken to avoid tangling these catheters in the pacemaker leads. Newly placed pacemaker leads are at risk of becoming dislodged by right-sided heart catheter insertion. For the patient who requires external defibrillation, electrical discharge to the pacemaker will be minimized if the defibrillator paddles are placed in an anteroposterior position.

Many newer pacemakers have a programmable option that makes magnet application ineffective. For this reason, knowledge of the patient's pacemaker dependency state and programming of the device may be required. Some pacemakers respond to magnet application only with a brief period of asynchronous pacing. Therefore, it is recommended that continuous telemetry be available during the surgical procedure.

There is no industry-wide standard response to either EMI or magnet application. It is therefore important that data regarding the individual pacemaker response to EMI and magnet application be obtained from the pacemaker manufacturer. However, in general, the recommendations outlined earlier are effective.

Management of Automatic Implantable Cardioverter-Defibrillators

Automatic ICDs (AICDs) are used for secondary prevention in the patient who has survived aborted sudden cardiac death. These devices are also effective in the primary prevention of sudden cardiac death for the patient with prior MI and advanced left ventricular dysfunction (LVEF 30% to 40%) and patients with nonischemic cardiomyopathy (LVEF ≤30% to 35%).

Electrocautery may affect AICDs in the same manner as it does pacemakers; the electromagnetic signal produced by electrocautery may be interpreted as intrinsic cardiac events. This phenomenon can lead to inhibition of pacing. In addition, if the EMI is interpreted by the AICD as a rapid ventricular rate, the AICD may deliver unnecessary and undesired shocks. Although the frequency of such an occurrence is small, the results of AICD shock delivered during a surgical procedure can be devastating. Therefore, it is recommended that AICDs be deactivated preoperatively if the use of electrocautery is a possibility. Continuous electrocardiographic monitoring and ACLS, including an external defibrillator, should be available when the AICD is deactivated. The AICD should be deactivated by one of two techniques. Either a magnet may be placed over the AICD for the duration of electrocautery, or the device can be deactivated with the use of the programmer. Magnet application over the pulse generator disables the device, preventing it from detecting tachyarrhythmias. For most AICDs, magnet application only temporarily deactivates the device, preventing it but some AICDs can be permanently deactivated with magnet application. Magnet application does not affect pacing functions of the AICD. Therefore, electrocautery may inhibit pacing from an AICD. Most patients with AICDs have significant left ventricular dysfunction with ischemic heart disease. These patients require close observation during the perioperative period.

INVASIVE HEMODYNAMIC MONITORING

Although attractive in theory, invasive pulmonary artery pressure monitoring has suboptimal sensitivity and specificity for the detection of perioperative myocardial ischemia. Numerous perioperative situations (e.g., intravascular volume overload, increased afterload) may result in increased pulmonary artery capillary wedge pressure without associated myocardial ischemia. Similarly, myocardial ischemia may be present without changes in pulmonary artery capillary pressure. **No evidence indicates that routine perioperative pulmonary artery catheterization, even when used to optimize perioperative hemodynamics in elderly high-risk patients who undergo elective or urgent major surgery, offers any advantage when compared with standard care** [⦿ *Sandham et al, 2004*]. My approach has been to assess the need for invasive hemodynamic monitoring on an individual basis. Clinical situations in which perioperative invasive hemodynamic monitoring may facilitate management include severe left ventricular dysfunction or fixed cardiac output in patients who undergo surgical procedures associated with significant fluid administration and decompensated CHF in patients who undergo major surgical procedures.

CONGESTIVE HEART FAILURE

CHF is a syndrome in which cardiac output is insufficient for the body's needs. It is the only major cardiovascular disorder that is increasing in incidence, prevalence, and overall mortality. CHF currently affects up to 2% of the U.S. population, and it has a prevalence of 6% to 10% in persons more than 65 years old. As the population of the United States ages, the incidence of chronic CHF in patients who undergo noncardiac surgical procedures will be likely to increase. The many possible causes include myocardial dysfunction related to ischemia, MI, hypertension, valvular and pericardial disease, and cardiomyopathy. CHF may also be precipitated by noncardiac causes that increase the demand for cardiac output. Common examples seen in the perioperative period include anemia, fever, and hypoxia. This section focuses on myocardial dysfunction, which is present in many patients with perioperative CHF.

Pathophysiology

Once valvular lesions, pericardial disease, and noncardiac conditions that increase the demand for cardiac output are ruled out, a primary myocardial abnormality is usually the cause of CHF. Approximately 70% of cases are related to left ventricular systolic dysfunction, and the remaining 30% are related to left ventricular diastolic dysfunction.

Impaired left ventricular contractility is the cause of left ventricular systolic dysfunction. It is associated with a decreased LVEF. Preload and cardiac volume subsequently increase as compensatory responses to increase cardiac output, but as left ventricular function deteriorates, cardiac output cannot increase. Increasing cardiac volume and ventricular pressure result in elevation of the left atrial pressure with subsequent pulmonary venous congestion. Decreased left ventricular contractility leads to decreased cardiac output.

In patients with primary left ventricular diastolic dysfunction, the main abnormality is reduced ventricular compliance. These patients usually have normal or enhanced left ventricular contractile function. The ventricular myocardium is less compliant than normal; increases in preload result in marked elevation of left ventricular end-diastolic pressure with a subsequent rise in pulmonary venous pressure and pulmonary venous hypertension. Left ventricular diastolic dysfunction is characterized by marked sensitivity to changes in intravascular volume. Patients are at risk for marked elevation of ventricular filling pressure in the setting of intravascular volume overload and for hypotension as a consequence of decreased ventricular pressure when intravascular volume is depleted. If patients subsequently develop ventricular systolic dysfunction, these responses become even more dramatic. The most common cause of ventricular diastolic dysfunction is left ventricular hypertrophy resulting from hypertension. Other less common causes include myocardial infiltrative processes such as amyloidosis and restrictive cardiomyopathy.

Risk for the Development of Perioperative Congestive Heart Failure

Goldman and associates found the preoperative presence of symptoms and signs of CHF to be the best predictor of the development of perioperative CHF. A history of CHF, which was absent in most of the patients who did develop the condition perioperatively, was a less powerful predictor [❶ *Goldman et al, 1978*]. In a study of patients at higher risk (i.e., those with hypertension or diabetes), Charlson and colleagues found that the risk for postoperative CHF was limited to patients with preoperative symptomatic cardiac disease (e.g., previous MI, valvular disease, or CHF). Patients with diabetes were at greatest risk, particularly if they had overt cardiac disease. Intraoperative fluctuations of the mean arterial blood pressure (increases or decreases of >40 mm Hg) were related to increased rates of postoperative CHF. Mangano and associates found that postoperative myocardial ischemia and a history of cardiac arrhythmia and diabetes predicted the development of postoperative CHF. CHF requiring hospital admission was found to be a significant indicator of subsequent risk in patients 65 years old or older who underwent noncardiac surgical procedures during the year following their hospital admission for CHF. For this group, the perioperative and 30-day mortality rate following noncardiac surgery was 11.7% compared with 6.6% for patients who had a history of coronary artery disease but not CHF.

When Does Perioperative Congestive Heart Failure Occur?

In a review of cases of perioperative CHF that occurred during the 1950s and 1960s, Cooperman noted that most cases developed within 1 hour of the cessation of anesthesia, the majority during the first 30 minutes. In a high-risk population of patients with diabetes or hypertension, most of those who developed perioperative CHF did so on the day of the surgical procedure or on the second postoperative day. I believe that the risk for postoperative CHF is greatest during two periods. The risk is significantly increased in the immediate postoperative period, probably as a result of hypertension or hypotension, myocardial ischemia, intraoperative fluid administration, sympathetic stimulation, cessation of positive pressure ventilation, and hypoxia. The second peak occurs 24 to 48 hours postoperatively and may be related to the reabsorption of interstitial fluid, myocardial ischemia, and, in some patients, the effects of withdrawal from long-term oral CHF medications.

General Approach to Diagnosis of Perioperative Congestive Heart Failure

In the perioperative period, appropriate CHF therapy is facilitated by determining whether CHF is caused by systolic ventricular dysfunction, diastolic ventricular dysfunction, or a combination of both. Although a cardiac imaging study (e.g., echocardiogram, radionuclide ventriculogram, or standard left ventricular angiogram) is necessary to definitively diagnose the presence of left ventricular systolic dysfunction, many clues to the diagnosis of CHF can be found in patients' histories, physical examinations, chest radiographs, and ECGs. CHF in patients with histories of MI, cardiomegaly, or S_3 strongly suggests the presence of left ventricular systolic dysfunction. In contrast, CHF in patients with hypertension, S_4, normal heart size on chest radiographs, evidence on ECGs of left ventricular hypertrophy, and no history of MI is suggestive of left ventricular diastolic dysfunction. Considerable overlap occurs, however; patients with CHF may have both systolic and diastolic components to their myocardial dysfunction. Interstitial pulmonary edema may be found in both varieties and does not aid in discrimination. Although the absence of left ventricular systolic dysfunction in patients with CHF suggests that diastolic dysfunction is the cause, a diagnosis of left ventricular diastolic dysfunction ideally requires invasive documentation of increased pulmonary capillary wedge pressure or elevated left ventricular end-diastolic pressure.

Approach to Patients with Compensated Chronic Congestive Heart Failure Who Require Noncardiac Surgical Procedures

In patients with compensated chronic CHF, effort is directed at identifying destabilizing factors (e.g., fluid overload, anemia, fever) that may occur in the perioperative period, preventing these conditions if possible, and rendering immediate treatment if they occur. The need for invasive hemodynamic monitoring also must be assessed. Finally, patients' CHF medical regimens must be converted to appropriate parenteral regimens until oral intake can be resumed.

Perioperative cardiac mortality depends most on patients' clinical status at the time of surgery. The risk of CHF is greatest if signs of CHF are present at the time of surgery or during the week before the surgical procedure. Patients with chronic CHF are evaluated to determine whether the condition is compensated. If patients are thought to be decompensated, the surgical procedure is delayed if possible, and attempts are made to achieve medical stabilization. Because the risk imposed by CHF is greatest in patients who have pulmonary edema within 7 days of surgery, I often delay elective surgical procedures for at least 1 week after CHF stabilization.

For patients with decompensated CHF who require emergency or semiemergency surgical procedures, invasive hemodynamic monitoring may aid in further preoperative cardiac stabilization. Because the risk of postoperative CHF extends beyond the immediate surgical period, invasive hemodynamic monitoring is usually continued for 48 to 72 hours postoperatively.

Use of Long-Term Congestive Heart Failure Medications in the Perioperative Period

Several medications used to treat chronic CHF may cause electrolyte or metabolic abnormalities in the perioperative period. Diuretics may induce intravascular volume depletion, which can predispose patients to hypotension if they are given vasodilator anesthetic agents or spinal anesthesia. Therefore, I monitor for orthostatic changes in blood pressure and pulse during the preoperative physical examination in all patients who receive diuretics. If orthostatic changes are documented, it is important that intravascular volume be replenished preoperatively. A similar approach is followed for patients who are being treated with vasodilators.

Preoperative serum potassium levels are obtained in all patients who are receiving diuretics, and these values are corrected before the surgical procedure if necessary. Although hypokalemia may cause ventricular ectopy, acute potassium loss is probably more arrhythmogenic than is chronic potassium loss. Hypokalemia that does not resolve with potassium supplementation suggests the presence of hypomagnesemia, which also must be corrected before a surgical procedure is undertaken. The hyperkalemia that sometimes accompanies the use of potassium-sparing diuretics may cause heart block and other abnormalities of cardiac conduction. Another potential cause of hyperkalemia in the perioperative period is aldosterone antagonists. Their use has increased in patients with CHF because these drugs have been shown to decrease mortality when they are used on a long-term basis in patients with NYHA class III or IV heart failure.

For patients who receive digoxin, serial blood levels are measured if renal function declines, and the dose is adjusted accordingly. Clinical trials documented that although digoxin does not decrease mortality, it does decrease CHF-related symptoms and increases exercise tolerance. Evidence indicates that withdrawal of digoxin may result in clinical deterioration. In a small study, Uretsky found the full effect of digoxin withdrawal on exercise tolerance 12 weeks following digoxin discontinuation. An initial decline in exercise tolerance was reported at 2 weeks. Although this study was not designed to assess functional capacity less than 2 weeks following digoxin withdrawal, it has been my practice to avoid discontinuation of digoxin in the perioperative period. Therefore, the drug is continued in patients who have been receiving long-term oral digoxin therapy, and it is given intravenously when oral intake is suspended. Cardiovascular drugs that may increase digoxin levels in the perioperative period include quinidine, verapamil, and amiodarone.

For patients who receive maintenance therapy with ACE inhibitors or angiotensin receptor blockers (ARBs), I often continue to administer the medications until the time of operation and then give the oral agents again as soon as possible in the postoperative period. Patients' left ventricular function, degree of compensation, dependence on ACE inhibitors or ARBs, and risk for perioperative CHF determine the need for parenteral ACE inhibitors postoperatively until oral intake can be resumed. Patients with moderate to severe ventricular dysfunction who are at high risk for perioperative CHF are given intravenous ACE inhibitors (enalapril, at 0.625 to 1.25 mg every 6 hours) until oral ACE inhibitors can be resumed. No parenteral ARBs are available.

Many patients, particularly those who cannot tolerate ACE inhibitors or ARBs, take the combination of nitrates and hydralazine as vasodilator therapy for CHF. During the time that patients are unable to take oral medications, topical or intravenous nitrates are given. Because of the short duration of action and risk for hypotension, I do not use parenteral hydralazine as a substitute for oral hydralazine. If CHF decompensates while patients maintained on nitrates and hydralazine are unable to take oral medications, I may discontinue the nitrates and use intravenous nitroprusside for its preload- and afterload-reducing properties. In some cases, if the contraindication to ACE inhibitors or ARBs is not well defined, I attempt to administer intravenous enalaprilat. In patients who are unable to receive ACE inhibitors or ARBs, perioperative CHF therapy is centered on diuretics, preload reduction with nitrates, preload and afterload reduction with nitroprusside, digoxin if indicated, and intravenous inotropic agents such as dopamine, dobutamine, and milrinone.

β-Blockers decrease symptoms and mortality in patients with NYHA class II and III heart failure as a result of left ventricular systolic dysfunction and have become standard therapy in this patient group. These drugs are initiated when the patient has been clinically compensated for at least 2 to 4 weeks. Their use in the patient whose CHF is not compensated can provoke further decompensation. Although there are no established guidelines regarding the use of these drugs in the perioperative period, my approach is to continue them if possible. If a noncardiac operation necessitates their interruption, I follow the practice guidelines of the ACC/AHA, which suggest that if β-blockers are interrupted for a period in excess of 72 hours, they be reinitiated at 50% of their previous dose if the patient is still deemed to be a candidate for their use. The dose is then cautiously increased generally no sooner than at 2-week intervals.

Treatment of Acute Congestive Heart Failure in the Perioperative Period

Numerous factors may lead to the new onset of CHF or the decompensation of otherwise stable CHF in the perioperative period. Myocardial ischemia or MI, perioperative volume overload, hypertension with a subsequent increase in afterload, occult valvular heart disease (e.g., aortic stenosis, mitral regurgitation), renal failure, anemia, sepsis, pulmonary embolus, pneumonia, and the new onset of atrial fibrillation or flutter with decreased cardiac output may provoke perioperative CHF. In addition, the stress of surgery in a patient receiving an inadequate medical CHF regimen may precipitate acute CHF in patients with otherwise stable chronic CHF in the nonoperative setting. Medical regimens may be inadequate because of inappropriate medication or the inability to replace orally administered drugs taken on a long-term basis with intravenous equivalents.

Treatment is directed at the primary cause of the acute episode of CHF. If volume overload is present, diuretics are administered. If patients are found to have left ventricular systolic dysfunction, inotropic agents are given to increase myocardial contractility and cardiac output. Intravenous inotropic agents such as dobutamine and dopamine are effective in the short term but must be used cautiously in patients with acute myocardial ischemia or MI because they may increase myocardial oxygen demand and exacerbate myocardial ischemia. Digoxin is less helpful in the treatment of acute

CHF in patients with left ventricular systolic dysfunction but may be beneficial for patients whose CHF is provoked by atrial fibrillation. It slows the atrial fibrillation ventricular response, thereby prolonging ventricular filling time and decreasing myocardial oxygen demand.

Vasodilator medical therapy may also be used in the perioperative period. Intravenous nitroprusside is the agent of choice for immediate blood pressure control and reduction of afterload in patients with CHF who exhibit hypertension or increased systemic vascular resistance. It is also of benefit when acute perioperative CHF is associated with aortic or mitral regurgitation. It decreases afterload and serves to decrease the regurgitant fraction in patients with these valvular lesions. Its use is limited by the need for continuous blood pressure monitoring and the risk of cyanate toxicity when it is administered for more than a short period.

Patients who require long-term parenteral vasodilator therapy, enalaprilat, which is an ACE inhibitor administered intravenously, is effective in reducing preload and afterload. When patients resume oral intake, oral ACE inhibitors or oral ARBs may be substituted. Nitrates are beneficial in the treatment of perioperative CHF when myocardial ischemia contributes to the condition or when reduction in preload is desired. β-Blockers and calcium channel antagonists should not be given to patients with acute perioperative CHF caused by left ventricular systolic dysfunction, but they may prove helpful in patients with left ventricular diastolic dysfunction by promoting left ventricular relaxation and increased compliance. When patients who have perioperative CHF in the absence of acute myocardial ischemia do not respond to the alleviation of precipitating factors and provision of medical therapy directed at normalizing intravascular volume and cardiac output, the presence of acute pulmonary embolism, sepsis, or other noncardiac causes must be considered.

THE PATIENT WITH CONGENITAL HEART DISEASE

Major risk factors for complications following noncardiac surgery in adults with congenital heart disease are the presence of cyanosis, pulmonary hypertension, and current therapy of CHF (Table 7-5) [● *Warner et al, 1998*]. Procedures most strongly associated with complications in this group are surgical procedures of the respiratory or nervous system. Data are lacking to guide the management of the patient with congenital heart disease who requires noncardiac surgical procedures. Patients with cyanotic congenital heart disease may have hyperviscosity secondary to an increased hematocrit and may be at risk for perioperative bleeding. Preoperative phlebotomy when the hematocrit exceeds 63% may decrease this risk. Patients with right-to-left intracardiac shunts are at risk for paradoxical embolism. Care must be taken to filter air from intravenous lines.

TABLE 7-5	Perioperative Complications in Adults with Congenital Heart Disease
Congenital Heart Lesion	**Perioperative Complication**
Atrial septal defect	Atrial arrhythmias
	Right ventricular failure
Bicuspid aortic valve	Bacterial endocarditis
Pulmonary hypertension	Hypotension with decreased cardiac output if systemic vascular resistance is lowered
Tetralogy of Fallot	
Unrepaired	Decreases in systemic vascular resistance increase right-to-left shunting
	Increases in systemic vascular resistance decrease cardiac output
	Bacterial endocarditis
	Rhythm and conduction abnormalities
Repaired	Rhythm and conduction abnormalities

Adapted from Webb G, Burrows F: The risks of noncardiac surgery. J Am Coll Cardiol 18:323-325, 1991.

MANAGEMENT OF CARDIAC MEDICATIONS IN THE PERIOPERATIVE PERIOD

Perioperative continuation of patients' long-term cardiac medications is often challenging. Many oral medications have no parenteral substitutes. The stress of surgery may render patients' long-term cardiac medical regimens inadequate during the perioperative period. Finally, few controlled studies have evaluated the use of cardiac medications during and after noncardiac surgical procedures. Several guidelines are helpful in attempting to maintain patients' long-term medical therapeutic regimens in the perioperative period.

β-Adrenergic blockers are used in the treatment of myocardial ischemia, arrhythmias, hypertension, and left ventricular systolic dysfunction. Patients who receive β-blockers on a long-term basis should be given oral doses on the morning of their surgical procedure. Long-acting agents such as atenolol and sustained-release metoprolol provide β-blockade for as long as 24 hours. Patients' long-term β-blocker regimens are then restarted 24 hours postoperatively if oral intake has resumed. For patients whose gastrointestinal tracts are not functional at that time, the administration of intravenous β-blockers (e.g., propranolol, 0.5 to 2 mg every 4 to 6 hours) is begun and is continued for as long as the usual long-term oral β-blocker is tolerated. This regimen is often effective for patients who are receiving β-blockers for coronary artery disease or cardiac arrhythmias but may require alteration in patients who take these drugs for hypertension or CHF. For the patient with hypertension, labetalol may be given intravenously by either of two methods: repeated intravenous injection with an initial 20-mg infusion over a 2-minute period, with additional infusions of 20 to 80 mg given at 10-minute intervals until desired blood pressure is achieved or a total of 300 mg is given. The other approach—slow, continuous infusion—is achieved by continuous infusion at 2 mg/minute. The short-acting intravenous β-blocker esmolol (at a loading infusion of 500 μg/kg/

minute for 1 minute followed by a continuous infusion of 50 to 300 μg/kg/minute) may also be used to control blood pressure in the postoperative period. Patients whose blood pressure is not controlled with these agents may require supplemental antihypertensive agents in addition to intravenous β-blockers until oral medications are resumed. For the patient receiving β-blockers for treatment of chronic CHF, I try to avoid discontinuation of β-blockers in the perioperative period unless the patient's clinical status deteriorates, as manifested by hypoperfusion, or the patient requires intravenous positive inotropic agents. In these cases, I temporarily discontinue the β-blocker but reinstitute it as soon as the patient is stabilized in an effort to reduce the risk of significant deterioration.

Nitrates are commonly used by patients with ischemic heart disease. Patients who are stable while receiving nitrates on a long-term basis typically are given their oral nitrate preparations on the morning of the surgical procedure. Topical nitroglycerin ointment (0.5 to 2 inches) is then applied every 8 hours until oral nitrates are resumed. This approach helps to maintain a nitrate-free period to decrease the risk of development of nitrate vasotolerance. Nitrates may cause excessive preload reduction and hypotension, which may be exacerbated by intravascular volume depletion and the simultaneous use of other vasodilator medications or anesthetic agents. In some patients, hypotension may occur unpredictably with the initial administration of nitrates. For this reason, I recommend that nitrates, given to decrease the likelihood of perioperative myocardial ischemia, be initiated well before the surgical procedure. Intravenous nitroglycerin should be considered when nitrates are used to treat perioperative myocardial ischemia.

Intravenous nitroprusside is effective in controlling perioperative hypertension, but the need for continuous blood pressure monitoring and the risk of cyanate toxicity render its use impractical for more than a few days. Intravenous methyldopa and enalaprilat, given three to four times daily, are effective in controlling postoperative hypertension, are well tolerated, and may be used without continuous blood pressure monitoring in stable patients. These drugs are useful adjuncts for controlling hypertension in the perioperative period.

Intravascular volume depletion may occur in patients receiving long-term diuretic therapy, and the condition places them at risk for hypotension when anesthetic agents that produce vasodilation are administered. Intravascular volume depletion is suggested by the presence of orthostatic changes in the blood pressure and heart rate and should be corrected with fluid administration, preoperatively if possible. Patients who take diuretics may also have hypokalemia or hyperkalemia resulting from potassium-sparing agents. Serum potassium levels should be checked in these patients before the surgical procedure. Investigators have suggested that a chronic serum potassium level of 3 mmol/L or higher is acceptable for anesthesia and surgery, and chronic asymptomatic hypokalemia as low as 2.5 mmol/L may be adequate in patients who are at low risk for cardiac complications. Hypokalemia has been shown to increase the incidence of cardiac arrhythmias in patients taking digoxin; therefore, perioperative hypokalemia should be corrected in this patient group.

Calcium channel antagonists are used to treat angina, hypertension, and arrhythmias. Sustained-release preparations of calcium channel antagonists that patients have been using may be given on the morning of the surgical procedure, in an effort to achieve effective drug levels for the next 24 hours. Patients who are capable of oral intake the day after the surgical procedure may resume oral calcium channel antagonists. Problems exist, however, in substituting appropriate parenteral formulations for patients who cannot resume oral calcium channel antagonists at this time. The few calcium channel antagonists that are available for parenteral administration often have their primary effect on the cardiac conduction system, rather than on hypertension or angina. Intravenous verapamil has potent negative chronotropic effects and can induce heart block. Intravenous diltiazem is indicated primarily to control the ventricular response in patients with atrial fibrillation and to convert PSVT to sinus rhythm in patients who have AVNRT. No parenteral preparations of nifedipine or amlodipine exist.

In patients who receive calcium channel antagonists for their antianginal effects, topical or intravenous nitrates may be substituted until oral intake resumes. In patients who take calcium channel antagonists for hypertension, intravenous α-methyldopa or enalaprilat is often effective until oral medications are resumed.

Digitalis glycosides may be given orally on the morning of the surgical procedure and then intravenously on a daily basis until patients' long-term oral regimens are resumed. The intravenous administration of these agents increases their bioavailability as much as 20%, and the maintenance parenteral dose may have to be reduced appropriately.

ACE inhibitors are used to treat hypertension and left ventricular systolic dysfunction. Enalaprilat is the only agent of this class available for parenteral administration and is given intravenously every 6 hours.

The abrupt withdrawal of centrally acting antihypertensive agents, as occurs in the perioperative period, may result in a *discontinuation syndrome* characterized by sympathetic overactivity and rebound hypertension. Symptoms may resemble those of pheochromocytoma. Clonidine is the prototype drug of this class. The discontinuation syndrome may occur 18 to 72 hours after clonidine is withdrawn, but it is rare in patients who receive less than 1.2 mg of clonidine daily. This syndrome may be aggravated by the simultaneous use of β-blockers, which may block peripheral vasodilatory β-receptors and leave vasoconstrictor α-receptors unopposed. The syndrome may be terminated by resumption of clonidine therapy. If that is not possible because patients cannot resume oral intake, rebound hypertension may be controlled with intravenous nitroprusside or labetalol. Clonidine withdrawal syndrome may be prevented by slow tapering of clonidine preoperatively. When this is not feasible, transdermal clonidine may be given in the perioperative period. Transdermal clonidine requires approximately 48 hours to achieve therapeutic drug levels. Therefore, it should be given well in advance of the surgical procedure and should first be administered simultaneously with oral clonidine for approximately 48 hours. The transdermal preparation maintains therapeutic clonidine levels for as long as 7 days.

Clopidogrel is a thienopyridine antiplatelet agent administered along with aspirin typically for a minimum of 4 weeks to patients who have had coronary stenting with a bare metal stent. Evidence indicates a possible beneficial effect on the reduction of stent thrombosis in this group with up to 9 months of post–stent placement clopidogrel use. For the patient who has received a drug-coated stent, clopidogrel, along with aspirin, is administered for at least 1 year. This drug is also used in the treatment of patients with acute coronary syndromes. Clopidogrel may increase the risk of bleeding during or immediately following major surgical procedures. Because its effect on platelets and bleeding may last for 5 days, many surgeons request at least a 5-day period between the discontinuation of clopidogrel and subsequent major surgery.

Statins are often used to treat hypercholesterolemia. Because of evidence that suggests their use in the perioperative period may be associated with a reduction in perioperative cardiac complications, I typically attempt to continue statins in the perioperative period. For patients who meet the National Cholesterol Education Program guidelines for statin use but are not receiving a statin at the time of preoperative evaluation, I use the preoperative evaluation as an opportunity to consider adding a statin to their medical regimen. At this time, there is no prospective data from randomized trials to support the use of perioperative statins to lower periop-erative risk in the patient who otherwise does not meet the criteria for long-term statin therapy.

Selected Readings

2005 American Heart Association Guidelines for Cardiopulmonary Resuscitation and Emergency Cardiovascular Care: Part 7.3: Management of symptomatic bradycardia and tachycardia. Circulation 112(24 Suppl): IV1-203, 2005. Epub 2005 Nov 28. Available at http://circ.ahajournals.org/cgi/content/full/112/24_suppl/IV-67

Auerbach A, Goldman L: Assessing and reducing the cardiac risk of noncardiac surgery. Circulation 113:1361-1376, 2006.

Ballantyne JC, Kupelnick B, McPeek B, Lau J: Does the evidence support the use of spinal and epidural anesthesia for surgery? J Clin Anesth 17: 382-391, 2005. **A**

Bonow RO, Carabello BA, Chatterjee K, et al: ACC/AHA 2006 guidelines for the management of patients with valvular heart disease: A report of the American College of Cardiology/American Heart Association Task Force on Practice Guidelines (Writing Committee to Develop Guidelines for the Management of Patients with Valvular Heart Disease). Available at http://www.acc.org/clinical/guidelines/valvular/index.pdf. **C**

Charlson ME, MacKenzie CR, Gold JP, et al: Risk for postoperative congestive heart failure. Surg Gynecol Obstet 172:95-104, 1991.

Cooperman LH, Price HL: Pulmonary edema in the operative and postoperative period. Am Surg 172:883-891, 1970

Dajani AS, Taubert KA, Wilson W, et al: Prevention of bacterial endocarditis: Recommendations by the American Heart Association. Circulation 96:358-366, 1997.

Eagle K, Berger PB, Calkins H, et al: ACC/AHA guideline update for perioperative cardiovascular evaluation for noncardiac surgery: A report of the American College of Cardiology/American Heart Association Task Force on Practice Guidelines (Committee to Update the 1996 Guidelines on Perioperative Cardiovascular Evaluation for Noncardiac Surgery). 2002. American College of Cardiology Web site. Available at http:/www.acc.org/qualityandscience/clinical/guidelines/perio/update/periupdate_index.htm. **C**

Eagle KA, Guyton RA, Davidoff R, et al: ACC/AHA 2004 guideline update for coronary artery bypass graft surgery: A report of the American College of Cardiology/American Heart Association Task Force on Practice Guidelines (Committee to Update the 1999 Guidelines for Coronary

Artery Bypass Graft Surgery). Circulation 110:e340-437, 2004. Erratum in Circulation 111:2014, 2005. Available at http://www.acc.org/clinical/guidelines/cabg/cabg.pdf

Fleisher LA, Beckman JA, Brown KA, et al: ACC/AHA guidelines on perioperative cardiovascular evaluation and care for noncardiac surgery: A report of the American College of Cardiology/American Heart Association Task Force on Practice Guidelines [Writing Committee to Revise the 2002 Guidelines on Perioperative Cardiovascular Evaluation for Noncardiac Surgery]. J Am Coll Cardiol 50:e159-241, 2007.

Fleisher LA, Beckman JA, Brown KA, et al: ACC/AHA 2006 guideline update on perioperative cardiovascular evaluation for noncardiac surgery: Focused update on perioperative beta-blocker therapy. A report of the American College of Cardiology/American Heart Association Task Force on Practice Guidelines (Writing Committee to Update the 2002 Guidelines on Perioperative Cardiovascular Evaluation for Noncardiac Surgery). J Am Coll Cardiol 47:2343-2355, 2006. Available at http://www.acc.org/clinical/guidelines/perio_betablocker.pdf. **C**

Fuster V, Ryden LE, Cannom DS, et al: ACC/AHA/ESC 2006 guidelines for the management of patients with atrial fibrillation: A report of the American College of Cardiology/American Heart Association Task Force on Practice Guidelines and the European Society of Cardiology Committee for Practice Guidelines (Writing Committee to Revise the 2001 Guidelines for the Management of Patients with Atrial Fibrillation). J Am Coll Cardiol 48:e149-e246, 2006. Available at www.acc.org. **C**

Goldman L, Caldera DL, Nussbaum SR, et al: Multifactorial index of cardiac risk in noncardiac surgical procedures. N Engl J Med 297:845-850, 1978. **A**

Grines CL, Bonow RO, Casey DE Jr, et al: Prevention of premature discontinuation of dual antiplatelet therapy in patients with coronary artery stents: A science advisory from the American Heart Association, American College of Cardiology, Society for Cardiovascular Angiography and Interventions, American College of Surgeons, and American Dental Association, with representation from the American College of Physicians. J Am Dent Assoc 138:652-655, 2007.

Hernandez A, Whellan D, Stroud S, et al: Outcomes in heart failure patients after major noncardiac surgery. J Am Coll Cardiol 44:1446-1453, 2004.

Howell SJ, Sear JW, Foex P: Hypertension, hypertensive heart disease, and perioperative cardiac risk. Br J Anaesth 92:570-583, 2004. **C**

Kertai M, Bountioukos M, Boersma E, et al: Aortic stenosis: An understated risk factor for perioperative complications in patients undergoing noncardiac surgery. Am J Med 116:8-13, 2004. **B**

L'Italien GJ, Cambria RP, Cutler BS, et al: Comparative early and late cardiac morbidity among patients requiring different vascular surgery procedures. J Vasc Surg 21:935-944, 1995. **B**

Lee TH, Marcantonio ER, Mangione CM, et al: Derivation and prospective validation of a simple index for prediction of cardiac risk of major noncardiac surgery. Circulation 100:1043-1049, 1999.

Mangano DT, Browner WS, Hollenberg M, et al: The Study of Perioperative Ischemia Research Group: Association of perioperative myocardial ischemia with cardiac morbidity and mortality in men undergoing noncardiac surgery. N Engl J Med 323:1781-1788, 1990.

McFalls EO, Ward HB, Moritz TE, et al: Reduction of postoperative mortality and morbidity with epidural or spinal anesthesia: Results from overview of randomised trials. BMJ 321:1493, 2000.

McFalls EO, Ward HB, Moritz TE, et al: Coronary-artery revascularization before elective major vascular surgery. N Engl J Med 351:2795-2804, 2004. **A**

Paul SD, Eagle KA, Kuntz K, et al: Concordance of preoperative clinical risk with angiographic severity of coronary artery disease in patients undergoing vascular surgery. Circulation 94:1561-1566, 1996. **B**

Polanczyk CA, Goldman L, Marcantonio E, et al: Supraventricular arrhythmia in patients having noncardiac surgery: Clinical correlates and effect on length of stay. Ann Intern Med 129:279-285, 1998.

Rodgers A, Walker N, Schug S, et al: Reduction of postoperative mortality and morbidity with epidural or spinal anaesthesia: Results from overview of randomised trials. BMJ 321:1493, 2000.

Sandham JD, Hull RD, Brant RF, et al: A randomized, controlled trial of the use of pulmonary-artery catheters in high-risk surgical patients. N Engl J Med 348:5-14, 2004. **A**

Uretsky BF, Young JB, Shahidi F, et al: Randomized study assessing the effect of digoxin withdrawal in patients with mild to moderate chronic congestive heart failure: Results of the PROVED trial. J Am Coll Cardiol 22:955-962, 1993.

Warner M, Lunn R, O'Leary P, Schroeder D: Outcomes of noncardiac surgical procedures in children and adults with congenital heart disease. Mayo Clin Proc 73:728-734, 1998. **C**

Wilson W, Taubert KA, Gewitz M, et al: Prevention of infective endocarditis: Guidelines from the American Heart Association: A guideline from the American Heart Association Rheumatic Fever, Endocarditis and Kawasaki Disease Committee, Council on Cardiovascular Disease in the Young, and the Council on Clinical Cardiology, Council on Cardiovascular Surgery and Anesthesia, and the Quality of Care and Outcomes Research Interdisciplinary Working Group. J Am Dent Assoc 138:739-745, 747-760, 2007. Published online April 19, 2007. Available at http://circ.ahajournals.org.

8 Perioperative Assessment and Management of Patients with Pulmonary Diseases

GREGORY C. KANE, MD
BARTOLOME R. CELLI, MD

The goal of the preoperative assessment for patients with pulmonary disease is to prevent morbidity and mortality among these patients as they undergo surgical procedures, to perform risk stratification in those patients who appear likely to experience complications, and to prepare the patient and surgical team for potential pulmonary problems in the postoperative period. On occasion, the preoperative assessment may indicate an unacceptable degree of risk for an elective surgical procedure. The assessment can be achieved by a thorough medical evaluation in concert with specific testing to asses cardiopulmonary function. The purpose of this chapter is to review the approach to the preoperative evaluation and thus allow the practitioner to maximize outcomes, to identify and minimize risks, and to prepare for postoperative challenges.

▌EFFECTS OF SURGERY

The function of the respiratory system is invariably affected during and after surgical procedures [❸ *Tisi, 1979*; ❸ *Breslin, 1981*; ❸ *Jackson, 1988*]. Despite a better understanding of the

---

Levels of Evidence:

❹—Randomized controlled trials (RCTs), meta-analyses, well-designed systematic reviews of RCTs. ❸—Case-control or cohort studies, nonrandomized controlled trials, systematic reviews of studies other than RCTs, cross-sectional studies, retrospective studies. ❺—Consensus statements, expert guidelines, usual practice, opinion.

pathophysiologic changes that occur during anesthesia and surgery, bronchoaspiration, atelectasis, pneumonia, pulmonary edema, exacerbation of underlying chronic obstructive pulmonary disease (COPD), respiratory failure, and pulmonary embolism remain the most frequent causes of postoperative morbidity and important reasons for mortality in this population [❾ Bartlett et al, 1973; ❽ Pontoppidan, 1980]. This chapter is devoted to the understanding of how respiratory function is altered by nonthoracic surgery, how to identify the patient at risk for complications, and what to do to prevent complications.

DEFINITION AND INCIDENCE OF POSTOPERATIVE PULMONARY COMPLICATIONS

The true definition and incidence of postoperative pulmonary complications depend on the diagnostic threshold of the investigator observing for such complications and the criteria used to define them. Using a constellation of clinical symptoms or signs (fever, cough, change in sputum, or leukocytosis), roentgenographic changes, and arterial blood gas determinations, the incidence has been reported to be as low as 9% to as high as 76% [❾ Hall et al, 1991; ❽ Pontoppidan, 1980]. All series agree that the incidence of pulmonary complications is much higher for procedures that are close to the diaphragm (upper abdominal), in which it ranges from 30% to 80%, than for procedures of the lower abdomen and the extremities [❾ Hall et al, 1991; ❽ Pontoppidan, 1980]. It is still customary to assess patients undergoing a major abdominal procedure by way of a thorough cardiovascular evaluation, with relatively little attention given to the respiratory system. More recent publications have addressed respiratory complications in such patients. A simple pulmonary evaluation easily detects patients at high risk for postoperative pulmonary complications. This is important because available interventions can reduce the incidence of postoperative pulmonary complications in high-risk groups and can also shorten hospital stays and cut costs.

EFFECTS OF ANESTHESIA ON PULMONARY FUNCTION AND PATHOGENESIS OF POSTOPERATIVE PULMONARY COMPLICATIONS

With the administration of general anesthesia, there is a small but significant drop in functional residual capacity (FRC) that is not related to the sedatives used as premedication [**O** *Laws, 1968*]. In nonabdominal or nonthoracic surgical procedures, these changes return to normal in the postoperative period, whereas they persist and may worsen after abdominal (especially upper abdominal) and thoracic procedures. Studies have documented the development of decreased diaphragmatic contractility that is not caused by alterations in the muscle itself, but most likely results from reflex inhibition of the respiratory drive arising from sympathetic vagal or splanchnic abdominal receptors [**O** *Dureuil et al, 1986;* **O** *Ford et al, 1983;* **O** *Rovina et al, 1996*]. This alteration in diaphragmatic function is not influenced by pain because its control by epidural anesthesia does not influence diaphragmatic excursion measured by ultrasonography. Diaphragmatic dysfunction can persist for days postoperatively and can contribute to decreased lung volumes [**O** *Simmoneau et al, 1983*].

The mechanical consequences of the alterations induced by anesthesia and diaphragmatic paresis are decreases in FRC, expiratory reserve volume, inspiratory capacity, vital capacity, and expiratory flows. These decreases, which range from 20% to 50% of preoperative values, may last for up to 2 weeks. Postoperatively, the pattern of breathing is modified, with an increase in respiratory rate and a decrease in tidal volume without a real change in minute ventilation. As a result of the drop in FRC, the shallow rapid breaths, and a decrease in sighs, the patient breathes with the end-tidal point at less than the closing volume. This situation is especially problematic in elderly patients or those with COPD, in whom the closing volume is already close to the resting FRC. In other words, many of the dependent areas of the lung close during tidal breathing. As the air in these unventilated areas is absorbed and the alveoli collapse, more dramatic atelectasis may result [❻ *Ford and Guenter, 1984*]. Because there is a decrease in mucus clearance and an increase in bacterial colonization, the risk of infection is elevated.

Immediately postoperatively and paralleling the change in mechanics is a 10% to 30% drop in arterial oxygen tension (PaO_2) believed to result from a ventilation/perfusion mismatch. The best explanation is that the atelectatic areas continue to be perfused but not ventilated. Because some small areas of atelectasis are not easily seen on chest roentgenograms, the concept of *microatelectasis* has emerged. In the absence of previous compromise in gas exchange, there is no alteration in the concentration of carbon dioxide. As expected, these events remain silent in the patient at low risk, but they may result in significant pulmonary complications in patients at high risk. In these latter patients, the increased work of breathing needed to maintain adequate blood gases places further strain on the respiratory muscles. When the energy demand is greater than the supply, respiratory failure may result.

CHOICE OF ANESTHESIA AND EFFECT ON POSTOPERATIVE PULMONARY COMPLICATIONS

The effect of anesthetic choice on the incidence of postoperative complications has been an area of debate, but studies have contributed to a growing consensus. **A review of these studies suggested a lower rate of pulmonary complications such as pneumonia (39% reduction) and respiratory depression (59% reduction) for patients who receive neuraxial blockade (e.g., spinal or epidural anesthesia), as opposed to general anesthesia** [❻ *Rodgers et al, 2000*]. This risk reduction does not appear to apply to all patients (unselected) undergoing general surgical procedures because a randomized trial did not confirm an improved outcome for patients with obesity, diabetes, or coronary artery disease [**◑** *Rigg, 2002*].

RISK FACTORS FOR POSTOPERATIVE PULMONARY COMPLICATIONS

Risk factors may roughly be divided into respiratory conditions and nonpulmonary conditions (Fig. 8-1).

Respiratory Factors

Because the respiratory system is invariably affected during abdominal surgery, the possibility of postoperative pulmonary complications is higher in patients with clinical or subclinical pulmonary disease. The easiest and still the best way to detect underlying pulmonary disease is a careful medical history, with a review of the patient's smoking history. The most important entities associated with increased postoperative pulmonary complications are COPD (emphysema and chronic bronchitis) and asthma.

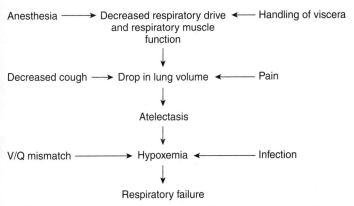

Figure 8-1 • Pathophysiology of the events leading to postoperative pulmonary complications. V/Q, ventilation/perfusion.

Smoking

Investigators have shown an association between the amount of cigarette smoking and related bronchial epithelial abnormalities and the incidence of postoperative pulmonary complications in asymptomatic smokers [❸ *Chalon et al, 1975;* ❸ *McAlister et al, 2003;* ❸ *Warner et al, 1984*]. Cigarette smoking is the single most important factor in the genesis of airflow obstruction. A history of 20 pack-years seems to be the cutting point at which the risk of postoperative pulmonary complications increases when compared with nonsmokers [❸ *Chalon et al, 1975*], although the risk seems to increase further with the number of pack-years [❸ *McAlister et al, 2003*]. When this history is coupled with airflow obstruction seen during pulmonary function testing and with cough associated with sputum production, the risk for postoperative pulmonary complications is even higher, and intervention to reduce the risk becomes necessary. Cessation of smoking for only a few days before the procedure is inadequate to decrease risk. Available data indicate that 6 to 8 weeks of abstinence are needed before pulmonary epithelial changes become evident. The length of time that smokers may need to discontinue their habit to maximize the postsurgical outcome has been further examined. In a prospective study of 200 patients, the complication rate for persons who had quit for more than 6 months compared with those who had quit for only 2 months was further reduced (11.1% versus 14.5%) [❹ *Warner et al, 1989*]. Perhaps difficult to explain, the rate was exceedingly high (57%) for patients who had quit for less than 8 weeks. Patients who continued to smoke had a 33% complication rate. This finding may be a consequence of a temporary increase in sputum production and cough that often occurs during the first 2 months of smoking cessation. Perhaps some of the patients who continued to smoke believed that they were in good health and at low risk for complications. A longer time quitting (>6 months) seems to be associated with the lowest rate of complications [❹ *Warner et al, 1989*].

Not well studied but potentially important is the role of elevated carboxyhemoglobin levels in heavy smokers. This level can oscillate between 3% and 10% in chronic smokers. Levels such as this have been shown to impair exercise performance and oxygen delivery. Smoking cessation, even if it occurs hours before surgery, could have potential benefits through this mechanism.

Also in need of further investigation are the findings of a European trial designed to evaluate an intensive smoking cessation program versus usual care on outcome after orthopedic procedures. The intensive smoking cessation program included sophisticated counseling, pharmacologic therapy, and careful follow-up. Patients were either enrolled in the intensive smoking cessation program or received usual care with simple advice to quit smoking. Investigators found a remarkably lower rate of any postoperative complication in the patients enrolled in the intensive program (18% versus 52%), as well as a much lower rate of wound complications (5% versus 31%) [❶ Moller et al, 2002]. The study used an intention-to-treat analysis. To avoid one wound-related complication, only four patients would need to be enrolled in such a program, regardless of actual smoking cessation. These data indicate a dramatic opportunity to reduce the rate of wound complications for patients undergoing orthopedic procedures. The significance of these complications can be dramatic when prosthetic devices are involved. Based on these data, elective orthopedic procedures should be considered only after an intensive trial of smoking cessation. The application in other surgical populations remains to be determined.

Chronic Obstructive Pulmonary Disease

Patients with COPD are at increased risk for postoperative pulmonary complications [❶ Chalon et al, 1975; ❷ Warner et al, 1984]. This concept was confirmed in a retrospective analysis of 107 patients with severe airflow obstruction who were undergoing several types of surgical procedures. The overall incidence of complications was 32%, with 5% mortality [❶ *Kroenke et al, 1992*]. In contrast, patients with restrictive pulmonary diseases in whom flows and cough are preserved have a lower risk. A history of cigarette smoking, chronic cough, phlegm production, pulmonary infections, or previous surgical experience provides useful information. The physical examination can also help to detect hyperinflation, with the presence of increased posteroanterior diameter and use of accessory muscles providing clues to severe obstruction and lung overinflation. In 2003, McAlister and coworkers observed that when the simple distance between the top of the thyroid cartilage to the suprasternal notch at the end of expiration was 4 cm or less, patients had an odds ratio of 2 for the development of postoperative pulmonary complications. **Decreased breath sounds, pulmonary crackles, wheezes, rhonchi, and prolongation of the expiratory phase of respiration have been shown to be indicators of increased pulmonary risk [❶ *Lawrence et al, 1996*]. A useful bedside test to assess the risk of perioperative pulmonary complications is the *cough test*, in which the patient is asked to inspire deeply and to cough. Development of recurrent coughing suggests an increased risk of postoperative pulmonary complications [❶ *McAlister et al, 2005*].** For the patient with COPD, spirometry is a valuable test before lung resection operations. **For nonpulmonary surgical procedures, the role or benefit of preoperative spirometry is unproven [❶ *Smetana et al, 2006*].** Despite a lack of prospective randomized data, some physicians find spirometry useful in evaluating patients with COPD to identify those at the highest risk for postoperative pulmonary complications. Spirometric studies performed include forced vital capacity (FVC), forced expiratory volume in 1 second (FEV_1), and possibly arterial blood gas determinations. An FVC lower than 70% of predicted and an FEV_1/FVC ratio lower than 50% of predicted have been associated with an increased risk for the development of postoperative pulmonary complications [● *Gracey et al, 1979*; ● *Stein and Cassara, 1970*]. Another test shown to be useful is the maximal voluntary ventilation. If the result obtained is lower than 50% of the predicted value, the possibility of postoperative pulmonary complications developing is significantly increased [● *Stein and Cassara, 1970*]. Perhaps the maximal voluntary ventilation test is valuable because it assesses the endurance of the respiratory system and the motivation of the patient, not just muscle strength or airflow. Finally, if the FVC is abnormal, arterial blood gas measurements help to determine the adequacy of the system to maintain normal PaO_2 and arterial carbon dioxide tension ($PaCO_2$). Three reports [● *Cain et al, 1979*; ● *McAlister et al, 2003*; ● *Stein and Cassara, 1970*] indicated that a $PaCO_2$ higher than 45 mm Hg is a predictor of important postoperative pulmonary complications. In our opinion, a high $PaCO_2$ does not absolutely contraindicate surgery, but rather points to the need to provide perioperative care with intense and careful postoperative support. Most hypercapnic patients tolerate surgery if the appropriate steps are taken.

Asthma

It is accepted that patients with poorly controlled asthma are at increased risk for postoperative pulmonary complications [● *Gold and Helrich, 1963*]. Nevertheless, even patients with severe, steroid-dependent asthma may undergo needed surgical procedures if an adequate plan is prepared and followed. The known risks for asthmatic patients who are undergoing anesthesia and abdominal surgery are bronchospasm, atelectasis, and cough. Cough may become an important factor in incisional pain and possible wound dehiscence. Although investigators have argued about avoidance of endotracheal intubation through the use of spinal anesthesia, "high" spinal anesthesia (above T6) may result in enhanced bronchospasm through blockade of sympathetic efferents that leave the vagal innervation of the bronchi unopposed. The risk in patients with poorly controlled asthma is more clearly related to the site of operation and to the duration of anesthesia than to the clinical severity of the asthma [❸ *Gold and Helrich, 1963*]. Well-controlled asthma is not a risk factor for postoperative pulmonary complications.

The best preparation for patients with poorly controlled asthma is to treat them until the clinical examination shows an absence of wheezing and their pulmonary function tests are optimized. Generally, these outcomes can be achieved with optimal inhaled therapy using an inhaled glucocorticoid alone or in combination with a long-acting β-agonist. Any asthmatic patient who is to undergo general anesthesia and who has required oral or systemic steroids during the last 6 months should receive parenteral steroids to prevent adrenal insufficiency [National Heart, Blood and Lung Institute Expert Panel, 1997]. Hydrocortisone, 100 mg intravenously every 8 hours starting 12 hours preoperatively, is often recommended and should suffice. The need for stress-dose steroids in asthmatic patients who are maintained on the highest dose of high-potency inhaled steroid formulations is controversial. Some studies suggested suppression of the hypothalamic-pituitary-adrenal axis in patients receiving high doses of fluticasone or budesonide (>750 μg inhaled steroid of these formulations daily) [❸ *Lipworth, 1999*].

Nonpulmonary Risk Factors

Nonpulmonary risk factors include those that affect respiratory function independent of the presence of previous pulmonary problems.

Site of Surgery

Surgical procedures associated with increased risk of pulmonary complications include aortic aneurysm repair, thoracic surgery, head and neck surgery, vascular surgery, esophageal resection, and abdominal surgery. **The risk for the development of postoperative pulmonary complications increases** with proximity to the diaphragm [❷ *Celli et al, 1984*]. Upper abdominal surgical procedures, such as those on the gallbladder, liver, spleen, stomach, small intestine, and pancreas, carry the highest risk, whereas procedures involving the lower abdomen and the extremities have a low risk. Besides the site, some evidence indicates that the type of incision may influence the frequency of postoperative pulmonary complications. In general, vertical laparotomies seem to carry a higher incidence of atelectasis and hypoxemia than do horizontal laparotomies [Halasz, 1964]. **Abdominal aortic aneurysm repair (open) and upper abdominal procedures carry a higher relative risk than other vascular or neurosurgical procedures** [❸ *Arozullah et al, 2001*].

Type of Surgery

The advent of laparoscopic surgery led to a reduction in perioperative pulmonary complications when compared with open cholecystectomy. This finding seems to result from less compromise of the respiratory muscles, with consequent higher vital capacity and PaO_2. In spite of these encouraging results, care must be taken not to extrapolate results from relatively low-risk patients to patients with severe airflow obstruction. The reason is that during laparoscopic surgery, significant amounts of carbon dioxide are used to distend the peritoneal cavity. The carbon dioxide is easily absorbed and exhaled in physiologically normal individuals, but the CO_2 load could become overwhelming to patients with poor gas exchange because of COPD. Until data are provided, it seems prudent to avoid this type of surgical procedure in patients with severe COPD, especially patients with carbon dioxide retention.

Duration and Type of Anesthesia

Emergency and lengthy surgical procedures (lasting >3 hours) are associated with increased pulmonary risk. In one study, the duration of the procedure was second to the site of operation as a risk factor for postoperative pulmonary complications

[**O** *Celli et al, 1984*]. It may be that the actual development of postoperative pulmonary complications does not depend on anesthesia time but rather on the procedure itself, which may be longer in those complicated cases that require more intra-operative manipulation of viscera.

Age

Age has been demonstrated to be an independent risk factor for postoperative pulmonary complications. The risk increases in relation to increasing age; the odds ratio for pulmonary complications is 2.09 for ages 60 to 69 years and 3.04 for ages 70 to 79 years. This increased risk is not a result of age-related comorbidities. With increasing age, some reflex activity of the upper airways may diminish, with a decrease in inspiratory and expiratory muscle forces [**O** *Rochester and Arora, 1983*], which may reduce the capacity to clear secretions. Furthermore, elderly individuals suffer from changes in lung mechanics, so that airway closure may occur even during tidal breathing. These changes are worsened in the supine position. Because FRC decreases during and after surgical procedures, older patients may experience significant closure of airways and alveoli with atelectasis, worsening of gas exchange, and possible respiratory failure.

Obesity

Although the obese patient may have reduced lung volumes and a spirometric pattern resembling restriction, **obesity has surprisingly not been definitively demonstrated to be a risk factor for perioperative pulmonary complications** [**O** *Smetana, 1999*].

Obstructive Sleep Apnea

Although evidence-based data are limited, obstructive sleep apnea is suspected to be associated with a trend toward increased postoperative pulmonary risk [**O** *Gupta et al, 2001*]. These complications include those related to airway management, the need for postoperative reintubation, and the risk of respiratory failure. In these patients, close postoperative observation and early institution of nasal continuous positive airway pressure (CPAP) may prevent the immediate postoperative complications of sleep apnea [❸ *Rennotte et al, 1995*]. Given the high and increasing prevalence of this disorder in the general population and the effects of anesthetic drugs on upper airway function, clinicians need to be vigilant in monitoring for postoperative problems in patients with sleep apnea [❸ *Robinson and Zwillich, 1985*].

When possible, the patient should be encouraged to lose weight preoperatively, but this is often not possible. In these patients, and more so in obese patients with sleep apnea or obesity-hypoventilation syndrome, postoperative analgesics and narcotics may exacerbate the underlying instability and may lead to hypercapnic respiratory failure.

Serum Albumin

A low serum albumin concentration has been shown to be a significant predictor of postoperative pulmonary complications [❹ *Gibbs et al, 1999*]. Although the studies that led to that finding varied in their definition of "low," the National Veterans Affairs Surgical Risk Study reported that a serum albumin less than 35 g/L was an important predictor of morbidity and mortality during the 30 days after the surgical procedure.

IDENTIFICATION OF THE HIGH-RISK PATIENT

Investigators have attempted to develop simple bedside assessment tools to help identify the patient at risk for postoperative pulmonary complications. The first study was conducted on a large group of patients (n = 1000) undergoing abdominal surgery [❸ *Hall et al, 1991*]. In that study, multivariate analysis showed that the best predictors of postoperative pulmonary complications were the classification of the American Society of Anesthesiologists (Table 8-1) and age older than 59 years. Unfortunately, the positive predictive value of 0.49 and the negative predictive value of 0.86 are too poor for clinical utility. Epstein and colleagues developed another cardiopulmonary risk index [❻ *Epstein et al, 1993*]. This index incorporates a modified version of the criteria first developed in 1977 by Goldman and associates with the respiratory factors believed to play a role in the genesis of postoperative pulmonary complications. Using a threshold value of 4, this index had a high positive (0.79) and negative (0.86) predictive value for postoperative pulmonary complications in patients undergoing thoracic surgery. Its validity in patients undergoing abdominal surgery remains to be determined.

Arozullah and colleagues developed a clinically useful risk assessment tool to predict the occurrence of postoperative pneumonia [❻ *Arozullah et al, 2001*]. The importance of this model must be emphasized because the study included data from 160,000 surgical procedures, and the prediction model was validated with a follow-up study. The prediction of pneumonia is important, given that 20% of patients who developed pneumonia died in the hospital. Table 8-2 shows the prediction model point system. Table 8-3 shows how the prediction model's rates for pneumonia correlated with the rates identified in the validation cohort.

One other study also attempted to identify factors associated with pulmonary complications after nonthoracic surgery.

TABLE 8-1	American Society of Anesthesiologists Classification of Anesthetic Risk
Class	**Characteristics**
I	Healthy
II	Mild to moderate systemic disease
III	Severe systemic disease
IV	Life-threatening systemic disease
V	Moribund

From New classification of physical status. American Society of Anesthesiologists. Anesthesiology 24:111, 1963.

TABLE 8-2	Preoperative History–Predicted Postoperative Pneumonia Point System	
Category	Risk Factor	Point Value
Type of surgical procedure	Abdominal aortic aneurysm	15
	Thoracic	14
	Upper abdominal	10
	Neck/neurosurgical	8
	Vascular other than AAA/ emergency	3
	GET/transfusion >4 U	4/3
Age	>80 yr/>70 yr/>60 yr/>50 yr	17/13/9/4
General health	Dependent/partially dependent	10/6
	Weight loss >10%	7
	Current smoker/drinker (>2/day)	3/2
History	Chronic obstructive pulmonary disease/stroke/altered MS	5/4
	Long-term steroid use	3

GET, General endotracheal anesthesia; MS, mental status.
Adapted from Arozullah A, Khuri SF, Henderson WG, Daley J: Development and validation of a multifactorial risk index. Ann Intern Med 135:847-857, 2001.

TABLE 8-3	Preoperative History–Predicted Postoperative Pneumonia Rate Correlation	
Risk Class (Points)	Rate of Pneumonia: Development Cohort	Rate of Pneumonia: Validation Cohort
1 (0–15)	0.24	0.24
2 (15–25)	1.19	1.18
3 (26–40)	4.0	4.6
4 (41–55)	9.4	10.8
5 (>55)	15.8	15.9

From Arozullah A, Khuri SF, Henderson WG, Daley J: Development and validation of a multifactorial risk index. Ann Intern Med 135:847-857, 2001.

McAlister and colleagues set out to determine the accuracy of preoperative assessment in predicting the occurrence of pneumonia, atelectasis, or mechanical ventilation before discharge. Although the study was prospective, patients underwent only selective preoperative studies, and the cohort was relatively small (272 patients). This feature is highlighted when the reader considers that only 22 patients (8%) developed postoperative complications. After multiple regression analysis, only three independent variables were associated with pulmonary complications. These were age greater than 65 years (odds ratio reported as 1.8), smoking history of at least 40 pack-years (odds ratio, 1.9), and maximum laryngeal height of 4 cm or less (odds ratio, 2.0). The small sample size and the lack of complete data on all patients make the conclusions of this study less compelling. Nonetheless, older smokers, whose respiratory mechanics are altered by advanced airflow obstruction and resultant hyperinflation, are at greatest risk for postoperative complications [❽ *McAlister et al, 2003*].

For the individual patient, the basic tool continues to be a good clinical examination. As stated before, the pulmonary history must be reviewed, with emphasis on those features that help to determine the presence of COPD or asthma. The patient's age, weight, and height help to determine whether these nonpulmonary risk factors are also present. The physician caring for the patient must know the site and organs to be handled during the surgical procedure and should discuss with the surgeon and anesthesiologist the possible duration of the procedure. For certain procedures, laparoscopic surgery may be the operation of choice. If these easily obtainable data suggest a high-risk patient, the evaluation should be complemented with a chest roentgenogram and spirometry. If the results of any of these tests are abnormal, arterial blood gas determinations are indicated. If the $PaCO_2$ is higher than 45 mm Hg, the incidence of surgical complications will be high, and the surgical procedure may be reconsidered unless it is really necessary.

Decreased exercise capacity has been shown to predict postoperative pulmonary complications after nonthoracic surgery. A simple way to determine exercise capacity is the ability to climb stairs. In a prospective study, Girish and co-workers determined an inverse correlation between the number of steps climbed and the development and severity of postoperative complications [❾ *Girish et al, 2001*]. In addition, the relationship also held true for hospital length of stay. Thus, an easy test to complete in anyone who is thought to be at risk from the history and the physical examination is to complete a stair climb. Less than two flights of stairs climbed should lead to a better evaluation of the patient and a consideration of intense interventions to prevent complications. If it is determined that the risk is high, measures must be taken that are known to decrease risk, including preoperative, intraoperative, and postoperative interventions that must be planned before the procedure.

APPROACHES TO DECREASE PERIOPERATIVE PULMONARY COMPLICATIONS

It is beneficial to discuss with the patient the type of procedure and its possible consequences. This has to be done in the context of the risk group into which the patient falls. If the patient smokes, he or she should stop as early as possible before the operation. Evidence indicates that the longer the patient stops before the surgical procedure, the more likely he or she is to benefit [❸ *Chalon et al, 1975*; ❸ *Warner et al, 1984*]. Six to 8 weeks may be the minimum needed to reverse some of the epithelial changes and some of the pulmonary functions such as closing volumes, small airway size, and tracheobronchial clearance of particles. Conversely, smoking cessation may lead to a decrease in the carboxyhemoglobin level, with the possible benefits described earlier. If the time between when the patient quits smoking and the surgical procedure is not long enough (<6 to 8 weeks), other steps can be taken to decrease the risk preoperatively. In patients with cough and phlegm in whom infected sputum is present, a course of antibiotics is indicated. Either ampicillin, at a dose of 250 mg orally four times daily, or doxycycline, 100 mg orally twice daily for 10 to 14 days, is a simple, narrow-spectrum selection with good efficacy.

Lung expansion techniques have been demonstrated to be beneficial in decreasing pulmonary complications

in the perioperative period, particularly for patients who undergo abdominal surgery [❶ Lawrence et al, 2006]. Modalities include incentive spirometry, cough, chest physical therapy, postural drainage, chest percussion, intermittent positive pressure breathing, and CPAP. No evidence favors one technique over another. It is our recommendation that the lung expansion technique selected be tailored to the patient's needs as well as the patient's ability to participate. There is also no evidence that combining lung expansion techniques offers any increased benefit.

Use of Bronchodilators in the Perioperative Period

In the patient with COPD, the bronchodilator regimen must be maintained until the day of the surgical procedure, preoperatively, and postoperatively. In asthmatic patients, bronchodilators should be administered as needed, and controller therapy (inhaled steroids or inhaled steroids in combination with long-acting dilators) should be maintained throughout the perioperative period.

Beta-Adrenergic Agonists

This group of drugs consists of the most effective bronchodilators that have the unique advantage of nebulization administration directly to the respiratory tract. An agent such as albuterol is administered as a standard solution at a dose of 2.5 mg diluted in 1.5 mL saline. This can be repeated every 4 hours throughout the procedure. In occasional cases of acute bronchospasm, either terbutaline, in a dose of 0.25 mL, or epinephrine, 0.3 mL of a 1:1000 solution administered subcutaneously, may be lifesaving. The latter medications should be avoided in patients with hypertension, a history of heart disease, narrow-angle glaucoma, or prostatic hypertrophy.

Theophylline

Although theophylline is not as effective a bronchodilator as the β-adrenergic agents, it also seems to improve diaphragmatic contractility [❻ Aubier et al, 1981; ❻ Siafakas et al, 1993].

If the patient is already receiving this therapy, a theophylline level should be determined. If the level is therapeutic (serum level between 5 and 15 μg/dL), an intravenous infusion of aminophylline can be started hours before the surgical procedure at a dose of 0.4 to 0.6 mg/kg/hour. The drug should be maintained until the patient can tolerate feedings, at which time it may be switched to the oral route. Care must be taken to monitor levels in patients with congestive heart failure, pneumonia, or liver dysfunction and patients receiving cimetidine or erythromycin. Besides nausea, patients with toxic levels may experience arrhythmias and seizures that seem to carry a poor prognosis.

Corticosteroids

In patients considered for emergency procedures (e.g., patients admitted for appendectomy) who manifest clinical evidence of bronchospasm (wheezes or labored breathing, or both) or whose pulmonary function tests show important airflow limitations with bronchodilator response, corticosteroids are indicated. Because it may take longer than 6 hours to achieve the initial effect, corticosteroids should be started at least 12 hours preoperatively. Either hydrocortisone, 2 mg/kg, or methylprednisolone, 20 to 60 mg every 6 hours, is an effective dose to be given intravenously in the perioperative period. These doses are not to be given indefinitely because they are high and should be tapered postoperatively to reach the 20- to 40-mg range of oral prednisone once the patient is eating again. We favor quick tapering (5 to 7 days) to avoid interference with wound healing.

POSTOPERATIVE CARE

Once the surgical procedure is completed, the patient enters a critical period in which he or she should be observed closely. During this time, good suctioning and lateral turning of the head help to prevent any possible aspiration. The airway needs to be patent, and adequate oxygenation and ventilation must be guaranteed. If the patient is at high risk, it may be more appropriate to maintain intubation until it has been clearly determined that he or she is able to maintain spontaneous ventilation and the degree of consciousness is such that bronchial aspiration becomes unlikely. The capacity to maintain spontaneous ventilation can be determined by using the following parameters:

- Vital capacity of at least 15 mL/kg body weight
- Inspiratory and expiratory forces greater than −20 and 25 cm H_2O, respectively
- Capacity to respond to and obey commands
- Arterial blood gases with normal Pa_{CO_2} (<45 mm Hg) and pH while breathing spontaneously
- Low alveolar-arterial oxygen difference

Evidence indicates that postoperative pain management with epidural analgesia is associated with a reduced incidence of postoperative pulmonary complications [❸ *Rodgers et al, 2000*]. The patient should receive a judicious regimen of analgesics, enough to control pain but not at a dose at which the respiratory centers may be inhibited. Similarly, bandages that restrict thoracic and abdominal excursions should be avoided.

For the patient who has undergone abdominal surgery and has postoperative nausea or vomiting, inability to tolerate oral intake, or symptomatic abdominal distention, evidence indicates that decompression of the stomach with a nasogastric tube results in a decreased incidence of perioperative atelectasis and pneumonia [❸ *Nelson et al, 2005*]. **For the patient without such triggering conditions, routine use of a nasogastric tube is not indicated.**

As soon as possible, the patient should be moved out of bed because the upright position alone increases FRC by 10% to 20%. At the same time, the respiratory program begun preoperatively should be resumed. In the high-risk patient, we employ incentive spirometry at one third to one half the preoperative vital capacity and deep breathing exercises as outlined. The maneuvers should be used intensely (every hour) throughout the first 72 hours after the procedure. Classic studies have demonstrated that, in patients with upper abdominal procedures, either form of therapy begun and continued postoperatively was effective in decreasing the incidence of postoperative pulmonary complications when compared with untreated controls. Furthermore, intervention is justified because the lower incidence of postoperative pulmonary complications in the treated patients resulted in a shortening in length of stay [○ *Celli et al, 1984*]. The use of intermittent positive pressure breathing was evaluated. The results indicated that intermittent positive pressure breathing was effective in preventing postoperative pulmonary complications, but its higher cost and the relatively high incidence of abdominal distention made this the least preferred form of therapy. Currently, the use of this therapy has fallen out of practice in most medical centers. The use of CPAP may increase as more studies document its effectiveness. Unfortunately, the possible risk of bronchial aspiration and bloating still needs to be evaluated before the widespread use of CPAP is advocated. If the patient was receiving inhaled bronchodilators, their use should be continued. Intravenous theophylline may be switched to oral preparations as soon as the patient is tolerating oral intake.

Pulmonary complications are a major cause of perioperative morbidity. Risk factors for complications include age greater than 60 years, the presence of COPD, and a history of congestive heart failure. The surgical categories associated with the greatest risk include thoracic surgery, abdominal surgery, neurosurgery, head and neck surgery, vascular surgery, aortic surgery, emergency surgical procedures, and surgical procedures that last longer than 3 hours. Evidence-based interventions demonstrated to decrease perioperative pulmonary complications include the following: lung expansion maneuvers;

nasogastric decompression of the stomach with a nasogastric tube in the patient with nausea, vomiting, inability to tolerate oral intake, or symptomatic abdominal distention (referred to as selective nasogastric decompression); and postoperative pain management.

Selected Readings

Arozullah A, Khuri SF, Henderson WG, Daley J: Development and validation of a multifactorial risk index. Ann Intern Med 135:847-857, 2001. **B**

Aubier M, DeTroyer A, Sampson M, et al: Aminophylline improves diaphragmatic contractility. N Engl J Med 305:249–252, 1981. **B**

Bartlett RH, Brennan ML, Gazzaniga AB, Hanson EL: Studies on the pathogenesis and prevention of postoperative pulmonary complications. Surg Gynecol Obstet 1367:925–933, 1973. **B**

Bermudez M, Rodriguez K, Celli B: Is weight an independent risk factor in the development of postoperative pulmonary complications after abdominal surgery? Am Rev Respir Dis 135:A211, 1987.

Breslin EH: Prevention and treatment of pulmonary complications in patients after surgery of the upper abdomen. Heart Lung 10:511–519, 1981. **B**

Buchwald H, Avidor Y, Braunwald E, et al: Bariatric surgery: A systematic review and meta-analysis. JAMA 292:1724-1737, 2004.

Cain HD, Stevens PM, Adanija R: Preoperative pulmonary function and complications after cardiovascular surgery. Chest 76:130–135, 1979. **B**

Celli BR, Rodriguez K, Snider GL: A controlled trial of intermittent positive pressure breathing, incentive spirometry, and deep breathing exercise in preventing pulmonary complications after abdominal surgery. Am Rev Respir Dis 130:12-15, 1984. **A**

Chalon J, Tayae MA, Ramanathan S: Cytology of respiratory epithelium as a predictor of respiratory complications after operation. Chest 67:32–35, 1975. **B**

Dureuil B, Viires N, Contineau JP, et al: Diaphragmatic contractility after upper abdominal surgery. J Appl Physiol 61:1775–1780, 1986. **B**

Epstein SK, Faling LJ, Daly BD, Celli BR: Predicting complications after pulmonary resection: Preoperative exercise testing vs. a multifactorial cardiopulmonary risk index. Chest 104:694-700, 1993. **B**

Ford GT, Whitelaw W, Rosenal TW, et al: Diaphragmatic function after upper abdominal surgery in humans. Am Rev Respir Dis 127:431–436, 1983. **B**

Ford GT, Guenter CA: Toward prevention of postoperative pulmonary complications. Am Rev Respir Dis 130:4–5, 1984. **B**

Gibbs J, Cull W, Henderson W, et al: Preoperative serum albumin level as a predictor of operative mortality and morbidity: Results from the National VA Surgical Risk Study. Arch Surg 134:36-42, 1999. **A**

Girish M, Trayner E, Dammann O, et al: Symptom-limited stair climbing as a predictor of post-operative cardiopulmonary complications after high-risk surgery. Chest 120:1147-1151, 2001. **B**

Gold MI, Helrich M: A study of the complications related to anesthesia in asthmatic patients. Anesth Analg 42:283–293, 1963. **B**

Gracey DR, Divertie MB, Didier EP: Preoperative pulmonary preparation of patients with chronic obstructive pulmonary disease. Chest 76:123–129, 1979. **A**

Guidelines for the diagnosis and management of asthma. Expert Panel Report 3. 2007. Available at www.nhlbi.nih.gov/guidelines/asthma/index.htm **C**

Gupta RM, Parvizzi J, Hanssen AD, Gay PC: Postoperative complications in patients with obstructive sleep apnea syndrome undergoing hip or knee replacement: A case controlled study. Mayo Clin Proc 76:897-905, 2001. **B**

Hall JC, Tarala RA, Hall J, Mander J: A multivariate analysis of the risk of pulmonary complications after laparotomy. Chest 99:923-927, 1991. **B**

Jackson C: Preoperative pulmonary evaluation. Arch Intern Med 148:2120–2127, 1988. **B**

Kroenke K, Lawrence VA, Theroux JF, Tuley MR: Operative risk in patients with severe obstructive pulmonary disease. Arch Intern Med 152:967-971, 1992. **B**

Lawrence VA, Dhanda R, Hilsenbeck SG, Page CP: Risk of pulmonary complications after elective abdominal surgery. Chest 110:744-750, 1996. **B**

Lawrence VA, Cornell JE, Smetana G: Strategies to reduce postoperative pulmonary complications after noncardiothoracic surgery: Systematic review for the American College of Physicians. Ann Intern Med 144:596-608, 2006. **B**

Laws AK: Effects of induction of anesthesia and muscle paralysis on functional residual capacity of the lungs. Can Anesth Soc J 15:325–331, 1968. **B**

Lipworth BJ: Systemic adverse effects of inhaled corticosteroid therapy: A systematic review and meta-analysis. Arch Intern Med 159:941-955, 1999. **B**

McAlister FA, Bertsch K, Man J, et al: Incidence of and risk factors for pulmonary complications after nonthoracic surgery. Am J Respir Crit Care Med 171:514-517, 2005. **B**

McAlister FA, Khan NA, Strauss SE, et al: Preoperative factors identified patients at risk for pulmonary complications after non-thoracic surgery. Am J Respir Crit Care Med 167:741-744, 2003. **B**

Moller AM, Villebro N, Pederson T, Tonnesor H: Effect of preoperative smoking intervention on postoperative complications: A randomized clinical trial. Lancet 359:114-117, 2002. **Ⓐ**

National Heart, Blood and Lung Institute Expert Panel, National Institutes of Health: Guidelines for the Diagnosis and Management of Asthma. Expert panel report 2. NIH publication no. 97-4051. Bethesda, MD, National Institutes of Health, 1997.

Nelson R, Tse B, Edwards S: Systematic review of prophylactic nasogastric decompression after abdominal operations. Br J Surg 92:673-680, 2005. **Ⓑ**

Pasulka PS, Bistrian BR, Benotti PN, Blackburn GL: The risks of surgery in obese patients. Ann Intern Med 104:540-546, 1986.

Pontoppidan H: Mechanical aids to lung expansion in non-intubated surgical patients. Am Rev Respir Dis 122:109–119, 1980. **Ⓑ**

Putensen-Himmer G, Putensen C, Lammer H, et al: Comparison of postoperative respiratory function after laparoscopy or open laparotomy for cholecystectomy. Anesthesiology 77:675-680, 1992.

Qaseem A, Snow V, Fitterman N, et al: Risk assessment for and strategies to reduce perioperative pulmonary complications for patients undergoing noncardiothoracic surgery: A guideline from the American College of Physicians. Ann Intern Med 144:575-580, 2006.

Ramsey-Stewart G: The perioperative management of morbidly obese patients (a surgeon's perspective). Anaesth Intensive Care 13:399-406, 1985.

Rennotte MT, Baele P, Aubert G, Rodenstein DO: Nasal continuous positive airway pressure in the perioperative management of patients with obstructive sleep apnea submitted to surgery. Chest 107:367-374, 1995. **Ⓑ**

Rigg JR, Jamrozik K, Myles PS, et al: Epidural anesthesia and analgesia and outcome of major surgery: a randomized trial. Lancet 359: 1276-1282, 2002. **Ⓐ**

Robinson RW, Zwillich CW. The effect of drugs on breathing during sleep. Clin Chest Med 6:603-614, 1985. **Ⓑ**

Rochester DR, Arora N: Respiratory muscle failure. Med Clin North Am 67:573–597, 1983. **Ⓑ**

Rodgers A, Walker N, Schug S, et al: Reduction of postoperative mortality and morbidity with epidural or spinal anesthesia: Results from overview of randomized trials. BMJ 321:1493, 2000. **Ⓑ**

Rovina N, Bouros D, Tzanakis N, et al: Effects of laparoscopic cholecystectomy on global respiratory muscle strength. Am J Respir Crit Care Med 153:458-461, 1996. **Ⓑ**

Siafakas NM, Stobou A, Stathopolou M, et al: Effect of aminophylline on respiratory muscle strength after upper abdominal surgery; a double blind study. Thorax 48:693–697, 1993. **Ⓑ**

Simmoneau G, Vivien A, Sartene R, et al: Diaphragm dysfunction induced by upper abdominal surgery. Am Rev Respir Dis 128:899–903, 1983. **B**

Smetana G: Preoperative pulmonary evaluation. N Engl J Med 340:937-944, 1999. **B**

Smetana G, Lawrence VA, Cornell JE: Preoperative pulmonary risk stratification for noncardiothoracic surgery: Systematic review for the American College of Physicians. Ann Intern Med 144:581-595, 2006. **B**

Stein M, Cassara E: Preoperative pulmonary evaluation and therapy for surgery patients. JAMA 211:787–790, 1970. **A**

Tisi GM: Preoperative evaluation of pulmonary function: Validity, indications and benefits. Am Rev Respir Dis 119:293–310, 1979. **B**

Warner MA, Divertie MB, Tinrer JH: Preoperative cessation of smoking and pulmonary complications in coronary artery bypass patients. Anesthesiology 60:380–383, 1984. **B**

Warner MA, Offord KP, Warner ME, et al: Role of preoperative cessation of smoking and other factors in postoperative pulmonary complications: A blinded prospective study of coronary artery bypass patients. Mayo Clin Proc 64:609-616, 1989. **A**

Gastrointestinal Complications in the Postoperative Period

JOHN A. EVANS, MD
DAVID G. FORCIONE, MD
LAWRENCE S. FRIEDMAN, MD

Many patients who undergo general surgery experience gastrointestinal problems in the postoperative period. Procedures in which the peritoneal cavity is entered have a profound effect on gastrointestinal function. Moreover, patients with preexisting or quiescent gastrointestinal disease may be at risk for a recurrence or exacerbation of the underlying disease. The first section of this chapter deals with perioperative management of patients with acute and chronic gastrointestinal diseases, the second section reviews common gastrointestinal problems that may occur in any patient undergoing a surgical procedure, and the third section discusses specific complications of surgery on the gastrointestinal tract.

PERIOPERATIVE MANAGEMENT OF GASTROINTESTINAL DISEASES

Gastroesophageal Reflux Disease

Gastroesophageal reflux is common in the general population and is a frequent cause of esophagitis in the perioperative period. The pathogenesis involves an increased frequency of

---

Levels of Evidence:

🅐—Randomized controlled trials (RCTs), meta-analyses, well-designed systematic reviews of RCTs. 🅑—Case-control or cohort studies, nonrandomized clinical trials, systematic reviews of studies other than RCTs, cross-sectional studies, retrospective studies. 🅒—Consensus statements, expert guidelines, usual practice, opinion.

transient relaxations of the lower esophageal sphincter or, to a lesser extent, incompetence of the lower esophageal sphincter. The latter mechanism appears to account for gastroesophageal reflux in critically ill ventilated patients. Contributing factors in the perioperative period include prolonged recumbency, abdominal surgery, and possibly the use of a nasogastric tube and percutaneous gastrostomy. Complications of severe and long-standing gastroesophageal reflux disease include the following: ulceration and bleeding; strictures in the distal esophagus (peptic stricture); Barrett's metaplasia of the esophageal mucosa with an associated increased risk of adenocarcinoma; pulmonary aspiration of refluxed gastric contents; and other extraesophageal complications such as laryngitis, asthma, and dental erosions.

Diagnosis

The clinical presentation of gastroesophageal reflux disease consists of pyrosis (heartburn), water brash (salivary secretion of salty fluid), and regurgitation. Regurgitation and aspiration may lead to asthma, morning hoarseness, and nocturnal choking.

The diagnosis of gastroesophageal reflux generally can be made on the basis of a careful history. If necessary, the following studies may be helpful, depending on the clinical problem: barium swallow, upper endoscopy, 24-hour esophageal pH monitoring, and esophageal manometry.

Management

Patients with known or suspected gastroesophageal reflux and esophagitis preoperatively should be maintained on standard antireflux therapy throughout the perioperative period. This includes elevation of the head of the bed, a low-fat diet, avoidance of meals before bedtime, and avoidance of caffeine, peppermint, chocolate, citrus juices, alcohol, and cigarettes. The patient should be instructed to avoid large meals, especially before and during recumbency. Drugs that decrease the lower esophageal sphincter pressure, such as calcium antagonists, sedatives, anticholinergic agents, and theophylline, should be avoided if possible.

Proton pump inhibitors are the most effective agents for raising gastric fluid pH and act by blocking the sodium-potassium/adenosine triphosphatase channel on gastric parietal cells (Table 9-1). Proton pump inhibitors are also the most effective agents for eliminating reflux symptoms and for healing esophagitis. Intravenous formulations of pantoprazole and lansoprazole are available in the United States. Clinical RCTs have demonstrated the efficacy of intravenous proton pump inhibitors in reducing gastric volume and in raising gastric pH. In the perioperative period, such therapy reduces the risk of aspiration. Of the five available oral proton pump inhibitors, esomeprazole, the S-isomer of omeprazole, may provide the greatest duration of gastric acid reduction. Whether this advantage translates into improved outcomes in the perioperative period is uncertain. In patients with severe gastroesophageal reflux and erosive esophagitis, therapy with proton pump inhibitors is preferred. In the absence of esophagitis, intravenous H_2-receptor antagonists may be adequate. Antacids (<30 mg orally 1 and 3 hours after meals and at bedtime) and sucralfate also are of benefit in protecting esophageal mucosa against peptic injury but are less convenient in postoperative patients. In randomized studies, sucralfate has been shown to be less effective in terms of the rate of complete healing and time to complete healing than both H_2-receptor antagonists and proton pump inhibitors in patients with moderate to severe reflux esophagitis.

If symptoms cannot be controlled with acid-reducing agents alone, the addition of a prokinetic drug such as metoclopramide (5 to 20 mg orally or intravenously) before meals and at bedtime may help by increasing lower esophageal sphincter pressure and enhancing gastric emptying. Unfortunately, metoclopramide has a high frequency of side effects (e.g., drowsiness, confusion, muscle spasm, and galactorrhea). Use of cisapride, a 5-hydroxytryptamine$_4$ (5-HT$_4$) agonist that

TABLE 9-1	Drugs Used in the Treatment of Peptic Ulcer Disease		
Drug	**Oral Dose**	**Intravenous Dose**	**Side Effects**
Sodium-Potassium/Adenosine Triphosphatase Inhibitors			
Omeprazole	20–40 mg qd/bid	Not available	Few reported (e.g., drug interactions)
Esomeprazole	20–40 mg qd/bid	20–40 mg qd	As for omeprazole
Pantoprazole	20–40 mg qd/bid	40 mg qd	As for omeprazole
Rabeprazole	20–40 mg qd/bid	Not available	As for omeprazole
Lansoprazole	15–30 mg qd/bid	30 mg qd	As for omeprazole
H_2-Receptor Antagonists			
Cimetidine	300 mg qid or 400 mg bid	300 mg q6h	Mental confusion, drug interactions (phenytoin, theophylline)
Ranitidine	150 mg bid or 300 mg qhs	50 mg q8h	Few reported (rare hepatitis)
Famotidine	20 mg bid or 40 mg qhs	20 mg q12h	Few reported
Nizatidine	150 mg bid or 300 mg qhs	Not available	Few reported
Defense-Enhancing Agents			
Sucralfate	1 g qid	Not available	Constipation and binding of other oral drugs
Aluminum hydroxide	15 to 30 mL four to eight times per day	Not available	Inconvenience and diarrhea
Magnesium hydroxide	Several times per day	Not available	Constipation
Prostaglandin Analogue			
Misoprostol	200 μg qid	Not available	Diarrhea, abdominal cramping
Triple Therapy for *Helicobacter pylori* (10–14 days)			
Omeprazole Two of the following:	20 mg bid	PO only	Few
Metronidazole	500 mg bid	PO only	Diarrhea, pseudomembranous colitis
Clarithromycin	500 mg bid		
Amoxicillin	1 g bid		

TABLE 9-1	Drugs Used in the Treatment of Peptic Ulcer Disease *(Continued)*		
Drug	**Oral Dose**	**Intravenous Dose**	**Side Effects**
Quadruple Therapy for *Helicobacter pylori* (2 wk)			
Bismuth subsalicylate	2 tablets qid	PO only	Diarrhea, pseudomembranous colitis
Metronidazole	250 mg tid	PO only	Nausea, indigestion, neuropathy, disulfiram effect
Tetracycline	500 mg qid	PO only	Diarrhea, pseudomembranous colitis
Proton pump inhibitor	Twice daily	PO only	Few
Alternative Regimen for Relapse or Persistent Infection			
Levofloxacin +	500 mg qd	PO only	Diarrhea, pseudomembranous colitis
Proton pump inhibitor +	Twice daily	PO only	Few reported
One of the following:			
Amoxicillin	1 g bid	PO only	Diarrhea, pseudomembranous colitis
Clarithromycin	500 mg bid	PO only	

bid, twice a day; qd, every day; qhs, at bedtime; qid, four times a day; PO, by mouth; tid, three times a day.

acts as a gastric prokinetic agent, is restricted because of the risk of cardiac dysrhythmias. Preliminary evidence suggests that tegaserod (6 mg orally twice daily), a $5\text{-}HT_4$ receptor partial agonist, also has prokinetic properties that may be useful in decreasing acid reflux.

Peptic Ulcer Disease

Peptic ulcer disease is common, occurring in up to 10% of the U.S. adult population. The classic history in a patient with a duodenal ulcer is of epigastric pain between meals or at night that is temporarily relieved by food or antacids. In contrast, the pain of gastric ulcer is more likely to be exacerbated by food. In addition, gastric ulcer is more likely than duodenal ulcer to be associated with anorexia and weight loss. However, it is difficult to differentiate a duodenal from a gastric ulcer on the basis of symptoms alone. Ulcer pain is often intermittent, and many individuals with peptic ulcer disease may have atypical symptoms or none at all.

Peptic ulcer disease is generally caused by either *Helicobacter pylori* or the long-term use of nonsteroidal anti-inflammatory drugs (NSAIDs) and is curable by eradication of *H. pylori* or discontinuation of the NSAID. In patients with a history of peptic ulcer disease, certain conditions that are common in the perioperative period may favor an acute recurrence (exacerbation) of an ulcer or may retard ulcer healing. For example, central nervous system trauma or surgery may be associated with gastric acid hypersecretion, and hypotension or anoxia may impair gastric mucosal defenses. Indeed, such factors are known to be risk factors for the development of stress ulcerations in any critically ill patient (see later). Whether patients with a previous peptic ulcer in whom *H. pylori* has not been eradicated are at increased risk of an exacerbation of their ulcer disease in the perioperative period is uncertain. **However, in patients with an active ulcer, perioperative stresses may lead to an increased risk of complications of ulcer disease, including hemorrhage and perforation** [❶ *Pollard et al, 1996*]. Therefore, in a patient with previous ulcer disease, it seems prudent to test for and, if present, eradicate *H. pylori* preoperatively.

Perioperative Management

DIAGNOSTIC CONSIDERATIONS

Ulcer disease should be suspected in patients with a history of peptic ulcer disease, ulcer-like pain, anemia, a positive test result for fecal occult blood, or overt gastrointestinal bleeding. The diagnosis of ulcer disease may be confirmed by either a barium radiograph or upper endoscopy. Endoscopy is more sensitive and specific than double-contrast upper gastrointestinal radiography, especially in patients with severe duodenal deformity resulting from chronic peptic ulcer disease. In addition, a rapid urease test or histologic evaluation with an immunostain can be performed on an antral biopsy specimen obtained at endoscopy to detect *H. pylori*. Additional measures to detect *H. pylori* include serologic testing (to detect immunoglobulin G antibody to *H. pylori*), radiolabeled urea breath testing, and an *H. pylori* fecal antigen enzyme-linked immunosorbent assay. Each of these assays has some limitations. The serologic test cannot distinguish active infection from remote exposure and clearance. The breath test is cumbersome and is not widely available. As the newest assay, the fecal antigen test is limited somewhat by a lack of data with regard to timing of antigen clearance following pharmacologic eradication of *H. pylori*. However, the fecal antigen test is convenient.

Ulcer-like pain in the absence of a demonstrable ulcer or other defined gastrointestinal disorder (e.g., cholelithiasis, gastroesophageal reflux disease, irritable bowel syndrome) is referred to as *functional* or *nonulcer dyspepsia* and is more common than peptic ulcer disease. The causes of functional dyspepsia are unclear but may include subtle gastroduodenal motility disturbances and reduced gastric accommodation. Patients with functional dyspepsia are not thought to be at increased risk of ulcer disease, perioperatively or otherwise, and the role of *H. pylori* in functional dyspepsia is uncertain. Meta-analyses have demonstrated a small but significant symptomatic benefit following *H. pylori* eradication in patients with functional dyspepsia.

Because gastric ulcers, even those that appear benign, may actually be malignant, it is important to perform endoscopic biopsies of these lesions to exclude malignancy. At least six biopsies are taken from the ulcer edge and one from the crater; a specimen for cytology also should be obtained. Repeat endoscopy, generally after 8 weeks of therapy, should be performed to ensure that a gastric ulcer has healed completely following therapy.

In general, elective surgery should be postponed in patients with an active, untreated ulcer. Because ulcers can heal significantly in 2 to 4 weeks, it is preferable to wait for at least partial healing with standard therapy before proceeding with surgery.

Treatment

With available drug therapy for ulcer disease, rigid dietary guidelines are no longer considered necessary. The single controllable nondrug determinant of ulcer healing is cigarette smoking, which should be restricted. Most available ulcer drugs result in 6- to 8-week healing rates of 80% to 90%. The main differences in the drugs relate to cost and side effect profiles (see Table 9-1).

Because of the role of H. pylori in the pathogenesis of peptic ulcer disease and ulcer recurrence, therapy to eradicate H. pylori from the stomach should be employed routinely when the organism is detected in a patient with an ulcer. Currently, the most commonly used triple-drug therapy for H. pylori consists of a proton pump inhibitor twice daily, amoxicillin 1000 mg twice daily, and clarithromycin 500 mg twice daily. Eradication rates in excess of 90% can be achieved with a 10- to 14-day course of therapy. Seven-day courses of antibiotics also appear to be cost effective but do not lead to eradication rates as high as with 10-day or 14-day regimens. For patients with persistent H. pylori infection after treatment, a quadruple-drug regimen consisting of bismuth subsalicylate two tablets four times daily, metronidazole 250 mg three times daily, tetracycline 500 mg four times daily, and a proton pump inhibitor twice daily is recommended. Recent data suggest that a 10-day course of levofloxacin 500 mg daily with a proton pump inhibitor twice daily and amoxicillin or clarithromycin also may be effective. Potential drawbacks to the use of multiple drugs to cure H. pylori infection and to heal ulcers include poor compliance, adverse reactions, and resistance to metronidazole and clarithromycin. In addition, patients must be cautioned not to take metronidazole with alcohol because of a disulfiram-like reaction. Nevertheless, in practice, side effects have not been a frequent problem.

Ulcers caused by NSAIDs are treated by discontinuation of the NSAID and use of a proton pump inhibitor for 4 to

8 weeks. If an NSAID must be continued, a proton pump inhibitor should also be taken twice daily. Alternatively, a selective cyclooxygenase-2 inhibitor may be considered.

Complications and Their Management

Several serious complications of peptic ulcer disease may occur and may, in fact, themselves be indications for surgical intervention.

BLEEDING

More than one half of all hospital admissions for gastrointestinal bleeding result from peptic ulcer disease. Peptic ulcer bleeding usually manifests as melena or hematemesis. Most bleeding ulcers are treated successfully with endoscopic therapy (e.g., electrocoagulation, injection of epinephrine, or placement of hemostatic clips). Treatment with a proton pump inhibitor reduces the risk of recurrent bleeding and the need for surgery but does not decrease the risk of mortality. (Diagnosis and management are discussed in the later section "Evaluation and Management of the Patient with Postoperative Gastrointestinal Bleeding.") It is difficult to apply a rigid set of indications for emergency surgery because the age of the patient and the presence of comorbid conditions play a large role in determining the outcome. Approximate indications for surgery include transfusion of 4 to 8 U of blood in the first 24 hours after admission and recurrent bleeding despite endoscopic interventions (see following sections). When bleeding is controlled successfully by conservative (nonoperative) measures and *H. pylori* is detected, therapy to eradicate *H. pylori* should be initiated and has been shown to decrease the risk of recurrent ulcer bleeding.

PERFORATION

The clinical presentation of a perforated peptic ulcer is with the sudden onset of severe abdominal pain that quickly generalizes to the entire abdomen and is followed by hypotension and fever. Acute peritonitis typically is accompanied by a rigid, boardlike abdomen, absent bowel sounds, and leukocytosis.

Free air under the diaphragm may be seen on an erect chest radiograph.

Treatment of a perforated ulcer is usually surgical and consists of closure of the perforation, possibly combined with a proximal gastric vagotomy. Rarely, a nonoperative approach may be considered if an upper gastrointestinal contrast series with meglumine diatrizoate (Gastrografin) shows no free leakage into the peritoneal cavity.

Ulcers may also penetrate posteriorly into the pancreas, resulting in acute pancreatitis with severe back pain and hyperamylasemia. Posterior penetration may respond to medical therapy with nasogastric decompression and gastric acid suppression with a proton pump inhibitor.

GASTRIC OUTLET OBSTRUCTION

Severe or recurrent ulcer disease may lead to gastric outlet obstruction, with a clinical presentation of vomiting, epigastric pain, weight loss, and early satiety. The diagnosis may be made by an upper gastrointestinal barium radiograph or upper endoscopy. A malignant cause of obstruction must be excluded.

Medical therapy, which is successful in no more than one fourth of patients with gastric outlet obstruction, consists of nasogastric suction, nutritional support, and aggressive anti-ulcer therapy. Endoscopic balloon dilation of the stenotic pylorus and placement of a stent may be considered. Many patients ultimately require surgical procedures for relief of the obstruction and for treatment of the ulcer diathesis.

Inflammatory Bowel Disease

Intestinal inflammation may result from a variety of infectious agents, ischemia, and radiation. The two main disease entities that constitute idiopathic inflammatory bowel disease are ulcerative colitis and Crohn's disease. The peak age of onset is in the second to third decades, although the disorders may occur at any age. Patients with inflammatory bowel disease may require surgical treatment for specific complications of their intestinal disease (e.g., intestinal obstruction, fistula, or cancer), for extraintestinal complications (e.g., cholelithiasis or nephrolithiasis), or for an unrelated condition.

Ulcerative Colitis

Ulcerative colitis is characterized by chronic inflammation of the colonic mucosa. The clinical presentation is typically with diarrhea, rectal bleeding, and rectal urgency. Involvement of the rectum is almost universal, and inflammation may extend proximally without interruption to a variable extent to involve the descending colon or occasionally the entire colon (pancolitis). The natural history is one of waxing and waning disease activity. Rarely, severe acute exacerbations of ulcerative pancolitis may be complicated by toxic megacolon or colonic perforation. Factors that account for flares in disease activity are poorly understood; in particular, whether surgical stress will lead to an acute exacerbation of ulcerative colitis is unpredictable.

Crohn's Disease

Crohn's disease is characterized by intestinal inflammation that is transmural (through all layers of the bowel wall), discontinuous, and in any segment of the gastrointestinal tract, most commonly the terminal ileum, colon, or both. Small intestinal involvement in particular is often complicated by the formation of strictures and fistulas, and colonic disease is often associated with perineal inflammation including fistulas and sinus tracts. Rectal involvement is less common in colonic Crohn's disease than in ulcerative colitis. The clinical presentation of Crohn's disease is often characterized by abdominal pain, diarrhea that may be nonbloody or bloody, fever, an inflammatory abdominal mass, and weight loss. Complications resulting from small intestinal inflammation include gallstones and kidney stones from bile salt malabsorption and malignancy. As in ulcerative colitis, the course is marked by exacerbations and remissions, and the effect of surgery on disease activity is unpredictable.

Perioperative Management

It is important for the medical consultant to confirm a diagnosis of ulcerative colitis or Crohn's disease and to determine the extent and severity of the disease at the time surgical treatment is planned. If necessary, diagnostic studies may include upper and lower barium radiographs and colonoscopy with biopsy. In about 10% of cases of chronic colitis, a distinction between ulcerative colitis and Crohn's colitis may not be possible, and the designation *indeterminate colitis* may apply. Serologic tests (antineutrophil cytoplasmic antibodies in ulcerative colitis and anti-*Saccharomyces cerevisiae* antibodies in Crohn's disease) may help to classify some such patients. In a patient with a recent flare in disease activity, stool cultures and examination for ova and parasites and *Clostridium difficile* toxin may be indicated to exclude superimposed infectious colitis. It is important to ask about systemic symptoms, including fever, arthritis, rash, ocular symptoms, jaundice, and weight loss, which may require further evaluation and treatment. Objective indicators of disease activity such as the hemoglobin level, hematocrit value, erythrocyte sedimentation rate, C-reactive protein, and serum albumin level should be obtained. In general, unless a surgical procedure is being performed for medically intractable inflammatory bowel disease, every effort should be made to control disease activity before elective surgery is undertaken. **It is important to consider the potential for perioperative NSAIDs to exacerbate disease activity in patients with inflammatory bowel disease** [❸ *Bonner et al, 2004*].

Drug Therapy for Ulcerative Colitis

Sulfasalazine, up to 4 to 6 g/day orally in three or four divided doses, or a related 5-aminosalicylate is the drug of choice for mild to moderately active ulcerative colitis. The major limitation of sulfasalazine is a high rate of side effects, which are most commonly dose related, including headache and indigestion, and less frequently idiosyncratic, such as fever, rash, pneumonitis, hepatitis, and pancreatitis. Alternative oral 5-aminosalicylate (mesalamine) compounds are as effective as sulfasalazine and cause fewer side effects, but they are more costly. Sulfasalazine or another aminosalicylate is often used to maintain remission in ulcerative colitis. Corticosteroids (e.g., oral prednisone, intravenous hydrocortisone, or methylprednisolone sodium succinate [Solu-Medrol]) may be added in acute exacerbations to obtain more rapid control of symptoms, although there is no role for corticosteroids in the maintenance therapy of ulcerative colitis. Corticosteroids are the drugs of choice for severe and fulminant attacks of ulcerative colitis. In patients with severe colitis unresponsive to high-dose intravenous corticosteroids, intravenous cyclosporine may be tried; clinical response to this agent is usually rapid (within 1 week). Patients who do not respond to cyclosporine require colectomy.

For patients with disease limited to the rectum or rectosigmoid colon, mesalamine or hydrocortisone retention enemas may be effective both in treatment of acute attacks and in maintenance of remission. Mesalamine is also available in a suppository formulation for use in limited rectal disease.

For patients with ulcerative colitis who receive maintenance therapy with sulfasalazine or mesalamine, there is no reason to add corticosteroids perioperatively. Oral sulfasalazine or mesalamine may be discontinued for several days and reinstituted when the patient is able to resume oral intake. If the patient is not able to take a drug orally, intravenous corticosteroids (e.g., hydrocortisone, 100 mg every 8 hours) may be necessary in the immediate postoperative period if the colitis appears to be flaring.

In all patients who have received oral prednisone preoperatively, appropriate "stress" doses of corticosteroids (e.g., hydrocortisone, 100 mg intravenously every 8 hours) must be administered perioperatively to prevent adrenal insufficiency. In patients with quiescent ulcerative colitis who have received no maintenance therapy preoperatively, it is generally not necessary to institute anti-inflammatory therapy in the peri-operative period unless the disease flares.

Drug Therapy for Crohn's Disease

Drug therapy for active Crohn's disease is similar to that for ulcerative colitis. In general, sulfasalazine and mesalamine are the drugs of choice for mildly to moderately severe Crohn's colitis, but sulfasalazine is less effective than corticosteroids in the treatment of small intestinal Crohn's disease. Corticosteroids are indicated for severe Crohn's disease, regardless of the site of involvement. Budesonide is an alternative to oral prednisone for the treatment of moderately active Crohn's ileocolitis. This agent is administered orally, undergoes extensive first-pass metabolism by the liver, and thus results in fewer corticosteroid-associated side effects. Budesonide and high-dose oral mesalamine therapy (e.g., 3 g/day) may have a role in maintaining remission. Because budesonide can suppress the adrenal axis in 60% of patients, patients receiving long-term budesonide therapy should be given stress doses of corticosteroids perioperatively.

Patients who have been taking prednisone preoperatively must continue to receive corticosteroids before, during, and after the procedure, in appropriate doses. Antibiotics (metronidazole and fluoroquinolones), which are often used to treat Crohn's colitis or perineal disease, and immunosuppressants (e.g., azathioprine, 6-mercaptopurine, and methotrexate), which may be used in disease refractory to corticosteroids alone, may be discontinued during the time the patient is unable to take medications orally. Patients with Crohn's disease who have been receiving corticosteroids and immunosuppressants may be immunocompromised and at risk for infectious complications in the perioperative period.

Some patients with Crohn's disease, particularly those with severe corticosteroid-dependent or corticosteroid-refractory Crohn's disease, and those patients with nonhealing enterocutaneous and perianal fistulas, may be treated with biologic therapy, specifically infliximab, a chimeric tumor necrosis factor-α antibody. **Limited data suggest that perioperative use of infliximab may be safe, but the increased risk of serious infections associated with use of this agent requires that patients undergoing both elective and nonelective surgical procedures be monitored closely** [❿ *Bibbo and Goldberg, 2004*].

Systemic Disease

About 4% of patients with ulcerative colitis and occasional patients with Crohn's colitis may have primary sclerosing cholangitis or, rarely, chronic hepatitis, which may occasionally lead to cirrhosis with portal hypertension and esophageal varices. Primary sclerosing cholangitis is a fibrosing inflammatory disorder of bile ducts. Affected patients may have hypoprothrombinemia resulting from malnutrition or liver disease and thrombocytopenia secondary to hypersplenism. Crohn's disease in particular may also be associated with renal disease and amyloidosis. **Patients with inflammatory bowel diseases have a threefold increased risk of developing venous thromboembolism and should routinely receive perioperative prophylaxis with pneumatic compression stockings and subcutaneous injection of a low-molecular-weight heparin** [❿ *Bernstein et al, 2001*] (see Chapter 6).

Intraoperative Considerations

Vigorous bowel preparation for abdominal surgery in patients with ulcerative colitis and Crohn's disease may occasionally lead to toxic megacolon and should be avoided. Elective bowel resection for inflammatory bowel disease should not be combined with other intra-abdominal procedures because of increased morbidity and mortality. However, intraoperative assessment of the status of inflammatory bowel disease during laparotomy for another reason is worthwhile; consideration should be given to intraoperative liver biopsy if liver biochemical test abnormalities have been noted. In all patients with chronic diarrhea, careful attention should be paid to intravascular volume, renal function, and electrolyte abnormalities. In addition, blood transfusions may be required in the patient with anemia caused by chronic blood loss. In patients with inflammatory bowel disease and chronic liver disease, it may be best to avoid nasogastric tubes, if possible, because of the presence of large esophageal varices. Such patients also require careful intravenous fluid replacement, because fluid overload may increase portal hypertension and may lead to variceal bleeding.

Complications and Their Management

TOXIC MEGACOLON

One of the most serious complications of severe inflammatory bowel disease in the postoperative period is toxic megacolon. The clinical presentation is with fever, tachycardia, and abdominal distention, with dilation of the colon to more than 6 cm. In the postoperative period, the clinical picture may be particularly confusing because postoperative ileus is common. Anesthetics, immobilization, use of sedatives and narcotics, hypokalemia, and intestinal surgery itself may predispose the patient with inflammatory bowel disease to toxic megacolon. Supportive treatment includes high-dose intravenous corticosteroids, broad-spectrum antibiotics, nasogastric suction, and correction of electrolyte abnormalities. In some patients, a trial of intravenous cyclosporine may be worthwhile. If the patient does not improve within 48 to 72 hours, emergency subtotal colectomy should be considered because of a high risk of colonic perforation and peritonitis in the unoperated patient.

MALNUTRITION

Patients with severe inflammatory bowel disease are at particular risk for malnutrition because of decreased caloric intake, malabsorption, maldigestion, enteric protein loss, and chronic inflammation. In the severely malnourished patient, elective surgical procedures should be postponed until profound nutritional deficiencies are corrected. In less severely malnourished patients, it may be appropriate to administer nutritional support in the perioperative period without postponing elective surgery, although the value of nutritional support in this setting is uncertain. Perioperative nutritional support may be administered by oral infusion of an elemental diet through a small-bore feeding tube or, if necessary, by total parenteral nutrition through a central venous line. Total bowel rest is often beneficial in controlling a flare of inflammatory bowel disease, and nutritional repletion is important for wound healing in the postoperative patient (see also Chapter 4).

Corticosteroid Use

Concern is often raised about an adverse effect of intravenous corticosteroids on wound healing and predisposition to postoperative infection, although the magnitude of the latter risk is uncertain. In addition, the clinician needs to be alert to other effects of corticosteroid use, including hyperglycemia, hypokalemia, fluid retention, and hypertension. The patient who has received long-term corticosteroid therapy is also at risk of osteoporosis, glaucoma, and cataracts.

Acute and Chronic Pancreatitis

Acute Pancreatitis

Acute pancreatitis is associated with a mortality rate as high as 10% and should lead to postponement of all but emergency surgery. The more common causes of acute pancreatitis include gallstones, alcohol, certain drugs, hyperlipidemia, and trauma (Box 9-1). (Postoperative pancreatitis is discussed later.)

The clinical presentation of acute pancreatitis is with boring epigastric abdominal pain, localized abdominal tenderness with signs of peritoneal irritation, nausea and vomiting, fever, hyperamylasemia, and, occasionally, hypotension or shock. Severe acute pancreatitis, which occurs in only a minority of patients, may affect multiple organs and may lead

Box 9-1	CAUSES OF ACUTE PANCREATITIS

Ethanol
Gallstones
Abdominal surgery
Toxins (e.g., organophosphorus)
Trauma
Idiopathic
Hypertriglyceridemia
Hypercalcemia
Drugs: Furosemide, hydrochlorothiazide, sulfonamides, tetra-
    cyclines, valproic acid, azathioprine/6-mercaptopurine,
    L-asparaginase, estrogens
Pancreas divisum
Ischemic (hypoperfusion, vasculitis)
Viral infections
Endoscopic retrograde cholangiopancreatography
Pancreatic or ampullary neoplasm
Hereditary pancreatitis
Penetrating peptic ulcer disease
Obesity
End-stage renal disease
Sphincter of Oddi dysfunction
Postoperative status

to acute respiratory distress syndrome, hypocalcemia, disseminated intravascular coagulation, acute tubular necrosis,
and fat necrosis. Several clinical and biochemical parameters
early in the course may be used to provide a rough estimation of prognosis (Box 9-2).

Radiologic evaluation of acute pancreatitis should include
plain radiographs of the abdomen to look for evidence of intestinal ileus and pancreatic calcifications resulting from
chronic pancreatitis. Chest radiographs should be obtained to
look for pleural effusions and interstitial lung edema. Computed tomography following administration of intravenous

Box 9-2	FACTORS ASSOCIATED WITH INCREASED MORTALITY IN ACUTE PANCREATITIS (RANSON'S CRITERIA)

AT ADMISSION

Age >55 yr
White blood cells >16,000/mm^3
Glucose >200 mg/dL
Lactate dehydrogenase >350 U/L
Aspartate aminotransferase >250 U/L

DURING INITIAL 48 HR

Hematocrit decrease of >10 mg/dL
Blood urea nitrogen increase of >5 mg/dL
Calcium <8 mg/dL
Partial pressure of arterial oxygen <60 mm Hg
Base deficit >4 mEq/L
Fluid sequestration >6 L

contrast material (generally after the first week of illness) may be used to assess the severity of pancreatitis; look for evidence of pancreatic necrosis, pseudocyst, and abscess; and guide needle aspiration in cases of pancreatic necrosis to determine whether infection, an absolute indication for surgical débridement, is present.

MANAGEMENT

Treatment of acute pancreatitis is largely supportive and includes volume resuscitation, parenteral analgesics and antiemetics, avoidance of oral intake, nasogastric suction in patients with vomiting or ileus, intravenous administration of a proton pump inhibitor or H_2-receptor antagonist, and careful monitoring of hemodynamics and renal function. Most patients recover uneventfully. In severe cases, monitoring of arterial oxygenation and the pulmonary capillary wedge pressure is desirable. Early use of endoscopic retrograde cholangiopancreatography with sphincterotomy is beneficial in patients with acute gallstone pancreatitis with evidence of biliary obstruction (dilated ducts or jaundice) and when cholangitis is also present. In patients with prolonged cases of acute pancreatitis, enteral nutrition should be administered. Serial computed tomographic scans should be obtained to monitor for the development of a pseudocyst or abscess, which may require percutaneous, endoscopic, or surgical drainage. Surgical débridement may be necessary in cases of pancreatic necrosis but should be delayed until the third to fourth week of illness if possible.

Chronic Pancreatitis

Surgery may be required in a patient with chronic pancreatitis as part of the treatment of the underlying disease, for a complication, or for an unrelated condition. Complications of chronic pancreatitis include the following: malnutrition; pseudocysts, which can rupture, bleed, become infected, or cause intestinal obstruction; obstruction of the intrapancreatic portion of the common bile duct; and thrombosis of the splenic or portal vein, with resulting gastroesophageal varices. Pancreatic ascites may best be managed by endoscopic placement of a stent across the disrupted pancreatic duct.

MANAGEMENT

Pancreatic enzyme replacement (e.g., pancrelipase, two to three tablets orally three times a day with meals and one or two with snacks) may improve the maldigestion and malnutrition that often accompany chronic pancreatitis. Frequently, chronic pancreatitis may lead to narcotic addiction because of a large requirement for analgesic medications to control chronic pain. Medication doses required for induction of anesthesia may be increased in such patients. When there is evidence of pancreatic duct obstruction with proximal dilation, the chronic pain of pancreatitis may respond to a drainage operation such as a longitudinal pancreaticojejunostomy, sometimes with resection of the pancreatic head. Similarly, endoscopic or surgical decompression of a large pseudocyst may result in pain relief. Pancreatic enzyme supplementation with an uncoated formulation to suppress pancreatic secretion, often given with oral bicarbonate, an H_2-receptor antagonist, or a proton pump inhibitor, may lead to pain relief in some patients. Total or subtotal pancreatectomy as a means of pain control is associated with unpredictable results. Neurolysis of the celiac ganglion is less effective in relieving the pain of chronic pancreatitis than the pain of pancreatic cancer.

GASTROINTESTINAL COMPLICATIONS IN THE POSTOPERATIVE PERIOD

Constipation

Causes

Constipation is common in bedridden postoperative patients; it is usually mild and self-limited and often multifactorial in origin. Many drugs used in the perioperative period may contribute to constipation (Box 9-3). Several common metabolic disorders that may occur postoperatively may contribute to constipation, including hypokalemia, hypercalcemia, acidosis, and uremia. Diabetes mellitus and hypothyroidism are additional metabolic causes of constipation. In some cases, mechanical disorders that may lead to constipation should be considered, including fecal impaction, intestinal tumors, volvulus, hernias, and strictures from ischemia, radiation, diverticulitis, or surgical procedures. Anorectal disorders that may lead to constipation include painful hemorrhoids, fissures, perirectal abscess, ulcerative proctitis, and rectal prolapse. Intestinal ileus and colonic pseudo-obstruction are common following gastrointestinal surgery (see later) and may account for constipation. Occasionally, extraperitoneal causes such as acute pancreatitis and retroperitoneal hemorrhage must be considered.

Box 9-3	DRUGS THAT MAY CAUSE CONSTIPATION

ANALGESICS

Opiates (e.g., morphine, codeine)
Opioids (e.g., fentanyl, pethidine, tramadol)
Nonsteroidal anti-inflammatory drugs (e.g., diclofenac, naproxen)

PSYCHIATRIC DRUGS

Antidepressants
Tricyclic antidepressants (e.g., amitriptyline, doxepin)
Monoamine oxidase inhibitors (e.g., phenelzine)
Selective serotonin reuptake inhibitors (e.g., fluoxetine, paroxetine)
Anxiolytics (e.g., trazodone, diazepam, chlordiazepoxide)
Antipsychotics (e.g., thioridazine, prochlorperazine, thiothixene)

ENDOCRINE AGENTS

Calcium supplements
Pamidronate, alendronate
Bromocriptine

GASTROINTESTINAL AGENTS

Proton pump inhibitors
Cholestyramine
Sucralfate
Others (5-acetylsalicylate agents, octreotide)

CARDIOVASCULAR DRUGS

Amiodarone
Disopyramide
Encainide
Flecainide
Clonidine
Guanfacine
Calcium antagonists (e.g., nifedipine)

ONCOLOGIC AND HEMATOLOGIC AGENTS

Vinblastine
Vincristine
Leuprolide
Iron supplements

OTHERS

Phenytoin
Anticholinergic agents (e.g., trihexyphenidyl, benztropine, amantadine)

Adapted from Lamparelli MJ, Kumar D: Investigation and management of constipation. Clin Med 2:415-420, 2002. Copyright 2002, Royal College of Physicians. Adapted by permission.

Postoperative Management

The management of constipation in the postoperative patient begins with discontinuation of predisposing medications when possible, especially opiate analgesics, and correction of any metabolic abnormalities that may be present. Resumption of normal physical activity and dietary intake, including adequate fluids and bulk, often helps. Various laxatives are available for the short-term treatment of constipation, as long as mechanical obstruction has been excluded. Bulk agents such as psyllium (e.g., Metamucil, 1 tbsp orally twice a day) and cellulose derivatives are generally the first line of therapy; it is important that they be accompanied by adequate fluid intake. Emollient agents such as docusate sodium (e.g., docusate, 100 mg twice a day) and lubricants such as mineral oil (15 to 45 mL orally twice a day) can be used to soften hard stool in the colon. Occasionally, saline cathartics such as magnesium citrate (200 mL orally every day), stimulant laxatives such as senna derivatives, osmotic agents such as lactulose (30 mL orally twice a day) or polyethylene glycol (Mira-Lax, 1 tsp/8 ounces of fluid/day), or a secretory agent such as lubiprostone (24 μg orally twice daily) may be needed.

Intestinal Pseudo-obstruction and Obstruction

Postoperative Ileus and Intestinal Obstruction

Abdominal surgery has a profound inhibitory effect on gastrointestinal motility as a result of sympathetic hyperactivity and inhibition of normal intestinal migrating myoelectric complexes; the resulting adynamic ileus often involves both the small and large bowel. In the immediate postoperative period, nasogastric suction traditionally has been used to prevent bowel distention and abdominal discomfort until intestinal function returns. **However, the need for routine nasogastric intubation in all patients undergoing abdominal surgical procedures has been questioned** [❶ *Nelson et al, 2005*]. Care should be taken to avoid hypokalemic alkalosis from the continuous suctioning of acidic gastric contents. Occasionally, postoperative ileus may be markedly prolonged, especially in the seriously ill patient who has undergone extensive surgical procedures. Nonmechanical causes of prolonged ileus are listed in Box 9-4. In the patient with an apparently prolonged postoperative ileus, it is necessary to exclude mechanical intestinal obstruction caused by adhesions, gut herniation, anastomotic stricture, or volvulus. An upright, plain abdominal radiograph is likely to demonstrate air-fluid levels in patients with either an ileus or mechanical intestinal obstruction; only mechanical obstruction is associated with dilated bowel above the level of obstruction and absent bowel gas below this level. Barium radiographs of the gastrointestinal tract may be necessary to determine the level of obstruction. A barium enema should be performed before an upper gastrointestinal series and small bowel follow-through to avoid inspissation of barium in the colon if there is an obstructing colonic lesion. Treatment of persistent mechanical intestinal obstruction is usually surgical.

Colonic Pseudo-obstruction

Colonic pseudo-obstruction, often referred to as *Ogilvie's syndrome,* is a particular form of intestinal pseudo-obstruction characterized by colonic ileus and dilation without obstruction,

Box 9-4	FACTORS THAT CONTRIBUTE TO PROLONGED POSTOPERATIVE ILEUS

UNDERLYING MEDICAL CONDITIONS

Sepsis
Collagen vascular diseases
Amyloidosis
Diabetes mellitus
Thyroid disease
Peritonitis
Ischemic bowel disease
Electrolyte disturbances (e.g., hypokalemia)

INTRAOPERATIVE BOWEL MANIPULATION

Open surgical procedure
Type of anesthesia

DRUGS (see Box 9-3)

most commonly involving the cecum and ascending colon. The clinical presentation is with abdominal distention, usually with abdominal pain, nausea, and vomiting. Bowel sounds may be normal or high pitched, and rebound tenderness may be present. The pathogenic factors are much the same as those for postoperative constipation (Box 9-5); drugs that inhibit gut motility (see Box 9-3) are frequently implicated. The exact cause of Ogilvie's syndrome is unclear, although an imbalance in sympathetic and parasympathetic tone is thought to be at the root of the problem. Patients undergoing spinal surgery or procedures during which the retroperitoneum is entered are at increased risk. The differential diagnosis of colonic pseudo-obstruction includes colonic volvulus, fecal impaction, ischemic colitis, typhlitis (neutropenic colitis), and mechanical obstruction.

POSTOPERATIVE MANAGEMENT

Management of intestinal or colonic pseudo-obstruction consists of nasogastric suction, rectal tube insertion, discontinuation of narcotic and anticholinergic medications, treatment

Box 9-5	FACTORS THAT CONTRIBUTE TO COLONIC PSEUDO-OBSTRUCTION

Age
Alcoholism
Drugs
  Narcotics
  Antidepressants
  Anticholinergics
  Clonidine
  Phenothiazines
Metabolic causes
  Electrolyte imbalance
  Acid-base disturbances
  Hypothyroidism
  Diabetes mellitus
Uremia
Sepsis
Surgery
Inflammatory processes (e.g., pancreatitis and cholecystitis)
Malignancy
Infection
Nonoperative trauma
Radiation therapy
Respiratory failure
Cardiovascular disease
Respiratory disease

From Vanek VW, Al-Salti M: Acute pseudo-obstruction of the colon (Ogilvie's syndrome): An analysis of 400 cases. Dis Colon Rectum 29:203-210, 1986. With kind permission from Springer Science and Business Media.

of infection, and correction of any metabolic abnormalities. **The parasympathomimetic agent neostigmine, 2 mg given intravenously over 1 to 3 minutes, has been shown to be effective in reversing acute colonic pseudo-obstruction** [❹ *Paran et al, 2000; Ponec et al, 1999; Stephenson et al, 1993*]. Evidence for the usefulness of prokinetic agents such as metoclopramide, erythromycin, bethanechol, and serotonin receptor agonists, such as tegaserod, is limited. Clinical response is determined by following serial abdominal examinations and radiographs.

COMPLICATIONS AND THEIR MANAGEMENT

Postsurgical pseudo-obstruction usually resolves with medical management within 3 to 6 days. The most feared complication of Ogilvie's syndrome is progressive dilation, leading to mucosal ischemia and colonic perforation with peritonitis. The risk of perforation increases greatly when the cecal diameter is more than 12 cm and when the duration of dilation exceeds 6 days. If colonic dilation does not resolve with conservative measures including neostigmine within 48 to 72 hours, consideration should be given to colonoscopic decompression with placement of a colonic tube; rarely, surgical decompression may be necessary.

Gastroparesis

Postoperative gastroparesis is seen particularly after vagotomy, in diabetic or uremic patients, or in patients with peptic ulcer disease and gastric outlet obstruction. Risk factors also include malnutrition and a Whipple procedure (pancreaticoduodenectomy) for malignancy [McCallum and George, 2001]. The clinical presentation is with abdominal distention and bloating. A succussion splash on physical examination and an enlarged gastric bubble on an abdominal radiograph are characteristic. When necessary, gastric outlet obstruction can be confirmed by an upper gastrointestinal series or upper endoscopy, whereas gastroparesis or delayed gastric emptying in the absence of mechanical obstruction can be demonstrated by a gastric emptying scintiscan after a meal containing a radiolabeled marker. Management of acute postsurgical gastric dilation includes nasogastric suction, an intravenous H_2-receptor antagonist or proton pump inhibitor, and a trial of intravenous metoclopramide or possibly erythromycin when mechanical obstruction has been excluded. Cisapride has been linked to cardiac toxicity and is no longer generally available. Gastric electrical stimulation techniques to improve gastroparesis are under investigation. Underlying causes should be sought and treated.

Nausea and Vomiting

Contributing Factors

Nausea and vomiting are common in the postoperative period and may represent an important sign of an underlying pathologic condition or a nonspecific, self-limited occurrence. Postoperative nausea and vomiting has numerous causes (Box 9-6). Drugs that may cause nausea and vomiting include general anesthetics, opiate analgesics, and digitalis, all of which act directly on the chemoreceptor trigger zone in the brain. The occurrence of postoperative vomiting is related to the duration of anesthesia, the amount of anesthetic used, and the types of anesthetics and associated drugs used (e.g., use of neostigmine to reverse the effects of nondepolarizing muscle relaxants). Postanesthetic nausea and vomiting are most likely to occur and tend to be most severe in women, obese patients, and those with a history of motion sickness. Nausea and vomiting are particularly associated with abdominal, gynecologic, urologic, ophthalmologic, and middle ear surgical procedures. Other contributory factors include postoperative ileus, gastroparesis, and mechanical intestinal obstruction. Other intra-abdominal processes associated with nausea and vomiting include peritonitis, acute pancreatitis, and acute cholecystitis. Nausea and vomiting may also result from food intolerance on resumption of oral feedings after prolonged total parenteral nutrition.

The temporal relationship between vomiting and oral intake may be helpful in the differential diagnosis. Vomiting immediately after a meal may result from pyloric channel edema and spasm caused by ulcer disease. Vomiting that occurs several hours after a meal may result from gastric outlet obstruction or a gastric motility disorder. The content of the emesis may also provide diagnostic clues: vomiting undigested food suggests achalasia or an esophageal diverticulum, whereas vomiting old digested food usually results from gastroparesis or gastric outlet obstruction. The presence of bile in the emesis implies a patent pylorus.

In most cases, nausea and vomiting in the postoperative period are self-limited. When symptoms are prolonged and severe, diagnostic studies, including an upper gastrointestinal

---

Box 9-6 FACTORS THAT CONTRIBUTE TO POSTOPERATIVE NAUSEA AND VOMITING

Length of anesthesia
Type of surgery (abdominal, gynecologic, urologic, ophthalmologic, middle ear)
Female gender
History of motion sickness
Postoperative ileus or pain
Gastroparesis
Refeeding after prolonged disuse of gastrointestinal tract
Metabolic factors
    Uremia
    Hyperglycemia/hypoglycemia
    Electrolyte disturbances
    Dehydration
Drugs
    General anesthetics
    Opiate analgesics
    Digitalis
Mechanical causes
    Intestinal obstruction
    Gastric outlet obstruction (e.g., pyloric channel ulcer)
Inflammatory processes
    Peritonitis
    Acute pancreatitis
    Acute cholecystitis

series, upper endoscopy, gastric emptying scan, and ultrasonography, may be necessary.

Perioperative Management

The cornerstone of treatment for postoperative nausea and vomiting is the elimination of precipitating causes, including contributing drugs. Intestinal obstruction and infection should be sought and treated. Intravenous hydration is critical, and nasogastric suction may be useful. Antiemetic drugs and proton pump inhibitors may be of benefit, but gastric prokinetic agents must be avoided if intestinal obstruction is present. The prokinetic agent metoclopramide (5 to 20 mg intravenously or orally four times a day 30 minutes before meals and at bedtime if the patient is eating) promotes gastrointestinal motility. The patient receiving metoclopramide must be monitored closely for side effects, including dystonic reactions, tremor, and mental confusion. When administered toward the end of a surgical procedure, ondansetron (4 mg intravenously), droperidol (1.25 mg intravenously), and dexamethasone (4 mg intravenously) have each been shown to decrease the frequency of postoperative nausea and vomiting. Combination therapy may be required in some patients. The 5-hydroxytryptamine receptor antagonists (5-HT$_3$) with activity similar to that of ondansetron include granisetron, tropisetron, and dolasetron. A newer class of antiemetics, neurokinin-1 receptor antagonists such as aprepitant, show promise for the treatment of postoperative nausea and vomiting. Droperidol has been associated with cardiac arrhythmias. Phenothiazines such as prochlorperazine are no longer routinely recommended.

Complications and Their Management

Vomiting in the postoperative period may lead to a variety of complications. Metabolic consequences of vomiting include hypokalemia, metabolic alkalosis, and sodium depletion.

Mechanical injury to the esophagus can result from retching or vomiting, including Mallory-Weiss (mucosal) tears at the gastroesophageal junction and, rarely, esophageal perforation with mediastinitis (Boerhaave's syndrome). Vomiting can lead to wound dehiscence and delayed healing of suture lines. The recumbent, often sedated postoperative patient is at particular risk of aspiration of the vomitus, with resulting pneumonia. Some evidence indicates that the risk of aspiration is increased further in patients receiving intravenous H_2-receptor antagonists, proton pump inhibitors, or oral antacids because of increased gastric pH and proliferation of intragastric bacteria (see later).

Diarrhea

Diarrhea is common in the postoperative period and may be caused by numerous factors.

Drugs

Drugs are a frequent cause of postoperative diarrhea (Table 9-2). Common pharmacologic causes of diarrhea in the postoperative period include magnesium-containing antacids, antibiotics, digitalis, quinidine, theophylline, and laxatives. Frequently, diarrhea can result from nutritional additives such as sorbitol. Oral caloric supplements may also cause diarrhea. Diarrhea can be expected to resolve when the offending drug is discontinued or when a caloric supplement is diluted or administered at a slower rate.

ANTIBIOTIC-ASSOCIATED DIARRHEA

Antibiotic-associated diarrhea is a major cause of diarrhea in postsurgical patients. The mild diarrhea that frequently occurs in postsurgical patients receiving antibiotics is thought to be caused by alteration of colonic bacterial flora and usually resolves promptly with discontinuation of the antibiotic. Of all patients with antibiotic-associated diarrhea, 15% to 25% have a positive stool assay for *C. difficile* toxin, which may

TABLE 9-2	Drugs That May Cause Diarrhea		
Antineoplastic	**Central Nervous System**	**Cardiovascular**	**Other**
Cytarabine	Alprazolam	Angiotensin-converting enzyme inhibitors (e.g., enalapril, captopril)	Antibiotics
Dactinomycin	Ethosuximide		Bumetanide
Doxorubicin	Fluoxetine		Cimetidine
Estramustine	Lithium		Clofibrate
Etoposide	Meprobamate	β-Blockers (e.g., propranolol)	Colchicine
Floxuridine (FUDR)	Valproic acid	Bretylium	Furosemide
Fluorouracil		Chlorpropamide	Gemfibrozil
Interferon		Digitalis	Glipizide
Methotrexate		Ergot derivatives	Lovastatin
Procarbazine		Guanethidine	Magnesium
		Hydralazine	Misoprostol
		L-Dopa	Olsalazine
		Methyldopa	Phosphorus
		Procainamide	Probucol
		Quinidine	Sulfasalazine
		Reserpine	Thyroxine
		Tocainide	

result in pseudomembranous colitis. The diarrhea of pseudomembranous colitis usually begins within a few days of the start of antibiotic therapy but may occur up to 6 weeks after completion of a course of either oral or intravenous antibiotics. The diarrhea is often profusely watery and may occasionally be grossly bloody. Patients with diabetes, sepsis, or cancer or those who have received preoperative bowel preparation or gastric acid suppressive therapy, especially a proton pump inhibitor, are at increased risk of pseudomembranous colitis. Any antibiotic except vancomycin may lead to pseudomembranous colitis; cephalosporins, ampicillin, clindamycin, and aminoglycosides were implicated most commonly in the past. In more recent outbreaks of C. difficile–associated diarrhea, administration of fluoroquinolones has been the most important risk factor. The diarrhea is usually positive for occult blood and is accompanied by fever, leukocytosis, and cramping abdominal pain. Less commonly, hematochezia, abdominal tenderness, and volume depletion occur; toxic megacolon may ensue. In elderly patients, *C. difficile* infection has been associated with subclinical protein-losing enteropathy in the absence of overt diarrhea. More recent outbreaks have been associated with a virulent form of *C. difficile* that produces high levels of toxin and with high morbidity and mortality rates (Loo et al, 2005).

The diagnosis of pseudomembranous colitis is often made in the appropriate setting by the detection of a *C. difficile* toxin in the stool. Two toxins (A and B) are involved in the pathogenesis of *C. difficile*. An assay for *C. difficile* toxin is positive in 90% to 95% of cases of pseudomembranous colitis when up to three stool specimens are tested. The standard tissue culture assay detects both toxins A and B and is slightly more sensitive than immunoassays, but the latter are much faster and are preferred. The diagnosis can also be confirmed on sigmoidoscopy by the demonstration of characteristic yellow-white plaquelike membranes on a boggy, erythematous base. In some cases, the rectum and even sigmoid colon are spared, and only right-sided pseudomembranous colitis is detectable on colonoscopy. Occasional patients with antibiotic-associated diarrhea and a negative *C. difficile* assay have pseudomembranous colitis caused by other toxigenic bacteria, such as *Clostridium perfringens*.

Management of Pseudomembranous Colitis. Treatment consists of withdrawing the offending antibiotic and starting oral metronidazole, 250 mg every 8 hours for 10 to 14 days [◉ *Bartlett, 2002*]. Alternatively, oral vancomycin, 125 mg every 6 hours, may be used, but it is more expensive than metronidazole and has been associated with the emergence of resistant *Enterococcus faecium* in some hospitals. Conversely, reports of resistance to metronidazole have begun to appear, with rates higher than 20% in some outbreaks. Antimotility agents such as diphenoxylate and atropine (Lomotil) or loperamide should be avoided. The relapse rate after therapy is about 20%; relapses usually respond to a second course of therapy. In the occasional patient with multiple relapses, it is necessary to treat with prolonged and tapering courses of oral vancomycin or novel therapies such as capsules containing the yeast *Saccharomyces boulardii*. A *C. difficile* toxoid vaccine for patients with recurrent *C. difficile*–associated diarrhea is under study. Severe cases of pseudomembranous colitis with intestinal ileus precluding oral drug administration may be treated with metronidazole, 500 mg intravenously every 8 hours. Occasionally, toxic megacolon develops and requires surgical treatment; an increased risk of toxic megacolon is associated with the use of corticosteroids, laxatives, or antimotility agents, total parenteral nutrition, immunosuppression, and prolonged hospitalization.

Fecal Impaction

In the immobile, medicated postoperative patient who has frequent, small, liquid stools or continuous oozing of liquid stool, the diagnosis of paradoxical diarrhea caused by a fecal impaction must be considered. The passage of liquid stool results from overflow around a large obstructing fecal mass, often in the rectum. The diagnosis usually can be made by rectal examination and a plain abdominal radiograph. Treatment is by manual disimpaction and tap water enemas. Occasionally, mineral oil given orally or rectally is helpful to loosen hard stools. After disimpaction, the patient should be given stool softeners and bulk laxatives.

Ischemic Colitis

Postoperative diarrhea may be caused by ischemic colitis, often resulting from ligation of the inferior mesenteric artery after aortoiliac reconstruction, abdominal aneurysmectomy, or abdominoperineal resection. Ischemic colitis caused by nonocclusive mesenteric ischemia may also occur in the setting of diminished cardiac output caused by congestive heart failure, cardiac arrhythmias, intravascular volume depletion, or cardiac surgery. Most patients are more than 50 years of age and have underlying atherosclerosis. The clinical presentation is with acute diarrhea, often containing gross blood, and abdominal pain, usually in the left lower quadrant and accompanied by nausea, vomiting, fever, chills, and leukocytosis. Peritoneal signs may not be clinically evident initially, and careful and repeated abdominal examination is necessary to monitor for the development of colonic infarction. Occasionally, the onset of ischemic colitis is subacute, with lesser degrees of abdominal pain and bleeding over days to weeks and sparing of the rectum because of collateral blood flow; resolution usually occurs within 2 to 4 weeks, occasionally with formation of a postischemic stricture.

Sigmoidoscopic or colonoscopic examination characteristically shows submucosal hemorrhage, mucosal bleeding, and ulceration. Abdominal radiographs may show colonic dilation and "thumbprinting" resulting from submucosal hemorrhage and edema. Barium enema is generally avoided because of the risk of perforation but classically shows sawtooth ulcerations and narrowing of the colonic lumen in the affected area, most commonly the sigmoid colon or splenic flexure. Angiography is generally not necessary for diagnosis.

MANAGEMENT

Treatment of ischemic colitis consists of bowel rest, nasogastric suction, intravenous fluids, optimization of the cardiac status, and intravenous broad-spectrum antibiotics. Digitalis preparations must be used with caution in patients with ischemic colitis because they may cause mesenteric vasoconstriction. Ischemic colitis is usually self-limited but occasionally progresses to colonic infarction with peritonitis. Surgical intervention may be required in cases of suspected infarction or perforation. Healing may lead to stricture formation, which may require endoscopic therapy or surgical treatment to relieve obstruction.

Infections

The usual infectious causes of diarrhea (e.g., *Escherichia coli, Salmonella, Shigella, Campylobacter*, and *Yersinia*) are encountered rarely when diarrhea develops in the postoperative period. Giardiasis, amebiasis, and opportunistic infections may also be seen. In immunocompromised hosts, such as patients with the acquired immunodeficiency syndrome, organisms such as *Mycobacterium avium* complex, *Cryptosporidium*, and *Isospora belli* should also be considered.

Consequences of Surgical Procedures

Diarrhea may be an expected, usually temporary, occurrence after certain types of gastrointestinal operations. It is often the first sign of the resumption of bowel activity. In some cases, diarrhea may represent a complication of a gastrointestinal operation and may require specific treatment, even reoperation.

TRUNCAL VAGOTOMY

Diarrhea is a well-described complication of truncal vagotomy, usually for peptic ulcer disease. The pathogenesis is unknown. Increased gastric emptying and decreased intestinal transit times may contribute to postvagotomy diarrhea. Therapy with octreotide, oral cholestyramine, which binds bile acids, or verapamil may be helpful.

ILEAL RESECTION

Large ileal resections (>100 cm) can lead to luminal bile salt deficiency resulting in fat malabsorption and colonic secretion caused by hydroxy fatty acids, which are released by the action of colonic bacteria on unabsorbed dietary triglycerides. Steatorrhea and malabsorption resulting from ileal resection are managed by limiting dietary fat intake and supplementing the diet with medium-chain triglycerides and fat-soluble vitamins. Shorter ileal resections (<100 cm) may cause diarrhea as a result of stimulation of colonic secretion by unabsorbed bile salts (choleraic diarrhea). By binding intestinal bile salts, oral cholestyramine (4 g four times a day) may control choleraic diarrhea (see also "Complications of Small Intestine Resection and Bypass").

CHOLECYSTECTOMY

Cholecystectomy can also lead to choleraic diarrhea as a result of loss of the gallbladder reservoir for bile and continuous delivery of bile to the intestine. Other mechanisms appear to be involved as well, and this explains the inconsistent response to therapy with cholestyramine.

PANCREATIC SURGERY

Some degree of pancreatic insufficiency, with resulting diarrhea and steatorrhea, is frequent after Whipple's procedure (pancreaticoduodenectomy) and is invariable after major pancreatic resections. Treatment with pancreatic enzyme supplements usually results in symptomatic improvement and decreased steatorrhea.

BLIND LOOP SYNDROME

A blind loop syndrome with overgrowth of intestinal bacteria and malabsorption may occur after partial gastrectomy with a Billroth II anastomosis or after intestinal bypass procedures. The blind loop syndrome is treated with intermittent courses of a broad-spectrum oral antibiotic.

UNMASKING OF UNDERLYING DISEASES

Surgery may cause diarrhea by leading to expression of a previously latent underlying gastrointestinal disease. For example, gastric resection may unmask celiac disease or intestinal lactase deficiency. As discussed earlier, nongastrointestinal surgical procedures may be associated with a flare of underlying inflammatory bowel disease.

Evaluation of the Patient with Postoperative Diarrhea

The evaluation of the patient with postoperative diarrhea should begin with a review of medications and other factors (e.g., radiation history, recent antibiotic use, nature of surgery) that may provide clues to the cause of diarrhea. Often, unnecessary diarrhea-inducing medications can be stopped. Rectal examination should be performed to exclude the possibility of overflow diarrhea around a fecal impaction. The stool should be examined for blood and fecal leukocytes and assayed for *C. difficile* toxin. Conversely, routine stool cultures for enteric pathogens have a low yield in nosocomial cases of acute diarrhea and are not routinely indicated. If these studies are unrevealing, sigmoidoscopy can be performed to look for evidence of colitis. Further testing can be pursued as appropriate to the clinical setting and may include colonoscopy, barium radiography, video capsule endoscopy, and tests for malabsorption (see earlier for specific therapy).

Gastrointestinal Bleeding

Gastrointestinal bleeding is a serious postsurgical problem with a mortality rate of up to 10%; in some subgroups, the mortality rate is 50% to 90% [◉ *Hiramoto et al, 2003*]. As in the nonsurgical patient, the first priority of management is to resuscitate the patient hemodynamically. When the patient is stable, an orderly search for the cause of bleeding can be undertaken, and in some cases specific therapy directed toward the underlying lesion can be administered. Common causes of gastrointestinal bleeding in the postoperative period are considered individually, and a general approach to the management of postoperative gastrointestinal bleeding follows.

Stress Gastropathy and Ulceration

OCCURRENCE

In the past, stress ulcers were a common cause of postoperative gastrointestinal hemorrhage; they are still nearly universal in critically ill patients. In contrast to chronic peptic ulcers, stress ulcers are likely to be asymptomatic, multiple, superficial (with a low risk of perforation), and located in acid-producing areas of the stomach (fundus and body). Bleeding from stress ulcers occurs 3 to 7 days postoperatively in a minority of patients, generally arises from superficial capillaries, and is thus rarely exsanguinating. However, the occurrence of significant bleeding increases the mortality rate considerably in critically ill patients. Risk factors for bleeding from stress ulcers include central nervous system injury (Cushing's ulcer), extensive burns involving more than 35% of the body surface area (Curling's ulcer), hypotension, uremia, sepsis, coagulopathy, and respiratory failure with the need for mechanical ventilation. With improvements in intensive care, the risk of serious bleeding from stress ulcers in patients in a medical intensive care unit has decreased since the early 1990s from approximately 20% to only 3.5%. **However, patients with risk factors for stress ulceration should still receive prophylactic treatment, which has been shown to decrease the bleeding risk by 50%** [● *Hiramoto et al, 2003*].

THERAPY

Prophylactic therapy against stress ulceration is more effective than treatment of actively bleeding ulcers, because mortality from acute bleeding may be as high as 80%. The standard approach to prophylaxis has been neutralization of the gastric luminal pH, most commonly by intravenous administration of an H_2-receptor antagonist or oral or intravenous administration of a proton pump inhibitor. Proton pump inhibitors are preferred because they are more potent and reliable acid suppressors than H_2-receptor antagonists. Sucralfate and antacids are no longer used routinely for stress ulcer prevention in the postoperative setting, although in the past, sucralfate was thought to be associated with lower rate of late-onset (after 4 days) pneumonia than were H_2-receptor antagonists. H_2-receptor antagonists are more effective in maintaining a steady gastric pH when they are given as a continuous infusion after an initial priming dose than when given as intermittent boluses, but both approaches are equally effective in preventing bleeding.

Oral proton pump inhibitors are well tolerated, have few side effects, and, when administered in a single daily dose, may reduce the frequency of clinically significant gastrointestinal bleeding by as much as 25% when compared with ranitidine, probably because of improved gastric acid suppression. Proton pump inhibitors can interfere with the metabolism of some orally administered medications.

Intravenous proton pump inhibitors act rapidly to suppress gastric acid production. Use of an intravenous formulation is attractive, particularly in postoperative patients who require prolonged mechanical ventilation. Intravenous proton pump inhibitors reduce the risk of recurrent gastrointestinal bleeding compared with placebo but have not been compared rigorously with oral proton pump inhibitors. Currently, the three intravenous proton pump inhibitors available in the United States are lansoprazole, pantoprazole, and esomeprazole.

Occasionally, angiographic, endoscopic, or surgical intervention is required to control bleeding from stress ulceration. In some cases, oversewing of bleeding sites may be accompanied by an acid-reducing operation.

REACTIVATION OF CHRONIC PEPTIC ULCER DISEASE

It is likely that surgical procedures promote exacerbation of chronic peptic ulcer disease (see also the earlier discussion of peptic ulcer disease). Reactivated peptic ulcer disease may easily be confused with stress ulceration in the postoperative period. Investigators have hypothesized that surgery may alter the balance between aggressive and defensive factors and may lead to reactivation of chronic ulcer disease. The role of *H. pylori* in this setting is unclear. Risk factors for ulcer bleeding include older age, use of NSAIDs, anticoagulation, and long-term corticosteroid use. Recurrent peptic ulcers in the postoperative period are often painless, and bleeding may occur in the absence of typical pain. As discussed earlier in the section on peptic ulcer disease, perioperative prophylaxis with a proton pump inhibitor is recommended for patients with a history of the disease, although the efficacy of such prophylaxis is unproved. When present, *H. pylori* should be eradicated with appropriate therapy. In patients who have bled from an ulcer, every effort should be made to avoid NSAIDs. If an NSAID is necessary, a proton pump inhibitor twice daily should be prescribed, or a selective cyclooxygenase-2 inhibitor should be considered, in combination with a proton pump inhibitor, in high-risk patients.

Mallory-Weiss Tears

Factors that predispose to Mallory-Weiss tears in the postoperative period include retching, vomiting, and coughing, with resulting high intra-abdominal pressures and large pressure gradients across the gastroesophageal junction. Mallory-Weiss tears account for fewer than 5% of cases of postoperative bleeding, are generally self-limited, and respond to control of nausea and vomiting with the use of nasogastric suction, antiemetics, and gastric acid suppression. Endoscopic intervention may occasionally be required.

Esophagitis

Esophagitis resulting from gastroesophageal reflux disease is discussed earlier in the section on gastroesophageal reflux disease. Postoperative patients are also at risk for the development of infectious esophagitis caused by *Candida albicans*, herpesvirus, and cytomegalovirus, which may cause bleeding. Predisposing factors include antibiotics, immunosuppression (including acquired immunodeficiency syndrome), diabetes, debility, and malnutrition. Symptoms of esophagitis such as substernal burning, dysphagia, and odynophagia may be minimal or absent. Moreover, oral thrush is absent in half of all persons with *Candida* esophagitis. The diagnosis of infectious esophagitis may be confirmed by endoscopy with brush cytologic studies, potassium hydroxide stain, biopsy, and culture. Treatment of *Candida* esophagitis consists of oral nystatin (500,000 U orally four times daily) or fluconazole (100 to 200 mg orally daily), which is preferred over itraconazole or ketoconazole. In refractory cases, low-dose (500 mg total) intravenous amphotericin can be used. For herpes esophagitis, intravenous acyclovir (250 mg/m^2 intravenously every 8 hours, then 200 to 400 mg orally five times daily) should be prescribed. For cytomegalovirus, ganciclovir (5 mg/kg intravenously every 12 hours) is given; foscarnet is an alternative. Nystatin and fluconazole are generally well tolerated; ketoconazole may cause hepatitis, nausea, and vomiting and interferes with the metabolism of some drugs; amphotericin may cause shaking chills, fever, arthralgias, phlebitis, hypokalemia, and abnormal renal function; and acyclovir may cause renal failure and mental status changes.

Moribund postoperative patients with long-standing nasogastric tubes are at risk for esophageal ulcerations caused by pressure necrosis. Treatment includes removal of the tube if possible and therapy to suppress gastric acid secretion.

Anticoagulant-Induced Small Intestinal Hemorrhage

Patients who bleed from the gastrointestinal tract while receiving anticoagulants and who have a normal endoscopic evaluation of the upper gastrointestinal tract and colon may be found to have an anticoagulant-induced small bowel hemorrhage. A characteristic "stacked-coin" appearance of the intestine may be seen on a plain radiograph of the abdomen or on a small bowel barium radiograph. Enteroscopy, video capsule endoscopy, or arteriography may be helpful in localizing the bleeding site. Identification of a specific underlying structural lesion (e.g., arteriovenous malformation) is more likely if the degree of anticoagulation is not excessive than if the patient is overly anticoagulated.

Ischemic Colitis

See "Ischemic Colitis" in the earlier section on diarrhea.

Pseudomembranous Colitis

See "Antibiotic-Associated Diarrhea" in the earlier section on diarrhea.

Mesenteric Ischemia and Infarction

See "Ischemic Colitis" in the earlier section on diarrhea.

Colonic Diverticulosis and Angiodysplasia

Colonic diverticulosis and angiodysplasia are frequent causes of lower gastrointestinal bleeding in older persons, although the risk of bleeding is not particularly increased in the perioperative period, except perhaps in renal transplant recipients. Although controversial, patients with aortic stenosis appear to be at increased risk of bleeding from colonic angiodysplasia. The pathogenesis is thought to relate to the combination of acquired von Willebrand syndrome and colonic mucosal ischemia from low cardiac output.

Intra-abdominal Hemorrhage

Postoperative bleeding in the gastrointestinal tract may result from breakdown of a surgical anastomosis with erosion into an adjacent blood vessel. Insufficient surgical hemostasis, failure to ligate a major vessel or cauterize smaller vessels, and unrecognized surgical injury to other organs can all lead to bleeding in the postoperative period. Severe postoperative hemorrhagic pancreatitis may also cause retroperitoneal and intra-abdominal hemorrhage (see also "Acute Pancreatitis" later).

Evaluation and Management of the Patient with Postoperative Gastrointestinal Bleeding

Gastrointestinal bleeding in the postoperative period may manifest as hematemesis, melena, hematochezia, a fall in the hemoglobin level, or hypotension and shock. In the bleeding postoperative patient, it is first necessary to assess the magnitude of blood loss and hemodynamic instability. Orthostatic hypotension greater than 10 mm Hg indicates a 20% or greater reduction in blood volume and may be associated with syncope, lightheadedness, nausea, and sweating. Pallor and cool, clammy skin are signs of shock that correspond to a 30 to 40% or greater reduction in blood volume.

Intravascular volume should be restored initially with intravenous isotonic solutions, such as normal saline or Ringer's lactate solution. Peripheral intravenous or central access must be adequate to allow infusions of large volumes. Volume management is aided by central venous pressure or, when appropriate, pulmonary capillary wedge pressure monitoring, especially in massively bleeding patients and those with multiorgan failure. Vital signs and urine output must be monitored closely in all patients.

Patients with signs of shock or those at risk for complications of hypoxemia, including angina, mesenteric ischemia, or respiratory compromise, should receive transfusions of red blood cells as soon as possible. Those who are actively bleeding or are likely to bleed again should also receive red blood cell transfusions early in resuscitation. Whole blood can be used for massive bleeding. In general, an attempt should be made to sustain a systolic blood pressure of at least 100 mm Hg and a hemoglobin level of 9 to 10 mg/dL. Fresh frozen plasma should be used to correct coagulopathy when associated with active bleeding. Transfusion of platelets should be considered if the platelet counts drop to less than 30,000/mm^3. Calcium supplementation may be necessary if the serum calcium level falls because banked blood is anticoagulated with calcium-binding agents.

An initial evaluation during the resuscitative phase can be made to locate the probable site of bleeding. Hematemesis usually indicates upper gastrointestinal bleeding proximal to the ligament of Treitz. Melena also usually signifies an upper gastrointestinal tract source, but a small intestinal or even an ascending colonic source is also possible. Hematochezia usually signifies lower gastrointestinal bleeding, but in about 10% of cases, hematochezia may be the result of massive upper tract bleeding.

EMPIRICAL THERAPY TO STOP ACTIVE BLEEDING

Most gastrointestinal bleeding stops spontaneously. In upper tract bleeding, the efficacy of gastric lavage with iced saline is unproven, but it allows assessment of the rapidity of bleeding and clears the stomach before endoscopy. Room temperature tap water may be preferable to cold saline, which may impair coagulation.

H2-Receptor Antagonists and Proton Pump Inhibitors. The rationale for drug therapy to stop upper gastrointestinal tract bleeding is that gastric acidity may inhibit platelet aggregation as well as ulcer healing. Antacids are of no apparent benefit as sole therapy for active bleeding. H_2-receptor antagonists also have not been shown to be of benefit in several controlled studies of active gastrointestinal bleeding. Intravenous and high-dose oral proton pump inhibitors are beneficial for the prevention of recurrent upper gastrointestinal bleeding caused by peptic ulcer disease. These agents also appear to play a role in arresting acute ulcer bleeding, reducing transfusion requirements, decreasing the risk of rebleeding, and reducing the need for surgical treatment, although they may not affect mortality. However, administration of a proton pump inhibitor is not a substitute for endoscopic therapy of a bleeding ulcer (see later). Use of these drugs may also be indicated for treatment of gastropathy or esophagitis.

Octreotide. For upper gastrointestinal bleeding caused by gastroesophageal varices, therapy to reduce splanchnic blood flow should be considered. The somatostatin analogue octreotide acts by inhibiting the release of glucagon and causing splanchnic arteriolar constriction, which, in turn, reduces portal venous pressure. Octreotide may be administered by intravenous bolus in a dose of 50 µg/hour followed by a 5-day infusion of 50-250 µg/hour.

PREVENTION OF REBLEEDING

As discussed earlier, empirical therapy with an H_2-receptor antagonist or proton pump inhibitor to prevent recurrent bleeding is indicated in patients with bleeding from stress ulcers and peptic ulcers. In patients with chronic peptic ulcer disease associated with *H. pylori*, eradication of *H. pylori* has been associated with a decreased rate of recurrent bleeding.

Diagnosis and Therapy

ENDOSCOPY

Endoscopy is the most reliable means of establishing the source of upper gastrointestinal bleeding. This procedure can be performed in most patients in the postoperative period, even soon after surgery, once the patient is hemodynamically stable. Barium radiography may be contraindicated in the postsurgical patient with an intestinal ileus.

The most common causes of postoperative upper gastrointestinal bleeding are duodenal and gastric ulcer, gastric stress ulcers, and Mallory-Weiss tears. Making a specific diagnosis is useful prognostically and for the selection of appropriate therapy. Early randomized trials to investigate whether urgent endoscopy had any effect on transfusion requirements, length of hospital stay, need for surgery, or morbidity and mortality showed no benefit to diagnostic endoscopy. However, none of these studies stratified patients on the basis of lesions at high risk for recurrent bleeding, nor did they evaluate the possible benefit of the numerous therapeutic endoscopic interventions now available. Studies have shown that endoscopic therapy with bipolar electrocautery, thermal coagulation (heater probe), injection of vasoconstricting agents, or hemoclip placement in patients with a visible or spurting vessel in a peptic ulcer base improves patient survival and decreases the transfusion requirement and need for surgery. Similarly, band ligation is an effective method for stopping bleeding from esophageal varices, and when repeated at regular intervals to the point of variceal obliteration, it leads to a decrease in re-bleeding rates and probably an improved long-term survival rate. Long-term administration of a nonselective β-blocker such as propranolol or nadolol also reduces the risk of recurrent variceal bleeding.

ANGIOGRAPHY

Angiography may be useful for persistent or severe upper gastrointestinal bleeding undiagnosed by endoscopy. Angiography may be preceded by a technetium-99m–sulfur colloid–labeled red blood cell scan to confirm that the bleeding rate is rapid enough for angiographic detection and to provide a guide to the localization of the bleeding site. A bleeding rate of at least 0.5 mL/minute is required for angiographic visualization of a bleeding site. Angiography is especially useful in the evaluation of arterial bleeding, bleeding from Mallory-Weiss tears, and bleeding from erosive gastropathy. Angiography may further allow therapeutic interventions, such as embolization of the left gastric artery with autologous clot, polyvinyl alcohol, coils, or gelatin sponge particles when massive bleeding is caused by stress gastropathy.

LOWER GASTROINTESTINAL TRACT BLEEDING

The most common causes of lower gastrointestinal bleeding are diverticular disease, angiodysplasia, polyps, carcinoma, and inflammatory bowel disease. Diagnostic evaluation of lower gastrointestinal tract bleeding should begin with placement of a nasogastric tube to exclude an upper gastrointestinal source. If there is any suspicion of an upper gastrointestinal tract source, upper gastrointestinal endoscopy should be performed. Once an upper source is excluded, consideration can be given to colonoscopy. In cases of massive bleeding, colonoscopy may be difficult or impossible, but it has become the test of choice in less severe bleeding after peroral (or nasogastric tube) administration of a colonic lavage solution. Colonoscopic techniques to control bleeding can be used, including electrocoagulation, thermal coagulation, polypectomy, and hemoclip placement.

When colonoscopy is not possible or diagnostic, mesenteric arteriography, possibly after a radiocolloid-labeled blood cell scan (as previously described), may be useful in identifying bleeding from diverticula or angiodysplasia. Intra-arterial infusion of vasopressin may control the bleeding in some cases.

SMALL INTESTINAL BLEEDING

If evaluation of both the upper and lower gastrointestinal tract produces normal results, consideration must be given to a small intestine source of bleeding, including arteriovenous malformations, a small intestine ulcer, a Meckel diverticulum, or a vascular neoplasm. Diagnostic studies may include a small intestine enteroclysis examination, which is a careful barium contrast study through peroral intubation of the small intestine, or peroral enteroscopy. In younger patients, a Meckel (technetium-99m pertechnetate) scan can be obtained. Video capsule endoscopy is a relatively new imaging modality that involves the ingestion of a pill-sized camera to visualize the entire small bowel. The ability of video capsule endoscopy to detect disease in the small intestines compares favorably to that of enteroscopy. However, its use in postoperative patients should be undertaken with care. A standard bleeding scan followed by angiography also may be helpful in patients with small intestinal bleeding. As a last resort, exploratory laparotomy with intraoperative enteroscopy may be necessary.

Jaundice

Jaundice is common in the postoperative period. The cause is usually multifactorial, but the pathophysiologic mechanisms may be grouped into four major categories (Table 9-3): (1) increased bilirubin load to the liver; (2) intrahepatic disease; (3) preexisting liver disease; and (4) extrahepatic obstructive disease.

In the postoperative period, hemolysis of transfused blood and resorption of hematomas account for the major portion of the increased load of bilirubin delivered to the liver. Similarly, medications administered in the postoperative period may induce hemolysis. Jaundice is particularly common in patients who have undergone extensive surgical procedures and have received multiple transfusions; the hyperbilirubinemia is primarily indirect, occasionally as high as 20 mg/dL. In patients undergoing cardiac surgical procedures, risk factors for postoperative jaundice include preoperative serum bilirubin elevation, elevated right atrial pressure, cardiac valve replacement, and the use of intra-aortic balloon counterpulsation.

Ischemic liver injury is a common cause of postoperative jaundice. The origin is multifactorial, likely related to a

TABLE 9-3	Causes of Postoperative Jaundice	
Increased Hepatic Bilirubin Load	**Intrahepatic Parenchymal Disease**	
Hemolysis after Transfusions	**Anesthetics**	
Hematoma	Enflurane	Desflurane (rarely)
Underlying hemolytic anemia	Halothane	Sevoflurane (rarely)
	Isoflurane	
Preexisting Liver Disease	**Antibiotics**	
Gilbert's syndrome*	Amoxicillin-clavulanic acid	Penicillins
		Rifampin
Dubin-Johnson syndrome†	Chloramphenicol	Sulfonamides
	Erythromycins	Tetracycline
	Isoniazid	
	Nitrofurantoin	
Extrahepatic Obstruction	**Other Drugs**	
Common bile duct stone	Androgens	Phenothiazines
Cholecystitis	Estrogens	Phenytoin
Pancreatitis	Fluconazole	Sulindac
Biliary stricture, leak, or tumor	Methyldopa	
	Other Causes	
	Parenteral nutrition	
	Viral hepatitis	
	Sepsis	
	Ischemic hepatitis	

*Unconjugated hyperbilirubinemia resulting from a congenital defect in the hepatic uptake of bilirubin.
†Conjugated hyperbilirubinemia resulting from a congenital defect in secretion of bilirubin from hepatocytes.
From Faust TW, Reddy KR: Postoperative jaundice. Clin Liver Dis 8:151-166, 2004.

reduction in splanchnic, portal venous, and hepatic artery blood flow during anesthesia. Ischemic hepatitis, or shock liver, may occur in the setting of shock, massive trauma, or hyperthermia. Persons with chronic passive congestion caused by right-sided heart failure are at particular risk. Ischemic hepatitis is characterized by greatly elevated aminotransferase levels (often >5000 units/L), bilirubin levels as high as 20 mg/dL or more within 2 to 10 days of surgical procedures, and a rapid return of aminotransferase levels toward normal within 5 to 7 days. Serum lactate dehydrogenase levels are characteristically high, in contrast to viral hepatitis.

Because of the routine screening of donated blood, acute hepatitis C is rarely seen now. The frequency of hepatitis C following blood transfusions, once as high as 12%, is now 1 per 2,000,000 units transfused. When it occurs, acute hepatitis C is frequently subclinical or indolent but is associated with up to an 85% risk of chronic hepatitis, with the potential to progress to cirrhosis. Since the development of sensitive serologic screening tests of donor blood, hepatitis B also has become an uncommon cause of transfusion-associated hepatitis. Even rarer are cases of transfusion-associated hepatitis D (Delta), Epstein-Barr viral infection, and cytomegalovirus disease (except in transplant recipients).

Hepatic parenchymal disease may be caused by certain general anesthetics (e.g., halothane), as well as several other drugs (see Table 9-3). Halothane is rarely used these days, and halothane-induced hepatitis is rare, with a frequency of 1 in 10,000 individuals, but it is potentially fatal.

Parenteral nutrition is a common cause of hyperbilirubinemia and elevated aminotransferase levels in postoperative patients. Fatty infiltration may result from intravenous infusions of concentrated glucose solutions and choline or carnitine deficiency, and intrahepatic cholestasis may result from intravenous infusions of amino acids and fat emulsions. Cholestasis, if prolonged, may lead to the development of cirrhosis, an indication for consideration of small intestinal and liver transplantation in patients with short bowel syndrome (see later). Sepsis may also induce intrahepatic cholestasis.

Extrahepatic biliary obstruction is a relatively uncommon cause of postoperative jaundice and may result from surgical injury to the biliary tree, retained common bile duct stones in patients who have undergone cholecystectomy, or acalculous cholecystitis (see the later discussion of cholecystitis). Occasionally, surgical procedures may unmask inherited disorders of bilirubin metabolism such as Gilbert's syndrome or Dubin-Johnson syndrome.

Management

Investigation of postoperative jaundice should include the following: an ultrasonographic examination to exclude evidence of extrahepatic obstruction (a dilated common bile duct, common hepatic ducts, or intrahepatic ducts); serologic studies for hepatitis A, B, and C; evaluation for hemolysis (reticulocyte count and examination of the peripheral blood smear); a review of the patient's medications for potential hepatotoxic agents; and exclusion of sepsis. As noted earlier, it is often not possible to attribute postoperative jaundice to a single cause, and several factors may be implicated. Fatty liver from total parenteral nutrition may be reversed with lecithin or choline supplementation, and cholestasis may be reversed with ursodeoxycholic acid or metronidazole.

Cholecystitis

Clinical Features

Acute cholecystitis is an uncommon but often overlooked complication after nonbiliary surgical procedures. Cholecystitis is classified as calculous (associated with stones in the biliary tree) or acalculous (no evidence of stones). Cholelithiasis may be common in patients undergoing renal transplantation, whereas patients who undergo cardiac transplantation and have cholelithiasis are at high risk of posttransplantation cholecystitis and should undergo pretransplant cholecystectomy. More than half the patients with postoperative cholecystitis have acalculous cholecystitis. Mortality rates of patients with acalculous cholecystitis range from 12% to 65%. Acute acalculous cholecystitis may follow abdominal or nonabdominal surgical procedures (especially orthopedic procedures), spinal cord injury, or bone marrow transplantation. Trauma and burns are also important risk factors.

Presentation

Postoperative acalculous cholecystitis usually manifests within 2 to 4 weeks of the surgical procedure. Patients are usually elderly, and in contrast to calculous cholecystitis, there is a male predominance. The clinical presentation is with fever, anorexia, epigastric and right upper quadrant pain and tenderness, nausea, vomiting, and a palpable abdominal mass. Patients may have leukocytosis and slight elevations in liver biochemical tests. Not infrequently, however, symptoms and signs may be masked, especially in comatose or obtunded patients. The diagnosis should be considered in any postoperative patient, even children, with unexplained fever. In postoperative acalculous cholecystitis, bile cultures are frequently positive for *E. coli, Pseudomonas, Klebsiella*, and *Staphylococcus aureus*. There is a high frequency of gangrene and perforation of the gallbladder, with mortality rates as high as 50%.

Pathogenesis

The pathogenesis of postoperative cholecystitis is unknown. Gallbladder stasis and local ischemia are important precipitating factors. Increased viscosity of bile may result from fever, fasting, and dehydration and may contribute to biliary stasis and cystic duct obstruction. Narcotic-induced ampullary contraction may also cause bile stasis, and positive pressure ventilation can increase common bile duct pressure. Hemolysis from multiple blood transfusions administered in the perioperative period may alter bile flow. Mucosal ischemia and necrosis can result from decreased vascular perfusion of the gallbladder as a result of hypotension or heart failure. Ischemia may also lead to cystic duct stenosis. Finally, activation of factor XII in the circulation can cause acute vasculitis of the gallbladder serosa and muscularis. In heart transplant recipients, a high rate of bile duct stones is thought to be the result of reduced bile flow and changes in serum lipids caused by cyclosporine, postoperative gallbladder stasis, rapid weight change, and hemolysis.

Management

A high index of suspicion is needed for early diagnosis. In some patients, typical findings of acute cholecystitis are evident on physical examination. In others, greater reliance must be placed on imaging studies. Abdominal ultrasound is usually the initial diagnostic test and may show a thickened gallbladder wall, an enlarged tender gallbladder, a pericholecystic fluid collection, or evidence of air within the gallbladder wall (emphysematous cholecystitis). Computed tomography may also show a thickened gallbladder wall with surrounding fluid. A gallbladder wall thicker than 3.5 mm is virtually diagnostic of acute cholecystitis. Hepatobiliary scintigraphy shows nonvisualization of the gallbladder in more than 90% of cases, although it has a higher rate of false-positive results than ultrasonography.

Management of postoperative cholecystitis consists of fluid and electrolyte replacement, administration of broad-spectrum antibiotics, and urgent cholecystectomy, if possible, once the diagnosis is confirmed. In patients who are poor surgical risks, percutaneous cholecystostomy is preferable to cholecystectomy. In patients with ascites or coagulopathy, endoscopic decompression with a stent placed in the cystic duct may be feasible.

Acute Pancreatitis

Acute pancreatitis may occur as a complication of both abdominal and nonabdominal surgical procedures. Postoperative pancreatitis has been recognized increasingly after heart surgery with cardiopulmonary bypass and is thought to result from ischemic injury to the pancreas secondary to hypoperfusion, which is more common with nonpulsatile bypass systems than with pulsatile systems. Other possible contributory factors include hypothermia, atheromatous or cholesterol emboli broken off during cannulation and cross-clamping of the aorta, venous sludging, and angiotensin-mediated selective blockade of pancreatic perfusion [❽ *Perez et al, 2005*]. Risk factors include a history of alcohol abuse, preoperative renal insufficiency, cardiac valve surgery, postoperative hypertension, and perioperative administration of calcium chloride.

A wide spectrum of pancreatic injury may result, ranging from minimal injury that is detectable only by biochemical testing to lethal necrotizing pancreatitis in less than 1% of patients. Clinical recognition may be difficult because abdominal pain, tenderness, and hyperamylasemia may be absent. The clinical course may be mild until a complication such as pancreatic necrosis or infection develops. The diagnosis must be considered in any postoperative patient with otherwise unexplained fever, leukocytosis, prolonged ileus, or multiorgan failure. In patients with suspected or confirmed acute pancreatitis, serial contrast-enhanced computed tomographic scans of the abdomen should be obtained to look for pancreatic necrosis or abscess.

Management

The prognosis is poor in postoperative patients with overt pancreatitis; mortality rates have been as high as 50%. Risk factors for a poor outcome after acute pancreatitis in nonoperative settings are probably those applicable to the postoperative patient with acute pancreatitis (see Box 9-2) and multiorgan failure. Treatment of acute pancreatitis includes eliminating oral intake and instituting nasogastric suction, intravenous fluids, analgesics as necessary, and enteral or parenteral nutrition in patients who are malnourished. Patients should be monitored closely for the development of a broad range of complications (see Box 9-2). Computed tomography may be particularly useful for identifying pancreatic necrosis, pseudocyst, or abscess. In patients with severe necrotizing pancreatitis, especially if infected, laparotomy with pancreatic débridement and drainage may need to be considered. Needle aspiration under endoscopic or radiologic guidance should be considered in clinically unstable patients.

Intestinal Ischemia and Infarction

A variety of factors in the perioperative period may contribute to an increased risk of intestinal ischemia and infarction. Intestinal ischemia may result from occlusive or nonocclusive processes involving the mesenteric circulation. Occlusive mesenteric vascular disease may be secondary to arterial thrombosis caused by advanced atherosclerosis. An embolus resulting from atrial fibrillation, valvular heart disease, a prosthetic heart valve, or angiography may also cause occlusive mesenteric vascular disease. Cholesterol crystal embolization may follow angiography or initiation of oral anticoagulation therapy. Mesenteric venous thrombosis, which may also lead to intestinal ischemia or infarction, may occur postoperatively or as a result of portal hypertension, peritonitis, abdominal abscess, trauma, neoplasms, antiphospholipid antibodies (lupus anticoagulant), antithrombin III deficiency, protein S or C deficiency, factor V Leiden mutation, prothrombin gene mutations, and oral contraceptive use. A final category of occlusive mesenteric vascular disease is vasculitis associated with systemic lupus erythematosus, polyarteritis nodosa, rheumatoid arthritis, and Henoch-Schönlein purpura. Nonocclusive mesenteric vascular disease may result from low-flow states induced by hypotension, cardiac arrhythmias, heart failure, dehydration, administration of vasopressor agents, splanchnic vasoconstriction by digoxin, and endotoxemia.

Acute Mesenteric Ischemia

CLINICAL FEATURES

The clinical presentation of acute mesenteric ischemia is with severe, periumbilical, colicky pain that is often out of proportion to abdominal tenderness. In patients with intestinal infarction, the pain may become more localized and associated with abdominal distention and decreased or absent bowel sounds. Anorexia, nausea, vomiting, diarrhea or constipation, tachycardia, hemoconcentration, and mild gastrointestinal bleeding often accompany the pain of intestinal ischemia. The progression may be slow, occurring over several weeks, as in mesenteric venous thrombosis, or acute and rapid, as after arterial embolization. Findings may include the following: leukocytosis; elevated blood phosphate, amylase, creatine kinase, and aspartate aminotransferase levels; and metabolic acidosis.

Abdominal radiographs often show air-fluid levels, bowel distention, and thick mucosal folds resulting from submucosal edema or blood (thumbprinting). Air in the bowel wall may be seen with intestinal infarction. Computed tomography may also show a thickened bowel wall.

The outcome of acute mesenteric ischemia varies from resolution to bowel infarction with intestinal gangrene and death. Progression of ischemia to bowel infarction is faster (as short as 6 hours) in patients in whom no collateral blood flow has been established. A high index of suspicion of progression to infarction must be maintained so that surgical treatment can be undertaken before completed infarction occurs. Mortality rates in patients with intestinal infarction approach 65%.

MANAGEMENT

Management of acute mesenteric ischemia consists of close observation of the patient and frequent assessment for intestinal infarction by serial abdominal examinations looking for signs of peritonitis. Supportive measures include intravenous hydration, correction of electrolyte imbalances, and administration of oxygen and broad-spectrum antibiotics, with careful attention to renal function. Avoidance of potentially harmful vasoconstricting drugs (e.g., digoxin and pressor agents) is also important. The decision to operate is often complicated by the patient's poor overall condition and the difficulty of distinguishing reversible ischemia from infarction.

When arterial embolus is suspected, immediate celiac and mesenteric arteriography and surgery with embolectomy are indicated. Surgical treatment should include resection of infarcted bowel, with a "second-look" operation in 24 to 48 hours to remove additionally infarcted bowel. Arterial or venous thrombosis may also require resection of infarcted bowel. In nonocclusive ischemia, intra-arterial infusion of a vasodilator such as papaverine, at a dose of 30 to 60 mg/hour, is recommended, although the efficacy of such an approach has not been established through controlled clinical trials.

Ischemic Colitis

See "Ischemic Colitis" in the earlier section on diarrhea.

Postoperative Abdominal Pain and Fever

The postoperative patient may present with acute abdominal pain and fever from a variety of causes, many of which are reviewed elsewhere in this chapter. Causes of abdominal pain and fever in the postoperative period include intra-abdominal abscess from anastomotic leakage, fistula formation with abscess, peritonitis from peritoneal soiling during surgery or wound dehiscence, acute pancreatitis, cholangitis from inadvertent bile duct injury, perforated peptic ulcer, acute acalculous cholecystitis, colonic volvulus (especially sigmoid and cecal) with a closed loop syndrome, pseudomembranous enterocolitis, acute appendicitis, diverticulitis, and acute intestinal ischemia or infarction. Intra-abdominal sepsis in the postoperative patient may be accompanied by hemoconcentration and even shock if there is third spacing of fluid, as is typical of severe pancreatitis, a closed loop such as volvulus, or severe pseudomembranous colitis with toxic megacolon.

Other medical disorders that may mimic an acute abdomen in the postoperative period include myocardial infarction, pneumonia, diabetic ketoacidosis, urinary tract sepsis, and acute fatty liver. Imaging studies such as computed tomography, ultrasonography, and hepatobiliary scintigraphy may be helpful in the differential diagnosis of postoperative abdominal pain and fever. Persistent abdominal pain, fever, and leukocytosis may require laparoscopy or laparotomy for definitive diagnosis.

COMPLICATIONS OF GASTROINTESTINAL SURGERY

Complications of Peptic Ulcer Surgery

Traditionally, the goal of peptic ulcer surgery has been to reduce gastric acid production, usually by removing the gastrin-producing cells of the antrum (antrectomy) and interrupting cholinergic stimulation to the parietal cells of the fundus (vagotomy). The gastric remnant is usually anastomosed from end to side to a loop of jejunum, with formation of a gastrojejunostomy (Billroth II) or, less often, a gastroduodenostomy (Billroth I). Because a complete vagotomy impairs gastric motility, highly selective (proximal) vagotomy (without antrectomy) was introduced. With the discovery of *H. pylori* and the recognition that its eradication cures peptic disease, the need for peptic ulcer surgery has decreased dramatically. Postgastrectomy syndromes may still be seen in patients who underwent ulcer surgery in the past or in the occasional patient who undergoes surgical treatment for a complication of ulcer disease (Table 9-4).

Ulcer Recurrence

Recurrence of peptic ulcer disease postoperatively occurs in approximately 5% of cases. Recurrence is more likely when the original operation was performed for duodenal ulcer

TABLE 9-4	Complications of Gastric Surgery
Early	**Late**
Wound infection	Ulcer recurrence
Anastomotic leak	Recurrent bleeding from ulcer
Bile duct injury	Gastric outlet obstruction
Delayed gastric emptying	Afferent loop syndrome
Anastomotic bleeding	Dumping syndrome
Anemia	Malabsorption
	Bile reflux gastritis
	Postvagotomy diarrhea
	Osteomalacia and osteoporosis
	Postgastrectomy carcinoma
	Pancreatitis

(3% to 10%) than for gastric ulcer (2%) and is less likely after antrectomy and vagotomy (1% to 4%) than after vagotomy alone (≤25%). Recurrent (stomal) ulcers occur most commonly at or just distal to the anastomosis.

Causes of ulcer recurrence include use of ulcerogenic drugs (e.g., aspirin, NSAIDs), inadequate vagotomy, inadequate gastric resection, retained gastric antrum, a long jejunal afferent loop, inadvertent gastroileal or gastrocolic anastomosis, poor gastric emptying, gastric neoplasm (mistaken preoperatively as a benign ulcer or newly occurring), undiagnosed Zollinger-Ellison syndrome, and persistent *H. pylori* infection. Most recurrent ulcers are attributable to the use of aspirin and other NSAIDs.

DIAGNOSIS

It is more common for patients with recurrent ulcers to present with hemorrhage than with pain; the bleeding is more often chronic than acute. A stomal ulcer may also cause symptoms of obstruction. Because upper gastrointestinal barium radiographs of the postoperative stomach are difficult to interpret, the diagnosis of a recurrent ulcer is best made by endoscopy. Surreptitious use of aspirin may be detected by a low platelet cyclooxygenase level. Fasting serum gastrin and calcium levels should be checked before any planned ulcer operation to screen for evidence of Zollinger-Ellison syndrome and a multiple endocrine neoplasia syndrome.

MANAGEMENT

Recurrent peptic ulcer disease has traditionally been treated with proton pump inhibitors, in some cases with continuation of full-dose therapy for life. Ulcerogenic drugs (aspirin and other NSAIDs) should be withheld. Treatment should include diagnosis and eradication of *H. pylori*. Surgical treatment, usually further resection and repeat vagotomy, may be indicated for complications (e.g., massive bleeding, obstruction) and should be considered carefully in patients with a refractory ulcer, because ulcers caused by aspirin and other NSAIDs tend to recur.

Afferent Loop Syndrome

The afferent loop syndrome appears to result from rapid gastric emptying and distention (by food-stimulated pancreatic and biliary secretions) of an incompletely draining, partially obstructed Billroth II afferent loop. Hypertonic meals or large volumes of orally ingested liquids may worsen the symptoms.

The disorder is characterized clinically by postprandial abdominal pain, early satiety, and bloating, which are relieved by vomiting that is bilious. The amount of vomitus is usually small. The symptoms are similar to those caused by distention of the proximal jejunum, which is another cause of postprandial abdominal pain and vomiting after peptic surgical procedures. The serum amylase level may be elevated. The diagnosis may be established by a barium radiograph or endoscopy. Therapy consists of surgical correction of the partially obstructed afferent loop.

Bile (Alkaline) Reflux Gastritis

Bile reflux gastritis is a poorly defined entity associated with early satiety, abdominal discomfort, and vomiting; it is thought to be caused by reflux of duodenal contents into the stomach after ulcer surgery. Endoscopic biopsies of the gastric mucosa often show histologic evidence of gastritis. It is not clear whether patients with bile reflux have abnormal bile or whether the stomach is abnormally sensitive to bile.

Medical therapy with agents such as sucralfate or cholestyramine is often unsatisfactory. Anecdotal evidence indicates that oral administration of ursodeoxycholic acid, a relatively nontoxic bile acid, may lead to symptomatic relief. A trial of a gastric prokinetic agent such as metoclopramide (10 to 20 mg with meals) may be attempted, although little evidence supports this intervention (grade D). In severe, refractory cases, surgical treatment may be necessary for correction of this disorder, with creation of a Roux-en-Y anastomosis, which diverts duodenal contents away from the stomach.

Dumping Syndrome

The dumping syndrome is characterized by postprandial vasomotor symptoms such as tachycardia, flushing, and palpitations in association with dyspeptic symptoms. The dumping syndrome is often divided arbitrarily into early and late phases.

Early dumping syndrome, occurring within 30 minutes of eating, is characterized by palpitations, tachycardia, diaphoresis, flushing, and dizziness with nausea, vomiting, and bloating. It is thought to result from rapid emptying of hyperosmolar gastric contents into the small intestine and consequent large fluid shifts that lead to contraction of plasma volume, release of vasoactive hormones, and triggering of autonomic reflexes by jejunal distention. *Late* dumping syndrome, occurring 90 minutes to 3 hours after eating, is characterized by similar symptoms and is thought to result from the rapid gastric emptying of carbohydrates into the proximal small intestine, followed by the sudden release of insulin in response to rapid increases in blood glucose, with subsequent hypoglycemia.

The dumping syndrome is generally managed by encouraging the patient to eat small, frequent meals and to avoid drinking liquids with solid food. The diet should be low in carbohydrates and lactose and high in protein and fat. In some cases, the somatostatin analogue octreotide, 25 to 100 μg subcutaneously three times a day, may be helpful. There are some case reports describing use of long-acting octreotide (monthly intramuscular depot injections) for this indication. Rarely, surgical revision to a Roux-en-Y gastrojejunostomy is necessary.

Postvagotomy Diarrhea

Chronic diarrhea may follow any ulcer operation; it is not clear whether the frequency is actually higher in patients who have had a vagotomy. The exact mechanism is unclear, but rapid gastric emptying and decreased intestinal transit time have been postulated, as have extragastric mechanisms such as increased intestinal bile acid concentrations. Symptoms are usually mild and may be controlled by antimotility medications or may resolve with time. Occasional patients respond to oral cholestyramine.

Late Complications

Late complications of ulcer surgery include the following:

- Hematologic complications, including iron deficiency anemia and vitamin B_{12} malabsorption
- Osteomalacia and osteoporosis
- Malabsorption and maldigestion
- Postgastrectomy carcinoma

Complications of Gastric Bypass

Bariatric surgery is discussed in Chapter 11.

Complications of Small Intestine Resection and Bypass

Volume Depletion and Electrolyte Abnormalities

Morbidity after small bowel resection is proportional to the length of bowel resected; it is especially high if less than 50 cm of jejunum or ileum remains. Combined ileal and colonic resection predisposes to greater volume and electrolyte depletion than does ileal resection alone, because of the loss of colonic compensation. Distal small intestinal resection is tolerated less well than proximal small intestinal resection because of the remarkable ability of the ileum to assume the absorptive function of the proximal small intestine (but not the reverse); 50% to 60% of the midjejunum can be resected with few long-term metabolic consequences, but resection of more than 30% of the ileum is poorly tolerated. A small bowel length of less than 200 cm is commonly used as an anatomic definition of short bowel syndrome. A more practical definition is loss of absorption resulting in the inability to maintain protein-energy, fluid, electrolyte, or micronutrient balances on a conventionally accepted normal diet. Voluminous diarrhea with electrolyte losses may result from the loss of the intestinal absorptive surface, shortened intestinal transit time, and acquired intestinal lactase deficiency. Resection of the distal ileum can lead to choleraic diarrhea, in which impaired bile salt absorption leads to stimulation of the colonic secretion of water and electrolytes. More extensive ileal resections may eventually result in steatorrhea caused by bile salt deficiency (see the following section). Other causes of diarrhea following intestinal resection include gastric acid hypersecretion (see the following section) and bacterial overgrowth resulting from loss of the ileocecal valve.

Other Metabolic Complications

Patients who have undergone small bowel resection are at increased risk of developing cholesterol gallstones, oxalate nephrolithiasis, and D-lactic acidosis. Gallstone disease appears to be related to supersaturation of hepatic bile in the setting of impaired small bowel enterohepatic recirculation of nonlithogenic bile acids. Cholecystectomy is necessary in symptomatic patients. Hyperoxaluria may develop with small bowel resection resulting from fat malabsorption. Oxalate is usually chelated by calcium in the colon. In patients with fat malabsorption, luminal calcium binds with long-chain fatty acids, thereby making oxalate available to be absorbed readily by the colon and excreted in the urine, where it may precipitate. Limiting oxalate-rich foods (tea, chocolate, cola beverages) and supplemental oral calcium may reduce the frequency of this complication. D-Lactic acidosis occurs in the setting of carbohydrate malabsorption and subsequent fermentation of carbohydrates by colonic bacteria to short-chain fatty acids and lactate. Patients may be treated with sodium bicarbonate. The efficacy of antibiotics in this setting is controversial.

Management

Treatment of volume depletion consists of replacement of fluid and electrolytes. Early implementation of total parenteral nutrition is essential in patients with short bowel syndrome, especially in the immediate postoperative period after massive resections, when fecal fluid losses may exceed 5 L/day. Proton pump inhibitors are used to reduce gastric acid and gastric fluid production. Diphenoxylate and atropine (Lomotil) (one to two tablets orally four times a day), loperamide (2 mg orally three to four times a day), or codeine (15 to 30 mg orally every 6 hours) can be used to prolong intestinal transit time and reduce diarrhea. Occasionally, deodorized tincture of opium (0.3 to 1 mL orally four times a day) may be necessary. The medications may be withdrawn gradually as the remaining intestine adapts to the resection. Octreotide (50 to 250 μg subcutaneously three times a day) may help to control massive diarrhea resulting from short bowel syndrome. Restriction of oral fat intake, especially long-chain fats, to less than 30 g/day and elimination of dietary lactose also may help. If bacterial overgrowth is suspected, a trial of broad-spectrum oral antibiotics may be instituted. Finally, cholestyramine in doses of 8 to 16 g/day orally may be effective in the treatment of bile salt–induced diarrhea resulting from limited ileal resection.

Malabsorption

As suggested previously, numerous mechanisms may be implicated in the pathogenesis of malabsorption after small bowel resection. The most obvious is loss of intestinal absorptive area. Although relatively long resections of the midjejunum are well tolerated, resection of even short segments of the specialized absorptive surfaces of the proximal or distal small bowel may lead to compromise of intestinal function. Decreased intestinal production of secretin and cholecystokinin, which stimulate exocrine pancreatic and biliary secretion, may contribute to malabsorption, as may poor mixing of gastric contents with pancreatic and biliary secretions as a result of altered anatomy. Other pathogenic factors include gastric hypersecretion, loss of the absorptive site of vitamin B_{12} resulting from terminal ileal resection, and bacterial overgrowth.

The result of these pathophysiologic processes may be a reduction in the absorption of electrolytes, minerals, vitamins, protein, carbohydrates, and fat, leading to malnutrition, immunocompromise, and infection. Diagnostic evaluation may include fecal fat quantitation, D-xylose absorption test, pancreatic function tests (e.g., secretin test), vitamin B_{12} levels, and breath tests or quantitative small intestinal cultures for bacterial overgrowth. In practice, however, therapeutic trials are often initiated empirically.

MANAGEMENT

Treatment consists of restriction of oral fat intake and replacement of long-chain fats with medium-chain triglycerides, supplementation of fat-soluble vitamins and trace elements, vitamin B_{12} injections in patients who have undergone ileal resection, oral broad-spectrum antibiotics if small bowel overgrowth is suspected (e.g., a rotation of one or more for the following: tetracycline 250 mg four times a day; metronidazole 250 mg three times a day, or ciprofloxacin 500 mg three times a day; rifaximin 400 mg three times a day 1 week out of 4), and, in the postoperative period, enteral hyperalimentation or total parenteral nutrition. Depending on the extent of the resection and adaptation of the remaining intestine, some patients may require long-term (home) enteral or parenteral alimentation. Cyclic (nocturnal) parenteral alimentation is preferable to continual administration. Small bowel transplantation may be considered in selected patients. Novel treatment strategies including the use of growth factors and glutamine are of uncertain benefit and are under investigation.

Gastric Acid Hypersecretion

The mechanism of gastric acid hypersecretion after small bowel resection is unclear. Probable mechanisms include elevated serum gastrin levels, resulting from decreased clearance of circulating gastrin or loss of a hormonal inhibitor, and reduced levels of intestinally produced inhibitors of gastric acid secretion, such as secretin, cholecystokinin, glucagon, vasoactive intestinal polypeptide, and gastric inhibitory peptide.

Ulceration may result from gastric acid hypersecretion. Other possible effects are intestinal mucosal damage, precipitation of bile salts, and deactivation of pancreatic enzymes with resulting diarrhea and malabsorption. Gastric acid hypersecretion is usually a transient phenomenon that occurs after extensive small bowel resection and is managed with a proton pump inhibitor.

Complications of Colectomy and Ostomies

Colostomy

With sigmoid colostomy, bowel function is often well preserved and stool is formed. The patient may be able to wear a small gauze pad instead of a pouch and to evacuate through irrigation enemas. Anal sphincter-saving surgical procedures should be performed in patients with low rectal carcinoma when feasible.

With a colostomy proximal to the splenic flexure, the discharge is often loose, even liquid, and malodorous because of the action of colonic bacteria. An appliance may be difficult to wear if the ostomy is above the belt line, and an ileostomy may in fact be preferable in some patients.

Ileostomy

PROBLEMS WITH CONVENTIONAL ILEOSTOMY

Conventional ileostomy requires the use of an appliance to control the frequent discharge of ileal effluent. Various problems may complicate the use of an ileostomy. Because of the loss of the resorptive surface of the colon, water and salt depletion may occur. Resulting changes in the composition of urine can lead to nephrolithiasis. Skin breakdown may result from sensitivity to adhesives or fungal infection. Treatment with a cortisone spray or an antifungal powder may be helpful. Odor may be a problem, particularly after the ingestion of certain types of foods. The odor can be treated by dietary modification or the use of special deodorants such as chlorine or sodium benzoate in the pouch. Leakage is rarely a problem with modern appliances and preoperative marking of proper stomal placement by an enterostomal therapist. Stomal obstruction, prolapse, or retraction may occur and may require surgical correction. Sexual dysfunction may result from neurologic impairment, depression, embarrassment, or rejection by a spouse or partner. Impotence is more common after colostomy, especially for rectal cancer, than after ileostomy. Problems of psychologic adjustment relate to the loss of self-esteem, a diminished sense of physical attractiveness, and rejection by a spouse or partner. Referral to a local ostomy chapter is important.

ILEAL POUCH–ANAL ANASTOMOSIS

With an ileal pouch–anal anastomosis, fecal elimination through the anus is preserved, and most patients ultimately have as few as five bowel movements per day. This operation cannot be used in patients with Crohn's disease. "Pouchitis," characterized by inflammation and bacterial overgrowth, is a frequent complication. This procedure should be performed only by experienced surgeons who are familiar with the technical intricacies of the procedure and the advantages and disadvantages of the various alternatives.

Diversion Colitis

Diversion colitis is an iatrogenic form of inflammatory bowel disease in which a bypassed or excluded segment of colon becomes inflamed. Diversion colitis may manifest with the passage of blood or mucus per rectum, although some patients are asymptomatic. It may be discovered within a few weeks of the colostomy procedure or years later and may involve the entire bypassed segment. Diffuse mild inflammation is seen on sigmoidoscopy. Histologically, one sees nonspecific mucosal and submucosal inflammation with surface ulceration and crypt abscesses. Biopsy may be helpful to distinguish diversion colitis from underlying Crohn's disease.

Treatment with the anti-inflammatory agents used to treat inflammatory bowel disease may, in fact, be helpful, although many patients show no improvement unless bowel continuity is restored surgically. Short-chain fatty acids, normally present in the fecal stream, are needed to maintain a healthy colonic mucosa, and enemas of short-chain fatty acids in the concentrations found in feces may lead to resolution of the inflammation.

Gastrointestinal Fistulas

Fistula formation is an important complication of gastrointestinal surgery. Anastomotic leakage can lead to communication between the gastrointestinal tract and other intestinal segments, other intra-abdominal structures such as the bladder, and the skin. Fistulas are commonly associated with abscesses along the fistulous tract. Enterocutaneous fistulas may develop as a consequence of surgical intervention but are more commonly related to malignant processes and may lead to large fluid, electrolyte, and protein losses, with consequent dehydration and malnutrition.

Clinical Presentation

Gastrointestinal fistulas commonly manifest with fever, leukocytosis, pain, and wound breakdown. The anatomy of the fistula may be defined by radiographs performed with meglumine diatrizoate (Gastrografin); barium can be used if there is no risk of leakage into the peritoneal cavity. Intestinal obstruction distal to the origin of the fistula should be excluded. Ultrasonography and computed tomography may be useful for localizing abscesses.

Management

Initial therapy for a gastrointestinal fistula consists of bowel rest, nasogastric suction, and correction of fluid and electrolyte abnormalities. Abscesses should be drained percutaneously or surgically. Intravenous broad-spectrum antibiotic therapy should be started pending culture results. Total parenteral nutrition should be started and advanced over 3 to 5 days. Nutritional support should be continued for 4 to 6 weeks before operative closure of a fistula is appropriate. Octreotide, 50 to 100 µg or more subcutaneously twice a day, may aid fistula healing by inhibiting exocrine secretions from the stomach, pancreas, and small intestine. Surgical therapy consists of resection of the fistula and involved segment of intestine; in patients with carcinoma or irradiated intestine, bypass of the involved segment may be all that is feasible. A trial of conservative management is especially important in patients with Crohn's disease in whom resection of a fistula is frequently complicated by recurrence. Spontaneous closure of a fistula is unlikely in the presence of epithelialization of the fistulous tract, intra-abdominal infection or abscess, neoplasia in the fistulous tract, active inflammatory disease of the bowel, a fistula output greater than 500 mL/24 hours, a fistulous tract diameter greater than 2 cm, intestinal obstruction beyond the origin of the fistula, or impaired blood supply to the involved segment of intestine. There is growing experience with fibrin glue to manage postoperative gastrointestinal-cutaneous fistulas.

Postcholecystectomy Syndrome

Postcholecystectomy syndrome is a term used to describe a wide variety of disorders and symptoms that may occur after cholecystectomy. Up to 15% of patients who undergo cholecystectomy continue to have or acquire distressing symptoms postoperatively. Such symptoms are more likely to develop when surgical procedures are performed for dyspepsia than for classic biliary pain. Persistence of symptoms postoperatively is also more likely when an uninflamed gallbladder is found at operation.

Nonbiliary causes of abdominal pain after cholecystectomy include irritable bowel syndrome, gastroesophageal reflux disease, diffuse esophageal spasm, gastritis, peptic ulcer disease, and pancreatitis. A high rate of psychiatric disturbances has been described in patients who complain of persistent pain but have no demonstrable organic disease or anatomic abnormality. Pain related to disease in the biliary tract after cholecystectomy may be caused by retained or recurrent common bile duct stones, bile duct strictures, bile stasis and recurrent stone formation in a long cystic duct remnant, and sphincter of Oddi dysfunction.

Evaluation

Exclusion of nonbiliary tract disease in patients with the postcholecystectomy syndrome may require upper gastrointestinal endoscopy, esophageal manometry and 24-hour pH monitoring, abdominal computed tomography, and other appropriate investigations as dictated by the nature of the symptoms. Magnetic or endoscopic retrograde cholangiopancreatography and endoscopic ultrasonography may be indicated to investigate the possibility of common bile duct and cystic duct stones, biliary strictures, and pancreatic abnormalities. Biliary scintigraphy may be used as a screening test to demonstrate partial or complete common bile duct obstruction. Sphincter of Oddi manometry may be performed to look for evidence of abnormal bile duct peristalsis and sphincter of Oddi dysfunction. Endoscopic sphincterotomy may provide relief of symptoms in carefully selected patients.

Selected Readings

Anonymous: NIH state-of-the-science statement on endoscopic retrograde cholangiopancreatography (ERCP) for diagnosis and therapy. NIH Consens State Sci State 19:1-26, 2002.

Apfel CC, Korttila K, Abdalla M, et al: A factorial trial of six interventions for the prevention of postoperative nausea and vomiting. N Engl J Med 350:2441-2451, 2004.

Apfel CC, Roewer N: Risk assessment of postoperative nausea and vomiting. Int Anesthesiol Clin 41:13-32, 2003.

Bardou M, Youbouti Y, Benhaberou-Brun, et al: Meta-analysis: Proton-pump inhibition in high-risk patients with acute peptic ulcer bleeding. Aliment Pharmacol Ther 21:677-686, 2005.

Bartlett J: Antibiotic associated diarrhea. N Engl J Med 346:334-339, 2002. **C**

Behm B, Stollman N: Postoperative ileus: Etiologies and interventions. Clin Gastroenterol Hepatol 1:71-80, 2003.

Bernstein CN, Blanchard JF, Houston DS, Wajda A: The incidence of deep venous thrombosis and pulmonary embolism among patients with inflammatory bowel disease: A population-based cohort study. Thromb Haemost 85:430-434, 2001. **B**

Bibbo C, Goldberg JW: Infectious and healing complications after elective orthopaedic foot and ankle surgery during tumor necrosis factor-alpha inhibition therapy. Foot Ankle Int 25:331-335, 2004. **B**

Bonner GF, Fakhri A, Vennamaneni SR: A long-term cohort study of nonsteroidal anti-inflammatory drug use and disease activity in outpatients with inflammatory bowel disease. Inflamm Bowel Dis 10:751-757, 2004. **B**

Buchman AL, Iyer K, Fryer J: Parenteral nutrition-associated liver disease and the role for isolated intestine and intestine/liver transplantation. Hepatology 43:9-19, 2006.

DiBaise JK, Young RJ, Vanderhoff JA: Enteric microbial flora, bacterial overgrowth, and short-bowel syndrome. Clin Gastroenterol Hepatol 4:11-20, 2006.

Dudnick RS, Martin P, Friedman LS: Management of bleeding ulcers. Med Clin North Am 75:947-965, 1991.

Faust TW, Reddy KR: Postoperative jaundice. Clin Liver Dis 8:151-166, 2004.

Fazel A, Verne G: New solutions to an old problem. J Clin Gastroenterol 39:17-20, 2005.

Gan SI, Beck PL: A new look at toxic megacolon: An update and review of incidence, etiology, pathogenesis, and management. Am J Gastroenterol 98:2363-2371, 2003.

Hanauer SB: Medical therapy for ulcerative colitis 2004. Gastroenterology 126:1582-1592, 2004.

Hiramoto JS, Terdiman JP, Norton JA: Evidence-based analysis: Postoperative gastric bleeding: Etiology and prevention. Surg Oncol 12:9-19, 2003. **C**

Kao LS, Flowers C, Flum DR: Prophylactic cholecystectomy in transplant patients: A decision analysis. J Gastrointest Surg 9:965-972, 2005.

Kovac A: Prevention and treatment of postoperative nausea and vomiting. Drugs 59:213-243, 2000.

Leontiadis GI, Sharma VK, Howden CW: Systematic review and meta-analysis: Proton pump inhibitor treatment for ulcer bleeding reduces transfusion requirements and hospital stay—results from the Cochrane Collaboration. Aliment Pharmacol Ther 22:169-174, 2005.

Loo VG, Poirier L, Miller MA, et al: A predominantly clonal multi-institutional outbreak of *Clostridium difficile*–associated diarrhea with high morbidity and mortality. N Engl J Med 353:2442-2449, 2005.

McCallum RW, George SJ: Review: Gastroparesis. Clin Perspect Gastroenterol 4:147-154, 2001.

Musher DM, Aslam S, Logan N, et al: Relativity poor outcome after treatment of *Clostridium difficile* colitis with metronidazole. Clin Infect Dis 40:1586-1590, 2005.

Nelson R, Tse B, Edwards S: Systematic review of prophylactic nasogastric decompression after abdominal operations. Br J Surg 92:673-680, 2005. ❸

O'Keeffe SJD, Buchman AL, Fishbein TM, et al: Short bowel syndrome and intestinal failure: Consensus definitions and overview. Clin Gastroenterol Hepatol 4:6-10, 2006.

Paran H, Silverberg D, Mayo A, et al: Treatment of acute colonic pseudo-obstruction with neostigmine. J Am Coll Surg 190:315-318, 2000. ❶

Pennazio M, Santucci R, Rondonotti E, et al: Outcome of patients with obscure gastrointestinal bleeding after capsule endoscopy: Report of 100 consecutive cases. Gastroenterology 126:643-653, 2004.

Perez A, Ito H, Farivar RS, et al: Risk factors and outcomes of pancreatitis after open heart surgery. Am J Surg 190:401-405, 2005. ❸

Pisegna JR, Martindale RG: Acid suppression in the perioperative period. J Clin Gastroenterol 39:10-16, 2005.

Pollard TR, Schwesinger WH, Page CP, et al: Upper gastrointestinal bleeding following major surgical procedures: Prevalence, etiology, and outcome. J Surg Res 64:75-78, 1996. ❸

Ponec RJ, Saunders MD, Kimmey MB: Neostigmine for the treatment of acute colonic pseudo-obstruction. N Engl J Med 15:1137-1141, 1999. ❶

Prajapati DN, Hogan WJ: Sphincter of Oddi dysfunction and other functional biliary disorders: Evaluation and treatment. Gastroenterol Clin North Am 32:601-618, 2003.

Ramsey PS, Podratz KC: Acute pancreatitis after gynecologic and obstetric surgery. Am J Obstet Gynecol 18:542-546, 1999.

Saunders MD, Kimmey MB: Systematic review: Acute colonic pseudo-obstruction. Aliment Pharmacol Ther 22:917-925, 2005.

Scharff JR, Longo WE, Vartanian SM, et al: Ischemic colitis: Spectrum of disease and outcome. Surgery 134:624-629, 2003.

Soll A: Consensus conference: Medical treatment of peptic ulcer disease. Practice guidelines: Practice Parameters Committee of the American College of Gastroenterology. JAMA 275:622-629, 1996.

Stephenson BM, Morgan AR, Drake N, et al: Parasympathomimetic decompression of acute colonic pseudo-obstruction. Lancet 342:1181-1182, 1993. ❶

Tenner S: Initial management of acute pancreatitis: Critical issues during the first 72 hours. Am J Gastroenterol 99:2489-2494, 2004.

Velayos FS, Williamson A, Sousa KH: Early predictors of severe lower gastrointestinal bleeding and adverse outcomes: A prospective study. Clin Gastroenterol Hepatol 2:485-490, 2004.

10 Management of the Surgical Patient with Liver Disease

JACQUELINE G. O'LEARY, MD, MPH

LAWRENCE S. FRIEDMAN, MD

Patients with liver disease who undergo surgical procedures have significantly increased morbidity and mortality, particularly if liver disease is overt preoperatively. Because patients with liver disease are frequently asymptomatic, the preoperative assessment must include a carefully performed history and physical examination to search for risk factors and evidence of a liver disorder. If signs of liver disease are present, further investigation into the cause and severity of the condition is indicated. Elective surgical procedures should be deferred in patients with acute necroinflammatory liver disease until the condition has resolved. Predicting how an individual patient will respond to the stresses of anesthesia and surgery is difficult. The liver is uniquely involved in numerous metabolic and synthetic processes, and management of perioperative problems in the patient with liver disease requires an understanding of both the multiple functions of the liver and the pathophysiologic processes that underlie the complications that may arise.

EFFECTS OF ANESTHESIA AND SURGERY ON THE LIVER

Changes in Liver Biochemical Test Levels

Most surgical procedures, whether performed using general or conduction (spinal or epidural) anesthetic techniques, are followed by elevations in serum liver biochemical test levels [❂ Friedman, 1999; Gholson et al, 1990; Keegan and Plevak, 2005]. In most cases, postoperative elevations of serum aminotransferase, alkaline phosphatase, or bilirubin levels are minor, transient, and of questionable significance. However, in patients with underlying liver disease, and especially those with compromised hepatic function, surgery can precipitate hepatic decompensation, which may result in increased morbidity and mortality. The role of anesthetic agents in causing minor postoperative hepatic dysfunction is unclear; none of the currently used anesthetic agents is a direct hepatotoxin.

The nature and extent of the surgical procedure may be more important contributors to postoperative hepatic dysfunction than the administration of anesthesia. The risk of hepatic dysfunction is greatest with biliary tract and upper abdominal surgery.

Hemodynamic Effects

Cirrhosis causes a hyperdynamic circulation with increased cardiac output, decreased systemic vascular resistance, and, in some patients, increased extravascular volume, increased or decreased intravascular volume, arteriovenous shunting, and decreased renal blood flow. At baseline, hepatic arterial and venous perfusion of the cirrhotic liver may be decreased: portal blood flow is reduced in patients with portal hypertension, and arterial blood flow can be decreased because of impaired autoregulation. The decreased hepatic perfusion makes the cirrhotic liver more susceptible to hypoxemia and hypotension. Decreased oxygen delivery to the liver during surgery is the single most important threat to hepatic function. All anesthetic agents, including those administered by the spinal or epidural route, reduce hepatic blood flow by 30% to 50% following induction. In fact, the type of anesthesia has never been correlated with outcome.

Additional factors that may contribute to decreased hepatic blood flow intraoperatively include hypotension, hemorrhage, hypoxemia, hypercarbia, congestive heart failure, vasoactive drugs, and intermittent positive pressure ventilation. Traction on abdominal viscera may cause reflex dilation of splanchnic capacitance vessels and may thereby lower hepatic blood flow.

Intravascular volume must be maintained to ensure hepatic and renal perfusion. However, excess crystalloid will extravasate and can lead intraoperatively to acute hepatic congestion, increased venous oozing during hepatic resections, and pulmonary edema and postoperatively to ascites, peripheral edema, and wound dehiscence.

Hypoxemia

Risk factors for intraoperative hypoxemia in patients with cirrhosis include ascites, hepatic hydrothorax, hepatopulmonary syndrome (the triad of liver disease, an increased alveolar-arterial gradient, and intrapulmonary shunting), hypoalbuminemia, and pulmonary hypertension. Hypoxemia also can be caused by aspiration. Ascites, encephalopathy, and anesthetic agents increase the risk of aspiration in patients with cirrhosis.

Hepatic Metabolism of Anesthetic Agents

Metabolism of anesthetic agents by the liver may result in the formation of toxic metabolites, especially in the presence of reduced hepatic blood flow and hypoxia. Occasional episodes of acute hepatitis associated with the administration of halothane, now rarely used in adults, are thought to be caused by immune sensitization to trifluoroacetylated liver proteins formed by oxidative metabolism of halothane by cytochrome

P-450 2E1 in genetically predisposed persons; such metabolism can be blocked experimentally by disulfiram. Hepatitis caused by isoflurane, desflurane, and sevoflurane, which undergo little hepatic metabolism, is rare. These anesthetic agents are good choices in patients with liver disease.

In many cirrhotic patients, the volume of distribution of drugs is increased. The action of anesthetic agents may be prolonged in patients with liver disease not only because of impaired metabolism, but also because of hypoalbuminemia (resulting in decreased drug binding), leading to impaired biliary clearance. Propofol is an excellent anesthetic choice in patients with liver disease, because it remains relatively short acting even in patients with decompensated cirrhosis.

Use of Other Perioperative Medications in Liver Disease

Sedatives, narcotics, intravenous induction agents, and neuromuscular blocking agents are generally tolerated in patients with compensated liver disease but must be used with caution in patients with hepatic dysfunction. Blood levels of narcotics that undergo high first-pass extraction by the liver increase as hepatic blood flow decreases. The sedative effects of benzodiazepines that undergo low first-pass extraction by the liver may be altered in liver disease, depending largely on their method of elimination. The elimination of drugs that undergo glucuronidation (e.g., oxazepam, lorazepam) usually is not affected by liver disease, whereas the elimination of those that do not undergo glucuronidation (e.g., diazepam, chlordiazepoxide) is prolonged in liver disease. In patients with decompensated liver disease, sedatives such as diazepam, narcotics such as meperidine, or induction agents such as phenobarbital may cause prolonged depression of consciousness and may precipitate hepatic encephalopathy even if they are used in standard doses; very small doses may be sufficient to achieve a therapeutic effect. In general, narcotics and benzodiazepines should be avoided in these patients; however, when necessary, remifentanil and oxazepam are the preferred narcotic and sedative, respectively, because the metabolism of these agents is unaffected by liver disease.

The volume of distribution of nondepolarizing muscle relaxants (e.g., pancuronium, atracurium, doxacurium, and vecuronium) is increased in patients with liver disease, and larger doses may therefore be required to achieve a given level of neuromuscular blockade. In addition, many of these agents are metabolized by the liver and excreted in bile, and their effect is prolonged in patients with liver disease. Atracurium and cis-atracurium are considered the preferred muscle relaxants in patients with liver disease because neither the liver nor the kidney is required for their elimination. Further, the duration of neuromuscular blockade produced by atracurium is not affected by decreased levels of plasma cholinesterase, which is synthesized by the liver. In contrast, hydrolysis of succinylcholine and mivacurium by plasma cholinesterase, which is normally rapid, is slightly prolonged in hepatic disease. Doxacurium, which is eliminated primarily by the kidney, is preferred for prolonged procedures such as liver transplantation.

OPERATIVE RISK IN PATIENTS WITH LIVER DISEASE

Problems in Estimating Surgical Risk

In a patient with liver disease, surgical risk depends on the type and severity of liver disease, the presence of comorbid conditions, and the nature of the surgical procedure. Certain conditions are associated with unacceptable surgical mortality and usually are considered contraindications to elective surgery (Box 10-1). When these contraindications are absent, the patient should undergo a thorough preoperative evaluation, and the patient's condition should be optimized before an elective surgical procedure is performed. Mortality and morbidity may increase when liver disease is present but unsuspected preoperatively, and therefore an assessment for

Box 10-1	CONTRAINDICATIONS TO ELECTIVE SURGERY IN PATIENTS WITH LIVER DISEASE

Fulminant hepatic failure

Acute viral hepatitis

Acute alcoholic hepatitis

Severe chronic hepatitis

Child-Turcotte-Pugh class C cirrhosis

Severe coagulopathy (prolongation of the prothrombin time by >3 seconds despite treatment with vitamin K: platelet count <50,000/mm^3)

Severe extrahepatic complications

Hypoxemia

Cardiomyopathy

Acute renal failure

possible liver disease should be part of every preoperative evaluation. Patients found to have advanced liver disease may benefit from alternative nonsurgical therapies when available and appropriate.

Estimating operative risk in patients with liver disease is difficult not only because of the problems inherent in assessing the severity of liver disease, but also because of the lack of large, prospective studies to guide the assessment of these patients. Most studies that have examined the risk of surgery in patients with liver disease have focused on patients with cirrhosis. Much less information has been published on the risk of surgery in patients with other forms of liver disease such as hepatitis. The available evidence is derived mostly from small, retrospective studies, many of which were published before the identification of the hepatitis C virus (HCV), recognition of nonalcoholic fatty liver disease (NAFLD), and the advent of modern hepatobiliary imaging. There is relatively little information on how the risk of surgery varies with the type of liver disease.

Preoperative Screening

Whether healthy, asymptomatic patients should undergo routine preoperative liver biochemical testing has been debated. When such screening has been undertaken, cases of subclinical hepatitis and even cirrhosis occasionally have been detected. Elevated serum aminotransferase levels have been found in 0.5% of asymptomatic U.S. Air Force basic trainees and as many as 9.8% of adults in the United States. Reliance on routine liver biochemical tests alone may be misleading, because patients with cirrhosis may have normal serum test results. In some cases, cirrhosis may be discovered after evaluation for characteristic symptoms such as fatigue or pruritus or on the basis of physical examination findings such as palmar erythema, cutaneous spider telangiectasias, hepatic encephalopathy, ascites, splenomegaly, testicular atrophy, or gynecomastia. Therefore, the importance of a thorough preoperative history and physical examination cannot be overemphasized. The evaluation should include careful history taking to identify risk factors for liver disease, including previous blood transfusions, tattoos, illicit drug use, sexual promiscuity, a family history of jaundice or liver disease, a personal history of jaundice or fever with anesthesia, quantitation of alcohol use, and a complete review of current medications (including over-the-counter medications and herbal preparations). Patients with a history of hepatitis should have testing for serum aminotransferase, alkaline phosphatase, bilirubin, and albumin levels, as well as prothrombin time and screening for hepatitis B surface antigen (HBsAg) and antibody to HCV (anti-HCV). If these studies are unrevealing, elective surgery should pose no increased risk. However, any patient found to have clinical or biochemical evidence of liver disease should undergo thorough investigation before having an elective surgical procedure.

A small proportion of patients discovered to have elevated serum aminotransferase levels will turn out to have viral hepatitis. If the hepatitis is acute, the patient may ultimately become symptomatic with jaundice. If these patients undergo surgical procedures and the liver disease becomes apparent postoperatively, hepatitis may be attributed erroneously to the anesthetic agent or the surgical procedure. Therefore, in asymptomatic, preoperative patients with significant liver biochemical abnormalities, elective surgical procedures should be postponed until the liver disease is evaluated and the course of the disease is observed. The extent to which liver biochemical test abnormalities should be evaluated depends on their nature and severity. Minor deviations from normal are not uncommon in asymptomatic patients but rarely lead to the detection of serious liver disease. When serum aminotransferase levels are at least 1.5 times the upper limit of normal on repeated occasions, diagnostic possibilities include NAFLD, metabolic liver disease (e.g., hemochromatosis or Wilson's disease), autoimmune liver disease, and celiac sprue, and appropriate biochemical and serologic testing may be needed. Liver biopsy may be necessary in patients with elevated serum aminotransferase levels, whereas abdominal ultrasonography, computed tomography, cholangiography (magnetic resonance cholangiopancreatography, endoscopic retrograde cholangiopancreatography, or percutaneous cholangiography), and liver biopsy may be necessary in patients with a cholestatic pattern of liver test abnormalities. The possibility of drug-induced liver dysfunction must be considered in all cases.

Acute Hepatitis and Fulminant Hepatic Failure

Acute hepatitis may be caused by drugs and toxins, viruses, autoimmune diseases, and genetic disorders and may be mimicked by vascular disease and acute biliary obstruction (Table 10-1). **Patients with acute hepatitis of any cause are thought to have an increased operative risk and perioperative mortality rate, and elective surgery during acute hepatitis is contraindicated, except in cases of biliary obstruction** [● *Gholson et al, 1990*]. This conclusion is based in large part on older studies, in which operative mortality rates of 10% to 13% were reported among patients who underwent laparotomy to distinguish intrahepatic from extrahepatic causes of jaundice. Today, such a distinction can almost always be made with a combination of serologic tests, imaging tests, and percutaneous liver biopsy. Nonetheless, it is appropriate to avoid all elective surgical procedures in patients with acute, even mild, viral hepatitis until the acute illness has resolved and, in most cases, the liver biochemical test levels have returned to normal.

Patients with *fulminant hepatic failure,* defined as the development of severe coagulopathy and hepatic encephalopathy within 8 weeks of the onset of acute hepatitis, are gravely

TABLE 10-1	Causes of Acute Hepatitis	
	Cause	**Initial Diagnostic Test**
Drugs and Toxins	Drug-induced	History
	Toxin-induced (including alcohol)	History
Viruses	HAV	IgM anti-HAV
	HBV	HBsAg
	HCV	anti-HCV
	HDV	anti-HDV
	HEV	anti-HEV
	CMV	CMV antigenemia
	EBV	Monospot
	HSV	Culture
Autoimmune Disorders	Autoimmune hepatitis	ANA, ASMA, IgG level
Genetic Disorders	Wilson's disease	Serum ceruloplasmin level
Other Causes	Vascular disease	Abdominal ultrasonography with Doppler or magnetic resonance imaging
	Acute biliary obstruction	Abdominal ultrasonography

ANA, antinuclear antibody; anti-HCV, antibody to hepatitis C virus; anti-HDV, antibody to hepatitis D virus; anti-HEV, antibody to hepatitis E virus; ASMA, anti–smooth muscle antibody; CMV, cytomegalovirus; EBV, Epstein-Barr virus; HAV, hepatitis A virus; HBsAg, hepatitis B surface antigen; HBV, hepatitis B virus; HCV, hepatitis C virus; HDV, hepatitis D virus; HEV, hepatitis E virus; HSV, herpes simplex virus; IgM anti-HAV, IgM antibody to hepatitis A virus.

ill and are unlikely to survive surgery other than liver transplantation.

Chronic Hepatitis

Chronic hepatitis refers to a group of disorders characterized by inflammation of the liver persisting for more than 6 months, although some patients have an acute clinical presentation. Numerous viral, genetic, autoimmune, metabolic, and drug-induced causes of chronic hepatitis have been identified (Table 10-2). Regardless of the cause, the histopathologic findings are classified by the grade of necroinflammatory activity and the stage of fibrosis according to one of various scoring systems; the METAVIR scoring system is shown in Table 10-3. If a patient is found preoperatively to have chronic hepatitis, treatment of the underlying disease can often reduce

TABLE 10-2	Causes of Chronic Hepatitis	
	Cause	**Initial Diagnostic Test**
Drugs	Examples include nitro-furantoin, isoniazid	History
Viruses	HBV	HBsAg
	HCV	anti-HCV
	HDV	anti-HDV
Autoimmune Disorders*	Autoimmune hepatitis	ANA, ASMA, IgG level
Metabolic Disorders	Nonalcoholic steatohep-atitis	History
Genetic Disorders	Hemochromatosis	Iron saturation, serum ferritin level
	Wilson's disease	Serum ceruloplasmin level
	α_1-Antitrypsin deficiency	Serum α_1-antitrypsin level
Other	Celiac sprue	Serum transglutaminase antibody

*Primary biliary cirrhosis and primary sclerosing cholangitis are in the differential diagnosis of chronic hepatitis but generally manifest as cholestatic liver disease.
ANA, antinuclear antibodies; anti-HCV, antibody to hepatitis C virus; anti-HDV, antibody to hepatitis D virus; ASMA, anti–smooth muscle antibody; HBsAg, hepatitis B surface antigen; HBV, hepatitis B virus; HCV, hepatitis C virus; HDV, hepatitis D virus.

TABLE 10-3	METAVIR Histologic Grading and Staging Classification of Chronic Hepatitis				
	INFLAMMATORY ACTIVITY			**DEGREE OF FIBROSIS**	
Grade	Portal	Lobular	Stage	Fibrosis	
0	None or minimal	None	1	No fibrosis or limited to expanded portal tracts	
1	Portal inflammation	Inflammation, no necrosis	2	Periportal fibrosis or portal-to-portal septa with intact architecture	
2	Mild limiting plate necrosis	Focal necrosis	3	Septal fibrosis with architectural distortion	
3	Moderate limiting plate necrosis	Severe focal cell damage	4	Cirrhosis	
4	Severe limiting plate necrosis	Bridging necrosis			

Data from Bedossa P, Poynard T: An algorithm for the grading of activity in chronic hepatitis C. Hepatology 24:289-293, 1996.

necroinflammatory activity and, in some cases, reverse fibrosis. Therefore, depending on the urgency of the surgical procedure, preoperative treatment of the underlying liver disease may reduce a patient's perioperative risk.

Operative Risk

Surgical risk in patients with chronic hepatitis correlates with the clinical, biochemical, and histologic severity of the disease. A patient's perioperative risk may be linked to the grade of inflammation, although little is known about the predictive value of hepatic inflammation alone. Most data about risk stratification relate to the fibrosis stage. **The few published studies of the risk of surgery in patients with mild to moderate chronic hepatitis without cirrhosis suggest that such patients are at low risk for complications** [❿ *Cheung et al, 2003; Runyon, 1986*]. However, medical therapy should be optimized preoperatively. Patients with biochemically and histologically severe chronic hepatitis have an increased surgical risk, particularly when hepatic synthetic or excretory function is impaired, portal hypertension is present, or bridging or multilobular necrosis is found on a liver biopsy specimen

Cirrhosis

Cirrhosis is characterized by parenchymal necrosis, nodular regeneration of remaining hepatocytes, and fibrosis with resulting disorganization of the hepatic lobular architecture and distortion of the vasculature. The most important complication of cirrhosis is portal hypertension, which results from functional obstruction of sinusoidal blood flow and may lead to bleeding from esophageal varices, splenomegaly with pancytopenia (hypersplenism), ascites, and hepatic encephalopathy. Ultimately, decompensated cirrhosis, which may manifest as worsening portal hypertension, deteriorating hepatic synthetic function, renal failure (hepatorenal syndrome), hypoxia (hepatopulmonary syndrome), and nutritional wasting, may ensue. Although the results of conventional liver biochemical tests (serum aminotransferase and alkaline phosphatase levels) correlate poorly with the degree of liver impairment in cirrhotic patients, hepatic dysfunction may be quantified somewhat by a low serum albumin level and prolongation of the prothrombin time, resulting from decreased synthesis of hepatic proteins, and elevation of the serum bilirubin level. Hepatic metabolism of drugs may be altered. In addition, the risk of infection is increased because of depressed activity of the reticuloendothelial system.

Operative Risk

Surgical risk is increased in patients with cirrhosis, but the risk is often difficult to estimate precisely. Perioperative mortality in cirrhotic patients correlates with the severity of cirrhosis, that is, with the degree of hepatic decompensation. **Although the optimal measure of hepatic decompensation remains unclear, some retrospective studies demonstrated that perioperative mortality and morbidity in patients with cirrhosis correlated well with the Child-Turcotte-Pugh class of cirrhosis and the model for end–stage liver disease (MELD) score** (Table 10-4) [❽ *Ziser et al, 1999; Malinchoc et al, 2000*]. The Child-Turcotte-Pugh scoring system, originally

TABLE 10-4	Child-Turcotte-Pugh Scoring System		
Points	1	2	3
Encephalopathy*	None	1–2	3–4
Ascites	None	Easily controlled	Poorly controlled
INR	<1.7	1.7–2.3	>2.3
Albumin (g/dL)	>3.5	3–3.5	<3
Bilirubin (mg/dL)	<2	2–3	>3
Score 5–6: Class A			
Score 7–9: Class B			
Score 10–15: Class C			

*According to Trey C, Burns DG, Saunders SJ: Treatment of hepatic coma by exchange blood transfusion. N Engl J Med 274:473–481, 1966.

INR, International normalized ratio.

From Shah VH, Kamath PS: Portal hypertension and gastrointestinal bleeding. *In* Feldman M, Friedman LS, Brandt LJ (eds): Gastrointestinal and Liver Disease Pathophysiology/Diagnosis/Management, 8th ed. Philadelphia, Saunders Elsevier, 2006, p 1918.

designed to predict mortality following portosystemic shunt operations, divides cirrhotic patients into three classes of severity on the basis of five easily assessed parameters. Several studies found a strong correlation between the Child-Turcotte-Pugh class and operative mortality in patients undergoing non-portosystemic shunt operations. In patients with cirrhosis who have undergone surgical procedures, the Child-Turcotte-Pugh class has been shown to predict perioperative mortality, with respective perioperative mortality rates of approximately 10%, 30%, 80% in patients with class A, B, and C cirrhosis. In addition to predicting perioperative mortality, the Child-Turcotte-Pugh class correlates with the frequency of postoperative complications, which include liver failure with worsening encephalopathy, bleeding, infection and sepsis, renal failure, hypoxia, and intractable ascites; in many cases, multiple complications develop. Ascites is also associated with an increased risk of abdominal wall herniation and wound dehiscence.

In patients with cirrhosis who undergo surgical procedures, other variables shown to predict complications are liver disease other than primary biliary cirrhosis, elevated serum creatinine level, chronic obstructive pulmonary disease, preoperative infection, preoperative upper gastrointestinal bleeding, high American Society of Anesthesiologists (ASA) class, intraoperative hypotension, and complicated operations [❽ *Ziser and Plevak, 1999*].

Although there are no prospective studies showing improved surgical outcome after preoperative interventions to improve hepatic function, a widely accepted guideline is that elective surgical procedures are well tolerated in patients with Child-Turcotte-Pugh class A cirrhosis, permissible with preoperative preparation in patients with Child-Turcotte-Pugh class B cirrhosis (except those undergoing extensive hepatic resection or cardiac surgery), and contraindicated in patients with Child-Turcotte-Pugh class C cirrhosis. However, even in patients with Child-Turcotte-Pugh class A cirrhosis, the risk of perioperative morbidity is increased when they have associated portal hypertension, as assessed by measurement of the hepatic venous pressure gradient. Preliminary observations suggest that postoperative morbidity may be reduced by preoperative placement of a transjugular intrahepatic portosystemic shunt (TIPS), but a TIPS can result in other complications, such as encephalopathy, and is not a routine preoperative measure. Surgery in patients with Child-Turcotte-Pugh class B or C cirrhosis is a major endeavor that requires careful consideration and preparation. Because the prognosis is thought to relate to the Child-Turcotte-Pugh class at the time of operation, meticulous preoperative preparation of the patient may reduce surgical risk.

In addition to correlating with the Child-Turcotte-Pugh classification, the risk of surgery is substantially greater for emergency procedures than for elective surgery, and for abdominal surgery (particularly biliary tract procedures), cardiac surgery, and hepatic resection than for other types of surgery (Table 10-5) (see later). Some studies have not confirmed the predictive value of the Child-Turcotte-Pugh classification, in part because few Child-Turcotte-Pugh class C patients were included, nor has any study validated the predictive value of the Child-Turcotte-Pugh class prospectively. Common causes of death following abdominal surgical procedures in patients with cirrhosis include hemorrhage, sepsis, and hepatorenal syndrome.

Respiratory compromise in patients with liver disease may result from hepatopulmonary syndrome, restrictive lung disease (caused by ascites or pleural effusions), pulmonary hypertension (which can be associated with cirrhosis), or immune-mediated lung disease (which can be associated with autoimmune liver diseases). The hepatopulmonary syndrome often manifests with orthodeoxia (a decline in oxygen saturation with standing). Severe hypoxemia (partial pressure of oxygen <60 mm Hg) associated with liver disease generally is considered a relative contraindication to surgery (except for

TABLE 10-5	Risk Factors for Surgery in Patients with Chronic Liver Disease
Type of Surgery	Emergency surgery
	Abdominal surgery (especially cholecystectomy, gastric resection, or colectomy)
	Cardiac surgery
	Hepatic resection
Patient Characteristics	Child-Turcotte-Pugh class (see Table 10-4)
	Ascites
	Encephalopathy
	Infection
	Malnutrition
	Anemia
	Elevated serum bilirubin level
	Hypoalbuminemia
	Portal hypertension
	Prolonged prothrombin time (>2.5 seconds) that does not correct with vitamin K
	Abnormal quantitative liver function tests (e.g., galactose elimination capacity)
	Hypoxemia
	Higher model for end-stage liver disease (MELD) score

liver transplantation, which may correct hepatopulmonary syndrome or restrictive lung disease from ascites). In a multivariate analysis, a diagnosis of chronic obstructive lung disease and surgical procedures of the respiratory tract were identified as risk factors for mortality in patients with cirrhosis who underwent operation. Administration of a higher than usual concentration of oxygen during anesthesia is recommended in all patients with cirrhosis.

A growing body of data has shown that the MELD score, based on the serum bilirubin level, serum creatinine level, and international normalized ratio (INR), is as accurate as the Child-Turcotte-Pugh class in predicting surgical mortality in patients with cirrhosis [❶ Teh et al, 2007] There is a linear increase in the postoperative 90-day mortality for each additional MELD point. The MELD score allows finer callibration of surgical risk than the Child-Turcotte-Pugh classification.

OPERATIVE RISK ASSOCIATED WITH SPECIFIC TYPES OF LIVER DISEASE

Chronic Hepatitis B

An estimated 400 million people worldwide and 1.25 million people in the United States are chronically infected with hepatitis B virus (HBV). Inactive carriers of HBV, who have normal serum aminotransferase levels and no hepatic inflammation, are not at increased risk for postoperative complications, but patients with chronic hepatitis B, with or without cirrhosis, may be at increased risk of operative morbidity, depending on the severity of hepatic inflammation and degree of hepatic dysfunction, as discussed previously.

There is a risk that exposure to blood, saliva, semen, or vaginal secretions of HBsAg-positive patients, especially those who are also hepatitis B e antigen (HBeAg) positive or have high serum HBV DNA levels, will infect medical and surgical personnel. This risk may be minimized by strict adherence to proper operating room protocol, use of disposable equipment, and appropriate decontamination and sterilization procedures. Moreover, all medical workers should receive a full course of recombinant hepatitis B vaccine (10 or 20 μg intramuscularly, depending on the specific preparation, at 0, 1, and 6 months). Because the vaccine failure rate is 5% to 10%, seroconversion should be confirmed by testing for the presence of antibody to HBsAg (anti-HBs) in serum 1 month after the third vaccine injection. For the rare unvaccinated medical worker who sustains an accidental needlestick exposure to HBV, the risk of infection ranges from 6% to 30%, depending on the infectivity of the source. For these exposed persons, hepatitis B immune globulin (0.06 mL/kg, or 5 mL, intramuscularly) should be administered immediately, and the vaccine series should be initiated. In previously vaccinated persons who sustain an accidental needlestick exposure to HBV, anti-HBs titers should be measured in serum, and, if the titer is less than 10 mIU/mL, a booster dose of the vaccine should be given. Although levels of anti-HBs following HBV vaccination decline over time and may fall to less than the seroprotective threshold, reexposure to HBV usually leads to an anamnestic response, or, in rare instances, subclinical infection. As a result, routine booster immunization of previously vaccinated persons who initially seroconverted to anti-HBs has not been recommended, except in immunocompromised persons.

Hepatitis C

One hundred seventy million people are infected with HCV worldwide, and in the United States 1.8% of the population is infected. Acute HCV infection is often asymptomatic, and serum aminotransferase elevations may be mild (100 to 300 U/L). Following acute HCV infection, up to 85% of patients progress to chronic infection. Patients with chronic HCV infection typically have elevated aminotransferase levels ranging from 1.3 to 3 times the upper limit of normal, although the serum aminotransferase levels may be within normal limits. The 15% of patients with acute HCV infection who clear the virus spontaneously and those with chronic HCV infection who achieve a sustained virologic response following treatment with PEG-interferon and ribavirin continue to have detectable antibody to HCV (anti-HCV) for life. Approximately 20% of patients with chronic hepatitis C progress to cirrhosis over 20 years; normal serum aminotransferase levels do not preclude the possibility of advanced fibrosis on a liver biopsy specimen. Of patients with cirrhosis caused by HCV, decompensated liver disease develops in 30% within 10 years. Host factors that favor progression to cirrhosis include male gender, alcohol use, age greater than 40 years at the time of acquisition of HCV infection, and human immunodeficiency virus (HIV) coinfection; other possible risk factors include increased hepatic iron concentrations and steatosis.

The impact of anti-HCV status on surgical outcome was studied retrospectively in U.S. veterans. Evidence suggests that anti-HCV positivity does not increase the risk of surgery [❿ *Cheung et al, 2003*]. Although mortality is likely unaffected, anti-HCV–positive patients may have higher peak serum aminotransferase levels postoperatively than do anti-HCV–negative patients [❿ *Murakami et al, 2004*].

A needlestick injury from an HCV-positive source can lead to HCV infection in a health care worker; the risk of transmission is approximately 4%. If symptomatic acute hepatitis C develops in the exposed worker, it usually occurs 4 to 12 weeks after exposure. Patients in whom jaundice develops are more likely to clear HCV spontaneously than are those who remain anicteric. Currently, the Centers for Disease Control and Prevention recommend serum alanine aminotransferase and anti-HCV testing at the time of and 4 to 6 months after the exposure. For earlier detection of HCV infection, testing with a sensitive assay for HCV RNA can be performed at 4 to 6 weeks after exposure. To date, a vaccine or alternative approach to postexposure prophylaxis of HCV infection has not been available outside clinical trials. Treatment with interferon-alfa for 4 weeks has been used after a needlestick injury, but the benefit of this approach is uncertain because the risk of HCV transmission by needlestick is low; studies of postexposure treatment of acute hepatitis C with PEG-interferon and ribavirin are ongoing.

Alcoholic Liver Disease

The spectrum of alcoholic liver disease includes fatty liver, acute alcoholic hepatitis, and cirrhosis. Even brief periods of heavy alcohol consumption may produce fatty liver, which usually is a mild, asymptomatic illness characterized by hepatomegaly and slight elevations of the serum aminotransferase, alkaline phosphatase, and γ-glutamyl transpeptidase levels. The diagnosis of fatty liver can be suspected on liver ultrasound study; however, ultrasonography is incapable of distinguishing fatty liver from alcoholic hepatitis reliably, and confirmation of the diagnosis of fatty liver requires liver biopsy. Alcohol-induced fatty liver without fibrosis usually resolves quickly with abstinence. Because liver function is preserved, elective surgical procedures are not contraindicated in patients with fatty liver; however, a period of abstinence from alcohol preoperatively is advisable for all patients with a histologic appearance of steatohepatitis or those who are suspected of recent excessive alcohol consumption. Alcoholic patients are at increased risk of perioperative alcohol withdrawal and hepatotoxicity with therapeutic doses of acetaminophen, even if they do not have liver disease. Surgery also should be postponed to allow correction of associated alcohol-induced nutritional deficiencies.

Alcoholic hepatitis is a serious necroinflammatory liver disease characterized histologically by hepatocyte swelling, infiltration of the liver with polymorphonuclear leukocytes, hepatocyte necrosis and, in many patients, Mallory's hyaline in hepatocytes. The broad range of clinical manifestations may include jaundice, fever, tender hepatomegaly, ascites, encephalopathy, gastrointestinal bleeding, and hepatorenal syndrome; the correlation between the clinical presentation and the histologic severity of inflammation and fibrosis is poor. Clinical and laboratory variables can be used to gauge prognosis in alcoholic hepatitis. A discriminant function (DF) can be calculated as follows:

$$4.6 \times (\text{prothrombin time} - \text{control prothrombin time}) + \text{serum bilirubin level}$$

A DF value greater than 32 is an indicator of severe disease, with a 30-day mortality rate of approximately 50%. The presence of hepatic encephalopathy is an additional important predictor of early death. **Glucocorticoid or pentoxifylline**

therapy for patients with a DF value greater than 32 decreases short-term mortality [⊘ *Ramond et al, 1992*].

Elective surgery in patients with alcoholic hepatitis is contraindicated. Patients with alcoholic hepatitis occasionally may be diagnosed incorrectly as having acute cholecystitis, a mistake that can have grave consequences if a laparotomy is performed. Mortality rates as high as 55% to 100% have been observed in patients with acute alcoholic hepatitis who have undergone open liver biopsy, portosystemic shunt surgery, or exploratory laparotomy. However, the studies that reported these results took place in the 1960s and 1970s, and advances in surgical technique and postoperative care since then may have improved the outcome in such patients. This possibility is illustrated by a report from 1984, in which operative liver biopsy findings were reviewed in 164 patients with alcoholic cirrhosis and bleeding varices who underwent emergency portacaval shunt surgery. Of these patients, 49 (30%) had histologic evidence of acute alcoholic hepatitis but had survival rates similar to those of the patients without alcoholic hepatitis.

Abstinence from alcohol, usually for 6 to 12 weeks, and clinical resolution of alcoholic hepatitis with return of the serum bilirubin level to normal are recommended before elective surgery is considered. However, severe alcoholic hepatitis may persist for many months, despite abstinence. We recommend that elective surgical procedures be delayed for at least 12 weeks before elective surgical procedures are performed. The severity of the underlying liver disease should be reassessed before a final recommendation for surgery is made.

Nonalcoholic Fatty Liver Disease

Patients with NAFLD but without significant hepatic fibrosis do not appear to have excessive mortality following elective surgical procedures. However, a trend toward increased mortality following hepatic resection has been observed in patients with moderate to severe steatosis (>30% of hepatocytes containing fat). Whether patients with steatohepatitis are at greater operative risk than those with simple steatosis is unknown.

NAFLD may be associated with a wide variety of conditions, most commonly diabetes, obesity, and hypertriglyceridemia (insulin resistance syndrome). NAFLD is relatively common in patients with morbid obesity who undergo gastric bypass surgery. **Unexpected cirrhosis presumably related to NAFLD may be discovered intraoperatively in up to 6% of patients who undergo a gastric bypass operation and is not thought to be a contraindication to the procedure** [❶ *Brolin et al, 1998*].

Wilson's Disease

Patients with Wilson's disease who have neuropsychiatric involvement may not be able to provide informed consent. Furthermore, surgical procedures can precipitate or aggravate neurologic symptoms. D-Penicillamine (a copper chelator commonly used for treatment) interferes with the cross-linking of collagen and may impair wound healing. As a result, the dose of D-penicillamine should be decreased preoperatively and during the first 1 to 2 postoperative weeks.

Hemochromatosis

Patients with hemochromatosis should be evaluated for complications, such as diabetes and cardiomyopathy, that could influence perioperative care. In the past, decreased survival following liver transplantation in patients with hemochromatosis as compared with other types of liver disease was attributed to underlying cardiomyopathy in many patients with hemochromatosis, but recent survival rates have improved because of better patient selection.

Autoimmune Hepatitis

Elective surgery is usually well tolerated in patients with autoimmune hepatitis in remission when liver disease is compensated. However, patients receiving long-term glucocorticoid therapy for autoimmune hepatitis should be given appropriate "stress" doses during the perioperative period (e.g., hydrocortisone sodium hemisuccinate, 100 mg intravenously every 8 hours beginning the night before the surgical procedure).

OPERATIVE RISK ASSOCIATED WITH SPECIFIC TYPES OF SURGERY

Biliary Tract Surgery and Obstructive Jaundice

Obstructive jaundice results from a stone, stricture, or tumor involving the extrahepatic bile ducts. Patients with cirrhosis are at increased risk of gallstone formation and associated complications as compared with noncirrhotic patients.

Operative Risk

Biliary tract surgery, including cholecystectomy, presents a particular problem in patients with cirrhosis, in part because of the increased vascularity of the gallbladder bed in patients with cirrhotic portal hypertension and the massive bleeding that may result from dissection of the gallbladder, even in the absence of overt coagulopathy. Coagulopathy and portal hypertension are relative contraindications to laparoscopic cholecystectomy. Evidence indicates that laparoscopic cholecystectomy can be performed safely in patients with Child-Turcotte-Pugh class A cirrhosis or a MELD score of 8 or less without portal hypertension. In contrast, open cholecystectomy in patients with cirrhosis carries a mortality rate of up to 25%. In an emergency, cholecystostomy, rather than cholecystectomy, is recommended in patients with poorly compensated cirrhosis and portal hypertension.

In patients with obstructive jaundice (generally without cirrhosis), perioperative mortality ranges from 8% to 28% and has not changed since the 1970s, although endoscopic has replaced surgical decompression as the preferred approach to urgent treatment. In this patient group, predictors of postoperative mortality include a hematocrit value less than 30%, an initial serum bilirubin level greater than 11 mg/dL (200 μmol/L), and a malignant cause of obstruction (Box 10-2). **When all three factors are present, the mortality rate approaches 60%; when no factors are present, the mortality rate is only 5%** [❸ *Dixon et al, 1983*]. Other predictors of poor surgical outcome include serum bilirubin level higher than 3 mg/dL (reflecting a malignant cause), elevated serum creatinine, hypoalbuminemia, and cholangitis.

Complications

Patients with obstructive jaundice are at increased risk of several perioperative complications, including infections (which result in part from bacterial colonization of the biliary tree, impaired Kupffer cell function, defective neutrophil function, and a high rate of endotoxemia), gastrointestinal bleeding caused by stress-related gastric mucosal disease, disseminated intravascular coagulation, delayed wound healing, wound dehiscence, incisional hernias, and renal failure. In addition, obstructive jaundice is thought to predispose to hypotension as a result of systemic vasodilation.

An increased frequency of postoperative renal failure has been recognized in patients with obstructive jaundice. The

Box 10-2	RISK FACTORS FOR OPERATIVE MORTALITY IN PATIENTS WITH OBSTRUCTIVE JAUNDICE

Hematocrit value <30%
Serum bilirubin level >11 mg/dL
Malignant cause of biliary obstruction
Azotemia
Hypoalbuminemia
Cholangitis

high frequency of renal failure may relate to increased absorption of endotoxin from the gut. In patients without liver or biliary disease, endotoxin absorption is limited by the detergent effect of bile salts on lipopolysaccharide (endotoxin); this protection is lost in patients with obstructive jaundice, in whom bile salt secretion is reduced. Renal vasoconstriction may be exaggerated in this setting by vasoactive mediators released as a result of renal oxidative stress induced by increased intravascular levels of bile salts.

Perioperative Volume Management

The risk of postoperative renal dysfunction appears to be reduced if intravascular volume and urine output are maintained during surgery. The use of preoperative blood transfusion should be considered in the patient with a hematocrit value lower than 30%. Close monitoring of intraoperative and postoperative fluid status is essential. If intravascular volume expansion is needed in patients with a low serum albumin level and a normal hematocrit value, 25% salt-poor albumin may be used. Aminoglycoside antibiotics and nonsteroidal anti-inflammatory drugs have a greatly increased potential for nephrotoxicity in jaundiced patients and should be avoided.

Prevention of Endotoxemia

Limited evidence suggests that the administration of bile salts or lactulose (30 mL orally every 6 hours for 3 days preoperatively) to patients with obstructive jaundice can prevent both endotoxemia and exaggerated renal vasoconstriction. Prophylactic administration of oral antibiotics also has been recommended in an effort to reduce the adverse effects of endotoxemia, although direct proof of the efficacy of this approach is lacking. Destruction of intestinal gram-negative organisms could actually prove detrimental, owing to systemic absorption of increased amounts of released endotoxin. Conversely, intravenous broad-spectrum antibiotics should be administered perioperatively to reduce the frequency of postoperative infections. Unfortunately, this approach does not affect mortality.

Biliary Decompression

No evidence indicates that preoperative transhepatic decompression of an obstructed biliary tree leads to a decrease in perioperative morbidity or mortality. Therefore, routine preoperative transhepatic decompression of an obstructed biliary system is not recommended. Endoscopic biliary drainage has the advantage of restoring enterohepatic circulation of bile acids while avoiding the complications of percutaneous puncture. Patients with cholangitis and choledocholithiasis who receive broad-spectrum intravenous antibiotics and undergo endoscopic drainage have lower mortality and morbidity rates than do patients who undergo immediate surgical decompression. However, for patients with a malignant cause of biliary obstruction, preoperative endoscopic drainage (e.g., external biliary drainage) has not been shown to improve subsequent surgical mortality.

Although endoscopic sphincterotomy is associated with an increased rate of complications in patients with cirrhosis, morbidity and mortality rates for this procedure are low even in patients with Child-Turcotte-Pugh class C cirrhosis when biliary decompression can be achieved. The main complication of endoscopic sphincterotomy in patients with Child-Turcotte-Pugh class C cirrhosis is bleeding. Endoscopic papillary balloon dilation is associated with a lower risk of bleeding than standard sphincterotomy and is preferred in patients with cirrhosis and coagulopathy; however, balloon dilation has been associated with a higher risk of pancreatitis in some studies.

Alternatives to Surgery

For patients who are poor surgical candidates or who have a limited life expectancy because of malignant disease, endoscopic biliary decompression and endoprosthesis (stent) insertion may be an excellent, albeit palliative, alternative to surgery. Percutaneous biliary decompression appears to be associated with higher rates of procedural morbidity and mortality than endoscopic decompression but may be required for proximal bile duct lesions or when an endoscopic approach is unsuccessful. A combined percutaneous-endoscopic approach to biliary stent placement may be effective if endoscopic stenting is unsuccessful.

Choledocholithiasis can be treated successfully by retrograde extraction after endoscopic sphincterotomy in up to 90% of cases. Of the remaining cases, approximately 80% can be managed successfully with endoscopic mechanical, laser, or electrohydraulic lithotripsy. Endoscopic stents also may be used as palliative treatment for large bile duct calculi that cannot be removed by nonoperative methods. In patients with an intact gallbladder, the risk of acute cholecystitis after endoscopic sphincterotomy for choledocholithiasis is only approximately 10% in the subsequent 5 years.

Patients with cholangitis caused by choledocholithiasis frequently improve with parenteral antibiotics, thereby allowing time to prepare for definitive therapy of the bile duct stones. Persons with severe cholangitis and those who do not respond promptly to intravenous antibiotics should undergo urgent endoscopic decompression. Endoscopic biliary decompression is highly effective therapy and is associated with significantly less morbidity and mortality than open surgical approaches. Ciprofloxacin is the drug of choice for severe cholangitis, based on its superior ability to penetrate an obstructed biliary system and its broad spectrum of activity against common biliary pathogens. In some patients, ampicillin, metronidazole, or both drugs should be added.

Cardiac Surgery

In patients with cirrhosis, the mortality associated with cardiac surgery is greater than with most other surgical procedures. **A Child-Turcotte-Pugh score of 7 or less or a MELD score of 8 or less suggests that cardiopulmonary** bypass can be accomplished safely in cirrhotic patients [❽ *Suman et al, 2004*].

Risk factors for hepatic decompensation following cardiac surgery include the total time of cardiopulmonary bypass, use of nonpulsatile as opposed to pulsatile cardiopulmonary bypass, and need for perioperative pressor support. Cardiopulmonary bypass can exacerbate underlying coagulopathy by inducing platelet dysfunction, fibrinolysis, and hypocalcemia.

In general, the least invasive options, such as angioplasty or minimally invasive revascularization techniques, should be considered in patients with advanced cirrhosis who require invasive intervention for cardiac disease.

Hepatic Resection

Hepatocellular carcinoma (HCC) is a well-established complication of liver disease. Chronic hepatitis B is thought to lead to HCC as a result of chronic necroinflammatory activity in the liver as well as integration of HBV DNA into the host genome. In endemic areas where HBV infection is acquired at or near birth, the 5-year cumulative frequency of HCC in cirrhotic patients is as high as 15%. Chronic hepatitis C can lead to HCC primarily by causing cirrhosis. After cirrhosis occurs, the risk of HCC is 1.4% to 6.9% per year. Like hepatitis C, most other forms of liver disease put patients at increased risk of HCC only after cirrhosis has occurred. Of all causes of liver disease, patients with hemochromatosis and cirrhosis have the highest risk of HCC. Screening for HCC with ultrasound and with serum α-fetoprotein testing every 6 months is recommended for all patients with cirrhosis and for noncirrhotic patients with chronic (replicative) hepatitis B as well as inactive HBV carriers who are more than 40 years old.

Patients with cirrhosis who undergo hepatic resection for HCC or other liver tumors are at increased risk of hepatic decompensation as compared with cirrhotic patients who undergo other types of surgical procedures. In addition to having severe underlying liver disease, these patients lose a substantial portion of functional hepatocellular mass as a result of hepatic resection at a time when their hepatic reserve is already compromised. In the past, cirrhosis was considered to be a contraindication to resection of hepatic tumors because mortality rates exceeded 50%. More recently, the perioperative mortality rate for hepatic resection has decreased to 0% to 8.7%. The improvement in outcomes has been attributed to better patient selection (including earlier detection of tumors), meticulous preoperative preparation, intensive intraoperative and postoperative monitoring, and improved surgical techniques. Despite better outcomes, 5-year recurrence rates are as high as 100%, and 5-year survival rates are no higher than 50%. The Child-Turcotte-Pugh classification is still the most widely used measure of operability, but studies have failed to confirm its value in predicting morbidity and mortality, in part because of selection bias and the small number of patients with Child-Turcotte-Pugh class B and C cirrhosis studied.

Although patients with Child-Turcotte-Pugh class A cirrhosis generally tolerate hepatic resection well, risk factors for postoperative morbidity include portal hypertension, thoracotomy, pulmonary disease, diabetes mellitus, malignancy, longer surgical time, the presence of active hepatitis, male sex, larger tumor size, and complex intrahepatic inflammatory disease. Increasingly, liver transplantation has been preferred over resection in patients with Child-Turcotte-Pugh class A cirrhosis and HCC, either one small (<5 cm) or up to 3 smaller (<3 cm each) tumors. However, the shortage of donor livers often precludes timely liver transplantation in these patients. Nonsurgical options for treating HCC include radiofrequency ablation, microwave ablation, ethanol injection, and chemoembolization. Radiofrequency ablation is utilized for tumors smaller than 5 cm in patients who are awaiting liver transplantation or who are not surgical candidates. To date, not enough evidence is available to recommend this technique for tumors larger than 5 cm in diameter, and a tumor adjacent to a blood vessel is not amenable to radiofrequency ablation. Chemoembolization is reserved for large HCCs that are not amenable to any other modality of therapy.

Other Types of Surgery

Repair of umbilical and groin hernias in patients with cirrhosis and ascites often can be accomplished at relatively low risk. Preoperative control of ascites is recommended. Although undertaken infrequently, peptic ulcer surgery is associated with increased postoperative complication and mortality rates in patients with cirrhosis, as compared with surgical treatment in noncirrhotic patients, and should be limited to the treatment of uncontrollable bleeding and perforation. Table 10-6 lists representative mortality and, when available, morbidity rates for various operations in patients with cirrhosis.

SPECIAL CONSIDERATIONS IN PERIOPERATIVE CARE

Coagulopathy

Pathophysiology

The liver synthesizes most of the factors (all except factor VIII) and inhibitors of the coagulation and fibrinolytic systems. In patients with liver disease, impaired hemostasis may result from a reduction in the levels of vitamin K–dependent clotting factors, caused by malnutrition and decreased hepatic protein synthesis, and an increase in plasma proteolytic activity, possibly caused by decreased hepatic clearance of proteases. Increased fibrinolytic activity and laboratory features of mild disseminated intravascular coagulation are common. The resulting pattern of hemostatic abnormalities consists of prolonged prothrombin time, low plasma fibrinogen level, normal or increased partial thromboplastin time, and prolonged thrombin time.

TABLE 10-6	Mortality Rates Associated with Surgery in Patients with Cirrhosis		
Type of Surgery	Number of Patients	Mortality (%)	Morbidity (%)
Laparotomy for trauma	17	44%	71%
Esophagectomy	18	16.7%	83.3%
Appendectomy	69	9%	NA
Transurethral resection of the prostate	30	6.7%	NA
Treatment of hepatic hydrothorax with talc	18	27.8%	57.1%
Surgery on the small intestine	14	57%	NA
Surgery on the stomach	82	51%	NA
Colorectal cancer surgery	72	13%	NA
Total knee arthroplasty	51	0%	39%

NA, not available. Data from Wahlstrom K, Ney AL, Jacobson S, et al: Trauma in cirrhotics: Survival and hospital sequelae in patients requiring abdominal exploration. Am Surg 66:1071-1076, 2000; Tachibana M, Kotoh T, Kinugasa S, et al: Esophageal cancer with cirrhosis of the liver: Results of esophagectomy in 18 consecutive patients. Ann Surg Oncol 7:758-763, 2000; Poulsen TL, Thulstrup AM, Sorensen HT, et al: Appendectomy and perioperative mortality in patients with liver cirrhosis. Br J Surg 87:1664-1665, 2000; Nielsen SS, Thulstrup AM, Lund L, et al: Postoperative mortality in patients with liver cirrhosis undergoing transurethral resection of the prostate: A Danish nationwide cohort study. BJU Int 87: 183-186, 2001; Milanez de Campos JR, Filho LO, de Campos Werebe E, et al: Thoracoscopy and talc poudrage in the management of hepatic hydrothorax. Chest 118:13-17, 2000; Wong R, Rappaport W, Witte C, et al: Risk of nonshunt abdominal operation in the patient with cirrhosis. J Am Coll Surg 179:412–416, 1994; Lehnert T, Herfarth C: Peptic ulcer surgery in patients with liver cirrhosis. Ann Surg 217:338–346, 1993; Gervaz P, Pak-art R, Nivatvongs S, et al: Colorectal adenocarcinoma in cirrhotic patients. J Am Coll Surg 196:874-879, 2003; and Shih LY, Cheng CY, Chang CH, et al: Total knee arthroplasty in patients with liver cirrhosis. J Bone Joint Surg Am 86:335-341, 2004.

Thrombocytopenia is common as a result of hypersplenism, folate deficiency, or alcohol-induced suppression of the bone marrow. Platelet function may also be abnormal.

Preoperative Preparation

The hemostatic stress of surgery requires that the patient undergo careful preoperative preparation as well as intraoperative monitoring of hemostatic parameters. Vitamin K, 10 mg given intramuscularly, usually corrects hypoprothrombinemia related to malnutrition or intestinal bile salt deficiency as a result of obstructive jaundice but not hypoprothrombinemia related to hepatocellular disease. Although an injection of vitamin K on 3 consecutive days is often recommended, one dose may be sufficient, and the effect is often evident within 6 to 12 hours.

When vitamin K repletion does not correct the coagulopathy, considerable hepatocellular dysfunction exists. In such patients, fresh frozen plasma (typically 6 to 8 U for severe coagulopathy) is the cornerstone of therapy. Correction of the prothrombin time to within 3 seconds of the normal control value is recommended. Unfortunately, the large quantities of fresh frozen plasma required to shorten a prolonged prothrombin time and the transient nature of the response limit the effectiveness of this therapy. A prolonged bleeding time also can be treated with diamino-8-D-arginine vasopressin (DDAVP). DDAVP shortens the bleeding time in patients with cirrhosis by releasing endogenous stores of von Willebrand multimers. Because cryoprecipitate contains large quantities of these multimers and is also rich in fibrinogen, intravenous infusion of 10 U of cryoprecipitate should be considered when hemorrhage cannot be controlled by other means. Recombinant activated factor VIIa is another option. Preoperative platelet transfusions are indicated when the platelet count is less than 100,000/mm^3; 8 to 10 U are given initially and are repeated postoperatively until the patient is hemodynamically stable. Hyperfibrinolysis may develop intraoperatively, especially during liver transplantation, or spontaneously in patients with advanced cirrhosis. Antifibrinolytic agents (ε-aminocaproic acid or aprotinin) are effective in decreasing transfusion requirements during liver transplantation, but their role in other surgical procedures remains unclear. The potential for thrombotic complications with these drugs is a concern.

Ascites

Pathophysiology

Preoperative assessment of fluid status and serum electrolyte levels is essential in the cirrhotic patient. Ascites in a patient with cirrhosis results from several factors: portal hypertension, decreased plasma colloid oncotic pressure owing to impaired hepatic synthesis of albumin and other serum proteins, leakage of protein-rich hepatic lymph caused by blockage of hepatic sinusoids and lymphatics, and hyperaldosteronism in part resulting from impaired hepatic metabolism of aldosterone. In addition, peripheral vasodilation, mediated by nitric oxide, leads to stimulation of the renin-angiotensin system with resultant renal vasoconstriction and avid sodium retention. Associated electrolyte abnormalities include hyponatremia, as a result of impaired free water clearance, and hypokalemic alkalosis, as a result of diuretic therapy and increased urinary or gastrointestinal losses of potassium.

Paracentesis

Preoperative evaluation in a patient with new or worsening ascites should include diagnostic paracentesis to exclude infection or malignancy and to differentiate spontaneous from secondary bacterial peritonitis (Table 10-7). **Routine admission paracentesis should be strongly considered for all patients with cirrhotic ascites because up to 20% of these patients are found to have spontaneous bacterial peritonitis** [◉ *Gines et al, 2004*]. The classic symptoms and signs of spontaneous bacterial peritonitis are abdominal pain,

TABLE 10-7	Laboratory Findings in Spontaneous and Secondary Bacterial Peritonitis	
Peritoneal Fluid	**Spontaneous**	**Secondary**
PMN count	>250 cells/mm^3	>250 cells/mm^3
PMNs >48 hr after procedure	Decrease	May increase
Lactate dehydrogenase	Normal	> Upper limit of normal of serum
Glucose	Equal to serum glucose	<50 mg/dL
Total protein	Often <1 g/dL	>1 g/dL
Gram stain (% positive)	Usually negative	Positive in 40%
Culture	Monomicrobial aerobes	Often polymicrobial aerobes, anaerobes, fungi

PMN, polymorphonuclear neutrophil. Data from Akriviadis EA, Runyon BA: Utility of an algorithm in differentiating spontaneous from secondary bacterial peritonitis. Gastroenterology 98:127–133, 1990.

fever, and increasing ascites, but up to 20% of patients with spontaneous bacterial peritonitis will have none of these findings. More subtle clues to the presence of ascitic fluid infection are worsening encephalopathy, renal function, or jaundice. Secondary bacterial peritonitis, typically resulting from gut perforation, in a patient with preexisting ascites can be present in the absence of physical findings characteristic of a surgical abdomen.

Because cultures of the ascites may be negative in a patient with spontaneous bacterial peritonitis, the diagnosis is based on an ascitic fluid neutrophil count greater than 250 cells/mm^3. When this criterion is met, empiric treatment with a third-generation cephalosporin provides effective coverage for nearly all the usual pathogens. Spontaneous bacterial peritonitis typically responds promptly to antibiotics, whereas secondary peritonitis requires definitive surgical therapy or abscess drainage.

Control of Ascites

To reduce the risk of postoperative wound dehiscence or abdominal wall herniation, it is advisable to control ascites medically before performing abdominal surgical procedures;

if necessary, the ascites can be drained at the time of laparoscopy or laparotomy. In patients with associated peripheral edema, rapid diuresis with higher doses of diuretics may be well tolerated, but in patients without peripheral edema, more gradual diuresis needs to be employed preoperatively to avoid precipitating renal insufficiency or encephalopathy. In patients with tense ascites, large-volume paracentesis of 5 L or more is generally well tolerated, irrespective of the presence of peripheral edema. Compared with diuretic therapy, large-volume paracentesis is faster and more effective. It also is associated with fewer renal and electrolyte abnormalities and less encephalopathy than is seen with diuretic therapy. Renal impairment following paracentesis may be prevented by the administration of intravenous 25% salt-poor albumin (10 g/L of fluid removed).

Medical therapy of ascites includes salt restriction to 2000 mg/day, spironolactone (beginning with 100 mg/day), and a loop diuretic such as furosemide (beginning with 40 mg/day). Combination therapy with furosemide and spironolactone may accelerate the onset of diuresis and reduces the frequency of hyperkalemia or hypokalemia. Fluid restriction is difficult to enforce and is generally unnecessary except when hyponatremia becomes severe (serum sodium <125 mEq/L). Chronic hyponatremia is generally well tolerated in cirrhotic patients and is not associated with seizures, except during alcohol withdrawal or when the decline in serum sodium is rapid. Ascites that is refractory to standard medical therapy often responds to placement of a TIPS.

Fluid and Electrolyte Replacement

If preoperative volume replacement is necessary, excessive salt administration should be avoided, and 25% salt-poor albumin, glucose solutions, and fresh frozen plasma should be used instead. Deficits in potassium and (especially in the alcoholic patient) phosphate and magnesium should be corrected. Careful monitoring of the patient's weight, intake and output, and urinary sodium concentration is essential, and, in some cases, the central venous pressure should be monitored.

Renal Dysfunction

Renal function should be monitored closely in surgical patients with cirrhosis and ascites. Serum creatinine, blood urea nitrogen, and creatinine clearance determinations may markedly overestimate the actual glomerular filtration rate in patients with cirrhosis because of muscle wasting and decreased urea synthesis. Furthermore, lean muscle mass may be difficult to estimate, particularly in edematous patients, thereby making calculation of drug doses challenging.

Pathophysiology

Patients with advanced liver disease have increased levels of endogenous vasodilators (e.g., nitric oxide and prostacyclin), which lead to peripheral vasodilation and a chronic hyperdynamic circulation. Among the clinical consequences of the hyperdynamic circulation is activation of the sympathetic nervous system and renin-angiotensin-aldosterone axis. During the compensated stage of cirrhosis, elevated levels of renal vasodilatory prostaglandins compensate for the vasoconstrictive influence of angiotensin. Inhibition of renal prostaglandin synthesis by nonsteroidal anti-inflammatory drugs is associated with decreased urinary sodium excretion and nephrotoxicity in some cirrhotic patients; therefore, these drugs should be avoided. Low urinary sodium excretion is the best predictor of susceptibility to the deleterious effects of nonsteroidal anti-inflammatory drugs.

Loss of vasodilatory compensation and a decrease in renal cortical blood flow are distinctive features of the *hepatorenal syndrome,* a frequent terminal event in patients with decompensated cirrhosis. This syndrome is characterized by oliguria, a very low rate of sodium excretion, hyponatremia, a progressive rise in the plasma creatinine concentration, and hypotension (unresponsive to volume expansion). The onset of renal failure is typically insidious but can be precipitated by an acute insult such as gastrointestinal bleeding or infection (e.g., spontaneous bacterial peritonitis).

It is important to distinguish the hepatorenal syndrome from other causes of renal failure (e.g., acute tubular necrosis and prerenal azotemia) because the treatment varies with the cause. Therapy of the hepatorenal syndrome can be attempted with the oral α-agonist midodrine (titrated to increase mean arterial blood pressure by 15 mm Hg), subcutaneous octreotide (100 μg three times daily), and intravenous 25% salt-poor albumin (50 to 100 g/day). Intravenous norepinephrine (titrated to increase mean arterial blood pressure by 10 mm Hg) in combination with intravenous albumin also has been used with success. In patients who fail to respond to medical treatment, a TIPS can be attempted as therapy for the hepatorenal syndrome. For many patients, the hepatorenal syndrome is a terminal event, and surgical procedures other than liver transplantation are unlikely to be performed in this setting.

Perioperative Management

Any potentially nephrotoxic drugs should be avoided in cirrhotic patients whenever possible. The use of aminoglycoside antibiotics in patients with liver disease is associated with an increased risk of nephrotoxicity; these drugs should be avoided in the perioperative period, when numerous other risk factors for renal dysfunction occur. The availability of newer antibiotics, including imipenem and aztreonam (1 to 2 g intravenously every 6 to 8 hours), provides effective non-nephrotoxic alternatives to aminoglycosides for the treatment of gram-negative infection. Third-generation cephalosporins are considered the drugs of choice for treating spontaneous bacterial peritonitis. Moxalactam should be avoided because of its association with serious bleeding disorders. As noted earlier, nonsteroidal anti-inflammatory drugs should be avoided.

Encephalopathy

Pathophysiology

Hepatic encephalopathy is a state of disordered central nervous system function characterized by disturbances in consciousness, behavior, and personality. The pathogenesis involves the shunting of portal venous blood into the systemic circulation, usually in the setting of hepatocellular dysfunction, and the entry into the central nervous system of potentially noxious agents, most notably ammonia, that escape normal hepatic detoxification.

Diagnosis

The diagnosis of hepatic encephalopathy may be obvious in the patient with confusion or stupor, hyperreflexia, asterixis, and an elevated serum arterial or venous ammonia level, but early or mild encephalopathy may escape detection unless a careful history (e.g., subtle personality changes, agitation, and "day-night reversal") or even psychometric testing and an electroencephalogram are obtained.

Treatment

The importance of recognizing the presence of hepatic encephalopathy preoperatively is that many factors known to precipitate or exacerbate encephalopathy are likely to occur with increased frequency in the perioperative period (Box 10-3). The treatment of encephalopathy preoperatively and the avoidance of precipitating factors intraoperatively and postoperatively should decrease the risk of worsening postoperative encephalopathy. Unless clinically overt encephalopathy can be controlled, all but emergency surgical procedures should be deferred. Treatment includes the following: removal of precipitating factors; mild restriction of protein to 60 to 80 g/day; and use of the oral, unabsorbable disaccharide lactulose (15 to 60 mL orally two to four times

---

Box 10-3	FACTORS THAT MAY PRECIPITATE HEPATIC ENCEPHALOPATHY

Gastrointestinal bleeding
High protein intake
Constipation
Azotemia
Hypokalemic alkalosis
Infection (especially spontaneous bacterial peritonitis)
Hypoxia
Central nervous system depressant drugs (e.g., narcotics and benzodiazepines)
Portosystemic shunt (TIPS or surgical shunt)
Progressive hepatocellular dysfunction

TIPS, transjugular intrahepatic portosystemic shunt.

---

a day, titrated to two to three soft stools daily) or, in some cases, oral neomycin (1 g orally twice a day) or rifaximin (200-400 mg orally three times daily). For patients unable to take medications by mouth, lactulose may be given by enema (300 mL lactulose with 700 mL tap water two to three times a day). Prophylactic treatment to prevent postoperative encephalopathy in non-encephalopathic patients with cirrhosis has been suggested but has not been evaluated prospectively. Bowel cleansing is performed routinely before abdominal operations and may help to prevent encephalopathy.

Gastroesophageal Varices

It is unknown whether surgery is a risk factor for variceal bleeding. For the patient with known moderately large or large varices, primary prophylaxis with either a nonselective oral β-adrenergic antagonist (e.g., propranolol, nadolol) or endoscopic band ligation should be instituted. In patients with grade 4 (largest) varices, primary prophylaxis with band ligation may be superior to β-blockade; however, for grade 3 varices and lower, the two approaches appear to be equivalent. Either method of primary prophylaxis reduces the risk of initial variceal hemorrhage and the mortality rate associated with variceal bleeding significantly. β-Blockade virtually eliminates the risk of variceal bleeding when the hepatic venous pressure gradient is reduced to less than 12 mm Hg. Because measurement of the hepatic venous pressure gradient is an invasive test, a decrease in heart rate is used as a surrogate marker of β-blockade. The dose of the β-blocker is titrated to reduce the resting pulse by 25% or to 55 beats/minute.

Any patient with actively bleeding varices must be treated and stabilized before an elective surgical procedure for an unrelated condition can be performed. Following such a bleeding episode, definitive treatment to reduce the risk of recurrent hemorrhage must be instituted. Effective therapies include variceal eradication by band ligation (usually in combination with a nonselective β-blocker), placement of a TIPS, or portosystemic shunt surgery.

Nutrition

Many patients with chronic liver disease experience severe protein-energy malnutrition, which may contribute to the development of complications and may adversely affect survival. In malnourished patients unable to tolerate enteral feeding, a period of preoperative parenteral nutrition may be beneficial. Parenteral nutrition is not without potentially serious hazards, such as those related to the central venous catheter itself (i.e., pneumothorax and catheter-related sepsis).

Enteral nutritional supplementation appears to improve immunocompetence and short-term prognosis in patients with cirrhosis. Limited evidence shows that perioperative nutritional support may reduce short-term operative mortality and morbidity, but the effect of this support on long-term survival is uncertain. Although oral supplementation is preferred, placement of a small-bore feeding tube may be necessary in patients with anorexia. Percutaneous endoscopic gastrostomy is contraindicated in patients with ascites and should usually be avoided in patients with any signs of portal hypertension because of the possibility of lacerating an abdominal wall varix.

The recommended nutritional supplement should provide total calories equal to 1.2 times the estimated resting energy expenditure and 1 g/kg/day of protein. Approximately 30% to 35% of total energy should be given as fat and the remainder as carbohydrate (usually 50% to 55%). In addition to vitamin K, supplementation of other fat-soluble vitamins (A, D, and E) may be necessary.

POSTOPERATIVE MONITORING

In the postoperative period, patients with liver disease need to be observed closely for signs of hepatic decompensation, including encephalopathy, coagulopathy, ascites, and worsening jaundice. The prothrombin time and serum bilirubin level are probably the best measures of hepatic function to follow. However, an elevated serum bilirubin without worsening coagulopathy can be expected in the immediate postoperative period, especially after complicated surgical procedures, multiple blood transfusions, bleeding, hemodynamic instability, or infection. Renal function must be monitored as well because of the risk of hepatorenal syndrome.

Hypoglycemia may occur in patients with end-stage cirrhosis or fulminant hepatic failure as a result of depleted hepatic glycogen stores. Serum glucose levels should be monitored closely when postoperative liver failure is suspected.

Selected Readings

Aranha GV, Sontag SI, Greenlee HB: Cholecystectomy in cirrhotic patients: A formidable operation. Am J Surg 143:55-60, 1982.

Bizouarn P, Ausseur A, Desseigne P, et al: Early and late outcome after elective cardiac surgery in patients with cirrhosis. Ann Thorac Surg 67: 1334-1338, 1999.

Brolin RE, Bradley LJ, Taliwal RV: Unsuspected cirrhosis discovered during elective obesity operations. Arch Surg 133:84-88, 1998. **B**

Capussotti L, Polastri R: Operative risks of major hepatic resections. Hepatogastroenterology 45:184-190, 1998.

Cheung RC, Hsieh F, Wang Y, et al: The impact of hepatitis C status on postoperative outcome. Anesth Analg 97:550-554, 2003. **B**

Dixon JM, Armstrong CP, Duffy SW, et al: Factors affecting morbidity and mortality after surgery for obstructive jaundice: A review of 373 patients. Gut 24:845-852, 1983. **B**

Friedman LS: The risk of surgery in patients with liver disease. Hepatology 29:1617-1623, 1999. **C**

Garrison RN, Cryer HM, Howard DA, et al: Clarification of risk factors for abdominal operations in patients with hepatic cirrhosis. Ann Surg 199:648-655, 1984.

Gholson CF, Provenza JM, Bacon BR: Hepatologic considerations in patients with parenchymal liver disease undergoing surgery. Am J Gastroenterol 85:487-496, 1990. **C**

Gines P, Cardenas A, Arroyo V, et al: Management of cirrhosis and ascites. N Engl J Med 350:1646-1654, 2004. **C**

Keegan MT, Plevak DJ: Preoperative assessment of the patient with liver disease. Am J Gastroenterol 100:2116-2127, 2005. **C**

Levitsky J, Mailliard ME: Diagnosis and therapy of alcoholic liver disease. Semin Liver Dis 24:233-247, 2004.

MacIntosh EL, Minuk GY: Hepatic resection in patients with cirrhosis and hepatocellular carcinoma. Surg Gynecol Obstet 174:245-254, 1992.

Malinchoc M, Kamath PS, Gordon FD, et al: A model to predict poor survival in patients undergoing transjugular intrahepatic portosystemic shunts. Hepatology 31:864-871, 2000. **B**

Mansour A, Watson W, Shayani V, et al: Abdominal operations in patients with cirrhosis: Still a major surgical challenge. Surgery 122:730-735, 1997.

Murakami S, Okubo K, Tsuji Y, et al: Changes in liver enzymes after surgery in anti-hepatitis C virus–positive patients. World J Surg 28:671-674, 2004. **B**

Nompleggi DJ, Bonkovsky HL: Nutritional supplementation in chronic liver disease: An analytical review. Hepatology 19:518-533, 1994.

Northrup PG, Wanamaker RC, Lee VD, et al: Model for End-Stage Liver Disease (MELD) predicts nontransplant surgical mortality in patients with cirrhosis. Ann Surg 242:244-251, 2005.

Ochs A, Rössle M, Haag K, et al: The transjugular intrahepatic portosystemic stent-shunt procedure for refractory ascites. N Engl J Med 332:1192-1197, 1995.

Perkins L, Jeffries M, Patel T: Utility of preoperative scores for predicting morbidity after cholecystectomy in patients with cirrhosis. Clin Gastroenterol Hepatol 2:1123-1128, 2004.

Ramond MJ, Poynard T, Rueff B, et al: A randomized trial of prednisolone in patients with severe alcoholic hepatitis. N Engl J Med 326:507-512, 1992. **A**

Runyon BA: Surgical procedures are well tolerated by patients with asymptomatic chronic hepatitis. J Clin Gastroenterol 8:542-544, 1986. **B**

Sarin SK, Lamba GS, Kumar M, et al: Comparison of endoscopic ligation and propranolol for the primary prevention of variceal bleeding. N Engl J Med 340:988-993, 1999.

Schepke M, Kleber G, Nurnberg D, et al: Ligation versus propranolol for the primary prophylaxis of variceal bleeding in cirrhosis. Hepatology 40:65-72, 2004.

Soper N: Effect of nonbiliary problems on laparoscopic cholecystectomy. Am J Surg 165:522-526, 1993.

Suman A, Barnes DS, Zein NN, et al: Predicting outcome after cardiac surgery in patients with cirrhosis: A comparison of Child-Pugh and MELD scores. Clin Gastroenterol Hepatol 2:719-723, 2004. **B**

Teh SH, Nagorney DM, Stevens SR, et al: Risk factors for mortality after surgery in patients with cirrhosis. Gastroenterology 132:1261-1269, 2007. **B**

Ziser A, Plevak DJ, Russell H, et al: Morbidity and mortality in cirrhotic patients undergoing anesthesia and surgery. Anesthesiology 90:42-53, 1999.

11 Bariatric Surgery: Preoperative Evaluation and Postoperative Care

JAMES FINK, MD

The latest statistics from the National Institutes of Health indicate that more than 50% of the U.S. population is overweight, more than 20% is obese, and 5% is classified as morbidly obese. Worldwide obesity includes about 1.7 billion persons, and the fastest growing subgroup are those with a Body Mass Index (BMI) greater than 35.

DEFINING AND CLASSIFYING OBESITY

The most accurate means for deciding on an individual's degree of obesity is by calculating the BMI (weight in kilograms divided by height in meters squared). **A normal BMI ranges from 18.5 to 25 kg/m². A BMI of 25 to 30 kg/m² is considered overweight, a BMI greater than 30 kg/m² is considered obese, a BMI of 40 to 50 kg/m² is considered morbidly obese, and a BMI greater than 50 kg/m² is considered superobese** (Table 11-1) [🅒 *Presutti et al, 2004*].

Obesity is associated with a host of comorbid conditions. Many of these conditions increase the complexity of weight loss surgery and also contribute to the risk of complications in the perioperative period (Box 11-1).

Levels of Evidence:

🅐—Randomized controlled trials (RCTs), meta-analyses, well-designed systematic reviews of RCTs. 🅑—Case-control or cohort studies, nonrandomized controlled trials, systematic reviews of studies other than RCTs, cross-sectional studies, retrospective studies. 🅒—Consensus statements, expert guidelines, usual practice, opinion.

TABLE 11-1	Definition and Classification of Obesity
Definition	**Body Mass Index (kg/m²)**
Normal	18.5–25
Overweight	25–30
Obese	>30
Morbidly obese	40–50
Superobese	>50

Adapted from Presutti RJ, Gorman RS, Swain JM: Primary care perspective on bariatric surgery. Mayo Clin Proc 79:1158-1166, 2004.

Box 11-1	OBESITY-RELATED COMORBIDITIES

Diabetes
Coronary artery disease
Hypertension
Osteoarthritis
Obstructive sleep apnea
Gastroesophageal reflux disease
Pulmonary insufficiency
Chronic venous stasis
Dysmenorrhea
Gallbladder disease
Skin infections

NONSURGICAL MANAGEMENT

Dieting, exercise, and medications have been the mainstays of treatment for obesity; however, there is little evidence in support of these methods. The 5-year failure rate approaches 100% for persons who diet to control weight. The reason is that few people can sustain a high dietary adherence level, and most do not exercise the recommended 150 minutes/week. Medications such as sibutramine (Meridia) and orlistat (Xenical) have afforded some weight loss. However, side effects such as insomnia, constipation, and increases in blood pressure, as well as steatorrhea and fecal incontinence, make these medications unattractive or contraindicated for certain patients. In addition, patients generally regain the lost weight on discontinuing these medications. **A recent systematic review further showed that little evidence exists to support the use of major commercial and self-help weight loss programs** [❾ *Tsai and Wadden, 2005*].

HISTORY OF BARIATRIC SURGERY

Surgical options for controlling obesity have been available since the 1960s. Bariatric surgery developed out of the observation that patients who had undergone partial gastrectomy for peptic ulcer disease remained underweight or had difficulty gaining weight. With this concept in mind, early attempts at weight loss surgery included the jejunoileal and jejunocolic bypass procedures. With these procedures, the majority of the small intestine was bypassed, leaving approximately 18 inches of absorptive small intestine intact. Unfortunately, patients who underwent these procedures experienced serious complications including intractable diarrhea and multiple nutritional deficiencies, as well as nephrolithiasis resulting from increased calcium oxalate absorption. Approximately 30% of patients developed liver abnormalities caused by steatosis that progressed to cirrhosis in 7% of patients following the jejunoileal procedure.

Since the early 1990s, the number of bariatric operations has been steadily growing. Today, more than 100,000 bariatric surgical procedures are performed annually in the United States. With the increasing prevalence of obesity, the improvements in safety and efficacy of current bariatric procedures, and evidence showing the benefits of weight loss on obesity-related comorbidities, these procedures qualify as more than just a passing fad.

CURRENT SURGICAL APPROACHES TO WEIGHT LOSS

Bariatric surgical procedures can be classified as restrictive or malabsorptive, or both (Figs. 11-1 to 11-6; Table 11-2). Today's bariatric procedures are safer, with more predictable short- and long-term complications, and most can be performed either as open operations or laparoscopically.

Restrictive Procedures

Vertical-banded gastroplasty and adjustable silicone banding are both strictly restrictive procedures. Both these procedures create a small proximal pouch 10 to 20 mL ($\approx$1 ounce) in size. The smaller stomach pouch is distended with a lesser amount

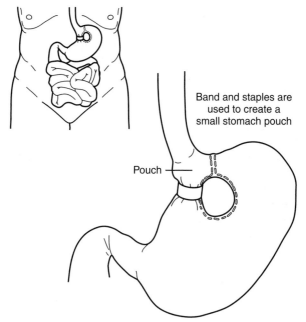

Band and staples are used to create a small stomach pouch

Pouch

Figure 11-1 • A band and staples are used to create a small stomach pouch.

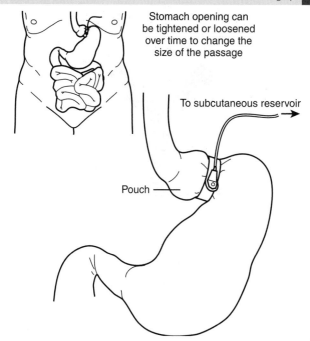

Stomach opening can
be tightened or loosened
over time to change the
size of the passage

To subcutaneous reservoir →

Pouch

Figure 11-2 • The stomach opening can be tightened or loosened over time to change the size of the passage.

TABLE 11-2	Current Surgical Approaches to Weight Loss		
Bariatric Surgery		**Restrictive**	**Malabsorptive**
Vertical-banded gastroplasty		Yes	No
Adjustable silicone gastric banding		Yes	No
Roux-en-Y gastric bypass		Yes	Yes (mild)
Biliopancreatic bypass with duodenal switch		Yes	Yes
Jejunoileal bypass*		No	Yes

*No longer a recommended bariatric surgical procedure.

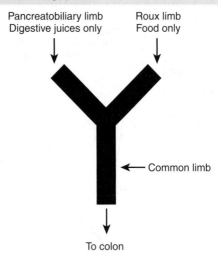

Pancreatobiliary limb
Digestive juices only

Roux limb
Food only

← Common limb

To colon

Figure 11-3 • Schematic view of Roux-en-Y stomach bypass. *(Adapted from Choban PS: Bariatric surgery for morbid obesity: Why, who, when, how, where, and then what? Cleve Clin J Med 69:897-903, 2002.)*

of food, to produce satiety. This restriction of caloric intake leads to weight loss. The pouch for vertical-banded gastroplasty is created using both a silicone ring or mesh band, to restrict the proximal stomach pouch outlet, and stapling. Adjustable gastric banding uses a silicone band placed around the proximal stomach and attached to a subcutaneous reservoir. Infusion of saline allows changes in the size and outlet of the proximal pouch. Weight loss with the adjustable silicone gastric banding appears to be more gradual than with vertical-banded gastroplasty; this finding may be related to the potential for less aggressive inflation of the band. In addition, function of this inflatable band may deteriorate over time.

Restrictive and Malabsorptive Procedures

Roux-en-Y gastric bypass is the most commonly performed bariatric procedure in the United States. This technique combines both a gastric restriction procedure, to create a small

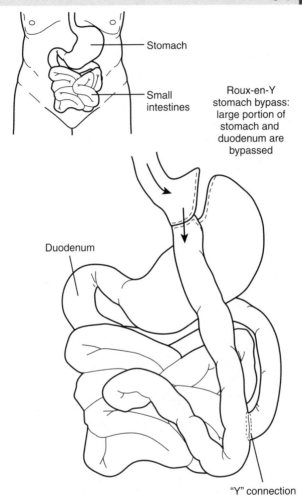

Figure 11-4 • Roux-en-Y stomach bypass. Large portions of the stomach and duodenum are bypassed.

proximal stomach pouch, and a bypass procedure, to promote malabsorption. The Roux-en-Y anastomosis allows food from the proximal stomach pouch to drain directly into the jejunum and thus bypasses the distal stomach, duodenum, and proximal portion of the jejunum. The small intestine is usually transected 10 to 15 cm beyond the ligament of Treitz. The distal segment becomes the "Roux" limb. This Roux limb varies from 75 to 200 cm in length, depending on the degree of malabsorption and weight loss desired. The longer the Roux limb, the shorter will be the common channel, and vice versa. The degree of malabsorption is related to the length of the common channel. The Roux-en-Y procedure produces more weight loss than do strictly restrictive procedures.

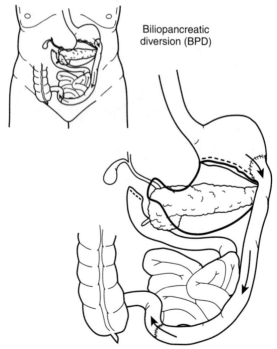

Figure 11-5 • Biliopancreatic diversion.

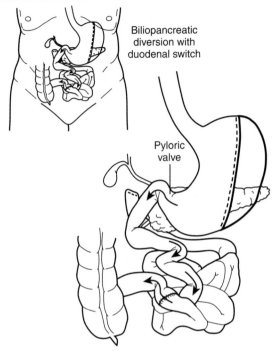

Biliopancreatic
diversion with
duodenal switch

Pyloric
valve

Figure 11-6 • Biliopancreatic diversion with duodenal switch.

The biliopancreatic bypass and biliopancreatic bypass with duodenal switch are similar to the Roux-en-Y gastric bypass in that they use both restriction and malabsorption to create weight loss. The biliopancreatic bypass procedures create a pouch by transecting the stomach; this pouch is larger than the 10- to 20-mL pouches seen with the other procedures. The malabsorptive component for these procedures is greater than in Roux-en-Y gastric bypass. The ileum is anastomosed to the remaining stomach or, in the case of the duodenal switch, is connected directly to a small segment of duodenum just distal to the pylorus (see Figs. 11-5 and 11-6). The duodenal switch is performed to decrease the incidence of stomal ulcer, and, by preserving the pylorus, it also helps to regulate the release of stomach contents into the intestine. The remainder of the duodenum and jejunum is then attached to the ileum just proximal (50 to 100 cm) to the ileocecal valve, to allow the pancreatic and biliary secretions to mix with the ileal contents before entering the colon.

PREOPERATIVE ASSESSMENT

Although preoperative requirements for bariatric surgical procedures vary, the medical consultant is certainly a key link in coordinating the preoperative screening and assessments for patients who are interested in these procedures. The current indications for bariatric surgery are a BMI of at least 40 or a BMI of 35 or greater in patients with co-morbid conditions (Box 11-2). In addition to these standard criteria, the medical consultant and patient will need to verify attempts at weight loss using diet, exercise, and medications for approximately 6 months during the last 2 years. The medical consultant may also have some insight into which patients would be at risk for maladaptive eating disorders or would be poor follow-up candidates. Additional assistance includes counseling and providing medical therapies as needed for cessation of tobacco use, a requirement for bariatric procedures. Depending on the patient's medical conditions and comorbidities, evaluation by subspecialists, including those in the fields of cardiology, pulmonology, and endocrinology, may also be requested before proceeding. The reasons for referral may include stress testing and evaluation of pulmonary hypertension, pulmonary function testing, and maximizing control of diabetes. Some surgical candidates are required to undergo a right upper quadrant ultrasound examination to identify possible cholelithiasis. Patients who have evidence of cholelithiasis are generally given a prophylactic cholecystectomy during the bariatric procedure. A psychiatric assessment is required and is usually performed

Box 11-2	PREOPERATIVE ASSESSMENT AND REQUIREMENTS FOR PROCEDURES

BMI >40, or BMI >35 with obesity-related comorbidities
Documented attempts at weight loss: diet, exercise, medications
Evaluation by cardiology, pulmonology, and endocrinology specialists
Tobacco cessation (must be ≥8 weeks before the procedure)
Right upper quadrant ultrasound to evaluate for cholelithiasis
Psychiatric assessment: specialists in eating disorders
Full disclosure of risks, benefits, expectations

BMI, body mass index.

by psychiatrists who specialize in eating disorders. Finally, before proceeding with the operation, patients must have a complete understanding of the risks and benefits, along with the preoperative and postoperative expectations, evaluations, and requirements.

Most weight loss surgical procedures are performed using a minimally invasive laparoscopic approach. Opinion suggests that for the obese patient, this method results in less depression of lung function and less postoperative pain than the laparotomy approach.

PERIOPERATIVE MANAGEMENT

Although the selection of anesthetic agents and their administration is the responsibility of the anesthesiologist, the medical consultant must know several important concepts. Anesthesia for these procedures has the potential to be hazardous because of the increased risk of difficult intubation and the potential for aspiration of gastric contents. **Neck circumference in the obese patient is an excellent predictor of problematic intubation; the reported incidence of difficult intubation in patients with a 40-cm neck circumference is 5%, and the probability of difficult intubation** in patients with a neck circumference of 60 cm is 35% [**⊙** *Brodsky et al, 2002*].

The obese patient may have undiagnosed pulmonary hypertension because of chronic hypoxia. Obstructive sleep apnea occurs in more than 70% of patients who undergo gastric bypass surgery. In addition to contributing to problems of pulmonary ventilation, obstructive sleep apnea may result in increased sensitivity to opioid and sedative medications.

Pharmacodynamic data regarding drug kinetics in the obese patient are not available for many medications utilized in the perioperative period. Use of total body weight may overestimate medication doses for those agents that are not lipophilic (e.g., vecuronium). **Highly lipophilic substances (e.g., barbiturates, benzodiazepines, succinylcholine) show significant increases in the volume of distribution compared with normal weight patients, and for these medications, weight-based medication dosing is often predicated on total body weight. Agents that are less lipophilic (e.g., vecuronium) are typically dosed based on ideal body weight** [**⊙** *Ogunnaike et al, 2002*].

▌ POSTOPERATIVE MANAGEMENT

Expected hospital stay following a bariatric surgical procedure is between 2 to 5 days. Two to 3 days following the procedure, before the initiation of enteral feeding, patients usually undergo an upper gastrointestinal radiographic series with contrast to evaluate for any leaks. If no leaks are identified, patients remain on a pureed diet for 4 weeks. Additional instructions may vary, but patients are often advised to refrain from lifting and from heavy work. They must not drive for 2 weeks following the procedure and should abstain from sexual intercourse for the first month postoperatively. Follow-up occurs at approximate intervals of 2 weeks, 1 month, 6 weeks, 3 months, 12 months, 18 months, and 2 years, with annual visits thereafter.

Twenty percent of patients may require admission to an intensive care unit or prolonged hospitalization. Intubation, vascular access, blood pressure monitoring, and potential difficulty in moving or turning these patients must be kept in mind. Morbid obesity is a significant risk factor for deep vein thrombosis (DVT) and pulmonary embolus (PE). The combined incidence of DVT and PE is 2%. **Evidence indicates that when low-molecular-weight heparin is used for DVT prophylaxis, the incidence of DVT is less when the dose of enoxaparin is 40 mg twice daily compared with 30 mg twice daily** [❶ *Scholten et al, 2002*]. **When unfractionated heparin is used, evidence indicates that weight-based dosing designed to keep factor anti-Xa levels at 0.11 to 0.25 U/mL is an effective approach to decrease the risk of perioperative DVT and PE in patients who undergo laparoscopic Roux-en-Y gastric bypass** [❶ *Shepherd et al, 2003*].

OUTCOMES OF WEIGHT LOSS SURGERY

Weight loss generally occurs at a rate of 10 pounds/month. A stable weight is usually achieved by 18 to 24 months after the procedure.

A meta-analysis evaluated the effectiveness of current bariatric procedures on weight loss and improving obesity-related comorbidities for up to 2 years postoperatively. Overall excess weight loss across all types of surgical procedures was approximately 61% at 2 years. The percentage of excess weight loss ranged from 47.5% for gastric banding to 70.1% for biliopancreatic diversions with duodenal switch. This percentage of excess weight lost is equivalent to approximately 30% to 40% of total body weight (excess weight = total preoperative weight − ideal weight). This analysis looked specifically at four obesity-related comorbid conditions: diabetes, lipid profile, hypertension, and obstructive sleep apnea. Of these patients, 85% had an improvement or resolution of their diabetes, and 70% had improved lipid profiles. The mean decreases in total cholesterol level, low-density lipoprotein, and triglycerides were 33, 29, and 79 mg/dL, respectively. Hypertension resolved or improved in 78% of patients, whereas 84% of patients with obstructive sleep apnea showed improvement or resolution of this condition.

The Swedish Obese Subjects (SOS) study compared patients at 2 years and 10 years after bariatric surgery. This study found that weight loss was significantly better for the bariatric surgery group as compared with controls at both 2 and 10 years. Patients who had undergone surgical procedures were able to keep their weight off, although the percentage of weight loss for these patients decreased from a maximum at 2 years, 23.4%, to that seen at 10 years, 16.1%. Overall, energy intake (kcal/day) was lower and physical activity was higher in the surgical group, and comorbidities, including diabetes, hypertriglyceridemia, low high-density lipoprotein, and hypertension, all remained improved through 10 years.

SHORT-TERM COMPLICATIONS

Operative mortality rates evaluated in different studies vary anywhere from 0.1% for restrictive procedures alone, to 0.5% for gastric bypass procedures, to 1% for biliopancreatic diversion with or without duodenal switch. Immediate postoperative complications include wound problems (infections, dehiscence, hernias, and seromas) in approximately 15% of patients. After upper abdominal operations, obese patients have a 45% incidence of atelectasis, which may prompt anesthesiologists or pulmonologists to use continuous positive airway pressure or bilevel positive airway pressure postoperatively. Laparoscopic bariatric surgery decreases these wound problems and reduces atelectasis and postoperative pain. Laparoscopic procedures are increasingly used more frequently for patients who weigh less than 350 lb (≤160 kg). DVT and PE affect 1% and 0.2% of these patients, respectively, despite preventive measures. All patients should receive prophylaxis for DVT and PE according to the 2004 American College of Chest Physicians guidelines with subcutaneous heparin or low-molecular-weight heparin and lower extremity compression devices. Dysphagia and vomiting occur in nearly 33% of patients who have a restrictive component to their procedure. Anastomotic leaks, band malfunction, and stomal and small bowel obstruction are also possible short-term complications.

LONG-TERM COMPLICATIONS

The *dumping syndrome* consists of postprandial sweating, weakness, hypoglycemia, and malaise and occurs in the majority of patients who have undergone a malabsorptive procedure. This syndrome most commonly occurs after eating foods high in sugar or fat and is believed to be related to fluid shifts from the intravascular space to the intestine. For this reason, these foods should be avoided by persons who have undergone gastric bypass. The condition is severe in approximately 1% of patients, but it generally disappears over time as the body adjusts to the malabsorption. Most bariatric surgeons believe that this is a favorable side effect that teaches patients to avoid maladaptive eating behaviors.

Nutritional deficiencies are a concern with all types of bariatric surgical procedures because of both decreased intake and absorption. Procedures that have a malabsorptive component and those with a shorter common channel are much more commonly associated with these deficiencies.

Vitamin and mineral deficiencies are particularly common because absorption of these substances occurs in the proximal small intestine, which is bypassed with these procedures. Fat-soluble (A, D, E, K) vitamin deficiencies are particularly common after biliopancreatic bypass procedures. Vitamin B_{12} and folate deficiencies have been implicated in hyperhomocysteinemia, seen in approximately 66% of patients who undergo bariatric surgical procedures. Iron deficiency is most commonly seen in menstruating women, with a prevalence ranging from 20% to 50%. The deficiency of iron is caused by two mechanisms: first, restrictive procedures limit the conversion of nonabsorbable ferric iron to absorbable ferrous iron that occurs when ferric iron is exposed to stomach acids and oxidation occurs; second, most iron absorption occurs in the duodenum and proximal jejunum, which is often bypassed with malabsorptive procedures. The duodenum and proximal jejunum are also the sites of most calcium absorption, a deficiency of that makes these patients susceptible to decreased bone mineral density. Protein malnutrition is also a potential complication of bariatric procedures.

Bariatric surgical patients have a 15% to 30% chance of needing a cholecystectomy within 3 years of the operation because of the increased formation of gallstones that results from weight loss. Although it is not well understood, the increased incidence of gallstones as a result of these procedures is thought to be related to increased concentrations of mucin, cholesterol, and calcium within the bile caused by a decrease in the enterohepatic circulation. Possible treatments for this complication include prophylactic cholecystectomy at the time of the original bariatric procedure or the use of ursodiol (300 mg twice daily) for the first 6 months postoperatively to reduce stone formation to approximately 2%.

Ulcers are a potential complication, particularly with use of nonsteroidal anti-inflammatory drugs. Strictures are also possible long-term complications and may require endoscopy with balloon dilation. Function of the inflatable gastric bands may deteriorate over time. Finally, the removal of excess skin, which remains after the weight loss occurs, may be considered cosmetic, and surgical correction of this condition may not be covered by insurance.

Postoperative Maintenance

Prevention and treatment of these long-term complications are accomplished by taking daily multivitamins and minerals. Ingesting 60 g/day of protein is recommended for malabsorptive procedures. Laboratory testing should be done every 3 months through the first year and at least annually thereafter. Included in the laboratory analysis should be complete blood count, electrolytes, liver function tests (particularly albumin), ferritin and iron studies, and vitamin B_{12} and folate determinations. Nonsteroidal anti-inflammatory drugs are contraindicated in patients who have undergone a bariatric procedure because of the potentially catastrophic consequences of ulcers. Female patients should not become pregnant in the first year following the procedure because nutritional deficiencies and adjustments will put their fetus at risk, and carrying a baby may compromise their surgical anatomy and incisions. In these patients, the medical consultant is instrumental in providing appropriate counseling and information on the use of contraception.

CONCLUSION

Bariatric surgery is proving to be a safe, effective, and increasingly popular method for combating obesity and its related comorbid conditions. The medical consultant will play an important role preoperatively in deciding which patients may be appropriate candidates for these procedures, by helping to document weight loss attempts, and in coordinating surgical clearance. Postoperatively, the medical consultant should be aware of possible short- and long-term complications and can provide support and knowledge for patients who have undergone these procedures.

Selected Readings

Berke EM, Morden NE: Medical management of obesity. Am Fam Physician 62:419-426, 2000.

Brodsky JB, Lemmens HJM, Brock-Utne JG, et al: Morbid obesity and tracheal intubation. Anesth Analg 94:732-736, 2002. ⓐ

Brolin RE: Bariatric surgery and long-term control of morbid obesity. JAMA 288:2793-2796, 2002.

Buchwald H, Avidor Y, Braunwald E, et al: Bariatric surgery: A systematic review and meta-analysis. JAMA 292:1724-1737, 2004.

Choban PS: Bariatric surgery for morbid obesity: Why, who when, how, where, and then what? Cleve Clin J Med 69:897-903, 2002.

Dansinger ML, Gleason JA, Griffith JL, et al: Comparison of the Atkins, Ornish, Weight Watchers and Zone Diets for weight loss and heart disease risk reduction: A randomized trial. JAMA 293:43-53, 2005.

Hocking MP, Duerson MC, O'Leary JP, Woodward ER: Jejunoileal bypass for morbid obesity: Late follow-up in 100 cases. N Engl J Med 308: 995-999, 1983.

MacGregor A: The story of surgery for obesity. American Society of Bariatric Surgery. Available at http://www.asbs.org

Mokdad AH: The spread of the obesity epidemic in the United States, 1991-1998. JAMA 282:1519-1522, 1999.

National Heart, Lung and Blood Institute and North American Association for the Study of Obesity: The Practical Guide to the Identification, Evaluation and Treatment of Overweight and Obesity in Adults. Bethesda, MD, National Institutes of Health, 2000.

Ogunnaike BO, Jones SB, Jones DB, et al: Anesthetic considerations for bariatric surgery. Anesth Analg 95:1793-1805, 2002. **C**

Presutti RJ, Gorman RS, Swain JM: Primary care perspective on bariatric surgery. Mayo Clin Proc 79:1158-1166, 2004. **C**

Scholten DJ, Hoedema RM, Scholten SE: A comparison of two different prophylactic dose regimens of low molecular weight heparin in bariatric surgery. Obes Surg 12:19-24, 2002. **B**

Schumann R, Jones S, Ortiz V, et al: Best practice recommendations for anesthetic perioperative care and pain management in weight loss surgery. Obes Res 13:254-266, 2005.

Shepherd MF, Rosborough TK, Schwartz M: Heparin thromboprophylaxis in gastric bypass surgery. Obes Surg 13:249-253, 2003. **B**

Sjöström L: Lifestyle, diabetes and cardiovascular risk factors 10 years after bariatric surgery. N Engl J Med 351:2683-2693, 2004.

Steinbrook R: Surgery for severe obesity. N Engl J Med 350:1075-1079, 2004.

Tsai AG, Wadden TA: Systematic review: An evaluation of major commercial weight loss programs in the United States. Ann Intern Med 142:56-66, 2005.

12 | Perioperative Management of Endocrine Disorders

KEVIN FURLONG, DO
INTEKHAB AHMED, MD
SERGE JABBOUR, MD

▌DIABETES MELLITUS AND HYPERGLYCEMIA

Diabetes mellitus is not uncommon in the surgical patient. It is estimated that 50% of diabetic patients will require some type of surgical procedure during their lifetime. Many surgical procedures, particularly cardiac and vascular, are necessitated by the complications of diabetes. An enlarging body of data reports that the aggressive management of diabetes and hyperglycemia results in improved outcomes. Studies have emerged showing the beneficial effects of improved glycemic control in patients who undergo surgery.

Investigators have shown that in general surgical patients with a blood glucose level greater than 220 mg/dL, infection rates were 2.7 times higher than the rates for similar patients with glucose levels lower than 220 mg/dL. In a study of surgical patients who required mechanical ventilation in the perioperative period, those treated with an intensive insulin regimen (continuous insulin to maintain glucose 80 to 110 mg/dL) had a 34% reduction in overall in-hospital mortality compared with a conventionally treated group (insulin administration only if glucose >215 mg/dL; target glucose, 180 to 200 mg/dL).

Levels of Evidence:

🅐—Randomized controlled trials (RCTs), meta-analyses, well-designed systematic reviews of RCTs. 🅑—Case-control or cohort studies, nonrandomized clinical trials, systematic reviews of studies other than RCTs, cross-sectional studies, retrospective studies. 🅒—Consensus statements, expert guidelines, usual practice, opinion.

Intensive insulin therapy has also been shown to reduce the need for prolonged ventilatory support, the duration of intensive care stay, the number of blood transfusions, the incidence of bloodstream infections, the need for dialysis, and the incidence of critical illness polyneuropathy. The benefit of intensive insulin therapy with continuous infusion insulin has been particularly evident in the patient who undergoes coronary artery bypass surgery. In this situation, implementation of intensive insulin therapy has been shown to decrease the risk of sternal wound infection, atrial fibrillation, recurrent myocardial ischemia, and death. For the patient without a prior history of diabetes who develops postoperative hyperglycemia, intensive control of serum glucose to achieve a mean concentration of 125 mg/dL has also been associated with a reduced rate of infection. **The available data clearly show that improved glycemic control in the hospitalized surgical patient leads to improvements in outcomes, even in those patients without previously diagnosed diabetes** [❷ *Van den Berghe et al, 2001*].

Preoperative Evaluation

Diabetic patients undergoing surgical procedures fall into a higher risk category than comparable patients without diabetes. Diabetic patients in general have a higher prevalence of cardiovascular, renal, and neurologic diseases, all of which can lead to increased perioperative morbidity and mortality. The prevalence and incidence of and mortality from all forms of cardiovascular disease are two- to eightfold higher in persons with diabetes than in persons without diabetes. Moreover, patients with diabetes have an increased risk of cardiac events once the diagnosis of cardiovascular disease has been established. Therefore, the American College of Cardiology/American Heart Association guideline for risk stratification before noncardiac surgery designates diabetes as a coronary risk equivalent, which means that patients with diabetes belong in the same risk category as patients with known cardiovascular disease. Diabetes is also the leading cause of end-stage renal disease in the United States. Renal insufficiency can lead to fluid balance difficulties, electrolyte abnormalities, increased insulin sensitivity, and an increased perioperative cardiovascular risk.

Furthermore, many diabetic patients suffer from peripheral or autonomic neuropathy, or both, which can lead to impaired angina recognition, increased risk of intraoperative hypotension and cardiac arrhythmias, and increased risk of decubitus ulcers with prolonged bed rest. These patients are also at increased risk of gastroparesis, which can make glycemic control difficult and can compromise a patient's nutritional status. Therefore, it is of utmost importance that all diabetic patients undergoing surgical procedures have a thorough preoperative evaluation by their internist or cardiologist.

Targets of Glycemic Control

The American College of Endocrinology and the American Association of Clinical Endocrinologists, together with key investigators of the major interventional studies, reviewed the available literature on inpatient diabetes management and outcomes. Based on their review, these organizations developed evidence-based glycemic targets for hospitalized patients with diabetes and hyperglycemia. These targets are in agreement with evidence-based targets set by the American Diabetes Association (ADA) and are as follows:

- For patients in the intensive care unit setting, results of a larger prospective study support an upper limit serum glucose of 110 mg/dL.
- In noncritical care units, observational data recommend a preprandial blood glucose of 110 mg/dL or less and a maximal blood glucose of 180 mg/dL.
- In pregnancy, it is recommended that preprandial blood glucose be 100 mg/dL or lower; 1-hour postprandial glucose

concentrations should be 120 mg/dL or lower; and during labor and delivery, blood glucose should be 100 mg/dL or lower.

Agents for Diabetic and Hyperglycemic Management

Although they are the mainstay of therapy for diabetes, oral diabetes agents are not well studied in the inpatient setting. Therefore, no specific evidence-based guidelines exist regarding their use in the hospitalized surgical patient. However, an understanding of their mechanism of action, side effects, and contraindications can lead to their appropriate and safe use in specific circumstances.

Biguanides

Metformin is the only approved biguanide in the United States. It decreases endogenous hepatic glucose production (main action), decreases intestinal glucose absorption, and increases peripheral glucose uptake and utilization. It generally does not produce hypoglycemia when it is used alone; however, episodes have occurred during caloric restriction, vigorous exercise, and concomitant use of other hypoglycemic agents. The drug is eliminated from the body by the renal route.

The drug's most worrisome potential side effect, albeit rare, is lactic acidosis. When this disorder occurs, it is fatal in 50% of cases. The risk of lactic acidosis increases with the level of kidney impairment and with hypoxic states, both of which occur more frequently in the inpatient setting. Radiologic studies involving the use of intravascular iodinated contrast materials can lead to acute deterioration of renal function and increase the risk of lactic acidosis. Therefore, metformin should be discontinued just before the procedure and withheld for 48 hours. It should be restarted only when renal function has been reevaluated and found to be normal.

Metformin should be temporarily discontinued before any surgical procedure and should be restarted when the patient's oral intake is resumed, renal function is normalized, and risk of hypoxia is no longer present. Metformin can also be problematic in the postoperative patient because of its propensity to cause gastrointestinal side effects such as nausea, vomiting, gas, and diarrhea.

Sulfonylureas

Sulfonylureas work by stimulating the pancreatic β cells to produce insulin. Various agents are available, all with different pharmacokinetic profiles. These drugs are all metabolized primarily by the liver, and their major side effect is hypoglycemia. Surgical patients often have variable oral intake, which increases the risk of hypoglycemia from these drugs. Therefore, we recommend that these agents be withheld the day of surgery and not restarted until the patient has resumed stable oral intake.

Meglitinides

Meglitinides work in a fashion similar to that of the sulfonylureas by stimulating the pancreatic β cells to release insulin. As with the sulfonylureas, the major side effect is hypoglycemia, although less severe and less common because of the shorter duration of action of the meglitinides. We recommend that these drugs be held starting on the day of surgery and resumed when the patient's oral intake is reestablished.

Thiazolidinediones

The thiazolidinediones work by decreasing insulin resistance in the periphery and in the liver. The results are increased glucose uptake by the muscle and decreased hepatic glucose output. These agents have limited utility for obtaining glycemic control in the hospitalized surgical patient because their mechanism of action is mediated by nuclear transcription, and their onset of action is quite slow (weeks). They can also cause fluid retention, which may precipitate exacerbations of congestive heart failure. These drugs should be avoided in patients with New York Heart Association class III and IV heart failure. They should also be avoided in hepatic insufficiency. The thiazolidinediones can lead to hypoglycemia when they are used with insulin or other agents that increase endogenous insulin secretion. These drugs should be withheld starting on the day of surgery and resumed when the patient's oral intake is reestablished.

5-α-Glucosidase Inhibitors

α-Glucosidase inhibitors work by delaying glucose absorption and therefore lowering postprandial hyperglycemia. They tend to have minimal effects on glycemic control and are not well suited to postoperative patients with variable oral intake. Furthermore, they cause abdominal pain, diarrhea, and flatulence in a large percentage of patients. These agents should be held starting on the day of surgery and resumed when the patient reestablishes oral intake.

In conclusion, each of these major classes of oral diabetes agents has significant limitations for use in the hospitalized surgical patient. These drugs offer little flexibility and may produce untoward side effects. A summary of these agents is provided in Table 12-1.

Subcutaneous Insulin

Insulin is the agent of choice to obtain glycemic control in the hospitalized surgical patient (Table 12-2). The components of the daily insulin requirement are classified as basal, nutritional or prandial, correction or supplemental, and illness or stress related. *Basal insulin* is defined as the amount of exogenous insulin per unit of time necessary to prevent hepatic gluconeogenesis and ketogenesis. Therefore, it is always required in patients with type 1 diabetes and in patients who lack endogenous insulin production. It may not be required in patients with type 2 diabetes or in those with only stress-induced hyperglycemia because these patients maintain some endogenous insulin production. In general, basal insulin accounts for approximately 40% to 50% of the total daily insulin requirement, and it can be provided by any one of several strategies such as continuous subcutaneous insulin infusion (i.e., insulin pump), once-daily injection of a long-acting

TABLE 12-1	Oral Agents Used in the Treatment of Type 2 Diabetes	
Drug Class and Agents	**Mechanism of Action**	**Contraindications and Cautions**

Sulfonylureas
  Chlorpropamide
  Tolbutamide
  Tolazamide
  Glipizide
  Glyburide
  Glimepiride
	Increase the secretion of insulin from β cells	Use with caution in patients with hepatic or renal insufficiency and in those with hypersensitivity to sulfonamides; most common side effect is hypoglycemia

Meglitinides
  Repaglinide
  Nateglinide
	Increase the secretion of insulin from β cells	Use with caution in patients with hepatic or renal insufficiency

Thiazolidinediones
  Pioglitazone
  Rosiglitazone
	Improve insulin action in the periphery and in the liver	Not indicated in NYHA class III and IV heart failure; use with caution in class I and II; use with caution if impaired hepatic function (ALT >2.5 times normal); avoid in fluid overloaded states

Biguanides Metformin	Decrease endogenous hepatic glucose production and increase peripheral glucose uptake	Do not use in patients at risk for lactic acidosis; do not use in female patients with serum creatinine >1.4 mg/dL and male patients with serum creatinine >1.5 mg/dL

α-Glucosidase inhibitors
  Acarbose
  Miglitol
	Inhibit intestinal α-glucosidase, thereby delaying glucose absorption	Contraindicated in inflammatory bowel disease, colonic ulceration, and intestinal obstruction

ALT, alanine aminotransferase; NYHA, New York Heart Association.

insulin (glargine), or multiple injections of an intermediate-acting insulin (NPH).

The *nutritional insulin requirement* is the amount of exogenous insulin necessary to prevent hyperglycemia associated with nutritional supplementation in any form (i.e., intravenous dextrose, total parenteral nutrition [TPN], partial parenteral nutrition, enteral feedings, and discrete meals). When the patient eats discrete meals without any other nutritional supplementation, the nutritional insulin requirement is referred to as the *prandial insulin requirement*. Its main effect is

TABLE 12-2   Insulin Formulations Used in the Treatment of Diabetes

Type of Insulin	Name: Generic (Proprietary)	Onset	Peak	Duration
Rapid-acting analogues	Lispro (Humalog) Aspart (NovoLog) Glulisine (Apidra)	5-15 min	1-2 hr	3-4 hr
Short-acting	Regular (Humulin R) (Novolin R)	30-60 min	2-4 hr	6-8 hr
Intermediate-acting	NPH (Humulin N) (Novolin N) Lente (Humulin L)	1-2 hr	4-8 hr	10-20 hr
Long-acting	Ultralente (Humulin U)	2-4 hr	Unpredictable	16-28 hr
Long-acting (true basal and 24-hr insulin)	Glargine analog (Lantus)	4-6 hr	Peakless	24-48 hr
Mixed insulin: 70% intermediate-acting insulin isophane suspension and 30% short-acting regular insulin	Humulin 70/30 Novolin 70/30	30-60 min	2-8 hr	10-20 hr
Mixed insulin: 75% intermediate-acting insulin lispro protamine suspension and 25% rapid-acting lispro insulin	Humalog Mix 75/25	5-15 min	1-4 hr	10-20 hr
Mixed insulin: 70% intermediate-acting insulin aspart protamine suspension and 30% rapid-acting aspart insulin	Novolog Mix 70/30	5-15 min	1-4 hr	15-18 hr

on peripheral glucose disposal into muscle after a carbohydrate load. Prandial insulin is best provided by using the rapid-acting insulin analogues, which are lispro, aspart, and glulisine. These insulin analogues have a very rapid onset of action and can physiologically match the normal insulin response to carbohydrate loads. Ideally, the dose should be given 0 to 15 minutes before meals. However, if it is uncertain how much the patient will eat, the dose can be given immediately after the completion of the meal. If regular insulin is used for prandial coverage, it should be given 30 to 45 minutes before the meal is consumed. It carries an increased risk of hypoglycemia when compared with the rapid-acting analogues because of its slower onset of action and longer duration of action.

Correction or supplemental insulin is insulin used to correct unexpected hyperglycemia that occurs before or between meals. The term may also refer to the insulin used to correct hyperglycemia in the patient who is allowed nothing by mouth (NPO). It is useful as a dose-finding strategy because appropriate changes can be made to the scheduled basal or nutritional insulin doses based on the amount of supplemental insulin used. Correction or supplemental insulin should not be confused with the concept of insulin titration and administration by a sliding scale. Sliding scales are used to treat hyperglycemia only after it has occurred and do nothing to prevent hyperglycemia. More important, these scales have been shown to be ineffective and possibly dangerous. *Illness- or stress-related insulin* is the amount of exogenous insulin necessary to prevent hyperglycemia from stress-induced counterregulatory hormones, glucocorticoids, pressors, or diabetogenic drugs. This amount varies among individuals and changes with the changing level of stress or illness. It is recommended that this stress- or illness-related insulin requirement be apportioned among the basal, nutritional, and correction dose insulin requirements.

Continuous Intravenous Infusion Therapy

Intravenous insulin infusion has many advantages over the subcutaneous route in the surgical patient. Its rapid onset of action and ease of titration allow for rapid control of hyperglycemia. This makes it the method of choice in patients with rapidly changing insulin requirements. This approach is also beneficial in patients with significant subcutaneous edema or impaired perfusion of subcutaneous sites. The medical literature supports the use of continuous intravenous insulin infusions for many clinical indications. Indications that have a high level of evidence include diabetic ketoacidosis and non-ketotic hyperosmolar state, critical illness, myocardial infarction or cardiogenic shock, and the postoperative period after cardiac surgical procedures. Indications that have a weaker level of evidence with respect to outcome data include patients with type 1 diabetes who are NPO, general perioperative care including organ transplantation, TPN, hyperglycemia during high-dose corticosteroid therapy, stroke, and use as a dose-finding strategy anticipatory to initiation of subcutaneous insulin therapy in type 1 or type 2 diabetes.

In their consensus conference, **the American College of Endocrinology and the American Association of Clinical Endocrinologists recommended evidence-based glycemic thresholds for initiating intravenous insulin infusion therapy** [❶ *Bode et al, 2004*]. These organizations recommended that for the surgical patient who is not critically ill, intravenous insulin infusion be initiated when serum glucose is greater than 180 mg/dL, with a target goal serum glucose of 90 to 140 mg/dL. For the critically ill surgical patient, it is recommended that intravenous insulin therapy be used when serum glucose exceeds 110 mg/dL, with a target glucose of 80 to 110 mg/dL.

Many different intravenous insulin administration protocols are available. Furthermore, glycemic targets may differ based on pragmatic considerations such as patient-to-nursing ratios and staff education. In general, regular insulin is typically mixed in a 1:1 ratio with 0.9% saline solution, and the infusion is given as a piggy back with other intravenous fluids. Frequent blood glucose monitoring is performed, and adjustments to the insulin infusion rate are made according to the hospital protocol.

Conversion from intravenous insulin infusion to subcutaneous insulin therapy should be attempted only after the patient's clinical status has stabilized; more specifically, the patient is no longer critically ill, is not receiving volume resuscitation and pressors, and has stabilized nutritional requirements. The patient's 24-hour insulin requirement can be estimated by extrapolating the average hourly rate necessary to achieve the goal serum glucose in the most recent 6- to 8-hour period. Eighty percent of the 24-hour requirement is then divided equally into basal and nutritional insulin. For example, suppose a patient has been maintained in the target glycemic range for the past 6 hours on an average of 2 U/hour. The total 24-hour requirement for that patient is 2 U/hour × 24 hours = 48 U of insulin. One then multiplies this number by 80%, which equals 38 U when rounding to the nearest unit. Therefore, 19 U would be given as basal insulin, and 19 U would be given throughout the day as nutritional or prandial doses.

When transitioning from continuous intravenous insulin infusion to subcutaneous insulin therapy, the first dose of subcutaneous insulin must be given before the intravenous insulin is stopped. If administering rapid-acting or short-acting insulin, one should wait 15 to 30 minutes before discontinuing the infusion. If intermediate-acting or long-acting insulin is given, one should wait 2 to 3 hours before discontinuing the insulin infusion.

A minority of patients receiving insulin infusions will not require standing subcutaneous doses of insulin on discontinuing the infusion. These patients typically have type 2 diabetes or stress-induced hyperglycemia and tend to require less than 0.5 U/hour of insulin.

Strategies to Achieve Glycemic Targets

In general, patients with diabetes should undergo surgical procedures in the early morning, to minimize the length of time that they are without oral intake. This approach helps to reduce wide glycemic excursions and the risk of hypoglycemia. Additionally, the patient's usual oral agents or insulin therapy doses are given the day before the surgical procedure, to ensure adequate glycemic control on the morning of the operation. Continuous intravenous insulin infusions can be used perioperatively to obtain glycemic targets. This is the preferred method of glycemic control when a prolonged postoperative NPO period is anticipated.

The specific strategy chosen by the clinician to achieve glycemic targets depends on the patient's metabolic and glycemic status at the time of surgery and the type of procedure planned. In general, patients can be categorized into those with endogenous insulin deficiency and those without it. Characteristics of patients who have or may have endogenous insulin deficiency include a history of any of the following: type 1 diabetes mellitus, pancreatectomy or pancreatic dysfunction, wide fluctuations in blood glucose levels, diabetic ketoacidosis, and insulin use for more than 5 years or a history of diabetes for longer than 10 years or both. Withholding basal insulin from these patients results in a rapid rise in blood glucose by 45 mg/dL/hour until ketoacidosis occurs. Therefore, these patients always need insulin. Patients without any of the aforementioned characteristics are assumed to have some degree of endogenous insulin reserve and may not require insulin in their perioperative management.

The nature and the duration of the surgical procedure also affect perioperative management. Patients undergoing minor surgical procedures of short duration and who require limited general, local, epidural, or spinal anesthesia may need only minimal changes in their diabetic regimen. These patients tend to have fewer glycemic excursions than patients undergoing longer procedures (>2 hours) under general anesthesia. Specific strategies to achieve glycemic targets are largely based on expert consensus opinion. There is a paucity of large RCTs comparing various strategies with respect to glycemic control and outcomes.

Patients with type 1 diabetes or those patients with endogenous insulin deficiency must always receive basal insulin to prevent iatrogenic ketoacidosis. If the surgical procedure is short and the patient will start eating after the procedure, he or she can receive 50% to 100% of the outpatient basal insulin dose (100% of glargine dose; 50% to 75% of intermediate-acting insulin dose the morning of the procedure because the intermediate-acting insulin formulations have a peak and can lead to hypoglycemia if given at full dose). Prandial doses of insulin should be omitted until the patient resumes eating. Blood glucose should be monitored frequently, and correction doses of regular insulin can be used to maintain glycemic targets. If blood glucose is not maintained within the target range despite correction doses, a continuous insulin infusion should be started. For longer, major surgical procedures or procedures associated with a prolonged postoperative NPO interval, a continuous intravenous insulin infusion should be used. In a patient treated with an insulin pump on a long-term basis, it is reasonable to continue the pump at the outpatient basal rate for short procedures in which the patient will be eating postoperatively. If the patient's blood glucose exceeds glycemic targets despite correction doses of insulin, a continuous intravenous insulin infusion should be started and the pump should be disconnected. We recommend consulting an endocrinologist for the perioperative management of patients with insulin pumps.

Patients with type 2 diabetes are a much more heterogeneous group than those with type 1 diabetes. Patients with type 2 disease have varying levels of insulin resistance and endogenous insulin reserve. As a result, the management strategy must be carefully tailored to match the patient's metabolic state and clinical condition. Patients with diet-controlled type 2 diabetes must be monitored for hyperglycemia perioperatively. These patients usually have sufficient endogenous insulin to prevent hyperglycemia while they are NPO.

When the patient is receiving oral diabetic medications, a general approach is to withhold the medication on the day of the surgical procedure. The medication should not be restarted until the patient's clinical situation stabilizes, oral intake has resumed at stable levels, and there are no contraindications to the specific agent. Insulin can be used in the interim to maintain glycemic targets. **For patients with type 2 diabetes who are being treated with long-acting insulin (glargine), the ADA recommends that they receive 50% to 100% of the total scheduled dose** [● *Clement et al, 2004*]. Because these patients may have adequate endogenous insulin reserve when they are NPO, we usually recommend 50% of the dose, to reduce the risk of hypoglycemia. Patients taking an intermediate-acting insulin should receive 50% to 75% of their normal morning dose on the day of the surgical procedure, and any short-acting prandial insulin should be withheld. Finally, patients who take mixed insulin on a long-term basis should receive 50% to 75% of the intermediate-acting component in the form of NPH insulin. For example, a patient taking 20 U of 70/30 insulin is receiving the equivalent of 14 U of NPH and 6 U of regular insulin. On the morning of the surgical procedure, this patient should receive 50% to 75% of the 14 U or 7 to 10 U of NPH. Correction doses of insulin can be used to maintain glycemic targets.

Postoperatively, patients can resume their preoperative insulin regimen if they have resumed stable oral intake. Further adjustment of insulin doses requires close monitoring of blood glucose levels and assessment of the patient's clinical circumstance. A summary of our recommendations can be found in Tables 12-3 and 12-4.

TABLE 12-3	Perioperative Management of Type 2 Diabetes*	
Outpatient Regimen	**Preoperative**	**Postoperative**
Diet controlled	Monitor BG	Monitor BG
	May need correction dose insulin or insulin infusion to obtain glycemic targets	Use correction dose insulin initially if higher than glycemic targets; may need a PO agent to control blood glucose at discharge
Metformin	Start holding the day of surgery	Restart when PO intake stabilizes, renal function is normal, and patient no longer at risk for hypoxia and lactic acidosis
Thiazolidinedione	Start holding the day of surgery	Restart after PO is established; do not restart if fluid overload is an issue; do not use in CHF or hepatic insufficiency
Sulfonylureas and meglitinides	Start holding the day of surgery	Restart after patient stabilized and PO intake resumed in stable amounts
Long-acting insulin	Give 50%–100% of normal basal dose the day of surgery	Continue insulin glargine; adjust dose based on BG
Intermediate-acting insulin	Give 50%–75% of dose the morning of surgery	Can resume basal doses postoperatively if necessary
Mixed insulins	Give 50%–75% of the long-acting component the morning of surgery	Do not resume mixed insulins until patient's condition has stabilized and PO intake is stable
Short-acting insulin	No doses the day of surgery if NPO	Restart when patient is eating; adjust doses based on results of BG monitoring and the amount of carbohydrate consumed
Rapid-acting insulin	No doses the day of surgery if NPO	Restart when patient is eating; adjust doses based on results of BG monitoring and the amount of carbohydrate consumed

*Intravenous insulin infusion is preferred for patients with wide glycemic excursions or a prolonged postoperative NPO period.

BG, blood gas; CHF, congestive heart failure; NPO, nothing by mouth; PO, oral.

TABLE 12-4	Perioperative Management of Patients with Type 1 Diabetes or Type 2 Diabetes with Intensive Insulin Management	

Outpatient Regimen	Day of Surgical Procedure	Postoperative
Insulin pump (Recommend consulting an endocrinologist to assist in management)	SP: Can continue pump at basal rate with frequent blood gas monitoring; can utilize correction boluses for hyperglycemia or stop the pump and start IV insulin infusion LP: IV insulin infusion	Continue insulin drip until patient has stabilized; can then convert back to insulin pump at basal rate; restart prandial boluses when patient resumes eating
LA insulin with SA or RA insulin	SP: Give full dose of the LA insulin in type 1 diabetes and 50% in type 2 diabetes; hold all SA and RA insulin while patient is NPO or utilize IV insulin infusion LP: IV insulin infusion	Continue insulin drip until patient has stabilized; convert back to SQ LA at previous dose if insulin requirement unchanged; if not, calculate new dose based on insulin drip requirement as stated in text; restart SA or RA when patient is eating
IA with SA or RA insulin	SP: Give 50%–75% of normal dose of IA the morning of surgery; hold all SA and RA insulin when NPO or utilize IV insulin infusion LP: IV insulin infusion	Continue insulin drip until patient has stabilized; convert back to SQ IA at previous dose if insulin requirement is unchanged; if not, calculate new dose requirement based on insulin drip rate as stated in text; restart SA or RA when patient is eating
Mixed insulins (Most type 1 diabetic patients do not take these insulins)	SP: Give 50%–75% of normal dose of morning IA component as separate injection of NPH LP: IV insulin infusion	Continue insulin drip until patient has stabilized; convert back to SQ mixed insulin at previous dose if insulin requirement unchanged; if not, calculate new dose requirement based on insulin drip rate as stated in text

IA, intermediate-acting; IV, intravenous; LA, long-acting; LP, long procedure (e.g., major procedure, typically using general anesthesia with duration of anesthesia longer than 2 hours); NPO, nothing by mouth; RA, rapid-acting; SA, short-acting; SP, short procedure (e.g., minor procedure of short duration utilizing limited general, local, epidural, or spinal anesthesia); SQ, subcutaneous.

One of the complications of diabetes management in the inpatient setting is hypoglycemia. This may be a result of decreased oral intake, interruption of tube feedings or parenteral nutrition, and the use of secretagogues or insulin. The correction of hypoglycemia is based on the cause. Adjustments should be made to the diabetic regimen to prevent further episodes of hypoglycemia.

Special Situations

Enteral Tube Feeding

Management of glycemic control for the patient requiring enteral tube feeding is dictated by the manner in which the tube feeding is administered. Continuous 24-hour tube feeding infusions provide the patient with a steady supply of carbohydrate; therefore, insulin needs to be present in a more continuous fashion to prevent hyperglycemia. Several options are available, none of which has been studied in large clinical trials. Basal insulin can be provided by a once-daily injection of long-acting insulin or twice-daily injections of an intermediate-acting insulin. Correction doses of a rapid-acting analogue are used to correct unexpected hyperglycemia. The major concern with this approach is the high risk of hypoglycemia if the tube feeding is interrupted; therefore, the basal insulin should be kept at no more than 40% of the total daily insulin requirement, and the blood glucose should be maintained at the high end of the target range. We prefer to use regular insulin every 6 hours with the addition of correction doses to correct for unexpected hyperglycemia. This offers flexibility and reduces the risk of hypoglycemia if the tube feeding is inadvertently discontinued. If the tube feeding is given during only a portion of the day, an intermediate-acting insulin should be given approximately 1 to 2 hours before the tube feeding is started. For example, if the tube feeding is given from 8 PM to 6 AM the patient would receive a dose of intermediate-acting insulin such as NPH at 6 or 7 PM.

Bolus tube feedings provide the patient with a discrete carbohydrate load; therefore, insulin needs to be provided in manner that optimally prevents postbolus hyperglycemia. The patient should receive rapid-acting insulin 0 to 15 minutes before or short-acting insulin 30 to 45 minutes before each bolus is given. The American College of Endocrinology recommends checking blood glucose 2 hours after giving an insulin bolus to determine the insulin effect. Dose adjustments should be made to keep postbolus blood glucose less than 180 mg/dL. Basal insulin can still be provided with once-daily long-acting or twice-daily intermediate-acting insulin.

Total Parenteral Nutrition

It is not uncommon for surgical patients to receive TPN during the postoperative period. TPN may increase the difficulty of achieving glycemic control. TPN has been shown to cause hyperglycemia in patients without a history of diabetes, and it worsens glycemic control in those with established diabetes. In one study of patients with type 2 diabetes, TPN necessitated the use of insulin in 77% of the patients who previously did not need insulin.

Glycemic targets for patients receiving TPN may be achieved most rapidly by using a separate continuous intravenous insulin infusion. Once glycemic control is obtained, the new total 24-hour insulin requirement can be calculated; 60% to 80% of this dose can be added to the next day's TPN, and the separate insulin infusion can be discontinued after the TPN is started. An alternative strategy for those with less dramatic hyperglycemia is to take 60% to 80% of the total subcutaneous insulin dose from the previous day and add that to the TPN bag in the form of regular insulin. Supplemental doses of insulin to correct for hyperglycemia should be continued every 4 to 6 hours. If frequent supplemental doses are used, the total supplemental dose should be added to the next day's TPN bag.

The Patient Receiving High-Dose Glucocorticoids

High-dose glucocorticoids can be problematic in the hospitalized patient because they affect carbohydrate metabolism and can lead to hyperglycemia. This effect worsens glycemic control in diabetic patients and can cause glucocorticoid-induced diabetes in patients without previously diagnosed diabetes. If the patient experiences wide glycemic excursions after high-dose steroids are instituted, a continuous insulin infusion should be used to obtain glycemic control. Once control is achieved, a new total daily insulin requirement can be calculated and apportioned among the basal, nutritional, and supplemental doses of subcutaneous insulin. Insulin requirements will be reduced as the steroid dose is tapered. Glucocorticoids often cause a blood glucose peak 4 to 12 hours after the dose is given. This delayed peak can be counteracted by giving intermediate-acting insulin with the steroid dose. Finally, alternate-day dosing of glucocorticoids may require only supplemental insulin on the days that they are given.

CORTICOSTEROIDS AND ADRENAL INSUFFICIENCY

Glucocorticoids play a vital role in the maintenance and regulation of immune and circulatory functions. The hypothalamic-pituitary axis (HPA) regulates adrenal release of glucocorticoids. Hypothalamic release of corticotropin-releasing hormone stimulates the pituitary to produce adrenocorticotropin hormone (corticotropin [ACTH]). ACTH, in turn, acts on the adrenal cortex to stimulate the synthesis and release of cortisol, which completes the cycle by exerting a negative feedback on corticotropin-releasing hormone and ACTH release. Most recent studies estimate glucocorticoid secretion to be approximately 8 to 12 mg/m^2/day of cortisol (the equivalent of 20 mg/day of hydrocortisone or 5 mg/day of oral prednisone), which is less than previously reported. Glucocorticoid levels exhibit diurnal variation, with a peak level occurring between 4 and 8 AM and minimal production during the evening. Synthesis of cortisol can increase five- to tenfold under conditions of severe stress, to a maximal level of approximately 100 mg/m^2/day [Jabbour, 2001]. Surgery is a well-studied physiologic stress that activates the HPA axis and results in increased ACTH and cortisol.

The most common cause of suppressed adrenal function is the use of exogenous steroids for a prolonged period of time. These agents can suppress the HPA axis; therefore, the patient who takes these drugs may not produce sufficient levels of ACTH and cortisol during physical or psychologic stress. If unrecognized or untreated, this condition can manifest as hypotension and shock with fatal consequences. To prevent this life-threatening complication, stress-dose steroids are given perioperatively to patients with documented or presumed HPA axis suppression.

Who Needs Stress-Dose Steroids?

Before initiating stress-dose glucocorticoid therapy in patients undergoing surgical procedures, physicians should screen patients who are suspected to have adrenal insufficiency. These patients can often be identified by taking a thorough history and physical examination, especially focusing on their medication history and the presence of other chronic illnesses. Illnesses associated with the long-term use of steroids include asthma, chronic bronchitis, rheumatoid arthritis, collagen vascular diseases, and inflammatory bowel disease; organ transplant recipients and patients who have had brain or spinal surgery are also at risk. Rarely, patients may also develop adrenal suppression from the use of topical corticosteroids for dermatologic disorders. This is more likely when the glucocorticoids are of higher potency, applied to large skin surface areas, and covered with occlusive dressings. Adrenal suppression may also occasionally occur with the use of potent inhaled glucocorticoids.

No well-established relationship exists among dose, duration of exogenous steroids, and suppression of the HPA axis. In general, oral glucocorticoids equivalent to 5 mg of prednisone or less given in a single morning dose for any duration of time, and any dose of glucocorticoids given for less than 3 weeks, do not cause clinically significant suppression of the HPA axis. Alternate-day glucocorticoids given in a morning dose produce less suppression of the HPA axis. Conversely, multiple daily doses or doses given in the evening tend to cause more HPA suppression. Table 12-5 shows the different available glucocorticoid preparations and their equivalencies.

Conversely, any patient who has taken more than 20 mg/day of prednisone or its equivalent for more than 3 weeks or who is clinically cushingoid should be assumed to have suppression of the HPA axis. Such patients do not need testing to evaluate the HPA axis and should be treated with stress doses of steroids perioperatively. Postoperatively, the patient will need to remain on replacement-dose steroids because it may take as long as 9 to 18 months for adrenal function to recover. Therefore, the response to provocative testing (i.e., cosyntropin stimulation test) generally normalizes 9 months or more after withdrawal from glucocorticoid therapy.

Patients receiving intermediate doses of steroids (between 5 and 20 mg of prednisone daily), or patients who are not

TABLE 12-5	Glucocorticoid Equivalencies	
Glucocorticoids	Equivalent Dose (mg)	Biologic Half-Life (hr)
Hydrocortisone (Cortef, Solu-Cortef)	20	8–12
Cortisone (Cortone)	25	8–12
Prednisone (Deltasone)	5	18–36
Methylprednisolone (Medrol, Solu-Medrol)	4	18–36
Dexamethasone (Decadron)	0.5	36–54

good historians about their glucocorticoid dose or duration of treatment, can be assessed by dynamic HPA axis testing. Cosyntropin (synthetic ACTH) stimulation testing assesses the ability of the adrenal gland to accelerate production of cortisol in response to a surge in ACTH levels. The test is performed as follows: Baseline cortisol levels are drawn, and then 0.25 mg of cosyntropin is administered intramuscularly or intravenously. Cortisol levels are repeated at 30 minutes and again at 60 minutes interval after the dose. Cortisol levels are expected to increase to more than 18 to 20 µg/dL after the stimulation test in nonstressed individuals [Oelkas, 1996]. Critically ill patients are expected to have higher cortisol levels (>25 µg/dL). Many experts believe that 0.25 mg of cosyntropin results in a supraphysiologic response of the adrenal and may miss subclinical or partial adrenal insufficiency. They favor using 1 µg of cosyntropin instead of 0.25 mg to assess the HPA axis. This recommendation has not gained widespread acceptance because it is cumbersome to make such a concentration from the original vial provided by the manufacturer. In the interpretation of either test, one should be aware of the cross-reactivity between all glucocorticoids (except dexamethasone) and the cortisol assay that may result in falsely high cortisol values. These agents should be held for at least 24 hours before the cosyntropin stimulation test is performed. Glucocorticoid coverage can continue during this time period by using dexamethasone.

Which Dose and Steroid Regimen to Use?

If a patient has documented or presumed HPA axis suppression, stress-dose steroids should be given before the surgical procedure. **Clinicians should replace glucocorticoids only in amounts equivalent to the normal physiologic response to the anticipated surgical procedure [◉ *Salem et al, 1994*].** Normally, the increase in ACTH and cortisol release starts with induction of anesthesia. Cortisol production remains elevated for approximately 2 days postoperatively and loses its normal diurnal variation. Thereafter, cortisol levels generally decline to the normal range and resume a diurnal pattern. Investigators have reported that up to 200 to 500 mg/day of cortisol can be secreted by the human body, depending on the severity of stress [Jabbour, 2001], although rates exceeding more than 200 mg are rare in the 24 hours after a surgical procedure. The following recommendations may serve as a guideline to estimate the patient's need for steroid coverage:

1. For minor surgical stress such as inguinal hernia repair, hand surgery, or any minor outpatient procedures, 100 mg of hydrocortisone is given intravenously with the induction of anesthesia, followed by the usual maintenance dose.

2. For major surgical stress such as cardiac surgery and neurosurgery, 100 mg of intravenous hydrocortisone is given before the induction of anesthesia and is continued at the same dose every 8 hours for at least the first 24 hours. When the major stress of the postoperative period is resolved, and the patient is stable and free of complications (fever, vomiting), hydrocortisone can be tapered during 3 to 5 days to the usual maintenance dose. Table 12-6 provides an example of a tapering schedule.

TABLE 12-6	Postoperative Steroid Tapering Regimen
Postoperative Day	**Recommendation**
Day 1	Hydrocortisone, 100 mg IV q8h, starting with induction of anesthesia
Day 2	If patient stable and major postoperative stress resolved, lower dose of hydrocortisone to 50 mg q8h
Day 3	Hydrocortisone, 25 mg q8h
Day 4	Hydrocortisone, 25 mg bid
Day 5	Maintenance dose (12–15 mg hydrocortisone/m²/day): 15–20 mg AM and 5–10 mg PM OR Switch to prednisone 5 mg every morning
bid, twice daily; IV, intravenously.	

In patients who have primary adrenal insufficiency (e.g., adrenal gland destruction by antibodies, infection, metastasis, hemorrhage), a mineralocorticoid (e.g., fludrocortisone, 0.1 mg/day) should be added to the maintenance regimen. There is no need to give patients fludrocortisone while they are receiving stress doses of steroids because hydrocortisone at doses more than 100 mg/day has a mineralocorticoid effect. In patients with secondary adrenal insufficiency, only glucocorticoids are necessary because mineralocorticoid secretion is normal.

HYPOTHYROIDISM

The most common cause of hypothyroidism in the United States is chronic autoimmune thyroiditis (Hashimoto's thyroiditis), which causes destruction of the thyroid gland. Other causes of primary hypothyroidism include surgical removal, treatment with radioactive iodine, drugs, or infiltration and replacement of the gland by tumor. Secondary hypothyroidism can be caused by pituitary and hypothalamic diseases. Patients classically present with fatigue, weight gain, constipation, cold intolerance, dyslipidemia, depression, and dry skin. Laboratory evaluation shows an elevated thyroid-stimulating hormone (TSH) concentration in primary hypothyroidism.

Myxedema coma is an extreme expression of hypothyroidism. It is characterized by coma, loss of deep tendon reflexes, cardiovascular collapse, and even death. This clinical presentation is frequently accompanied by hypothermia, hypoxia, hyponatremia, and hypoglycemia. It occurs mostly during or after the sixth decade, and 80% of the cases occur in women. More than 90% of cases have been reported to occur during winter months and are frequently associated with intercurrent illness or stressors such as burns, trauma, and nonthyroid surgery. Other common precipitating factors include pneumonia, other infections, and sedating drugs.

Approximately 50% of patients with myxedema coma have lapsed into coma after admission to the hospital, probably as the result of stress caused by diagnostic and therapeutic interventions encountered during hospitalization. Although mortality can be high, these abnormalities are reversible with thyroid hormone replacement therapy.

The impact of hypothyroidism on general surgery outcomes is unclear. Although some reports indicate that hypothyroidism increases the risk of perioperative complications and poor outcome, others do not. Because several studies suggested that hypothyroidism may increase anesthesia risk, we recommend that the hypothyroid patient be rendered euthyroid before an elective surgical procedure is performed.

Perioperative Management

Hypothyroid patients undergoing nonthyroid surgery can be broadly grouped into the following categories, based on their clinical and biochemical profiles:

1. Most patients with hypothyroidism on replacement therapy are euthyroid (clinically and biochemically) at the time of surgery. Euthyroidism can be confirmed by a normal TSH level. In patients with central hypothyroidism (reduced circulating thyroid hormone as a result of inadequate stimulation of a normal thyroid gland by TSH, which may be secondary to pituitary disease or tertiary resulting from hypothalamic dysfunction), TSH levels are not representative of thyroid function, and free thyroxine (T_4) should be obtained. Such euthyroid patients do not carry an increased risk of perioperative morbidity and do not require special treatment other than continuation of their usual thyroid hormone replacement. Most of these patients can take their replacement dose on the day of the operation, although it is optional because the half-life of T_4 is 6 to 7 days. During the postoperative period, patients can be given levothyroxine (LT_4) treatment orally or

intravenously on a regular basis. In the case of intravenous administration, 80% of the oral dose is given because almost 80% of orally administered LT_4 is absorbed in the proximal small intestine. If the patient is NPO and intravenous LT_4 is not available, one can easily skip the dose for several days because of the long half-life. Very few indications exist today for the use of triiodothyronine (T_3) treatment (myxedema coma and patients with thyroid cancer in preparation for radioactive iodine treatment). T_3 has a very short half-life (1.5 days); therefore, it may be necessary for patients to receive their usual dose on the day of the surgical procedure. In contrast to T_4, almost 100% of an oral dose of T_3 is absorbed.

2. Patients who are biochemically hypothyroid are at increased risk of having complications during the perioperative period [● *Mercado, 2003*]. Perioperative morbidity in these patients relates to cardiovascular depression refractory to catecholamine administration, hypothermia, airway difficulties from generalized edema, aspiration from delayed gastric emptying, and depressed mental status. Elective surgery in these patients should be postponed until patients are rendered euthyroid. Urgent surgery should not be postponed, but the patient should be managed expectantly for the complications described earlier.

3. The most challenging area involves the role of preoperative thyroid hormone replacement in patients undergoing coronary artery revascularization surgery. Investigators have reported that thyroid replacement therapy has induced myocardial ischemia. Therefore, it is prudent to operate before replacement therapy is started or after only partial replacement has begun. The dose can be slowly titrated upward after coronary artery blood flow has improved.

4. Patients with myxedema coma may be treated with either 200 to 400 μg of intravenous LT_4, followed by 50 to 100 μg daily. Concomitantly, 10 μg of intravenous T_3 every 8 hours

can be given to speed recovery. **Coexisting adrenal insufficiency in patients with severe hypothyroidism should be an important consideration because treatment of hypothyroidism without providing steroid replacement may precipitate adrenal crisis** [● *Mercado, 2003*]. Therefore, stress-dose steroids should be provided to these patients until adrenal insufficiency has been excluded. Other treatment points include rewarming with a warming blanket and correction of hyponatremia, hypovolemia, and hypoglycemia.

HYPERTHYROIDISM

Hyperthyroidism has many causes, the most common being Graves' disease. This is an autoimmune disorder in which TSH receptor antibodies abnormally stimulate the thyroid gland to produce excessive thyroid hormone. Other causes of hyperthyroidism include toxic multinodular goiters, toxic nodules, thyroiditis, and exogenous ingestion of LT_4.

Hyperthyroidism may be clinically overt, and patients may present with classic symptoms such as tachycardia, tremor, weight loss, heat intolerance, goiter, and ophthalmopathy. However, patients may also present in an atypical fashion. This presentation is known as apathetic or "masked" hyperthyroidism and is more common in the geriatric population. These patients may be asymptomatic, or they may complain only of fatigue. Occasionally, they present in atrial fibrillation without any other symptoms.

Laboratory investigation reveals a suppressed TSH with a high free T_4 or free T_3 concentration. Patients may also have subclinical hyperthyroidism, which is defined by a suppressed TSH but normal free T_4 and free T_3. Subclinical hyperthyroidism can manifest by increased nocturnal pulse rates, frequent atrial premature beats, or the onset of atrial fibrillation in elderly patients.

The greatest risk to undiagnosed or inadequately treated hyperthyroid patients undergoing surgery is thyroid storm, a rare but life-threatening complication. Thyroid storm is recognized by the onset of fever, tachycardia, delirium, and gastrointestinal disturbances that may progress to cardiovascular collapse and death. It is advisable to treat the patient based on clinical suspicion alone while waiting for confirmatory thyroid function tests. The laboratory value itself does not distinguish between usual hyperthyroidism and thyroid storm.

Patients with untreated or inadequately treated hyperthyroidism who are undergoing a major surgical procedure are at increased risk of perioperative complications, the most concerning being thyroid storm (fever, tachycardia, cardiovascular collapse). Excess T_4 and T_3 can cause extra heat production that leads to a slight rise in body temperature, which, in turn, activates heat-dissipating mechanisms. Perioperative tachycardia is common, and atrial fibrillation is present in 10% to 20% of patients. Hyperthyroid patients should be clinically and biochemically euthyroid before they undergo surgical procedures.

Perioperative Management

1. For an elective surgical procedure, patients with medically treated and adequately controlled hyperthyroidism should take their antithyroid medications on the morning of surgery. It is common for TSH values to remain suppressed as a result of prolonged hyperthyroidism in patients who have otherwise normalized their free T_4 and T_3 values on therapy. The TSH level in such cases will eventually increase (within few months) and should not be considered a contraindication to surgery.

2. If possible, patients with uncontrolled hyperthyroidism should have their surgical procedure postponed until they receive adequate medical therapy to reduce the risk of thyroid storm.

3. If a patient needs emergency surgery, therapy to block the systemic effect of excess thyroid hormone as well as agents to decrease thyroid hormone production may be started by administering β-blockers, antithyroid medication (thionamides) such as propylthiouracil (PTU) or methimazole (Tapazole), and iodine. Thionamides block thyroid hormone synthesis but do not affect the release of the preformed hormone. Iodine is the earliest effective agent used in the preoperative preparation of thyrotoxic patients. In supraphysiologic doses, iodine acts to decrease the synthesis of new thyroid hormone (the Wolff-Chaikoff effect) and to decrease the release of preformed hormones from the thyroid. This effect can be seen within 24 hours of iodine treatment and is maximal at approximately 10 days of treatment. Iodine should not be administered first, because supplemental iodine provides more substrate for thyroid hormone synthesis. This can result in an increased amount of thyroid hormone released from the thyroid gland and can potentially precipitate thyroid storm (the jod-basedow effect). This effect is mainly seen in patients with toxic nodules. One should wait at least 1 hour after administering the thionamide before initiating iodine therapy. Propylthiouracil may be administered as a loading dose of 1 g orally or by nasogastric tube and later followed by a dose of 150 to 200 mg orally or by nasogastric tube every 6 to 8 hours. Saturated solution of potassium iodide (SSKI) is the iodine most commonly used. It is given as oral drops in a dose of 4 to 8 drops every 6 to 8 hours. Patients with thyrotoxicosis are also at risk for adrenal insufficiency (coexistent Graves' disease and Addison's disease) and should receive stress doses of glucocorticoids. Moreover, glucocorticoids decrease the peripheral conversion of T_4 to T_3. For symptomatic treatment, propranolol has been the β-blocker of choice at doses of 10 to 40 mg four

times a day. However, cardioselective β-blockers can be used, especially in patients with asthma. Preoperative use of long-acting β-blockers such as atenolol confers a better heart rate control in the postoperative period.

4. Treatment of thyroid storm includes the administration of thionamides, iodines, steroids, β-blockers, antipyretics, nutritional support with dextrose and vitamins, and treatment of cardiac complications such as atrial fibrillation and high-output heart failure. This therapy should occur in a setting where continuous cardiac monitoring is available. Aspirin should not be used as an antipyretic agent in patients with thyroid storm, because it interferes with the protein binding of T_4 and T_3 and can increase free thyroid hormone concentrations. Methods to enhance thyroid hormone clearance may also be used, including cholestyramine to bind the hormone and clear it through the gastrointestinal tract. Rarely, charcoal hemoperfusion, hemodialysis, or plasmapheresis may be needed to increase thyroid hormone clearance.

EUTHYROID SICK SYNDROME

Thyroid function tests are notoriously difficult to interpret in patients who are chronically or critically ill. Many of these patients are receiving medications that may interfere with the results of thyroid function tests. For example, dopamine, dobutamine, and high-dose corticosteroids can suppress TSH. One of the more common thyroid function abnormalities encountered in critically ill patients is termed the *euthyroid sick syndrome* (low T_4, T_3, and TSH). These patients are thought to be euthyroid; however, some studies suggest that they may have acquired, transient central hypothyroidism. Treatment with LT_4 in these patients is of little benefit and in fact may be harmful. It is thought that these thyroid function changes may be protective by preventing excessive tissue catabolism.

Characteristic thyroid function alterations in the euthyroid sick syndrome are as follows:

- Low serum total T_3 resulting from decreased conversion of T_4 to T_3 by circulating inhibitors (e.g., free fatty acids, cytokines) or decreased binding of T_3 to thyroid binding globulin (TBG) or both
- Elevated reverse T_3 (rT_3) because conversion of T_4 to T_3 is reduced, leading to more conversion of T_4 to rT_3
- Low serum total T_4, because of decreased binding to TBG and reduction in the serum concentration of TBG and other binding proteins
- High uptake of T_3-resin and low to normal free T_4 index (calculated free T_4)
- Normal or low free T_4 as measured by most laboratories, but normal free T_4 measured by dialysis equilibrium
- Normal or low TSH, depending on the severity of sickness
- During recovery from sickness, transient rise in TSH (up to 20 mU/L) before TSH, T_4, and T_3 return to normal

PHEOCHROMOCYTOMA

Pheochromocytoma is an uncommon neuroendocrine tumor of the chromaffin cells that occurs in less than 0.2% of patients with hypertension. In approximately 10% of patients, the tumor is discovered incidentally during computed tomography or magnetic resonance imaging of the abdomen for unrelated symptoms. The classic triad of symptoms in patients with pheochromocytoma consists of episodic headache, sweating, and tachycardia, accompanied by paroxysmal hypertension. The presence of this triad has a sensitivity and specificity of more than 90%, although not all patients have the three classic symptoms, and patients with essential hypertension may present with similar symptoms. The diagnosis is made by detecting significantly elevated urinary metanephrines or catecholamines (24-hour urine collection). Alternatively, plasma free metanephrines can be measured, although false-positive results are common. Testing should always be done after interfering medications (tricyclic antidepressants, benzodiazepines, labetalol, sotalol) have been discontinued. **When urine or serum metanephrine or catecholamine levels suggest the presence of pheochromocytoma, the diagnosis is further established by magnetic resonance imaging of the adrenal glands, to localize the tumor** [◉ *Pacak et al, 2001*].

Perioperative Management

Patients with pheochromocytoma have excessive circulating catecholamines causing vasoconstriction that leads to both hypertension and hypovolemia. These patients may experience severe hypertensive crisis or hypotension. Removal of a pheochromocytoma can result in acute hypotension as a result of a sudden decrease in catecholamines. Therefore, the perioperative management of pheochromocytoma requires vital cooperation of multispecialty teams to avoid any preoperative, intraoperative, or postoperative complications. The goal of perioperative management is to minimize the risk of clinically significant hypertension or hypotension in the perioperative period. α**-Adrenergic blockers are initiated 10 to 14 days preoperatively to inhibit the peripheral vasoconstriction produced by pheochromocytoma-released catecholamines. Another approach is to treat the patient preoperatively with calcium channel antagonists to control hypertension and to use intraoperative nitroprusside for treatment of significant hypertension** [◉ *Ulchaker et al, 1999*]. Perioperatively, intravenous hydration with 0.9% saline is also essential to prevent hypovolemic shock and hypotension (mainly after removal of the tumor).

PITUITARY DISEASES

The perioperative management of patients with pituitary disease is complex and varies depending on the underlying disease. Therefore, an endocrinologist with expertise in pituitary disorders should be involved in the perioperative management of these patients. Key management concepts include the following:

- Patients who have a macroadenoma (>1 cm) can suffer from mass effect by tumor compression of adjacent structures, such as the optic chiasm; therefore, formal visual field testing should be performed preoperatively.
- Patients with macroadenomas should be screened for hypopituitarism, particularly central hypothyroidism (low free T_4 with low to normal TSH) and central adrenal insufficiency (low cortisol, either random morning value or after cosyntropin stimulation testing with low to normal ACTH). Replacement therapy with glucocorticoids and LT_4 should be initiated while waiting for the surgical procedure to be performed. Glucocorticoids should always be started before LT_4 therapy to prevent the onset of adrenal crisis.
- For pituitary surgery, glucocorticoids should be given perioperatively because normal ACTH-secreting cells can be damaged perioperatively, thus leading to adrenal insufficiency. Glucocorticoids are then tapered over a few days to a maintenance dose (e.g., prednisone, 5 mg/day), and the HPA axis is reassessed in 3 months by performing a cosyntropin stimulation test. The reason we wait 3 months is that it takes a few weeks to a few months for the adrenals to atrophy and therefore to lose their response to cosyntropin.
- Transient or permanent diabetes insipidus may occur perioperatively. Moreover, during the second postoperative week, a transient phase of syndrome of inappropriate antidiuretic hormone can result from release of stored antidiuretic hormone. This syndrome may cause clinically

significant hyponatremia. Careful assessment of the patient's volume status and frequent monitoring of serum electrolytes are essential.

- Patients with panhypopituitarism of whatever cause should always continue glucocorticoid therapy. Stress doses may need to be administered based on the level of expected stress and the patient's clinical condition. These patients should also continue to receive LT_4 therapy. TSH is useless for monitoring therapy in patients with central hypothyroidism; therefore, free T_4 should be followed to monitor adequacy of replacement.

CALCIUM DISORDERS

Calcium is essential to homeostasis and the function of multiple organ systems. It should be strictly maintained in the normal range before, during, and after surgical procedures. Abnormalities in calcium metabolism are mostly secondary to parathyroid disease, but they may be a harbinger of other underlying conditions, such as neoplasia or granulomatous diseases. Management strategies depend on the severity of clinical symptoms and the urgency of the underlying medical conditions. Patients who require urgent surgery can be taken to the operating room with careful intraoperative and postoperative monitoring, and calcium concentrations can be maintained with medical management. Elective surgery can be deferred until workup of the calcium derangement is complete. Rarely, patients require intensive care management secondary to cardiac arrhythmias.

HYPERCALCEMIA

The most common causes of hypercalcemia are hyperparathyroidism and malignancy. In malignant disease, mechanisms of hypercalcemia include parathyroid hormone (PTH)-related peptide-secreting neoplasms, $1,25(OH)_2D$-secreting lymphomas, and local osteolysis from bone metastasis. Other causes of hypercalcemia include milk-alkali syndrome, granulomatous diseases, and medications such as thiazide diuretics, lithium, and vitamins D and A.

Hypercalcemia affects multiple organ systems and leads to myriad clinical signs and symptoms. Most patients with hypercalcemia become symptomatic at the level of 12 mg/mL, and almost all patients at the level of 14 mg/mL or higher. Gastrointestinal symptoms result from smooth muscle relaxation and include constipation, anorexia, nausea, and vomiting. Increased calcium concentrations also have been shown to cause pancreatitis. Neurologically, patients with hypercalcemia can be lethargic, hypotonic, confused, or even comatose. Effects on the kidneys include polyuria, dehydration, and nephrolithiasis. Dehydration leads to proximal tubule resorption of sodium and calcium in an effort to expand the extracellular volume, but this paradoxically worsens hypercalcemia.

Hypercalcemia also affects cardiac conduction. Patients with elevated calcium concentrations have electrocardiographic changes marked by shortened QTc intervals. Cardiac arrhythmias and conduction problems generally are not associated with this phenomenon.

Diagnosis

Establishing the correct diagnosis is the essential first step in the treatment of hypercalcemia. A careful history and physical examination will often help to identify the underlying cause. Measurement of calcium and intracellular PTH will differentiate all causes of hypercalcemia into two main categories, PTH mediated and non–PTH mediated (malignancy and other causes). The presence of elevated calcium and PTH invariably establishes the diagnosis of primary hyperparathyroidism. Plasma $1,25(OH)_2D$ should be measured when sarcoidosis, other granulomatous disorders, and $1,25(OH)_2D$-secreting lymphomas are considered in the differential diagnosis.

Perioperative Management

Any management of hypercalcemia should be directed at the underlying pathophysiologic mechanism. The goal is to lower the serum calcium to a safe level. An assessment of the severity of the hypercalcemia is needed to guide therapy. Although there are no formal guidelines, a serum calcium level of 10.5 to 11.9 mg/dL (2.6 to 2.9 mmol/L) is regarded as mild hypercalcemia, a level of 12.0 to 13.9 mg/dL (3.0 to 3.4 mmol/L) is moderate, and severe hypercalcemia is a level of 14.0 mg/dL (3.5 mmol/L) or greater [Stewart, 2005].

Intravenous Fluids

Patients with moderate to severe hypercalcemia may be substantially dehydrated as a result of a renal water-concentrating defect (nephrogenic diabetes insipidus) induced by hypercalcemia and by decreased oral hydration resulting from anorexia, nausea, or vomiting. The dehydration leads to a reduction in the glomerular filtration rate that further reduces the ability of the kidney to excrete the excess serum calcium. Therefore, volume expansion should be the first goal of treatment. Although no randomized clinical trials have been conducted to guide this therapy, in general practice normal saline is administered at a rate of 200 to 500 mL/hour, depending on the baseline level of dehydration and renal function, the patient's cardiovascular status, the degree of mental impairment, and the severity of the hypercalcemia. Patients should have careful clinical monitoring for physical findings that are consistent with fluid overload.

Medications

1. Loop diuretics are used to increase the renal excretion of calcium. They should not be administered until after full hydration has been achieved because they can cause or worsen dehydration. Dehydration, in turn, leads to a decline in the glomerular filtration rate and the filtered load of calcium.

2. Intravenous bisphosphonates are by far the best studied, safest, and most effective agents for use in patients with hypercalcemia of any cause, especially for hypercalcemia of malignancy. These drugs work by blocking osteoclastic bone resorption. Bisphosphonate therapy should be initiated as soon as hypercalcemia is diagnosed, because a response requires 2 to 4 days, and the nadir in serum calcium generally occurs within 4 to 7 days after therapy is initiated. Approximately 60% to 90% of patients have normal serum calcium levels within 4 to 7 days, and responses last for 1 to 3 weeks. As compared with pamidronate, zoledronate has the advantage of rapid and simpler administration, whereas pamidronate is less expensive.

3. Glucocorticoids [Binstock and Mundy, 1980] have a role in the treatment of some patients, such as those with lymphomas resulting in elevated levels of $1,25(OH)_2$ vitamin D.

4. Calcitonin may result in a more rapid reduction in serum calcium levels than do other agents (the maximal response occurs ≤ 12 to 24 hours), but its value is questionable because the reductions are small (≤ 1.0 mg/dL [0.25 mmol/L]) and transient.

A review of the commonly used treatments is provided in Table 12-7.

Dialysis

In patients who have acute or chronic renal failure, aggressive saline infusion is not possible, and other therapies such as bisphosphonates should be used with caution, if at all. In these circumstances, dialysis against a dialysate containing little or no calcium is a reasonable and highly effective option for selected patients.

TABLE 12-7	Commonly Used Treatments for Hypercalcemia			
Intervention	Dose	Onset of Action	Calcium Response	Cautions
Intravenous fluids	200–500 mL/hr	Hours	Decreases by 1–3 mg/dL	Watch for fluid overload
Loop diuretics	20–40 mg	Hours	Decreases by 1–3 mg/dL	Give only after patient has been adequately hydrated.
Zoledronic acid	4 mg IV	1–3 days	Normalizes in 90% of patients	Can cause renal failure and flulike symptoms
Pamidronate	60–90 mg IV	1–3 days	Normalizes in 70% of patients	Can cause renal failure and flulike symptoms
Calcitonin	4–8 IU SQ or IM q12h	12–24 hr	Decreases by 1–2 mg/dL	May cause flushing and nausea

IM, intramuscularly; IV, intravenously; SQ, subcutaneously.

HYPOCALCEMIA

Hypocalcemia is common in older patients with multiple chronic illnesses. Common causes include idiopathic or auto-immune hypoparathyroidism, hypomagnesemia, vitamin D deficiency, acute pancreatitis, hyperventilation, and hypoparathyroidism from previous surgery or radiation to the neck. Before instituting any treatment for hypocalcemia, the diagnosis should always be verified, because many cases of hypocalcemia are the artifact of hypoalbuminemia. Management aimed at correcting calcium concentrations depends on the severity of the patient's symptoms. If symptoms are mild, oral calcium supplementation can be given; otherwise, intravenous calcium should be administered.

Patients with long-standing hypocalcemia may be asymptomatic. In acute hypocalcemia, the patient may present with perioral numbness, paresthesias, muscle cramps, and mild mental status changes such as irritability. As hypocalcemia becomes more severe, there can be neuromuscular and cardiac findings, including Chvostek's sign (elicited by tapping the facial nerve anterior to the ear, which produces spasm of the muscles of the face; it has been shown to be positive in 10% to 30% of people with normal calcium concentrations) and Trousseau's sign (positive when pressure on the wrist induced by inflation of a blood pressure cuff for 3 to 5 minutes or tapping on the median nerve induces carpal spasm), as well as mental status changes, seizures, tetany, hypotension, and acute heart failure.

Acute hypocalcemia decreases cardiac function by lengthening phase 2 of the cardiac action potential, which results in prolongation of the ST segment and the QT interval on the electrocardiogram. This finding is an independent risk factor for arrhythmias and cardiac death. Patients who present to the hospital in cardiac arrest often are severely hypocalcemic. Hypocalcemia can rarely lead to cardiac failure, and this can be reversed with administration of calcium.

Perioperative Management

Treatment should be given to every symptomatic patient and to patients with serum calcium of less than 7.6 mg/dL who may be at risk of developing complications. In general, symptomatic patients should be given parenteral calcium, whereas asymptomatic patients can be managed with oral calcium supplementation as follows:

1. Intravenous calcium: Calcium gluconate, 10 mL 10% weight/volume (90 mg of calcium) diluted in 50 mL of 5% dextrose or 0.9% sodium chloride can be given intravenously by slow injection (5 to 10 minutes) and can be repeated as necessary until symptoms disappear. If deemed necessary, a continuous infusion can be started by diluting 10 ampules of calcium gluconate in 1 L of 5% dextrose or normal saline at a rate of 50 mL/hour. The goal is to keep serum calcium in the low normal range. In the setting of hypocalcemia, one should always anticipate simultaneous abnormalities in magnesium concentrations because intravenous magnesium administration may be necessary to achieve normalization of calcium concentrations.

2. Oral calcium: Different calcium supplements are available on the market. The patient can be given 400 to 800 mg of elemental calcium every 8 to 12 hours. The goal is to keep the patient asymptomatic and to avoid any complications associated with hypercalciuria, especially in the absence of PTH or its function.

3. Vitamin D: In the setting of severe 25-hydroxyvitamin D deficiency, ergocalciferol (vitamin D_2) 50,000 U (every week for 8 weeks) can be given without any risk of toxicity. Patients with mild or moderate deficiency should receive 800 to 1200 IU/day of cholecalciferol (vitamin D_3). Serum calcium and urine calcium should be initially checked on a weekly basis and then at least every 6 months to ensure stabilization.

4. Use of thiazide diuretics in therapeutic doses is helpful especially when the hypocalcemia is secondary to hypoparathyroidism because thiazides enhance reabsorption of calcium from the kidney.

Selected Readings

American College of Endocrinology: Position statement on inpatient diabetes and metabolic control. Endocr Pract 10:5-9, 2004.

American Diabetes Association: Clinical practice recommendations 2005. Diabetes Care 28(Suppl 1):S24-S28, 2005.

Axelrod L: Perioperative management of patients treated with glucocorticoids. Endocrinol Metab Clin North Am 32:367-383, 2003.

Binstock ML, Mundy GR: Effect of calcitonin and glutocorticoids in combination on the hypercalcemia of malignancy. Ann Intern Med 93:269-272, 1980.

Bode BW, Braithwaite SS, Steed RD, et al: Intravenous insulin infusion therapy: Indications, methods, and transition to subcutaneous insulin therapy. Endocr Pract 10(Suppl 2):71-80, 2004. Ⓐ

Clement S, Braithwaite S, Magee MF, et al: Management of diabetes and hyperglycemia in hospitals. Diabetes Care 27:553-591, 2004. Ⓒ

Connery LE, Coursin DB: Assessment and therapy of selected endocrine disorders. Anesthesiol Clin North Am 22:93-123, 2004.

Furnary AP, Wu Y, Bookin SO: Effect of hyperglycemia and continuous intravenous insulin infusions on outcomes of cardiac surgical procedures: The Portland Diabetes Project. Endocr Pract 10(Suppl 2):21-33, 2004.

Glister B, Vigersky R: Perioperative management of type 1 diabetes mellitus. Endocrinol Metab Clin North Am 32:411-436, 2003.

Jabbour SA: Steroids and surgical patients. Med Clin North Am 85:1140-1147, 2001.

Krinsley JS: Effect of an intensive glucose management protocol on the mortality of critically ill adult patients. Mayo Clin Proc 79:992-1000, 2004.

Mercado DL: Perioperative medication management. Med Clin North Am 87:41-57, 2003. Ⓒ

Oelkas W: Adrenal insufficiency. N Engl J Med 335:1206-1212, 1996.

Pacak K, Linehan WM, Eisenhofer G, et al: Recent advances in genetics, diagnosis, localization, and treatment of pheochromocytoma. Ann Intern Med 134:315-329, 2001. Ⓒ

Salem M, Tainsh RE, Bromberg J, et al: Perioperative glucocorticoid coverage: A reassessment 42 years after emergence of a problem. Ann Surg 219:416-425, 1994. Ⓒ

Schiff RL, Welsh GA: Perioperative evaluation and management of the patient with endocrine dysfunction. Med Clin North Am 87:175-192, 2003.

Sherman SI, Ladenson PW: Complications of surgery in hypothyroid patients. Am J Med 90:367-370, 1991.

Stewart AF: Hypercalcemia associated with cancer. N Engl J Med 352:373-379, 2005.

Ulchaker JC, Goldfarb DA, Bravo EL, et al: Successful outcomes in pheochromocytoma surgery in the modern era. J Urol 161:764-767, 1999. ●

Umpierrez GE, Isaacs SD, Bazargan N, et al: Hyperglycemia: An independent marker of in-hospital mortality in patients with undiagnosed diabetes. J Clin Endocrinol Metab 87:978-982, 2002.

Van den Berghe G, Wouters P, Weekers F, et al: Intensive insulin therapy in critically ill patients. N Engl J Med 345:1359-1367, 2001. ●

Van den Berghe G: How does blood glucose control with insulin save lives in intensive care? J Clin Invest 114:1187-1195, 2004.

Vance ML: Perioperative management of patients undergoing pituitary surgery. Endocrinol Metab Clin North Am 32:355-365, 2003.

13 Perioperative Management of the Ophthalmologic Patient

MARVIN E. GOZUM, MD

Ophthalmic surgery is safer than general surgery. Early studies estimated ophthalmic surgery mortality anywhere from 0.06% to 0.18%, with the variations resulting from the type of ophthalmic surgical procedure and the anesthetic regimen. More recent surveys continued to reinforce that ophthalmic surgery is safe. Unstable medical disorders remain a principal cause of postoperative complications. Today, most ophthalmic procedures are performed in physicians' offices, outpatient surgical centers, and, less commonly, in-hospital settings.

When postoperative complications occur following ophthalmic surgical procedures, medical conditions are commonly at fault, whether from system medications in anesthesia, intubation, fluid load, or stresses caused by unresolved postoperative pain. Rarely, complications result from the systemic effects of topical eye drop medications or from systemic issues related to the globe.

This chapter focuses on two points: (1) perioperative consultations that establish a patient's suitability for surgery by identifying preexisting and new diseases, defining risk factors, and offering advice concerning risk reduction methods; and (2) postoperative care of the patient's chronic medical problems as well as any systemic complications occurring during or after the surgical procedure.

Levels of Evidence:

🅐—Randomized controlled trials (RCTs), meta-analyses, well-designed systematic reviews of RCTs. 🅑—Case-control or cohort studies, nonrandomized clinical trials, systematic reviews of studies other than RCTs, cross-sectional studies, retrospective studies. 🅒—Consensus statements, expert guidelines, usual practice, opinion.

RISK OF OPHTHALMIC SURGERY

Petruscak and associates evaluated the risk associated with more than 3000 ophthalmic procedures performed in the late 1960s and early 1970s. The most important risk factor contributing to the deaths of patients undergoing ophthalmic surgical procedures was the patient's preexisting medical condition [❻ *Petruscak et al, 1973*]. Mortality was found to correlate well with the American Society of Anesthesiologists risk classification. Quigley evaluated postoperative morbidity among 47,000 cases and found that the type of surgical procedure was related to a risk of untoward complications. Retinal detachment repair was associated with a small but significantly higher risk of mortality (0.23%) than cataract (0.1%) or muscle (0.01%) operations [❻ *Quigley, 1974*]. More recent studies continued to reinforce the general safety of various ophthalmic procedures relative to general surgery to within similar percentages [❻ *Adler and Kountz, 1990;* ❽ *Katz et al, 2001*].

PREOPERATIVE EVALUATION

Cardiovascular Risk Stratification

Patients should be evaluated in the same manner as general surgical patients, and all medical conditions should be optimally controlled. Perioperative cardiovascular risk is estimated by using criteria developed by the American Society of Anesthesiologists or the American College of Cardiology/American Heart Association.

Unless specified, ophthalmic procedures are often performed in the outpatient setting, in which advanced medical services are sparse or unavailable. Patients at moderate cardiovascular risk should preferably have procedures performed in facilities with advanced medical support, whereas patients at high cardiovascular risk should be considered for overnight inpatient hospitalization.

It is the consultant's job to estimate and recommend intervention for medical conditions that could complicate surgical procedures. With a patient's medical risks in mind, it is the anesthesiologist's or surgeon's role to decide whether to proceed with a procedure, but it is the patient who lives with the outcome. Rarely is ophthalmic surgery lifesaving, but optimal vision may weigh heavily on a patient's reason for being. Some procedures such as those of the retina or glaucoma are sight saving within a limited time frame, whereas cataract surgery can be postponed without disability. Therefore, in patients with optimally managed but high-risk medical disease, it is important to convey the possible outcomes to patients and to coordinate the patients' wishes with the objectives of the surgical team.

Preoperative Laboratory Testing

Cataract surgery remains the most common ophthalmic operation. **No evidence indicates that routine medical testing before cataract surgery increases the safety of the procedure** [◉ *Schein et al, 2000*]. For the patient with specific medical conditions, laboratory tests may be indicated, based on the patient's medical condition and its surgical impact. For example, patients with diabetes mellitus should have perioperative serum glucose monitoring by finger stick glucometer until they are allowed to eat postoperatively. Specific protocols for patients with diabetes mellitus can be followed, as discussed later.

For all other ophthalmic procedures, the need for preoperative laboratory testing is proportionate to coexisting medical disease, the likelihood of receiving general anesthesia, and intravenous or systemic medications. As a rule, the same evaluations may be ordered as for general surgical procedures.

PERIOPERATIVE ANTICOAGULANTS

Patients undergoing cataract surgery do not need to discontinue antiplatelet agents or reverse therapeutic anticoagulation [❽ *Dunn and Turpie, 2003*]. In general, antiplatelet agents and therapeutic anticoagulation need not be discontinued for most ophthalmic procedures. However, small amounts of bleeding can reduce surgical outcome considerably. Antiplatelet agents are preferably discontinued if the patient has no coexisting diseases requiring antiplatelet therapy, such as in the healthy geriatric patient taking daily aspirin. Warfarin is safely discontinued only in patients receiving prophylactic anticoagulation, such as in atrial fibrillation with no history of embolic stroke; otherwise, these patients should be therapeutically anticoagulated preoperatively. Surgeons will then make specific requests, on a case-by-case basis, to hold anticoagulation based on the type of procedure or a prior history of bleeding [❷ *Parkin and Manners, 2000*]. Patients who require that therapeutic anticoagulation be reversed may need intravenous unfractionated heparin or subcutaneous low-molecular-weight heparin to maintain anticoagulation while warfarin is discontinued.

OPHTHALMIC MEDICATIONS

A review of the topical ocular medications received by patients is part of the differential diagnosis when postoperative complications are evaluated. Eye drops may enter the nasolacrimal duct and may be systemically absorbed through the nasal mucosa or the gastrointestinal tract. β-Blockers can cause bradycardia (especially in the patient with cardiac conduction disease), bronchospasm, or congestive heart failure. Sympathomimetic agents and atropine cause tachycardia and aggravate underlying coronary artery disease. Summaries of the most common ophthalmic medications and their complications are given in Tables 13-1 and 13-2. The consultant

TABLE 13-1	Common Ophthalmic Drugs	
Trade Drug Class	**Name**	**Generic Name**
Eye Drops		
Nonselective β-blockers	Timoptic	Timolol
β$_1$-Specific β-blockers	Betoptic	Betaxolol
	Betagan	Levobunolol
Sympathomimetic agents	Propine	Dipivefrin
		Epinephrine
		Phenylephrine
Parasympathomimetic agents		Pilocarpine
		Carbachol
Anticholinergic agents	Mydriacyl	Tropicamide
	Cyclogyl	Cyclopentolate
		Scopolamine
		Homatropine
		Atropine
Diuretics Used for Ophthalmic Treatment		
Carbonic anhydrase inhibitors	Diamox	Acetazolamide
		Methazolamide
Osmotic diuretics		Intravenous mannitol 20% solution

TABLE 13-2	Systemic Complications of Eye Drops
Common Systemic Complications	**Implicated Drugs**
Congestive heart failure	β-Blockers, osmotic diuretics
Bradycardia	β-Blockers
Tachycardia	Sympathomimetic agents, anticholinergic agents
Hypotension	β-Blockers
Bronchospasm	β-Blockers (less with β$_1$-selective β-blockers and parasympathomimetic agents)
Skin flushing	Atropine
Depression, confusion	Anticholinergic agents, β-blockers, CAIs
Paresthesias	CAIs
Nausea, vomiting	CAIs, parasympathomimetic agents
Hyperglycemia	Glycerol
Metabolic acidosis	CAIs
Hypokalemia	CAIs
Urinary retention	Anticholinergic agents, osmotic diuretics
CAIs, carbonic anhydrase inhibitors.	Metabolic acidosis, electrolyte imbalance

should consider withholding diuretics in patients taking carbonic anhydrase inhibitors.

Sodium fluorescein is used in diagnostic fluorescein angiography of the fundus. This imaging study is as common an ophthalmic procedure as cataract surgery. Patients may experience allergic reactions similar to contrast dye reactions seen with conventional radiologic procedures. Common symptoms include nausea (occurring in 7% of patients) and urticaria (0.5% of patients). Severe reactions include wheezing, anaphylaxis, and arrhythmias.

TYPE OF ANESTHETIC

The final decision regarding the use of general or local anesthesia resides with the anesthesiologist and the surgeon. From a technical standpoint, general anesthesia offers greater immobilization of the patient and better surgical control. General anesthesia may offer benefits to patients who are unduly anxious, restless, or suffering from specific conditions (e.g., osteoarthritis) that prohibit lying comfortably in a supine position. Although data suggest that local anesthesia is equivalent to general anesthesia in terms of the risk of complications, the design of this research may have been flawed because sicker patients may have been selected to receive local anesthesia. No large-scale series have been repeated. A commonly held belief is that local anesthesia is safer for patients with borderline pulmonary status or those who have heart, liver, or kidney disease and who are susceptible to problems related to mechanical ventilation or anesthetics. In addition, blood pressure shifts are more likely with general anesthesia.

ANTIBIOTIC PROPHYLAXIS

The use of systemic antibiotic prophylaxis for patients at risk for endocarditis remains undefined. The eye is a sterile organ, and manipulation is unlikely to cause bacteremia. In

severe ocular infections such as endophthalmitis, procedures performed in infected or contaminated operative
fields or ruptured globes, or cases requiring general anesthesia, the possibility of bacteremia is plausible. In these cases,
I generally follow the recommendations of the American
Heart Association for patients at risk for endocarditis. Endocarditis prophylaxis typically is not required for cataract
surgery.

COMMON MEDICAL DISORDERS

In my more than 18 years of evaluating patients for ophthalmic procedures, I estimate that approximately 70% of patients
have had one or more of the following diseases: diabetes mellitus, hypertension, and coronary artery disease. Thus, most
common postoperative complications include severe hyperglycemia, diabetic ketosis, hypertension requiring urgent care
or emergency treatment, and unstable angina to myocardial
infarction. Mortality within 4 weeks postoperatively is rare.
The likelihood of morbidity is proportionate to the severity of
coexisting medical disease, however, and morbidity often occurs within the first 24 hours postoperatively.

COMMON PROBLEMS IN OPHTHALMIC SURGERY

Postoperative Nausea and Vomiting

Nausea and vomiting are common postoperatively, but these
problems are multifactorial and may be caused by, in order of
frequency: anesthesia, rising intraocular pressure, and, rarely,
in diabetic patients, impending ketoacidosis.

Postoperative Confusion

The evaluation of postoperative confusion should proceed as
in any patient with mental status changes. Especially among
geriatric patients, common causes are, in order of frequency:

anesthetic medication, systemic effects of anticholinergic eye drops, and cerebrovascular events.

Postoperative Bradycardia

Postoperative bradycardia is a physiologic reflex that produces a decrease in heart rate secondary to the vagotonic effects of traction on the extraocular muscles or pressure on the eye. This arrhythmia is more common in children. The oculocardiac reflex can result in asystole or arrhythmias, and this reflex should be kept in mind if a patient experiences intraoperative bradycardia. The consultant should evaluate the possibility of other reversible causes (such as β-blocker eye drops) while observing the patient. The effects of the reflex should resolve within several hours if the bradycardia has no other cause. Other arrhythmias may be triggered by perioperative drugs or undiagnosed coronary artery disease and should be managed and evaluated similarly to any new-onset arrhythmia.

Dehydration or Electrolyte Imbalance

Dehydration or electrolyte imbalance may be caused by the use of carbonic anhydrase inhibitors or osmotic diuretics in concert with a patient's existing diuretic regimen. When diuretics cannot be discontinued, close attention to electrolytes is warranted.

Metabolic Acidosis

Carbonic anhydrase inhibitors produce non–anion gap acidosis that is usually marked after the first few days of starting one of these drugs. This condition is often compensated and of little clinical concern.

Urinary Retention

Male patients who experience symptomatic urinary retention following ophthalmic surgical procedures often have some form of prostate disease. In patients with prostate disease, diuretics of all types should be used with caution.

High-Dose Corticosteroids

Patients who receive high-dose corticosteroids are at risk for steroid-related complications, most commonly glucose intolerance, gastritis, hypertension, and mental status changes. Patients receiving corticosteroids for more than 3 to 4 weeks should be considered for preoperative stress doses.

I recommend that patients receiving high-dose corticosteroids be evaluated with daily serum finger glucose checks

TABLE 13-3	Diabetes Mellitus	

Hold all insulin and oral agents* on operative day
Check fasting serum glucose level with electrolyte panel
Sliding scale insulin as follows:

Initial Fasting Serum Glucose Levels	Notes	Intravenous Fluid Administration
>400 mg/dL	Defer surgery until serum glucose is controlled	None until ~<300 mg/dL
>350 mg/dL	Give full AM long-acting insulin dose preoperatively; repeat q1h glucose checks and fast-acting insulin: 10 U Humulin Regular or Humalog insulin SC, until serum glucose <300 mg/dL	D₅W to run 50 mL/hr or keep vein open
200-350 mg/dL	Give two thirds of AM long-acting insulin dose preoperatively and 4 U Humulin Regular or Humalog insulin	D₅W to run 100 mL/hr preoperatively
100-200 mg/dL	Give two thirds of AM long-acting insulin dose preoperatively	D₅W to run 100 mL/hr preoperatively
>80 mg/dL	Give one half of AM long-acting insulin dose preoperatively	D₅W to run 100 mL/hr preoperatively
<80 mg/dL	Hold all forms of insulin; if serum glucose does not rise within 1 hr, consider deferring surgery	D₁₀W to run 100 mL/hr preoperatively

*Most oral hypoglycemic agents have half-lives in excess of 24 hours. Patients taking oral agents follow the same protocol for insulin coverage and intravenous fluids but *do not* receive long-acting insulin. Check all postoperative serum glucose levels. Check serum glucose levels every 4 hours until the time of operation.

D₅W, 5% dextrose in water; D₁₀W, 10% dextrose in water; SC, subcutaneously.

and alternate-day electrolyte determinations. Histamine (H_2)-blocker protection is started as prophylaxis against steroid-induced gastritis. In rare patients at risk for tuberculosis, a baseline chest radiograph should be obtained before steroids are initiated. If hyperglycemia accompanies corticosteroid use, appropriate diabetes management should be undertaken. Hyperglycemia frequently resolves as the corticosteroid doses are tapered.

Diabetes Mellitus and Glucose Management

The brief duration of most ophthalmic surgical procedures usually prevents severe derangement of diabetic glycemic control. For more than 10 years, I have used the simple protocol outlined in Table 13-3. In practice, Humulin Regular or Humalog administration or equivalent sliding scale insulin may be substituted for a patient's particular sensitivity for a sliding scale.

Selected Readings

Adler AG, Kountz DS: Eye surgery in the elderly. Clin Geriatr Med 6: 659-667, 1990. **C**

Bass EB, Steinberg EP, Luthra R, et al: Do ophthalmologists, anesthesiologists, and internists agree about preoperative testing in healthy patients undergoing cataract surgery? Arch Ophthalmol 113:1248-1256, 1995. **C**

Britman NA: Cardiac effects of topical timolol. N Engl J Med 300:562, 1979. **C**

Cavallini GM, Saccarola P, D'Amico R, et al: Impact of preoperative testing on ophthalmologic and systemic outcomes in cataract surgery. Eur J Ophthalmol 14:369-374, 2004. **A**

Dunn AS, Turpie AG: Perioperative management of patients receiving oral anticoagulants: A systematic review. Arch Intern Med 163:901-908, 2003. **B**

Hall DL, Steen WH, Drummond JW: Anticoagulants and eye surgery. Ann Ophthalmol 12:759, 1980. **C**

Katz J, Feldman MA, Bass EB, et al: Study of Medical Testing for Cataract Surgery Study Team: Adverse intraoperative medical events and their association with anesthesia management strategies in cataract surgery. Ophthalmology 108:1721-1726, 2001. **B**

Lama PJ: Systemic adverse effects of beta-adrenergic blockers: An evidence-based assessment. Am J Ophthalmol 134:749-760, 2002. **B**

Norregaard JC, Bernth-Petersen P, Bellan L, et al: Intraoperative clinical practice and risk of early complications after cataract extraction in the United States, Canada, Denmark, and Spain. Ophthalmology 106: 42-48, 1999. **B**

Parkin B, Manners R: Aspirin and warfarin therapy in oculoplastic surgery. Br J Ophthalmol 84:1426-1427, 2000. **C**

Petruscak J, Smith RB, Breslin P: Mortality related to ophthalmological surgery. Arch Ophthalmol 89:106,1973. **B**

Quigley HA: Mortailty associated with ophthalmic surgery: A twenty year experience at the Wilmer Institute. Am J Ophthalmol 77:517-524, 1974. **B**

Saitoh AK, Saitoh A, Taniguchi H, Amemiya T: Anticoagulation therapy and ocular surgery. Ophthalmic Surg Lasers 29:909-915, 1998. **B**

Schein OD, Katz J, Bass EB, et al: The value of routine preoperative medical testing before cataract surgery: Study of Medical Testing for Cataract Surgery. N Engl J Med 342:168-175, 2000. **A**

Vander Zanden JA, Valuck RJ, Bunch CL, et al: Systemic adverse effects of ophthalmic beta-blockers. Ann Pharmacother 35:1633-1637, 2001. **B**

Yannuzzi L, Rohrer K, Tindel L, et al: Fluorescein angiography complication survey. Ophthalmology 93:611-617, 1986. **C**

14 | Nonobstetric Surgery in the Pregnant Patient

BARBARA KNIGHT, MD
JANINE V. KYRILLOS, MD

Up to 2% of pregnancies are complicated by the need for nonobstetric surgical procedures, and more than 75,000 pregnant patients in the United States require surgery during their pregnancy each year. Most of these surgical procedures are performed to treat conditions that commonly occur in this age group such as traumatic injuries, appendicitis, cholecystitis, and breast masses. However, even major procedures such as craniotomy, cardiopulmonary bypass, and liver transplantation are occasionally indicated in the pregnant patient and usually result in good outcomes for mother and fetus. Newer and more efficient imaging can decrease the number of unnecessary surgical procedures; however, safer and more advanced techniques such as minimally invasive surgery can also increase the number of lower-risk procedures.

Clinicians caring for the pregnant patient must take several additional variables into account in the perioperative period. It is important to consider the perioperative needs of two patients, both the mother and the fetus. Evidence has indicated that exposure to anesthesia may lead to lower-birthweight babies. The adaptive anatomy and physiology in the mother may alter the presentation of common surgical conditions and may cause considerable difficulty in the diagnosis of

---

Levels of Evidence:

Ⓐ—Randomized controlled trials (RCTs), meta-analyses, well-designed systematic reviews of RCTs. **Ⓑ**—Case-control or cohort studies, nonrandomized controlled trials, systematic reviews of studies other than RCTs, cross-sectional studies, retrospective studies. **Ⓒ**—Consensus statements, expert guidelines, usual practice, opinion.

disorders requiring surgical intervention. There is often reluctance to obtain radiographs and to perform other diagnostic tests during pregnancy because of the potential risks to the fetus. This unwillingness may lead to delays in diagnosis and treatment of the underlying disease. Although pregnancy itself does not increase surgical maternal mortality, the often delayed interventions associated with pregnancy may lead to more complex surgical procedures, as well as intraoperative and postoperative problems for both mother and fetus.

ANATOMIC AND PHYSIOLOGIC CHANGES DURING PREGNANCY

An understanding of the physiologic and anatomic changes that occur during pregnancy is essential for the medical consultant. Much of the difficulty in diagnosing intra-abdominal disorders during pregnancy stems from changes in abdominal landmarks as the pregnancy progresses, as well as from the physiologic and laboratory changes normally seen during pregnancy (Tables 14-1 and 14-2). This section describes the major changes in pregnancy by system.

Hematologic Changes

Beginning in the first trimester and reaching a plateau at 34 weeks, blood volume significantly increases in the pregnant patient. The average increase in blood volume is 40% to 50%, with a range of a 20% to 100% increase based on the patient's size and parity. Because of the significant increase in blood volume, the pregnant patient can sustain substantial blood loss before manifesting the physical findings of tachycardia and hypotension. The rise in blood volume is a result of increases in plasma volume and red blood cell mass. Plasma volume increases more than red blood cell mass, and this situation causes *physiologic anemia of pregnancy,* which results in a decrease of hematocrit by 3% to 4% (but not below 30).

TABLE 14-1	Cardiac Changes in Normal Pregnancy That May Mimic Heart Disease

Symptoms

Reduced exercise tolerance
Dyspnea

Signs

Peripheral edema
Distended neck veins
Point of maximal impulse displaced laterally

Auscultation

Increased splitting of first and second heart sounds
Third heart sound (S_3 gallop)
Systolic ejection murmur along left sternal border

Chest Radiography

Straightening of left heart border
Heart position more horizontal
Increased cardiothoracic ratio
Increased pulmonary vascular markings

Electrocardiogram

15-beat elevation in heart rate
Flat or inverted T wave in leads III, V_1, and V_2
Q waves in leads III and aVF
15-degree left axis deviation (without hypertrophy)

Leukocyte counts also increase during pregnancy (see Table 14-2). Normal white blood cell counts in pregnancy range from 5000 to 12,000/mm³, with counts up to 16,000 in the third trimester. White blood cell counts as high as 25,000 to 30,000/mm³ can occur during labor. This finding can pose a problem when evaluating the patient for infection or inflammation.

Discrepancy exists over the effects of pregnancy on platelet counts. Although early studies suggested an increase in platelet counts, more recent studies demonstrated a slight decrease in platelet counts resulting from increased platelet destruction.

Clotting factors I (fibrinogen), VII, VIII, IX, and X are all increased during pregnancy and elevate the risk of thromboembolic disease (see Table 14-6). Although prothrombin

TABLE 14-2	Summary of Laboratory Changes in Pregnancy		
Laboratory Test	**Normal Range**	**Pregnancy Effect**	**Gestational Timing**
Sodium	135–145 mEq/L	Lowered 2–4 mEq/L	By midpregnancy
Potassium	3.5–4.5 mEq/L	Lowered 0.2–0.3 mEq/L	By midpregnancy
Creatinine	0.6–1.1 mg/dL	Lowered 0.3 mg/dL	By midpregnancy
Creatinine phosphokinase	26–140 U/L	Raised two- to fourfold	After labor (MB bands also)
Glucose (fasting)	65–105 mg/dL	Lowered 10%	Gradual fall
Fibrinogen	200–400 mg/dL	Raised 600 mg/dL	By term
Urea nitrogen	12–30 mg/dL	Lowered 50%	First trimester
Hematocrit	36%–46%	Lowered 4%–7%	Nadir at 30–34 wk
Hemoglobin	12–16 g/dL	Lowered 1.4–2.0 g/dL	Nadir at 30–34 wk
Leukocyte count	4000–10,000/mm^3	Raised 3500/mm^3	Gradual increase to term ($\leq$25,000/mm^3 in labor)
Platelets	150,000/mm^3	400,000/mm^3	Slight decrease

Adapted from Barclay ML: Critical physiologic alterations in pregnancy. *In* Pearlman MD, Tintinalli JE (eds): Emergency Care of the Woman. New York, McGraw-Hill, 1998, pp 303-312.[1]

time and partial thromboplastin time values decrease slightly, they remain within the normal prepregnancy range.

Cardiovascular Changes

Because the diaphragm is elevated, the heart is displaced to the left and upward. This change results in apparent enlargement of the cardiac silhouette on chest radiography and straightening of the left heart border. Electrocardiographic changes can also occur with a left axis shift, positional Q waves in leads III and aVF, and nonspecific ST segment/T-wave abnormalities.

Cardiac output increases 30% to 50% over nonpregnant levels as a result of increased stroke volume and heart rate. Systemic vascular resistance decreases, thus reducing diastolic blood pressure and mean arterial pressure by 5 to 10 mm Hg, and reaches a nadir at 16 to 20 weeks. Cardiac output is affected by maternal position. In the supine position, the enlarged uterus puts pressure on the vena cava and the aorta. Compression of the vena cava can lead to a 10% to 30% decrease in cardiac output. Therefore, whenever possible, the supine position should be avoided in the perioperative period. Beyond the first trimester, maternal hypotension and subsequent decreased uteroplacental perfusion can be avoided by placing a wedge under the right hip or tilting the operating table 15 degrees to the left.

Many of the normal cardiovascular changes in pregnancy can be mistaken for primary cardiovascular disease or congestive heart failure including mild tachycardia, jugular venous distention, peripheral edema, and a laterally displaced point of maximal impulse (see Table 14-1). As many as 80% to 90% of pregnant women have a third heart sound. Systolic ejection murmurs (<grade III) are heard in 96% of pregnancies, and diastolic murmurs, although much less common, can be heard in 18% of normal pregnancies (Fig. 14-1).

Pulmonary Changes

As pregnancy progresses and the uterus enlarges, the diaphragm is elevated by as much as 4 cm, and the ribs flare outward. This change causes a slight decrease in total lung capacity, although vital capacity is unchanged, and a 20% reduction in functional residual capacity. These anatomic alterations increase the risk of postoperative atelectasis, and the patient should be instructed on deep breathing exercises.

Minute ventilation increases by as much as 50% during pregnancy as a result of elevated tidal volume. The increase in minute ventilation leads to the hyperventilation (or dyspnea) of pregnancy, which produces mild respiratory alkalosis with compensatory metabolic acidosis. Normal blood gas values in pregnancy are a pH of 7.4 to 7.47, a partial pressure of arterial carbon dioxide (Pa_{CO_2}) of 30 to 32 mm Hg, and a normal to slightly elevated partial pressure of arterial oxygen (Pa_{O_2}). Serum bicarbonate values remain between 18 and 21 mEq/L. Therefore, a Pa_{CO_2} of 40 mm Hg can represent hypoventilation in the pregnant patient and a risk

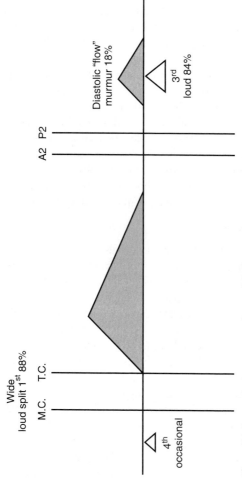

Figure 14-1 • Findings on auscultation of the heart in pregnancy. A_2 and P_2, aortic and pulmonary elements of the second heart sound; M.C., mitral closure; T.C., tricuspid closure. *(From Gabbe SG, Niebyl JR, Simpson JL [eds]: Obstetrics: Normal and Problem Pregnancies, 4th ed. New York, Churchill Livingstone, 2001.)*

of fetal hypoxia. The hyperventilation of pregnancy causes the pregnant patient to complain frequently of shortness of breath, dyspnea on exertion, or "air hunger."

Gastrointestinal Changes

Much of the problem in diagnosing intra-abdominal disorders in pregnant women stems from changes in abdominal landmarks as the pregnancy progresses, as well as from the physiologic changes normally seen in pregnancy. By the second trimester, the intestines and omentum are displaced superiorly and laterally by the expanding uterus, thereby making the gastrointestinal tract more vulnerable to penetrating injuries and the omentum less able to contain areas of peritonitis. The anterior abdominal wall is also elevated so that underlying inflammation is less likely to manifest with usual symptoms of peritoneal irritation.

Smooth muscle relaxing effects of elevated levels of progesterone and decreased levels of motilin cause delayed gastric emptying and decreased intestinal transit times. Delayed gastric emptying and relaxation of the lower esophageal sphincter lead to an increased risk of acid reflux and aspiration. Aspiration can be associated with chemical pneumonitis and superimposed bacterial pneumonia; therefore, patients should be given nonparticulate antacids (e.g., 30 mL sodium citrate) before induction of general anesthesia. If the surgical procedure is elective, adequate time should be given to allow for gastric emptying. Liver function tests remain normal, with the exception of elevated levels of alkaline phosphatase to two to four times normal values during the third trimester.

Renal Changes

The glomerular filtration rate increases during pregnancy by 50%, and the serum concentration of creatinine and blood urea nitrogen are proportionally decreased. Plasma levels of creatinine greater than 0.8 mg/100 mL and blood urea nitrogen greater than 14 mg/100 mL may indicate renal impairment. The increased glomerular filtration rate may cause medications to be excreted more rapidly, thus necessitating close monitoring of serum drug levels.

Dilation of the collecting system begins as early as the first trimester and causes hydronephrosis and hydroureter. This dilatation results in urinary stasis and asymptomatic bacteriuria, which increases the risk of urinary tract infections during pregnancy. Unnecessary urinary catheterization and the placement of Foley catheters should be avoided, to prevent the introduction of bacteria into the bladder.

Proteinuria does not change during pregnancy; 200 to 300 mg/24 hours are normally excreted. Urinary protein losses greater than 300 mg/24 hours suggest a disease process. Glucosuria is normal during pregnancy in more than 50% of women, but the patient should be monitored closely for signs and symptoms of diabetes.

GENERAL CONSIDERATIONS

Timing of Surgery

Timing of nonurgent surgical procedures is an important consideration in the pregnant patient to minimize the risk of complications. Common complications of surgery in this population include bleeding, aortocaval compression syndrome, delayed healing, infection, dehiscence, spontaneous abortion, preterm labor, and fetal morbidity. Because the most active phase of organogenesis occurs between 6 and 13 weeks' gestation, the fetus is most susceptible to teratogenic effects or spontaneous abortion at this time. Anesthesia is generally avoided during this trimester if at all possible. Furthermore, although no anesthetic agent has been linked specifically to premature labor, uterine manipulation, intra-abdominal infection, and decreased uteroplacental blood flow and oxygen delivery are predisposing factors to premature labor and delivery, especially in the advanced stages of gestation. Most surgeons try to avoid third trimester procedures. **For these reasons, surgery and anesthesia are thought to be safest during the second trimester** [⊙ *Goodman, 2002*].

Imaging

There is always concern about the use of radiologic studies during pregnancy, and this is the source of great anxiety to the pregnant patient. Used properly, diagnostic imaging is usually harmless to the fetus, and knowledge about the risks of exposure will help to allay fears and to ensure proper use (Table 14-3). Most single diagnostic radiologic procedures have shown no measurable increased risk for fetal harm. However, cumulative doses or exposure to therapeutic or prolonged fluoroscopic examinations may cause significant risk for miscarriage, fetal malformation, or mental impairment. Care should

TABLE 14-3	Fetal Radiation Dose from Common Diagnostic Radiologic Examinations	
Examination	Mean (mGy) Dose	Maximum (mGy) Dose
Abdomen CT*	8.0	49
Abdomen radiograph	1.4	4.2
Barium enema	6.8	24
Barium swallow	1.1	5.8
Chest CT scan*	0.06	1.0
Chest radiograph	<0.01	<0.01
Head CT scan*	<0.005	<0.005
Intravenous urogram; lumbar spine radiograph	1.7	10
Pelvis CT scan*	25	80
Pelvis radiograph	1.1	4
Skull/thoracic spine radiograph	<0.01	<0.01

*Doses are higher in newer spiral or multicut CT scans.
CT, computed tomography.
Data from the International Commission on Radiological Protection, United Kingdom, 1998. Publication 84. Copyright 1999, 2000, 2003, Annals of the International Commission on Radiological Protection.

be taken to establish the pregnancy status of all childbearing women before any radiologic procedure is performed. It is important to consult the radiologist to determine the most appropriate diagnostic test to minimize unnecessary exposure. It is often possible to find similar information using magnetic resonance imaging or ultrasound.

The risk of radiation injury depends on the stage of pregnancy and the dose of exposure. During organogenesis from weeks 3 through 8, the risk of malformation is increased, and from weeks 8 to 15 and later, the risk of cognitive impairment and mental retardation is increased (Table 14-4). The International Commission on Radiological Protection recommends, if medically prudent, confining radiologic procedures to women of childbearing age to the first 10 days after the beginning of menstruation, to avoid accidental radiation exposure. The unit of measure for the actual absorbed radiation dose is called a Gray (Gy; 100 mGy = 100 mrad). It is estimated that doses higher than 100 mGy can cause a decreased intelligence quotient (IQ), and doses greater than 1000 mGy may result in severe mental retardation and microcephaly. Exposure can be minimized with proper shielding and restricting examination to specific body parts.

In 1977, the National Council on Radiation Protection and Measurements recommended maintaining a total cumulative dose at a maximum of 50 mGy because the potential for fetal harm is negligible at this dose when compared with other risks of pregnancy. The Council also reported that the risk of malformations is substantially increased above control levels only at doses higher than 150 mGy. Table 14-5 gives risk estimates for cancer from prenatal radiation exposure.

Anesthesia

Anesthesia remains a significant cause of maternal mortality. **Failed intubation and pulmonary aspiration of gastric contents remain the two leading causes of maternal mortality associated with anesthesia** [● *Goodman, 2002*]. Pregnant

TABLE 14-4 Potential Health Effects (Other Than Cancer) of Prenatal Radiation Exposure

Radiation Dose to the Embryo/Fetus	Blastogenesis (≤2 wk)	Organogenesis		Fetogenesis	
		TIME POST CONCEPTION			
		(2–7 wk)	(8–15 wk)	(16–25 wk)	(26–38 wk)
<50 mGy	Noncancer health effects NOT detectable		Growth retardation possible	Noncancer health effects unlikely	
50–500 mGy	Incidence of failure to implant may increase slightly, but surviving embryos will probably have no significant (noncancer) health effects	Incidence of major malformations may increase slightly Growth retardation possible	Reduction in IQ possible (≤15 points, depending on dose) Incidence of severe mental retardation ≤20%, depending on dose		
>500 mGy	High risk of failure to implant but surviving embryos will probably have no significant (noncancer) health effects	Increased risk of miscarriage Substantial risk of major malformations such as neurologic and motor deficiencies Growth retardation likely	Depending on dose, increased risk of: Miscarriage Growth retardation Reduction in IQ (>15 points) Incidence of severe mental retardation >20% Incidence of major malformations	Depending on dose, increased risk of: Miscarriage Growth retardation Reduction in IQ (>15 points) Incidence of severe mental retardation >20% Incidence of major malformations	Incidence of miscarriage and neonatal death will probably increase depending on dose

Adapted from Centers for Disease Control and Prevention (CDC): Prenatal Radiation Exposure: A Fact Sheet for Physicians by the CDC. Available at http://www bt.cdc.gov/radiation/prenatalphysician.asp

TABLE 14-5	Estimated Risk for Cancer from Prenatal Radiation Exposure	
Radiation Dose	**Estimated Childhood Cancer Incidence*†**	**Estimated Lifetime‡ Cancer Incidence§ (exposure at age 10 yr)**
Background radiation exposure only	0.3%	38%
<50 mGy	0.3%–1%	38%–40%
50–500 mGy	1%–6%	40%–55%
>500 mGy	>6%	>55%

*Data published by the International Commission on Radiation Protection.
†Childhood cancer mortality is roughly half of childhood cancer incidence.
‡The lifetime cancer risks from prenatal radiation exposure are not yet known. The lifetime risk estimates given are for Japanese men who were exposed at age 10 years, from models published by the United Nations Scientific Committee on the Effects of Atomic Radiation.
§Lifetime cancer mortality is roughly one third of lifetime cancer incidence.
Centers for Disease Control and Prevention (CDC): Prenatal Radiation Exposure: A Fact Sheet for Physicians by the CDC. Available at http://www.bt.cdc.gov/radiation/prenatalphysician.asp

women are at increased risk for failed intubation when compared with nonpregnant patients because of the normal weight gain of pregnancy as well as airway mucosal edema and breast enlargement. The most important safeguard against aspiration is skillful intubation while cricoid pressure is applied. Without doubt, the major risks of anesthesia for the fetus are intraoperative maternal hypoxia, hypotension, and acidosis. **There is little support for the use of one anesthetic agent over another with regard to the risk of abortion, prematurity, or congenital malformations, as long as maternal hypoxia, hypotension, and acidosis are avoided** [◉ *Mazze and Kallen, 1989*]. Spinal and epidural anesthetic techniques are not without risk during pregnancy and may produce vasodilation with a subsequent decrease in uteroplacental blood flow that leads to fetal hypoxia.

Pulmonary aspiration of gastric contents is a major cause of morbidity in the pregnant patient undergoing general anesthesia because of the decreased competence of the lower esophageal sphincter. Beyond midpregnancy, all pregnant women should be considered to be at risk for a "full stomach," regardless of the interval since the last meal. The use of oral clear liquid antacids (Bicitra) or sodium citrate, administered 10 minutes before the induction of anesthesia, can be useful in buffering stomach acid and attenuating the risk of pulmonary irritation if aspiration occurs.

Risk of Thromboembolism

It is well established that pregnancy alone increases the risk of thromboembolic disease (Fig. 14-2 and Table 14-6). This factor further predisposes the pregnant patient to thromboembolism in addition to the already known perioperative

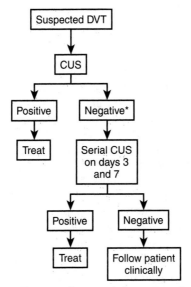

Figure 14-2 • Diagnosis of suspected deep venous thrombosis (DVT) during pregnancy. *, Consider contrast leg venography, computed tomography, or magnetic resonance imaging if isolated iliac vein thrombosis is suspected; CUS, compression ultrasound. *(From Chan WS, Ginsberg JS: Diagnosis of deep vein thrombosis and pulmonary embolism in pregnancy. Thromb Res 107:85-91, 2002.)*

TABLE 14-6	Changes in Clotting Factors with Pregnancy
Factor	**Change with Pregnancy**
I	↑150%
II	↔/↑
V	↔
VII	↑ 120%–200%
VIII	↑ 100%–300%
IX	Slight ↑
X	↑ 120%
XI	Slight ↓
XIII	Slight ↓
Plasminogen	↓
Fibrinopeptide A	↑
Fibrin monomers	↑

↓ decreased; ↑ increased; ↔ no change.
From Mercer BM, Garner P: Thrombophlebitis. *In* Gleicher N (ed): Principles and Practice of Medical Therapy in Pregnancy. Norwalk, CT, Appleton & Lange, 1992, pp 1284-1296.

risks. Therefore, during the perioperative period, thromboembolism prophylaxis is indicated for patients undergoing surgical procedures. **Heparin, 5000 U every 12 hours, is considered effective in average-risk patients** [◉ *Jilma et al, 2003*]. The clinical diagnosis of deep venous thrombosis (DVT) and pulmonary embolism (PE) is difficult during pregnancy because leg edema and dyspnea are common throughout the gestational period. Because the history and physical examination are at best 50% reliable, noninvasive or invasive testing is indicated when patients have acute onset of lower extremity swelling and tenderness. Duplex ultrasonography is a sensitive and specific test for proximal DVT involving the femoral and popliteal veins. If the test is initially negative, it may be repeated serially. Although venography remains the gold standard for assessing lower extremity thrombotic disease, it is infrequently performed. The use of limited venography excluding the iliac system, with lead apron shielding of the abdomen, lessens the radiation exposure to the fetus [Mercer and Garner, 1992]. The estimated radiation exposure for the fetus is 0.021 cGy, well within accepted radiation dose levels of less than 0.05 Gy.

PE is a major cause of maternal death. It may be difficult to diagnose, given the changes in physiology, which can cause tachycardia and dyspnea. A careful history and physical examination are essential to make a decision for further testing. A lower extremity ultrasound scan may reveal a thrombus, and no further study is required to begin anticoagulation. **If suspicion remains high, most institutions now use helical computed tomography (CT) or CT angiography to diagnose PE** [⊙ *Schuster et al, 2003*].

Investigators have shown that helical CT delivers an estimated mean fetal dose ranging from 3.3 to 130.8 mGy, depending on the trimester; the highest exposure occurs late in pregnancy when the fetus is larger and cannot be shielded as easily. Radiation exposure during the third trimester, however, poses the least risk of fetal harm. The dose of exposure during a ventilation/perfusion scan can be as high as 370 mGy; it exposes the fetus to a higher risk of radiation effects, and the study may not be adequate for diagnosis.

Patients with acute DVT or PE during pregnancy are treated with a continuous heparin infusion or low-molecular-weight heparin. After acute management with heparin, long-term anticoagulation is required. Because of the risk of teratogenesis with oral warfarin, subcutaneous heparin is the drug of choice for the continuation of anticoagulation. For patients with a previous history of DVT or PE, the recommended regimens for prophylaxis remain controversial because of the lack of controlled trials for this population. The American College of Chest Physicians conference guidelines recommend the use of subcutaneous heparin, 5000 U every 12 hours, as a method of preventing peripartum DVT in patients with a previous history of thromboembolism. **A large, systematic review of the use of low-molecular-weight heparin in pregnancy confirmed that this agent is safe and effective for treating and preventing thrombosis in pregnancy** [⊙ *Greer and Nelson-Piercy, 2005*].

Analgesia

Pregnancy and lactation present obvious concerns over the effects of drugs on the developing fetus and newborn. The U.S. Food and Drug Administration created a classification system for drugs based on the analysis of risk data (Tables 14-7 and 14-8). Acetaminophen appears to be safe to use during pregnancy and lactation in therapeutic doses. Aspirin consumption during pregnancy may produce adverse effects in the mother, including anemia, antepartum and postpartum hemorrhage, prolonged gestation, and prolonged labor. High doses of aspirin may be related to increased perinatal mortality, intrauterine growth retardation, and teratogenic effects. Regarding the use of aspirin and other nonsteroidal anti-inflammatory agents, there is a theoretic risk of premature closure of the ductus arteriosus in utero that would result in persistent pulmonary

TABLE 14-7	Current Categories for Drug Use in Pregnancy
Category	Description
A	Adequate, well-controlled studies in pregnant women have not shown an increased risk of fetal abnormalities.
B	Animal studies have revealed no evidence of harm to the fetus; however, there are no adequate and well-controlled studies in pregnant women.
	OR
	Animal studies have shown an adverse effect, but adequate and well-controlled studies in pregnant women have failed to demonstrate a risk to the fetus.
C	Animal studies have shown an adverse effect, and there are no adequate and well-controlled studies in pregnant women.
	OR
	No animal studies have been conducted, and there are no adequate and well-controlled studies in pregnant women.
D	Studies, adequate well-controlled or observational, in pregnant women have demonstrated a risk to the fetus. However, the benefits of therapy may outweigh the potential risk.
X	Studies, adequate well-controlled or observational, in animals or pregnant women have demonstrated positive evidence of fetal abnormalities. The use of the product is contraindicated in women who are or may become pregnant.

TABLE 14-8   Antiemetics and Analgesics in Pregnancy

Antiemetic	Pregnancy Category
Chlorpromazine (Thorazine)	C
Dimenhydrinate (Dramamine)	B
Diphenhydramine (Benadryl)	B
Droperidol (Inapsine)	C
Meclizine (Antivert)	B
Metoclopramide (Reglan)	B
Ondansetron (Zofran)	B
Prochlorperazine (Compazine)	C
Promethazine (Phenergan)	C
Trimethobenzamide (Tigan)	C

Narcotic Analgesic	Common Trade Names	Pregnancy Category
Butorphanol	Stadol	C
Codeine		C
Hydrocodone	Dilaudid	C
Hydromorphone	Vicodin	C
Meperidine	Demerol	C
Methadone	Dolophine, Methadose	C
Morphine	MS Contin, Kadian	C
Oxycodone	OxyContin, OxyIR	B
Note that Percocet (oxycodone plus acetaminophen) is class C		
Pentazocine	Talwin	C
Propoxyphene	Darvon, Darvocet	C

Non-Narcotic Analgesic	Common Trade Names	Pregnancy Category
Acetaminophen	Tylenol	B
Aspirin	Bayer, St. Joseph's	D
Celecoxib	Celebrex	C, contraindicated in third trimester
Diclofenac	Voltaren	C, contraindicated in third trimester
Ibuprofen	Advil, Motrin, Nuprin	B, contraindicated in third trimester
Ketoprofen	Oruvail	B, contraindicated in third trimester
Meloxicam	Mobic	C, contraindicated in third trimester
Naproxen	Naprosyn, Aleve	C, contraindicated in third trimester
Piroxicam	Feldene	C, contraindicated in third trimester
Sulindac	Clinoril	B, contraindicated in third trimester

hypertension in the newborn if the drug were used during the third trimester. Furthermore, the use of aspirin near term may affect hemostasis in the newborn and increase the risk of intracranial hemorrhage.

Morphine and meperidine are acceptable to use in the perioperative period. As with all narcotics, maternal and neonatal addiction is a possible consequence of inappropriate use. Respiratory depression in the newborn after the use of narcotic drugs in labor is time and dose dependent; however, some studies confirmed that meperidine causes less respiratory depression than morphine. Codeine derivatives have been associated with an increased risk of congenital anomalies.

Nausea and Vomiting

The pregnant patient is susceptible to postoperative nausea and vomiting (see Table 14-8). Adequate fluid and electrolyte balance may help symptoms and should be the first action. Pyridoxine (vitamin B_6) has been documented to have some efficacy in the treatment of nausea. In pharmacologic doses (25 mg three times daily) it is not known to be associated with a risk of birth defects. Antiemetics deemed safe in pregnancy are meclizine, diphenhydramine, metoclopramide, and ondansetron.

Fluid and Electrolytes

Because of increased circulating volume during pregnancy, careful attention should be paid to adequate hydration and proper electrolyte management perioperatively. Prevention of *supine hypotension syndrome* is well documented in many sources. The pregnant patient should be tilted 15 degrees on her left side to keep the pregnant uterus away from the vena cava to prevent this syndrome. Exacerbation of type 2 diabetes may occur at times of stress, including exposure to surgery, infection, and steroids. When these conditions cause significant hyperglycemia, insulin is most appropriate.

SURGICAL CONSIDERATIONS DURING PREGNANCY

Laparoscopy

Laparoscopy, which was once thought to be contraindicated during pregnancy, has been increasingly used since the 1990s. It is used most commonly for cholecystectomy, appendectomy, and adnexal mass assessment and exploration. The major advantages of laparoscopy are decreased postoperative morbidity including lower risk of wound complications, diminished postoperative maternal hypoventilation, less pain (and thus less fetal exposure to narcotics), and a shorter postoperative recovery time.

Possible disadvantages include injury to the pregnant uterus, decreased uterine blood flow resulting from excessive intra-abdominal pressures, and increased carbon dioxide absorption. A study from the Swedish Health Registry evaluated 2233 laparoscopic and 2491 open laparotomy cases from 2 million deliveries in Sweden from 1973 to 1993. No statistically significant differences between laparoscopy and open laparotomy were identified when the investigators compared birth weights, gestational duration, intrauterine growth retardation, congenital malformations, stillbirths, and neonatal death.

The Society of American Gastrointestinal Endoscopic Surgeons (SAGES) has recommendations concerning laparoscopic surgery during pregnancy. Highlights include minimizing pneumoperitoneum to 8 to 12 mm Hg, using an open technique to gain pneumoperitoneum, and monitoring maternal end-tidal carbon dioxide [SAGES, 2000]. As the pregnancy progresses, however, the size of the uterus often interferes with laparoscopic views and approaches. Therefore, after 28 weeks, open laparotomy may be indicated.

Acute Appendicitis

Acute appendicitis is the most common nonobstetric surgical problem in the pregnant patient. The incidence of appendicitis during pregnancy has been estimated to range from

0.06% to 0.1% of deliveries. The incidence of appendicitis is not increased in pregnancy, and the likelihood of its occurrence is equal in all three trimesters.

The diagnosis of appendicitis may be difficult because signs and symptoms may mimic other conditions commonly seen in a normal pregnancy. The most common presenting symptom is vague right lower quadrant abdominal pain. A long-held belief was that as pregnancy progressed, the location of the abdominal pain would migrate upward during gestation as the gravid uterus displaces the appendix. **A retrospective review demonstrated that, for all trimesters, the most common location for abdominal pain of acute appendicitis is the right lower quadrant** [❽ Mourad et al, 2000]. Muscle guarding and rebound tenderness may be elicited but are not specific to appendicitis. Symptoms of nausea, vomiting, and anorexia are also not reliable symptoms because they also occur commonly in normal pregnancy. In addition, fever and elevated white blood cell count are not reliable findings because leukocytosis is normal during pregnancy, although a leftward shift in the white blood cell count is more commonly seen in appendicitis. Following serial white blood cell counts may be of some benefit; an increasing count may be an indicator of acute appendicitis. Ultrasound has been used to aid in the diagnosis of acute appendicitis. The sensitivity of ultrasound in the pregnant patient is about the same as in the nonpregnant patient. CT is used in nonpregnant female patients to aid in the diagnosis of appendicitis, but currently there are no published studies on its use in pregnant patients.

The treatment of suspected acute appendicitis in the pregnant patient is emergency appendectomy. Because of the difficulty in diagnosis and the increased morbidity to the patient and fetus in the event of appendiceal perforation or rupture, a higher negative laparotomy rate of 30% to 33% is acceptable.

Both laparotomy and laparoscopy are used during pregnancy. Laparoscopic procedures are used more commonly in acute appendicitis because of the quicker recovery time, shorter hospital stay, and decreased pain. Laparoscopy is often performed at less than 20 weeks of gestation, when there is less chance of penetrating the uterus with the trochar (see the earlier discussion of laparoscopy). Laparotomy is still commonly performed in all trimesters for this indication.

Cholecystitis

Cholecystectomy for gallbladder disease represents the second most common surgical procedure performed in the pregnant patient. Its occurrence is estimated to be approximately 0.2 to 0.5 cases per 1000 pregnancies. It is estimated that between 3.5% and 10% of pregnant patients have asymptomatic gallstones. The rate of gallstone formation is increased in the pregnant patient secondary to decreased gallbladder contractility, higher residual gallbladder bile volume, increased viscosity of bile, and increased numbers of micelles in which cholesterol crystals precipitate. The risk of cholelithiasis increases with age and multiparity. Cholelithiasis is the most common cause of cholecystitis in the pregnant patient.

Presenting signs and symptoms of acute cholecystitis are similar to those in the nonpregnant patient. Common symptoms include nausea, vomiting, anorexia, dyspepsia, intolerance to fatty foods, and colicky right upper quadrant or epigastric pain that may radiate to the flank or the scapula. Biliary colic attacks are often characterized as acute in onset, triggered by fatty meals, and episodic. Physical examination may reveal a low-grade fever, right upper quadrant pain, and Murphy's sign (tenderness under the liver with deep inspiration).

Laboratory findings of acute cholecystitis are also similar to those in the nonpregnant patient. An increased white blood cell count with a left shift is commonly seen in cholecystitis, as well as elevated liver enzymes such as aspartate aminotransferase, alanine aminotransferase, alkaline phosphatase, and bilirubin.

Ultrasound is the diagnostic test of choice for evaluating biliary disease. It is 95% sensitive in detecting gallstones in pregnancy and also can show signs of inflammation such as distention of the gallbladder, pericholecystic fluid, and gallbladder wall thickening while exposing the fetus to no radiation.

Initial treatment of acute cholecystitis is typically medical. This includes nothing-by-mouth (NPO) status, intravenous hydration, intravenous antibiotics, correction of electrolyte imbalances, and pain management. Most patients respond to supportive care. Surgical intervention is reserved for patients who do not respond to medical management, have repeated bouts of biliary colic, or have complications such as obstructive jaundice, choledocholithiasis, or gallstone pancreatitis.

Surgical interventions, when indicated, include open and laparoscopic cholecystectomy. The timing and choice of procedure depend on gestational age and severity of symptoms. The spontaneous abortion rate with open cholecystectomy is 12% during the first trimester, 5.6% during the second trimester, and 0% in the third trimester [McKellar et al, 1990]. The risk of preterm labor in the second trimester is nearly 0%, and it is 40% during the third trimester. The optimal time for cholecystectomy is in the second trimester, when the risk of spontaneous abortion and preterm labor is the least [Curet et al, 1996]. Compared with open cholecystectomy, laparoscopic cholecystectomy is associated with shorter recovery time, less uterine manipulation, earlier ambulation, and a possibly lower incidence of preterm labor.

Endoscopic retrograde cholangiopancreatography is an alternative to surgical intervention. This procedure can be done to remove small biliary stones and for stent placement, techniques that may delay or obviate the need for cholecystectomy. The optimal time for this procedure is also the second trimester because the fetus is most sensitive to radiation in the first trimester.

Acute Intestinal Obstruction

Intestinal obstruction is the third most common reason for surgical laparotomy in the pregnant patient. Its is estimated to occur in approximately 1 to 3 in 10,000 pregnancies, similar to the incidence in the general population. The most common cause of intestinal obstruction is adhesion, which occurs in approximately 60% of cases. Patients with previous abdominal or pelvic surgical procedures, including cesarian delivery, and pelvic inflammatory disease are at increased risk of intestinal obstruction secondary to adhesions. Intestinal obstruction occurs most commonly in the third trimester. Volvulus occurs in approximately 25% of cases. Less common causes of bowel obstruction include intussusception, hernia, and neoplasm.

The signs and symptoms of intestinal obstruction are the same as in the nonpregnant patient. The classic triad of abdominal pain, vomiting, and obstipation is noted, although these symptoms may occur in normal pregnancy. As the disease progresses, patients may display signs of more severe sequelae such as perforation or ischemia. These signs include fever, tachycardia, localized abdominal pain, guarding or rebound tenderness, and leukocytosis.

Imaging includes upright and supine plain abdominal films. The sensitivity increases as serial films are performed. Serial films should reveal progressive changes that confirm the diagnosis of intestinal obstruction.

The initial treatment of intestinal obstruction in pregnancy is essentially the same as in the nonpregnant patient. Treatment includes nasogastric decompression, aggressive intravenous hydration, intravenous antibiotics, and timely surgical intervention when warranted. A low threshold for exploratory laparotomy is appropriate before perforation or necrosis occurs. If after 6 to 8 hours of medical therapy, there is no response, laparotomy should be performed. Aggressive therapy is appropriate because fetal loss rates following intestinal obstruction are between 20% and 26%, and maternal mortality can range from 6% to 20%.

Breast Mass or Breast Cancer

Pregnancy-associated breast cancer is defined as breast cancer that is diagnosed during pregnancy or within 1 year following pregnancy. The occurrence of pregnancy-associated breast cancer is approximately 1 in 10,000 to 1 in 3000 pregnancies.

It is becoming more common because more women are delaying childbearing until their late 30s or 40s. The typical presentation is a painless, palpable mass, with or without nipple discharge. As in the nonpregnant patient, ductal carcinoma is the most common tumor type.

Initial management of a breast mass is essentially no different from that in a nonpregnant patient. Low-dose mammography with fetal shielding can be performed, although this is typically avoided during the first trimester. Mammography may be of limited value because it has a high false-negative rate related to the increased density of the fibroglandular breast tissue during pregnancy. Ultrasound may be used and is helpful in differentiating between solid and cystic masses. Magnetic resonance imaging has been used to evaluate breast masses in the nonpregnant patient, but currently it is not recommended for use in pregnancy. Cystic lesions should be aspirated and evaluated for cytology. Tissue diagnosis is essential by core needle biopsy, open biopsy, or fine needle aspiration. These procedures can be done using local anesthesia to limit the risk to the fetus.

The mainstay of therapy for pregnancy-associated breast cancer is still surgical resection. Studies suggest that local control and adjuvant therapy can be tailored to the patient according to the stage of pregnancy and the stage of cancer. It is beyond the scope of this chapter to delineate possible treatment options. Needless to say, a combined approach with the patient, surgeon, oncologist, and maternal-fetal medicine specialist should ensure optimal treatment while minimizing the risk to the mother and fetus. Elective termination of the pregnancy is no longer routinely recommended because no improvement in survival has been demonstrated.

Ovarian Disease

Increased use of ultrasonography has led to the increased finding of adnexal masses during pregnancy. Most adnexal masses are incidental findings on ultrasound and spontaneously resolve as pregnancy progresses. In fact, more than 90% of first trimester, unilateral masses that are smaller than 5 cm resolve on their own.

As stated previously, the patient is usually asymptomatic when the diagnosis of adnexal mass is made. The exception is when rupture or torsion of the mass occurs. Rupture of the adnexal mass is rare and occurs in approximately 2% of cases. Torsion is much more common, especially during pregnancy, and it has a frequency of approximately 28%.

Treatment of an ovarian mass depends on the size of the mass, the gestational age, and complicating factors. Most simple ovarian cysts smaller than 6 cm in pregnant women spontaneously resolve. Serial ultrasound studies are warranted to follow the mass to resolution (most commonly) or progression. Asymptomatic adnexal masses discovered in the third trimester may be followed expectantly until delivery. Surgical intervention is indicated if the adnexal mass is enlarging as noted on serial ultrasound, contains solid and complex components or internal vegetations, is surrounded by abdominal ascites, or is fixed or if the patient has symptoms or ultrasonic findings of torsion or rupture. The second trimester is preferred for elective surgical treatment of ovarian masses in the pregnant patient.

Trauma

The incidence of trauma during pregnancy is approximately 7%. The most common cause of trauma is motor vehicle accidents, which account for 40% of all traumas in pregnancy. This is followed by falls (30%), direct assault on maternal abdomen (20%), and other causes (10%). Domestic violence is an increasingly recognized cause of trauma to the mother and fetus. The most common cause of fetal demise is death of the mother. The second most common cause of fetal death is abruptio placentae.

Primary treatment in pregnant patients who experience trauma consists of resuscitation and stabilization of the mother. Pregnancy should not alter evaluation and treatment of the mother. In 1998, the American College of Obstetricians and Gynecologists made the following recommendations for surgical exploration after trauma:

1. Penetrating abdominal injury
2. Clinical evidence of intraperitoneal hemorrhage
3. Suspected bowel perforation
4. Suspected injury to the uterus or fetus

In addition, cesarean delivery is indicated if the clinician notes nonreassuring fetal test results in a viable fetus that fails to respond to maternal resuscitative efforts.

Uncommon Disorders

Splenic Artery Aneurysm

Splenic artery aneurysm occurs in approximately 0.1% of all adults. It is estimated that 6% to 10% of splenic artery aneurysms will rupture, and 25% to 40% of those ruptures will occur during pregnancy, especially during the third trimester. Risk factors for rupture include portal hypertension and pregnancy. Maternal mortality for ruptured splenic artery aneurysm is 75%, and fetal mortality is up to 95%. Patients with a splenic artery aneurysm before rupture are fairly asymptomatic; vague epigastric pain, left upper quadrant pain, and left shoulder pain are among the most common complaints.

Radiologic studies for the diagnosis of splenic artery aneurysm include plain abdominal film, ultrasound, and angiography. On plain abdominal film, an oval calcification with a central lucent area is a very specific sign for aneurysm. In pregnancy, ultrasound evaluation with Doppler study is preferred to minimize radiation exposure to the fetus. Angiography is the gold standard when the patient is stable, but this procedure increases radiation exposure to the fetus.

Because of the high morbidity and mortality associated with ruptured aneurysm, treatment for pregnant women and women of childbearing age consists of elective splenic artery ligation and resection of the aneurysm with or without splenectomy. Treatment of suspected ruptured aneurysm is immediate laparotomy. Pneumococcal vaccine should be given 2 weeks before elective splenectomy and immediately following emergency splenectomy.

Hepatic Adenoma

Hepatic adenoma is a benign lesion that is associated with glycogen storage disease, diabetes, steroid uses, oral contraceptive use, and pregnancy. The exact incidence of hepatic adenomas in pregnancy is unknown.

The major complication of hepatic adenomas during pregnancy is spontaneous rupture. Ruptured adenoma carries a maternal and fetal mortality of approximately 60%. Symptoms include severe right upper quadrant pain with pain referred to the right shoulder. Laboratory findings include anemia, thrombocytopenia, and low fibrinogen levels.

Treatment of suspected ruptured hepatic adenoma is immediate laparotomy, control of hemorrhage, and resection of adenoma if possible. Because of the high mortality associated with ruptured hepatic adenoma, elective resection should be considered if the lesion is discovered during pregnancy. If elective resection is performed, the second trimester is optimal.

Pheochromocytoma

The incidence of pheochromocytoma is rare in pregnancy. Maternal and fetal mortality in undiagnosed pheochromocytoma is greater than 50%, and the greatest risk is from the onset of labor to 48 hours after delivery.

The typical signs and symptoms of pheochromocytoma include labile blood pressure, anxiety, diaphoresis, fever, headache, and palpitations. The diagnosis is made by measuring 24-hour urine for catecholamine, metanephrines, and vanillylmandelic acid.

Treatment depends on gestational age at diagnosis. When the diagnosis is made early in pregnancy, elective surgery with tumor removal is recommended and has shown a significant reduction in fetal mortality. Again, the second trimester is the optimal time for surgery. If the diagnosis is made in the latter part of pregnancy, cesarean delivery with simultaneous excision of tumor should be performed when fetal maturity is achieved. Blood pressure and cardiovascular condition should be optimized preoperatively.

CONCLUSION

In pregnant patients requiring nonobstetric surgical procedures, maternal and fetal morbidity and mortality do increase with a delay in diagnosis and treatment. In 2003, the American College of Obstetricians and Gynecologists reissued an opinion statement that recommended the following: "Although there are no data to support specific recommendations regarding nonobstetric surgery and anesthesia in pregnancy, it is important for nonobstetric physicians to obtain obstetric consultation before performing nonobstetric surgery." The decision to use fetal monitoring should be individualized, and each case warrants a team approach for optimal safety of the woman and her baby. Indeed, close communication among all specialists involved in the care of the pregnant patient—the internist, the obstetrician, the surgeon, and the anesthesiologist— ensures that both the mother and the fetus will have the best possible outcome.

Selected Readings

American College of Obstetricians and Gynecologists Committee on Obstetric Practice: ACOG Committee Opinion Number 284: Nonobstetric Surgery in Pregnancy. Obstet Gynecol 102:431, 2003.

Andersen B, Nielsen TF: Appendicitis in pregnancy: Diagnosis, management and complications. Acta Obstet Gynecol Scand 78:758-762, 1999.

Angelini DJ: Obstetric triage revisited: Update on non-obstetric surgical conditions in pregnancy. J Midwifery Womens Health 48:111-118, 2003.

Chesnutt AN: Physiology of normal pregnancy. Crit Care Clin 20:609-615, 2004.

Coleman MT, Trianfo VA, Rund DA: Nonobstetric emergencies in pregnancy: Trauma and surgical conditions. Am J Obstet Gynecol 177:497-502, 1997.

Curet MJ, Allen D, Josloff RK, et al: Laparoscopy during pregnancy. Arch Surg 131:546-551, 1996.

Czeizel AE, Pataki T, Rockenbaue M: Reproductive outcome after exposure to surgery under anesthesia during pregnancy. Arch Gynecol Obstet 261:193-199, 1998.

Faure EA: Anesthesia for the Pregnant Patient, Department of Anesthesia and Critical Care, University of Chicago. Available at http://acc-www.uchicago.edu/manuals/obstetric/obanesthesia.html

Goodman S: Anesthesia for nonobstetric surgery in the pregnant patient. Semin Perinatol 26:136-145, 2002. **C**

Graham G, Baxi L, Tharakan T: Laparoscopic cholecystectomy during pregnancy: A case series and review of the literature. Obstet Gynecol Surv 53:566-574, 1998.

Greer IA, Nelson-Piercy C: Low-molecular-weight heparins for thromboprophylaxis and treatment of venous thromboembolism in pregnancy: A systematic review of safety and efficacy. Blood 106:401-407, 2005. **B**

Holschneider CH: Surgical diseases and disorders in pregnancy. Curr Obstet Gynecol Diagn Treat 451-465, 2003.

International Commission on Radiological Protection (ICRP): Pregnancy and medical radiation. Annals of the International Commission on Radiological Protection. Publication 84. 30/1 December 2000.

Jilma B, Kamath S, Lip G: Antithrombotic therapy in special circumstances. I. Pregnancy and cancer. BMJ 326:37-40, 2003. **C**

Mazze RI, Kallen B: Reproductive outcome after anesthesia and operation during pregnancy: A registry study of 5405 cases. Am J Obstet Gynecol 161:1178-1185, 1989. **C**

McKellar DP, Anderson CT, Boynton CJ, Peoples JB: Cholecystectomy during pregnancy without fetal loss. Surg Clin North Am 70:1249-1262, 1990.

Mercer BM, Garner P: Thrombophlebitis. *In* Gleicher N (ed): Principles and Practice of Medical Therapy in Pregnancy. Norwalk, CT, Appleton & Lange, 1992, pp 1284-1296.

Mhuireachtaigh RN, Gorman DA: Anesthesia in pregnant patients for non-obstetrical surgery. J Clin Anesth 18:60-66, 2006.

Mourad J, Elliott JP, Erickson L, Lisboa L: Appendicitis in pregnancy: New information that contradicts long-held clinical beliefs. Am J Obstet Gynecol 182:1027-1029, 2000. ❸

Pearlman MD, Tintinalli JE, Lorenz RP: Blunt trauma during pregnancy. N Engl J Med 323:1609-1613, 1990.

Schuster ME, Fishman JE, Copeland JF, et al: Pulmonary embolism in pregnant patients: A survey of practices and policies for CT pulmonary angiography. AJR Am J Roentgenol 181:1495-1498, 2003. ❸

Sharp HT: Gastrointestinal surgical conditions during pregnancy. Clin Obstet Gynecol 37:306-315, 1994.

Society of American Gastrointestinal Endoscopic Surgeons (SAGES) Committee on Standards of Practice: SAGES guidelines for laparoscopic surgery during pregnancy. October 2000. Available at http://www.sages.org/sagespublication.php?doc=3

15 The Patient with Substance Abuse Going to Surgery

ELIZABETH TEPEROV, MD

Substance abuse is widespread in our society, and it is therefore crucial for the physician to be able to diagnose, prevent, and manage its many complications. The physician caring for these patients in the perioperative period may be asked to risk stratify, medically optimize, identify, and treat acute substance intoxication and withdrawal and help to manage complications related to abuse. Because some patients who require surgery may be unable or unwilling to admit to dependence, the medical consultant needs to be vigilant, especially in patients with unexplained cardiac, pulmonary, or mental status changes that may be a result of substance abuse. Substance abuse may be defined by the criteria given in the revised fourth edition of the *Diagnostic and Statistical Manual of Mental Disorders* (Box 15-1). This chapter discusses surgical patients who are dependent on alcohol, cocaine, opioids, benzodiazepines, tobacco, and marijuana.

Levels of Evidence:

Ⓐ—Randomized controlled trials (RCTs), meta-analyses, well-designed systematic reviews of RCTs. Ⓑ—Case-control or cohort studies, nonrandomized controlled trials, systematic reviews of studies other than RCTs, cross-sectional studies, retrospective studies. Ⓒ—Consensus statements, expert guidelines, usual practice, opinion.

Box 15-1	DSM-IV TR CRITERIA FOR SUBSTANCE ABUSE

A maladaptive pattern of substance use leading to clinically significant impairment or distress, as manifested by one (or more) of the following, occurring within a 12-month period:

1. Recurrent substance abuse resulting in a failure to fulfill major role obligations at work, school, or home.
2. Recurrent substance use in situations in which it is physically hazardous (e.g., driving an automobile when impaired by substance use).
3. Recurrent substance-related legal problems.
4. Continued substance use despite having persistent social or interpersonal problems caused or exacerbated by the effects of the substance.

From American Psychiatric Association: Diagnostic and Statistical Manual of Mental Disorders, 4th ed, text rev. Washington, DC, American Psychiatric Association, 2000. Reprinted with permission from the Diagnostic and Statistical Manual of Mental Disorders, copyright 2000. American Psychiatric Association.

PERIOPERATIVE CARE OF THE ALCOHOL-DEPENDENT PATIENT

Background

Alcohol is a major public health problem in the United States. *Alcohol abuse* is usually defined as the consumption of 60 g/day or more of alcohol, although smaller quantities can certainly be physically and psychologically harmful. Patients with alcoholism are frequent users of the health care system, particularly of surgical and trauma services. Alcoholic patients also have two to three times more postoperative complications than nonalcoholic patients. The most commonly encountered problems are infections, bleeding, alcohol withdrawal syndrome, and cardiac and respiratory dysfunction. Chronic abusers of alcohol are also noted to have diminished cellular immunity and exaggerated responses to surgical stress. **Some studies suggest that 1 month of abstinence** before surgical procedures is recommended to improve preoperative organ function and to decrease postoperative morbidity [**❸** *Tonnesen and Kehlet, 1999*].

Diagnosis of Alcohol Abuse

Physicians frequently fail to identify alcohol abuse. Of several screening tests for alcoholism, **the CAGE questions are still the easiest and most widely used** [**❹** *Ewing, 1984*]. CAGE is a mnemonic for the following questions:

1. Have you tried to *Cut* down on your drinking?
2. Are you *Angry or annoyed* when others criticize your drinking?
3. Do you ever feel *Guilty* about your drinking?
4. Do you ever take an *"Eye opener?"*

Two or more "yes" answers have an approximate 75% sensitivity and 95% specificity for alcohol dependence, although this may vary according to the prevalence of alcoholism in the population examined. Elevations of certain laboratory test results (e.g., γ-glutamyltransferase and aspartate aminotransferase levels and mean corpuscular volume) are sensitive for alcoholism but, unfortunately, are not very specific. Elevations of these markers may, however, raise the suspicion for alcoholism. A perioperative medical workup for suspected alcohol abuse should include a complete blood count with differential, a complete metabolic panel, prothrombin time, a fasting lipid panel, vitamin B_{12} and folate levels, urinalysis, an electrocardiogram (ECG) and chest radiograph, and a urine toxicology screen if additional substance abuse is suspected. Other tests, such as stool occult blood (Hemoccult), computed tomography of the brain, and ultrasound of the liver, should be ordered based on the clinical situation.

Medical Complications and Treatment

Patients who abuse alcohol are at an increased risk for various medical problems, including but not limited to: hepatitis, cirrhosis, portal hypertension, gastritis, pancreatitis, esophageal and gastric varices, peptic ulcer disease, cardiomyopathy, arrhythmias, hypertension, stroke, neuropathy, anemia, thrombocytopenia, carcinoma, and psychosis. **They are also at increased risk for medical complications in the perioperative period** [❿ *Tonnesen et al, 1992*].

Symptoms of Withdrawal

One of the most common complications that occurs when the alcoholic patient enters the hospital is *withdrawal*. It can be divided into four stages in ascending severity: autonomic hyperactivity, hallucinations, seizures, and delirium tremens. Mild to moderate signs and symptoms related to autonomic hyperactivity (e.g., tremulousness, irritability and sleep disturbance, nystagmus, hyperreflexia, nausea and vomiting, tachycardia, diaphoresis, and fever) start within hours, peak 24 to 48 hours after the last drink, and generally resolve within 24 to 36 hours.

The hallucinations that characterize the second stage are usually visual, but they may be tactile or auditory as well. They develop about 12 to 24 hours after cessation of alcohol use and usually resolve within 24 hours, but may persist up to 6 days.

Approximately 10% of patients progress from the second to the third stage and develop seizures. The seizures are usually generalized, tonic-clonic, single, and of short duration. Although seizures typically do not occur until after 12 to 48 hours of abstinence, they have been reported as early as 2 hours after the last use of alcohol.

Delirium tremens (also known as DTs) is the fourth and most severe stage of alcohol withdrawal syndrome. It peaks about 5 days after the last drink and consists of symptoms from any or all of the preceding categories in addition to delirium. A typical patient may present with confusion, prominent autonomic symptoms (e.g., temperature >101°F, blood pressure >140/90 mm Hg, pulse >100), and visual and auditory hallucinations. The normal duration is several days, but like the other complications, delirium tremens has been reported to last much longer in some people. The mortality may be as high as 15% in untreated patients. It is usually heavy, long-time drinkers who develop hallucinosis, seizures, and delirium tremens, although patients with concurrent acute medical illnesses are five times more likely to experience delirium tremens than are those without acute illnesses.

The signs and symptoms of alcohol withdrawal may begin within hours after the last drink, and they may not be fully resolved until after a week of abstinence. In the postoperative patient, the onset of withdrawal may be delayed for as long as 14 days because of the effects of anesthesia and narcotics. Agitated, critically ill patients with unknown alcohol histories must also be evaluated for other common causes of delirium in this setting, such as infection, bleeding, hypoxemia, hypotension, metabolic disturbances, or primary neurologic causes. Patients with suspected or presumed alcohol withdrawal should be placed in a setting where symptoms can be closely monitored, a minimum of every 4 hours while awake. Scales, such as the 19-item Clinical Institute Withdrawal Assessment (CIWA) that uses a calculated point score for various clinical features, have been developed to help medical providers objectively monitor the withdrawal state. The CIWA-Ar is a shortened, revised version that is probably the most commonly used alcohol withdrawal monitoring scale (Fig. 15-1). Although this assessment tool has been validated, care must be taken during the assessment because certain medical and psychiatric conditions may mimic alcohol withdrawal and may result in a false-positive alcohol withdrawal assessment. In addition, the use of certain medications (e.g., β-blockers) may blunt the symptoms and signs of alcohol withdrawal and may lead to underestimation of the severity of withdrawal.

Treatment of Withdrawal

All patients with symptoms of alcohol withdrawal should receive thiamine, folate, and multivitamins either orally or parenterally (Table 15-1). **Benzodiazepines, preferably those with**

Nausea and vomiting. Ask "Do you feel sick to your stomach? Have you vomited?"
Observation:
0–No nausea and no vomiting
1–Mild nausea with no vomiting
2–
3–
4–Intermittent nausea with dry heaves
5–
6–
7–Constant nausea, frequent dry heaves, and vomiting

Tremor. Ask patient to extend arms and spread fingers apart.
Observation:
0–No tremor
1–Tremor not visible but can be felt, fingertip to fingertip
2–
3–
4–Moderate tremor with arms extended
5–
6–
7–Severe tremor, even with arms not extended

Paroxysmal sweats
Observation:
0–No sweat visible
1–Barely perceptible sweating; palms moist
2–
3–
4–Beads of sweat obvious on forehead
5–
6–
7–Drenching sweats

Anxiety. Ask "Do you feel nervous?"
Observation:
0–No anxiety (at ease)
1–Mildly anxious
2–
3–
4–Moderately anxious or guarded, so anxiety is inferred
5–
6–
7–Equivalent to acute panic states as occur in severe delirium or acute schizophrenic reactions

Agitation
Observation:
0–Normal activity
1–Somewhat more than normal activity
2–
3–
4–Moderately fidgety and restless
5–
6–
7–Paces back and forth during most of the interview or constantly thrashes about

Tactile disturbances. Ask "Do you have any itching, pins-and-needles sensations, burning, or numbness, or do you feel like bugs are crawling on or under your skin?"

Observation:

0–None

1–Very mild itching, pins-and-needles sensation, burning, or numbness

2–Mild itching, pins-and-needles sensation, burning, or numbness

3–Moderate itching, pins-and-needles sensation, burning, or numbness

4–Moderately severe hallucinations

5–Severe hallucinations

6–Extremely severe hallucinations

7–Continuous hallucinations

Auditory disturbances. Ask "Are you more aware of sounds around you? Are they harsh? Do they frighten you? Are you hearing anything that is disturbing to you? Are you hearing things you know are not there?"

Observation:

0–Not present

1–Very mild harshness or ability to frighten

2–Mild harshness or ability to frighten

3–Moderate harshness or ability to frighten

4–Moderately severe hallucinations

5–Severe hallucinations

6–Extremely severe hallucinations

7–Continuous hallucinations

Visual disturbances. Ask "Does the light appear to be too bright? Is its color different? Does it hurt your eyes? Are you seeing anything that is disturbing to you? Are you seeing things you know are not there?"

Observation:

0–Not present

1–Very mild sensitivity

2–Mild sensitivity

3–Moderate sensitivity

4–Moderately severe hallucinations

5–Severe hallucinations

6–Extremely severe hallucinations

7–Continuous hallucinations

Headache, fullness in head. Ask "Does your head feel different? Does it feel like there is a band around your head?"

Do not rate for dizziness or lightheadedness; otherwise, rate severity.

0–Not present

1–Very mild

2–Mild

3–Moderate

4–Moderately severe

5–Severe

6–Very severe

7–Extremely severe

Orientation and clouding of sensorium. Ask "What day is this? Where are you? Who am I?"

Observation:

0–Oriented and can do serial additions

1–Cannot do serial additions or is uncertain about date

2–Date disorientation by no more than two calendar days

3–Date disorientation by more than two calendar days

4–Disoriented for place and/or person

Total score:_____(maximum = 67)   Rater's initials_____

For legend, see next page

Figure 15-1 • Revised Clinical Institute Withdrawal Assessment for Alcohol Scale. (*Adapted from Sullivan J, Sykora K, Schneiderman J, et al: Assessment of alcohol withdrawal: The revised Clinical Institute Withdrawal Assessment for Alcohol Scale [CIWA-Ar]. Br J Addict 84:1853-1857, 1989.*)

TABLE 15-1	Drug Treatment of Alcohol Withdrawal			
Medication	Loading Dose	Route	Subsequent Doses (q2-4h as Needed)	Maximum Doses
Chlordiazepoxide (Librium) Long t½	25–100 mg	PO or IV	25–50 mg	400 mg/24 hr
Diazepam (Valium) Long t½	5–20 mg	PO or IV	5–10 mg	100 mg/24 hr
Lorazepam (Ativan)* Intermediate t½	1–2 mg	PO, IV, or IM	1 mg	
Oxazepam (Serax)* Intermediate t½	15–30 mg†	PO	15–30 mg	

*May need to be administered more frequently because of shorter half-lives.
†Other sources suggest using 60 mg of oral oxazepam every 2 hours.
IM, intramuscularly; IV, intravenously; PO, by mouth; q, every; t½ half-life.

a long half-life, such as diazepam or chlordiazepoxide, are the first-line agents for treatment of withdrawal symptoms [● Mayo-Smith et al, 2004]. An agent with a shorter half-life, such as lorazepam or oxazepam, may be considered for use in patients with respiratory insufficiency, decreased mental status, or significant hepatic synthetic dysfunction, as evidenced by hypoalbuminemia, hyperbilirubinemia, and coagulopathy, but not isolated transaminase elevations. Although it was used in the past, oral ethanol is not recommended to treat alcohol withdrawal syndrome or to prevent alcohol withdrawal seizures.

Approach to Treatment Options

- *Symptom-triggered approach:* From 2 to 4 hours after initial loading doses are given, reassess the patient, and give additional doses only *as needed*. The goal of treatment is a comfortable patient who is easily awakened.

- *Front-loading approach*: Give high-dose benzodiazepines initially, to quickly achieve adequate sedation. Example: diazepam, 5 to 10 mg every 5 to 10 minutes intravenously, not to exceed 250 mg in 8 hours, or chlordiazepoxide, 200 to 400 mg orally once, then additional doses of 25 to 50 mg as needed. Doses should be held if the patient develops symptoms of sedation or respiratory depression.
- *Fixed-dosing schedule approach*: The option of giving benzodiazepines at specific intervals around the clock, with supplemental doses as needed, is *no longer routinely recommended*. Symptom-triggered therapy, as described earlier, has been shown to shorten the duration of detoxification and avoids unnecessary overmedication.
- *Tapering options*
  - Calculate the total dose required to suppress the withdrawal symptoms over the first 24 hours, then give that amount in four divided doses the following day.
  - In general, total duration of treatment should not exceed 10 days. Higher doses and longer courses of treatment (see Table 15-1) may be required in severe withdrawal states.
  - An aggressive (3-day) regimen, which reduces the total dose by 25% to 50% each day, will suffice as prophylaxis against alcohol withdrawal syndrome.
  - A more conservative (5- to 7-day) regimen, which is generally better psychologically tolerated by the patient, tapers the initial calculated 24-hour dose by a total of 25% over the first 3 days, then 25% to 50% per day on subsequent days.

Adjunctive and Alternative Therapy

- β-*Blockers* and α-*adrenergic agonists*: Medications such as propranolol, given 10 mg orally every 6 hours as needed, and clonidine, 0.5 mg orally two to three times per day as needed, may be helpful for autonomic hyperactivity symptoms. Because no data have shown that these drugs help to prevent delirium tremens or seizures, they should not be used as monotherapy, and patients need close monitoring for hypotension with both these agents. However, these drugs may be particularly useful as an adjunct to benzodiazepines in patients with baseline hypertension, tachycardia, or persistent anxiety.

- *Barbiturates*: Although barbiturates are still used, there are no controlled studies demonstrating the effectiveness of barbiturates over benzodiazepines for alcohol withdrawal symptoms.
- *Antipsychotics*: Haloperidol, given 0.5 mg intramuscularly, every 2 hours, may control agitation, but it should be used cautiously, and only in combination with benzodiazepines, because it can lower the seizure threshold.
- *Anticonvulsants*: Carbamazepine, used extensively in Europe, has been shown to reduce withdrawal symptoms and seizures in some studies. Its efficacy is not adequately established, however, and it is not currently recommended as a first-line treatment agent in the United States. Phenytoin alone is ineffective in preventing alcohol withdrawal seizures, but it can be added for patients who have a known underlying seizure disorder. Gabapentin, valproic acid, or magnesium in addition to benzodiazepines may be empirically given to a high-risk patient, such as someone with known previous alcohol withdrawal seizure or previous episodes of severely symptomatic alcohol withdrawal.
- *Anesthetics*: In severe refractory agitation despite adequate benzodiazepine treatment, a patient can be intubated for airway protection and started on continuous intravenous propofol.

Medical Complications of Alcohol Abuse

Encephalopathy

Korsakoff's syndrome is a memory disorder with antegrade and retrograde amnesia characterized by confabulation. The classic triad of Wernicke's encephalopathy is confusion, ataxia, and ophthalmoplegia. The ophthalmoplegia usually presents as nystagmus or gaze palsies. Wernicke's encephalopathy is caused by a systemic thiamine deficiency that disrupts normal cerebral glucose utilization. Only about one third of patients present with the classic triad defined earlier. Other findings may include pupillary meiosis, orthostatic hypotension, syncope, and hypothermia, and approximately 80% of patients have varying degrees of Korsakoff's psychosis. The clinical diagnosis can be supported by characteristic brain findings on magnetic resonance imaging.

Wernicke's encephalopathy is a medical emergency and has a 10% to 20% mortality rate if it is not treated with intravenous thiamine. Just 2 to 3 g thiamine will reverse the ophthalmologic findings, and the other symptoms usually resolve within 1 to 6 hours after treatment with parenteral thiamine is initiated. To prevent Wernicke's encephalopathy and Korsakoff's syndrome in high-risk patients, 100 mg of parenteral thiamine should be given during the first 24 hours of admission and before any carbohydrate-containing infusions or food. The concern is that administration of glucose to a thiamine-deficient patient may further deplete the body's limited reserve of thiamine and precipitate acute Wernicke's encephalopathy. Oral thiamine should be avoided while the patient is still intoxicated because of its decreased absorption in the presence of alcohol. After the serum alcohol levels decrease, the patient can be started on 50 mg of daily oral thiamine, which is continued for a minimum of several weeks. Longer courses are required if neurologic symptoms are present. Patients can also develop cognitive dysfunction that does not meet criteria for Korsakoff's syndrome, and is potentially reversible if alcohol use is stopped.

Patients with severe underlying liver disease also can develop hepatic encephalopathy. This is a broad category defined as reversible neurologic deficits associated with impaired liver function. Symptoms can range from minor agitation, difficulty with memory and concentration, nystagmus, asterixis, and clonus, to progressive lethargy, stupor, and coma. This diagnosis is mostly based on clinical suspicion. It can be supported by an elevated serum ammonia level, which is not very sensitive or specific, and confirmed by characteristic findings on an EEG. Only approximately 60% to 80% of patients with hepatic encephalopathy have elevated ammonia levels, and not all of them show a clinical response that parallels the normalization of the laboratory value.

The management of hepatic encephalopathy includes first identifying and correcting any common precipitating causes such as gastrointestinal bleeding, infection, oversedation with benzodiazepines, and electrolyte abnormalities. The objective of medical treatment is to decrease systemic ammonia levels. Approaches that can facilitate clearance or reduce production of ammonia include reversal of hypokalemia, restriction of dietary protein to 70 g/day, and institution of a bowel regimen for constipation. Lactulose, which is the first-line medication for hepatic encephalopathy, can be administered orally or rectally, depending on the severity of the symptoms, and should be titrated to about three soft bowel movements per day. Antibiotics such as neomycin, rifaximin, vancomycin, or metronidazole can decrease gastrointestinal ammonia absorption; however, their use is somewhat limited by side effects. Other options for treatment include acarbose, sodium benzoate, and ornithine aspartate, all of which interfere with enzymes involved in ammonia production.

Seizures

The peak period of risk for an alcohol withdrawal seizure is between 1 and 2 days after the last drink. Unless a patient has a known underlying seizure disorder, prophylactic anticonvulsants are not routinely used. Alcohol withdrawal seizures are typically grand mal, nonfocal, and one or two in number. When a seizure occurs more than 48 hours after the last drink or when the patient has a history of head trauma, a focal finding on the neurologic examination, or a focal seizure, the physician should consider other possible causes besides alcohol. Regardless, computed tomography or magnetic resonance imaging scan of the brain should be done in any patient who presents with new onset of seizures. As previously discussed, benzodiazepines are believed to be sufficient and effective prevention of alcohol-related seizures. A patient who has had a seizure should be observed in the hospital for at least 24 hours afterward. Long-term anticonvulsant therapy is not initiated for a seizure that is believed to be purely alcohol related.

Disorders Related to Volume Status, Electrolytes, and Vitamins

Patients suffering from alcohol withdrawal frequently develop metabolic derangements, which can complicate and prolong the withdrawal syndrome. Dehydration can be caused by fever, tachypnea, or diaphoresis. Depleted electrolytes can significantly increase morbidity. At baseline, levels of potassium, magnesium, and phosphorus may all be low secondary to poor nutrition. Potassium and magnesium are also lost through vomiting, diarrhea, malabsorption, and electrolyte shifts. Profound potassium depletion can cause life-threatening ventricular arrhythmias. Patients with significant hypomagnesemia are also at risk for arrhythmias, but these are related to prolongation of the Q-T or P-R interval. Very low serum phosphate levels can cause seizures, coma, and rhabdomyolysis. Hypoglycemia develops in advanced liver disease when ethanol disrupts gluconeogenesis. Once hepatic glycogen stores become depleted, the body is forced to break down fatty acids, and the result is systemic alcoholic ketoacidosis. Treatment of all these complications is supportive, with appropriate replacement of electrolytes, intravenous fluids, and glucose. Thiamine depletion is discussed earlier. The alcohol-dependent patient should also routinely receive a multivitamin secondary to malabsorption of folate and fat-soluble vitamins, such as vitamin K. Oral, subcutaneous, or intravenous vitamin K supplementation may be required to reverse alcohol-related coagulopathy.

Cardiovascular Complications

Cardiac complications of chronic alcohol use can include hypertension, cardiomyopathy, arrhythmias, and angina. Approximately one third of alcoholic patients have decreased ejection fractions, usually secondary to nonischemic dilated cardiomyopathy. This alcoholic cardiomyopathy generally occurs in people who consume more than 90 g/day of alcohol for more than 5 years. Congestive heart failure caused by alcohol abuse is essentially treated in the same way as heart failure of other causes. Atrial arrhythmias, including premature contractions, tachycardia, atrial flutter, and atrial fibrillation, commonly seen during an active binge, are referred to as the *holiday heart syndrome*. Although the patient should be closely monitored with telemetry, antiarrhythmic treatment is not indicated unless the atrial flutter or fibrillation persists or the patient develops hemodynamic compromise. Epidemiologic studies have shown that the long-term consumption of alcohol is associated with an increase in blood pressure. As mentioned earlier, treatment with a β-blocker or clonidine may be effective, especially if the patient is having active withdrawal symptoms. Patients with a history of alcohol abuse are also more likely to complain of angina. The mechanism is postulated to be either a result of increased coronary demand from a reduced ejection fraction or coronary vasospasm as a direct toxic effect of ethanol.

Pulmonary Complications

Alcoholic patients are more likely to develop postoperative pneumonia with higher mortality rates and longer admissions than in the general population. The specific contributing factors are thought to be poor dentition, malnutrition, aspiration, immune suppression, and frequent concurrent abuse of other substances such as tobacco. The isolated organisms and the treatments are generally the same as in community-acquired pneumonia, but alcoholic patients have an increased risk of developing anaerobic pneumonias and tuberculosis and are predisposed to complications of pneumonia such as empyema and acute respiratory distress syndrome.

Hepatic Complications

It is thought that only approximately 10% to 20% of patients with chronic alcoholism develop significant liver disease. The broad spectrum of disease includes fatty liver, alcoholic hepatitis, portal hypertension, and cirrhosis (see Chapter 10). An individual patient may be affected by more than one problem. Patients who have alcohol-related liver disease have been shown in multiple studies to have more perioperative complications. In fact, older studies from the 1970s reported mortality rates as high as 55% for patients undergoing open liver biopsy. Patients should be carefully questioned and examined for suggestive physical findings of advanced hepatic dysfunction such as jaundice, hepatomegaly or splenomegaly, ascites, edema, gynecomastia, varices, and abnormalities on laboratory tests and studies, as previously outlined. Individual patient risk for perioperative complications is multifactorial and is generally determined by the number and severity of comorbid medical conditions, the extent of liver disease, and the risk of the procedure. Various scoring systems, such as the MELD (Model for End-Stage Liver Disease) score and the Child-Turcotte-Pugh classification, have been developed and validated as preoperative risk assessment tools in patients with cirrhosis. Anesthesiologists should be notified of suspected or known alcohol abuse, so they can select less hepatotoxic anesthetics, sedatives, and analgesics to use in the operating room. Acute alcoholic hepatitis is a relative contraindication to surgery, and patients with this condition should have elective procedures postponed until they can be medically optimized and, if possible, encouraged to undergo preoperative detoxification programs.

Gastrointestinal Complications

Alcoholic patients with advanced liver disease are prone to developing esophageal and gastric varices and subsequent life-threatening bleeding (see Chapter 9). Alcohol is also the most common cause of acute pancreatitis in the United States; this disease usually occurs only after 4 to 7 years of heavy ethanol abuse. Twenty to 30% of these patients develop acute necrotizing pancreatitis, which has been reported to have a mortality rate as high as 30%. Alcohol also increases gastric acid secretion, and patients are prone to developing gastritis, ulceration, and bleeding complications. Perioperative acid suppression therapy should be initiated for patients with epigastric pain or suspected upper gastrointestinal bleeding. Patients with chronic alcohol use have also been found to have increased risk for gastrointestinal malignancies as compared with the general population.

Hematologic Complications

Anemias of various causes have been found in 10% to 60% of hospitalized patients with alcoholism (see Chapter 6). Microcytic anemia can be caused by gastritis, peptic ulcer disease, or malignancy and exacerbated by alcohol-related coagulopathy. Hemolytic anemia is usually the result of alcohol-related splenomegaly and sequestration. Nutritional folate deficiency can cause megaloblastic anemia. By an unknown mechanism, alcohol can also independently cause macrocytosis, with or without anemia, in the presence of normal folate levels. The increased risk for infection with chronic alcohol use and frequent comorbid conditions predispose patients with long-term alcoholism to anemia of chronic disease.

Thrombocytopenia, defined as a platelet count of less than 150,000/µL from direct bone marrow toxicity, is also common in alcoholic patients. A hospitalized patient with a forced period of abstinence from alcohol may subsequently develop *rebound thrombocytosis.* The platelet count usually rises after the fifth hospital day and may exceed 1 million/μL. Despite the level of elevation, there does not appear to be any association with thrombosis. In addition to quantitative platelet deficiencies, patients with chronic alcoholism tend to have abnormal platelet function because of decreased thromboxane A_2 release from platelets. Platelet number and function generally return to normal within 2 weeks of abstinence. (Indications for platelet transfusion are discussed in Chapter 6.)

Miscellaneous Complications

Possible alcohol-related endocrinopathies include hyperlipidemia, hypogonadism, testicular atrophy, gynecomastia in men, amenorrhea, sexual dysfunction, and premature menopause. Alcohol has been known to cause painful peripheral neuropathies and myopathies, characterized by elevated creatine phosphokinases and myoglobinuria. Women who consume more than 30 to 60 g/day of alcohol have an increased relative risk of breast cancer.

Drug Interactions

Chronic alcohol use causes an induction in the cytochrome P-450 system. As a result, these patients have an induced tolerance to other drugs also metabolized by this system, such as benzodiazepines and narcotics. In the perioperative period, these patients are likely to require higher doses of anesthetics, analgesics, and sedatives. As dysfunction progresses, the metabolism of these drugs slows down, and patients begin to become increasingly sensitive to equivalent doses. Very close monitoring is required postoperatively in a patient with chronic alcoholism to balance optimal pain management with oversedation and respiratory depression. Alternatively, if a patient is acutely intoxicated just prior to the operation, alcohol will competitively inhibit other compounds that rely on the microsomal system, and increased serum levels of these medications will result.

PERIOPERATIVE CARE OF THE COCAINE-DEPENDENT PATIENT

Background

Based on reports from the National Institutes of Health, the number of cocaine users in the United States is increasing at a rate of about 1 million people per year. In 2004, 34.2 million Americans older than 12 years reported using cocaine at least once, and 7.8 million reported using "freebase" or "crack," an extremely addictive, smokeable form of cocaine that produces almost instantaneous effects through rapid absorption into the pulmonary circulation. Cocaine can also be injected, snorted (nasally insufflated), or ingested. In terms of its mechanism of action, cocaine is an indirect sympathomimetic that increases circulating catecholamine levels. In the central nervous system, cocaine inhibits reabsorption of dopamine into sympathetic nerve terminals. The elevated levels of dopamine cause persistent neuronal stimulation and are believed to account for cocaine's addictive properties.

Long-term users of cocaine are also known to develop physiologic tolerance that requires escalating doses of the drug and increased frequency of use to achieve equivalent effects. To prevent withdrawal symptoms or unpleasant side effects of high doses of cocaine, many cocaine abusers self-medicate with other substances. The addition of cannabis increases plasma cocaine levels. Combining cocaine with heroin, called "speedballing," is reported to enhance the effects of both drugs. Of people who admit to cocaine abuse, 92% also report using alcohol. The concomitant use of cocaine and alcohol creates a potentially lethal metabolite known as cocaethylene. Its toxicity is greater than either parent drug, it has a longer half-life, and according to the National Institutes of Health reports, it has been linked to more deaths than any other two-drug combination. Cocaine is quickly metabolized and is detectable in the urine anywhere from several days to 2 weeks later, depending on extent of use. Because of individual differences in metabolism, serum cocaine levels are not helpful in predicting the severity of intoxication or morbidity, and people have been known to experience sudden cardiac death on their first use of the drug.

Symptoms of Cocaine Intoxication and Withdrawal

Patients who use cocaine report that it produces a sense of euphoria, increased energy and productivity, decreased appetite, and a decreased need for sleep. The higher the dose and the faster the route of absorption, the more intense the pleasurable effects are. An acutely intoxicated patient may present with dilated pupils, sinus tachycardia, fever, and elevated blood pressure. At higher doses, symptoms escalate to paranoia, violent behavior, auditory hallucinations, and tremor. Overdoses can be characterized by seizures, acidosis, pulmonary edema, and cardiac or respiratory arrest. As with alcohol, early withdrawal symptoms from cocaine may be masked by anesthesia and narcotic pain medications. In a postoperative patient with an unknown or inaccurate medical history, the initial signs of cocaine withdrawal can be subtle and nonspecific. A patient may complain only of depressed mood, fatigue, difficulty sleeping or increased need for sleep, anxiety, or myalgias. In time, these symptoms intensify, and the patient can develop extrapyramidal symptoms or acute psychosis, with characteristic features of severe paranoia, bizarre delusions, and tactile hallucinations, particularly of "bugs crawling under the skin," a phenomenon known as *formication*. At this time, the patient will also be experiencing strong cravings for the drug and may be anxious to leave the hospital, frequently against medical advice. Withdrawal from cocaine, although uncomfortable, is characterized mostly by these psychiatric symptoms and is generally not life-threatening. Moreover, because cocaine has a half-life of only approximately 30 to 90 minutes, most surgical procedures can be delayed until the acute intoxication period has passed.

Treatment of Cocaine Withdrawal

If possible, the actively withdrawing patient should be placed in quiet surroundings and be allowed to sleep and eat at will. Benzodiazepines may be required to control severe agitation and psychosis. If psychosis does not respond to a benzodiazepine, an antipsychotic with minimal anticholinergic side effects can be tried next. Multiple agents such as bromocriptine, amantadine, desipramine, fluoxetine, bupropion, and carbamazepine have all been tested in clinical trials, but unfortunately, to date, no medication has been proven effective for either the withdrawal symptoms or the treatment of cocaine addiction. As with other suspected substances of abuse, differential causes of acute mental status changes should be investigated in an acutely ill patient with an unknown or unreliable history. Cocaine withdrawal usually does not last longer than several days, so if symptoms of psychosis or agitation persist beyond that period, another diagnosis should be pursued.

Cardiovascular Complications

The most frequent presenting complaint in a patient addicted to cocaine is likely to be cocaine-related chest pain (Box 15-2). Cocaine can actually cause numerous cardiovascular problems by various mechanisms, and the nature and severity of the complications are affected by the dose, the chronicity of use, the individual's level of tolerance or sensitivity to the drug, and the presence of underlying heart disease. Cocaine's mechanisms of action in the cardiovascular system include inhibition of cellular sodium transport and an increase in catecholamine levels with resulting sympathetic activation. Rapid, appropriate diagnosis and treatment by the physician may be compromised by a patient's reluctance to admit to recent use of the drug, as well as by "atypical" presenting signs and symptoms. It is particularly important to suspect cocaine as a cause of myocardial ischemia in the young patient who presents with an acute coronary syndrome. A laboratory and radiologic evaluation of a

Box 15-2	MEDICAL COMPLICATIONS OF COCAINE USE

- Cardiac: Arrhythmias (tachycardia, sinus bradycardia, premature ventricular conduction, ventricular tachycardia, ventricular fibrillation), malignant hypertension, myocardial infarction, myocardial ischemia, congestive heart failure, hypertension, aortic rupture, pneumopericardium, sudden death, dilated cardiomyopathy, ventricular hypertrophy myocardial fibrosis, myocarditis
- Respiratory: Chronic rhinitis, osteolytic sinusitis, nasoseptal perforation, pneumonia, pulmonary barotrauma, hemoptysis, diffuse alveolar hemorrhage, asthma, interstitial pneumonitis, hypersensitivity pneumonitis, bronchiolitis obliterans-organizing pneumonia, "crack-lung," recurrent pulmonary infiltrates with eosinophilia, noncardiogenic pulmonary edema, pneumomediastinum, pneumothorax
- Neurologic: Seizures, intracranial hemorrhage, ischemic stroke headache, tics, ataxia, movement disorders
- Gastrointestinal (generally from cocaine ingestion): Delayed gastric emptying, ulcers, intestinal ischemia, colitis, hepatic necrosis
- Psychiatric: Insomnia, psychosis, weight loss, hallucination, anxiety, panic attacks, paranoia
- Renal: Acute rhabdomyolysis, acute renal failure, renal infarction, focal segmental glomerulosclerosis
- Miscellaneous: Fever, thrombocytopenia, sexual dysfunction, human immunodeficiency virus infection, and hepatitis B or C infection in injection drug users

patient suspected to have cocaine-related chest pain should include a urine drug screen, complete blood count, a basic metabolic panel (with special attention to glucose, electrolytes, and creatinine), arterial blood gas, urinalysis, creatinine kinase, troponin I, an ECG, and a chest radiograph.

It is generally accepted that cocaine-induced acute coronary syndromes are more likely to occur in persons with preexisting coronary artery disease, and the risk for cocaine-related myocardial infarction is higher in otherwise healthy cocaine users than in matched controls. Cocaine-related chest pain is believed to be caused by coronary vasoconstriction. Vasospasm can be diffuse or local and can occur in both diseased and normal coronary arteries, although it is usually more pronounced in the atherosclerotic vessels. Cardiac ischemia may develop anywhere from several minutes up to as long as 15 hours after last use of the drug. The major physiologically active metabolites (e.g., such as ethyl methyl ecgonine and benzoylecgonine [the compound detected by the standard urine drug screen]) are thought to account for prolonged, delayed, or recurrent episodes of chest pain that occur after the parent compound is fully hydrolyzed. Only approximately 50% of patients with cocaine-related cardiac ischemia present with typical anginal pain; therefore, the lack of a classic history of "unstable angina" should not be relied on as an effective method for triage of patients. Findings on the ECG in patients who are having acute coronary syndromes are frequently nonspecific or nondiagnostic; only approximately 8% of patients present with an acute injury pattern. Elevated levels of cardiac troponins have been found to have better correlation with myocardial injury than abnormalities on the ECG.

Despite their known benefit in acute myocardial infarction, as well as symptomatic relief of hypertension and tachycardia, β-blockers have traditionally been avoided out of concerns about unopposed α-adrenergic effects with subsequent coronary artery vasoconstriction. Because no large RCTs have been conducted in humans to determine whether the more selective β-blockers should truly be prohibited in the care of the patient with cocaine-induced myocardial ischemia, no evidence-based recommendations are currently available. Although some authors question the contraindication to β-blockade in patients who present with cocaine-related chest pain, most physicians would continue to withhold these medications in patients with a known history of cocaine abuse.

For management of cocaine-induced hypertension, nitrates and other direct acting vasodilators such as hydralazine or nitroprusside can be used. If arrhythmias develop following cocaine use, they are generally short lived and should resolve without any medical intervention. However, if the patient develops signs of associated hemodynamic compromise, he or she should be treated according to Advanced Cardiac Life Support Protocols (see Cardiology section). Cocaine addiction has been associated with accelerated coronary atherosclerosis, and the development of a hypercoagulable state. One hypothesis is that cocaine decreases levels of antithrombin III and protein C in chronic users. Other theories suggest increased platelet activation and aggregation, and increased production of thromboxane, and plasminogen activator inhibitor. Another less common cardiovascular complication of cocaine use is associated with the sudden and wide fluctuations in blood pressure from catecholamine excess. These dramatic escalations and precipitous drops are similar to those seen in pheochromocytoma, and can lead to aortic dissection and valvular damage. This in turn, increases the risk for aortic and mitral valve endocarditis, especially in patients who concurrently abuse injection drugs. Congestive heart failure will develop in some long-term cocaine users. The mechanisms include drug related interstitial myocardial fibrosis, left ventricular hypertrophy, systolic dysfunction, or a dilated cardiomyopathy. Arrhythmias such as sinus tachycardia, sinus bradycardia, supraventricular tachycardia, and ventricular fibrillation are commonly seen just after cocaine is systemically absorbed. The etiology is likely cocaine's similarity to the Class I antiarrhythmic drugs.

Patients who present for surgical procedures with active cocaine intoxication or very recent use should be monitored closely with telemetry. Surprisingly, studies have demonstrated a relatively low overall "rule-in" rate of about 6% for acute MI and a mortality rate for all cocaine-induced chest pain of less than 1%, despite documentation of coronary artery disease by subsequent cardiac catheterization in some of these patients. These studies also determined that of the patients who do suffer a myocardial infarction, only 36% develop complications such as CHF and arrhythmias, and 90% of these episodes developed within the first 12 hours after use. Life-threatening arrhythmias such as ventricular fibrillation or tachycardia were generally not seen, and therefore were presumed to have occurred prior to arrival to the Emergency Department. An explanation for the overall low mortality rate suggested by one author is that cocaine-related deaths tend to occur mainly in those abusers with severe underlying structural or electrophysiologic heart disease, a massive overdose, or a very prolonged history of cocaine abuse.

Pulmonary Complications

Smoking crack cocaine may lead to numerous pulmonary complications (Box 15-3). Acutely, cocaine can cause bronchospasm and can precipitate or worsen asthma exacerbations.

Box 15-3	TREATMENT OF COCAINE-RELATED CHEST PAIN AND CARDIAC ISCHEMIA

GENERALLY RECOMMENDED FIRST-LINE TREATMENTS
- Oxygen
- Aspirin (acutely, to reduce thrombus formation, and long term if evidence of coronary artery disease is present)
- Benzodiazepines (given in sedative doses, to reduce myocardial oxygen demand and to decrease anxiety)
- Nitrates (to relieve symptoms of chest pain)
- Morphine (to relieve pain and to decrease myocardial oxygen demand)
- Primary angioplasty, if available (treatment of choice in ongoing ischemia over fibrinolytics)

SECOND-LINE TREATMENTS OR CAUTIOUS USE

- Calcium channel blockers (theoretically to relieve vasospasm, but variable results seen in clinical trials)
- Intravenous heparin (risks and benefits need to be weighed in light of increased risk for intracranial hemorrhage and aortic dissection)
- Phentolamine (pure α-antagonist, no good studies, but recommended by the International Guidelines for Emergency Cardiovascular Care for cocaine-induced ischemia)
- Thrombolytics (as above, cautious use in patients with cocaine-induced ST segment elevation myocardial infarction, when angioplasty is not available)
- Bicarbonate "suggested" for use with wide complex tachycardia (for myocardial electrical stability with cocaine's sodium channel blocking properties)
- Lidocaine and magnesium (cautious use for arrhythmias, no evidence-based information about other antiarrhythmics such as lidocaine)
- Epinephrine use for asystole (controversial, owing to presence of already elevated catecholamine levels)
- General anesthesia (because of anesthesia's cardiac effects, regional anesthesia preferred if possible)

TREATMENTS TO AVOID

- Class Ia antiarrhythmics (owing to similar effects)
- β-Blockers (as above, generally avoided, but no good evidence; labetalol, with weak α-effects would theoretically be preferable, but in practice does not offer any advantage over propranolol because of high ratio of β-blocker to α-blocker effects)

Data from Ghuran A, Nolan J: Recreational drug misuse: Issues for the cardiologist. Heart 83:627-633, 2000; Hollander J, Henry T: Evaluation and management of the patient who has cocaine-associated chest pain. Cardiol Clin 24:103-114, 2006; Jones J, Weir W: Cocaine-associated chest pain. Med Clin North Am 89:1323-1342, 2005; Stouffer G, Sheahan R, Lenihan D, et al: Cocaine associated chest pain. Am J Med Sci 324:37-44, 2002.

Other symptoms reported by heavy users that do not usually require immediate medical attention include melanoptysis, hemoptysis, cough, and shortness of breath. Chronic cocaine use may lead to recurrent pneumonia, pulmonary barotrauma, diffuse alveolar hemorrhage, and "crack lung," an acute lung injury syndrome with pulmonary infiltrates, eosinophilia, fever, and characteristic histologic findings.

Neurologic Complications

Cocaine abusers have also been known to develop seizures, usually within 90 minutes of use and rarely also during the withdrawal phase. Diazepam or lorazepam is usually effective in terminating the seizure. Patients are also at higher risk for hemorrhagic stroke. Although these strokes typically occur in patients with ruptured berry aneurysms or arteriovenous malformations, the blood pressure fluctuations themselves are sufficient to cause cerebral hemorrhage, and no underlying vascular defect is necessary. Ischemic strokes associated with recent cocaine use are thought to be related to cerebral vasospasm.

PERIOPERATIVE MANAGEMENT OF THE OPIOID-DEPENDENT PATIENT

Background

Opioids are synthetic and natural substances derived from the opium poppy that all have effects similar to those of morphine. Heroin, morphine, codeine, oxycodone, meperidine, and fentanyl are the most commonly abused drugs in this class. Opioid dependence, from either illicit or increasingly prevalent prescription drug abuse, may result in many serious medical complications (Box 15-4). Up to 2% of opioid-dependent individuals die annually of complications from the drug, and 53% of individuals who ever try heroin become addicted to it. In certain areas of the United States, rates of infection with human immunodeficiency virus have been reported to be as high as 60% in patients who are

Box 15-4	MEDICAL COMPLICATIONS OF CHRONIC OPIOID DEPENDENCE

- Infections: Generally related to infectious drug use, including human immunodeficiency virus, endocarditis (usually right sided), septic thrombophlebitis, cellulites, abscess, necrotizing fasciitis, tetanus, tuberculosis, osteomyelitis, septic arthritis, viral hepatitis, methicillin-resistant *Staphylococcus aureus* infections, sepsis, pneumonia, septic emboli
- Cardiac: Drug-induced bradycardia, atrial and ventricular arrhythmias,* hypotension†
- Pulmonary: Noncardiogenic pulmonary edema, talcosis, severe or fatal asthma exacerbations
- Neurologic: Sedation, seizures, transverse myelitis, polyneuropathy
- Gastrointestinal: Nausea, ileus, constipation
- Pregnancy-related complications: Preeclampsia, miscarriage, infection, neonatal complications
- Urinary tract: Urinary retention, glomerulonephritis

*Rapid metabolism should render most cardiac arrhythmias short-lived. If they persist, conventional treatment is recommended with no special precautions. However, a patient who develops an arrhythmia should remain in a monitored environment for at least 24 hours.
†Although blood pressure may commonly be reduced during toxicity, hypotension leading to end-organ damage is rare.

addicted to intravenous heroin. Heroin can be injected, nasally insufflated, or smoked. The intravenous route is the most rapid and produces the highest drug concentrations.

Predictable physiologic tolerance (in which progressively larger doses are required to achieve effects and to avoid withdrawal) and physical dependence (when cessation or significant dose reduction precipitates withdrawal) develop after only 1 to 2 weeks of daily use. Patients appear to develop tolerance to most of the effects of opioids except constipation, which continues to worsen with increased use. In general, opioid metabolites can be detected in urine for 48 hours to several days, with the longer durations noted in more chronic users. The presence of 6-MAM, a specific metabolite of heroin, distinguishes its use. False-negative results on drug testing can occur because not all metabolites of all opioids are detected in routine urine drug screens. False-positive drug screens may occur in patients who are taking fluoroquinolones or rifampin or who consume large quantities of poppy seeds.

As with cocaine, preoperative opioid use generally does not complicate nonemergency operations because of the relatively short half-life of commonly abused opioids, and most procedures can be delayed until the patient is stabilized. However, with the increasing prevalence of use, especially the nonmedical use of prescription narcotics, the perioperative consultant should not only be able to recognize and treat opioid toxicity or withdrawal, but should also assist with acute pain management in patients addicted to opioids, or those enrolled in maintenance programs.

Opioid Toxicity

The major physiologic effects of opioids are on the central nervous system and the cardiovascular system. The characteristic signs of acute opioid intoxication or overdose may be analgesia, euphoria, varying degrees of lethargy (including coma), respiratory depression, bradycardia, hypotension, hypothermia, and miosis. An opioid antagonist such as naloxone should be given to any patient exhibiting signs of hemodynamic instability such as respiratory depression, bradycardia, or hypotension. An initial dose of 0.4 mg of naloxone may be sufficient to reverse the respiratory depression. This same dose may be repeated two or three times in the first few minutes if there is no improvement in symptoms, especially if the diagnosis is in doubt. Because naloxone is a short-acting antagonist, if a clinical response is seen, a continuous infusion of two thirds of the initial bolus dose each hour should be started promptly. The adult dose is typically 0.25 mg/hr to 6.25 mg/hr. The infusion should be continued for at least 12 hours and titrated according to the patient's medical status. If a patient is hemodynamically stable, it is preferable to *avoid* treatment with naloxone. Although rare, noncardiogenic pulmonary edema resulting from heroin toxicity can occur up to 24 hours after drug use. It can be severe and may require positive pressure ventilation or intubation. The exact cause is unknown, but administration of naloxone can acutely precipitate this complication. Of course, if the overdose was intentional, the patient should be evaluated by psychiatry before discharge.

Symptoms of Opioid Withdrawal

Withdrawal usually develops within 4 to 6 hours of the last injection, peaks at 24 to 48 hours, and lasts about a week. The time frames vary depending on the half-life of the individual drug. For heroin, withdrawal is typically evident 36 to 42 hours after discontinuation. Symptoms can include restlessness, difficulty sleeping, myalgias, abdominal cramping, nausea, vomiting, diarrhea, anxiety, yawning, increased diaphoresis, pupillary dilation, and increased lacrimation. The onset of withdrawal may occur shortly after admission or may be delayed until the postoperative analgesics are metabolized. A patient can be physically detoxified from opioids in as little as 1 week in an inpatient setting; without proper motivation and follow-up, however, the relapse rates are high.

Treatment of Opioid Withdrawal

Methadone Therapy

- Methadone is a common and effective treatment for narcotic withdrawal. It is a synthetic long-acting opioid, which is classified by the U.S. Drug Enforcement Administration (DEA) as a schedule II drug, carrying the highest potentials for dependence and abuse. As a pain medication, any physician with an active DEA license can prescribe methadone. However, its use for the treatment of addiction is highly restricted and requires special licensing in the United States. These regulations are waived for inpatients, because these patients frequently require methadone to improve compliance during hospitalization. Methadone is metabolized by the cytochrome P-450 system; therefore, it has many significant medication interactions, which must be carefully monitored throughout the admission.

- In the United States, methadone is approved for oral (liquid or pill), subcutaneous, or intramuscular use. Common side effects of methadone are increased sweating, constipation, and sexual dysfunction. Methadone has a biphasic pattern of elimination. The first phase lasts a total of about 6 to 8 hours and corresponds to the duration of its analgesic effects. The second phase, which lasts 30 to 60 hours, is sufficient to prevent withdrawal symptoms, but it does not provide any additional analgesia. For withdrawal prevention, it is usually administered at 20 to 40 mg divided into two doses per day. The initial dose can be estimated by standardized conversion tables of other narcotics to methadone; however, methadone is known to be highly variable among individuals, and some patients require doses greater than 100 mg/day. Although these recommended starting doses should be sufficient to prevent physical withdrawal symptoms, larger doses are frequently requested by the patient to control opioid craving. A patient started on methadone during a hospital admission should be able to tolerate a total dose reduction by 5 to 10 mg/day.

- Additional short-acting opioids will likely be required for acute pain management, especially in the postoperative setting, and are described in more detail later.

Other Opioid Replacement Options

- Sublingual buprenorphine (Subutex) is a mixed opioid agonist-antagonist that has been used with some success in patients with mild to moderate physical dependence. It has a longer half-life than methadone and can therefore be administered every 2 to 3 days. Although it is not as effective as methadone, buprenorphine is generally safer, it is more readily available on an outpatient basis, it has a low risk of illegal use, and an overdose with sublingual buprenorphine (Buprenex) carries less risk of respiratory depression. The dose range is 4 to 24 mg/day with a target dose of 16 mg/day. Adverse effects such as liver function test abnormalities are generally mild, but there have been case reports of lethal overdose of intravenous buprenorphine (a route of administration not commonly used in the United States) when the drug was simultaneously injected with intravenous benzodiazepines.

- Naltrexone, an opioid antagonist, is used in outpatient treatment programs. It is not feasible for the actively addicted hospitalized patient, however, because it can precipitate acute opioid withdrawal syndrome.

- In some countries such Switzerland and the Netherlands, heroin withdrawal is being treated with heroin maintenance programs. This is generally reserved for individuals who have failed other more conventional modalities. The literature from these centers reports some success in maintaining these patients in treatment programs and away from criminal activities.

Symptomatic Treatment–Only Options

Referral to a methadone program may be needed for patients who cannot be weaned from methadone and who were not in a program preoperatively. If methadone therapy is not feasible or desirable, detoxification can be accomplished with a combination of medications that help to suppress the physical discomfort associated with withdrawal. Unfortunately, these medications do little to prevent the associated psychological symptoms of opioid craving and therefore are less well tolerated than methadone.

Although clonidine is not approved by the Food and Drug Administration for this indication in the United States, this drug has been used to help with gastrointestinal and autonomic symptoms of opioid withdrawal, and it may be especially valuable in the surgical patient who has hypertension. The recommended initial doses are 2 μg/kg three times per day for 7 to 10 days, then taper over 3 days. The transdermal patch (Catapres-TTS) may also be used, although it should be overlapped with oral clonidine, because it takes several days to be fully effective. Patients need to be carefully monitored for hypotension and bradycardia. For short-acting opioids such as heroin, clonidine-assisted withdrawal can be completed in 4 to 6 days. In noncompliant patients, clonidine is a poor choice for continued outpatient therapy in light of its potential life-threatening toxicities as well as a risk of rebound malignant hypertension if the drug is abruptly discontinued. Withdrawal can also be treated symptomatically with antidiarrheals, antiemetics, antispasmodics, and nonsteroidal anti-inflammatory medications. Anxiolytics may also be required, but they must be used with caution because of their high risk of dependence.

Acute Pain Management for Methadone Maintenance Patients

- Opioid-dependent patients may report being enrolled in a methadone maintenance program preoperatively. This history should be confirmed before initiating "maintenance" inpatient therapy.
- Once the dose is established, methadone should be continued preoperatively at the outpatient dose, including the morning of surgery.
- As stated earlier, patients taking high doses should receive a preoperative ECG to assess for Q-T interval prolongation.
- To prevent withdrawal, other opioid analgesics should be used parenterally as a substitute for methadone while the patient is taking nothing by mouth (NPO). In patients who take very high doses of methadone, patient-controlled analgesia should be considered, with a constant basal rate to prevent withdrawal. Oral methadone should be restarted at home doses as soon as the patient is adequately tolerating fluids.

- Postoperatively, patients require treatment with additional short-acting opioids to control pain. Methadone should not be titrated upward for analgesic purposes in these patients, because its very long elimination half-life compared with its short analgesic half-life predisposes to toxicity from dose accumulation. Advice from the outpatient methadone treatment center should be requested if the methadone is to be restarted after more than 5 days.

For the patient who is receiving opioids for chronic pain management, the perioperative period is an inappropriate time to attempt a reduction in the dosage. In general, physicians tend to underdose with narcotic medications for the following reasons: concern for neurologic, respiratory, or cardiac depression; fear of creating iatrogenic drug abuse or causing a relapse in a former addict; "giving-in" to drug-seeking behavior; or the presumption that the current maintenance doses are sufficient for analgesia. All these fears are exacerbated in patients with a known history of substance abuse, or who are receiving chronic outpatient therapy, resulting in overall inadequate pain management. Investigators have observed for many years that opioid-addicted patients also appear to have decreased pain thresholds or hyperalgesia, and even higher than usual doses may be required because of opioid cross-tolerance. Patients taking methadone on a long-term basis should not be treated with mixed agonist-antagonist analgesics for pain, because these drugs provide no benefit over the traditional narcotic medications, and they may precipitate acute opioid withdrawal.

PERIOPERATIVE MANAGEMENT OF THE BENZODIAZEPINE-DEPENDENT PATIENT

Benzodiazepines, one of the most prescribed classes of drugs in the United States, have a significant abuse potential and may cause physiologic dependence and withdrawal. Substance abusers add benzodiazepines to enhance the "high" or to self-medicate for withdrawal symptoms of other illicit substances. Patients with benzodiazepine toxicity may present with lethargy, ataxia, and dysarthria. Fortunately, when benzodiazepines alone are abused, significant respiratory depression is uncommon.

The antidote for benzodiazepine overdose is flumazenil, a partial benzodiazepine agonist. The initial dose is 0.2 mg IV bolus, repeated at 0.3 to 0.5 mg doses until a clinical response is noted or the maximal dose of 3 mg is reached. Very cautious use of flumazenil is recommended, because chronic users who are physically dependent can develop withdrawal seizures. In these patients, any abrupt discontinuation of benzodiazepines can also precipitate withdrawal symptoms. These symptoms may include anxiety, irritability, depressed mood, insomnia, and sensitivity to light and sound, as well as fatigue, tremor, muscle cramps, myoclonic jerking, and, rarely, seizures or nonconvulsive status epilepticus. Patients can also experience severe rebound anxiety or insomnia if the medication was originally prescribed for these symptoms. Withdrawal reactions usually do not occur unless the patient has been taking benzodiazepines continuously for at least 3 months and may continue for several months after cessation. Both the dose and the duration of use affect the severity of withdrawal, so a patient taking a stable low dose on a long-term basis may be as symptomatic as someone who had recently started abusing high doses of the medication. Moreover, a patient who has been taking a benzodiazepine with a long half-life may not exhibit signs of withdrawal for up to a week after discontinuation of the drug. The anesthesiologist should be notified of known or suspected long-term benzodiazepine use, because these patients typically require less sedation during anesthesia, and they may require higher doses of opioid pain medications postoperatively.

There is also a syndrome of "pseudowithdrawal," which is difficult to distinguish from true benzodiazepine withdrawal.

This condition usually occurs in a patient who is psychologically unprepared for the medication to be tapered and who develops psychologically rather than physiologically mediated withdrawal symptoms.

If a benzodiazepine is being initiated in the hospital, either for anxiety or withdrawal from another substance such as alcohol, it should be titrated very cautiously in elderly patients, because they metabolize benzodiazepines more slowly and are at increased risk of toxicity related to drug accumulation. Withdrawal symptoms, especially seizures, tend to be worse with the shorter-acting agents: lorazepam, alprazolam, and oxazepam. If possible, patients should be switched to a benzodiazepine with a longer half-life such as diazepam or chlordiazepoxide. These longer-acting benzodiazepines can then be very slowly (not more than one fourth of the total daily dose/week) tapered over 6 to 12 weeks in the outpatient setting. Propranolol, at 20 mg every 6 hours, can be added to reduce the hypertension, tachycardia, and anxiety that may occur during benzodiazepine withdrawal. If the physician is reluctant to proceed with a long-term benzodiazepine taper in an addicted patient, another option is to use phenobarbital. Although it does help to reduce rebound anxiety, it is physically less well tolerated as a primary tapering agent.

PERIOPERATIVE MANAGEMENT OF THE PATIENT WHO SMOKES TOBACCO

Tobacco use clearly increases postoperative pulmonary complications. Patients with known chronic obstructive pulmonary disease, significant respiratory symptoms, or radiographic abnormalities should have appropriate preoperative evaluation. Smokers are also more likely than nonsmokers to develop perioperative cardiac events, infectious complications, and difficulty with bone and soft tissue healing. Although the optimal duration of preoperative abstinence is unknown, observational and physiologic studies have suggested that at least 2 to 3 months are required for full benefit.

Smoking cessation is frequently impeded by physical and psychological withdrawal symptoms. Withdrawal may manifest with symptoms of depressed mood, difficulty sleeping, irritability, restlessness, bradycardia, and increased appetite. These symptoms can begin as soon as several hours after the last cigarette, peak at about 24 to 48 hours, and on average, persist for about a month. It is also known that psychological dependence, manifested by cigarette craving, can continue much longer in people with a high level of nicotine dependence. Fortunately, many methods are currently available to help patients facilitate quitting, such as referrals to commercial clinics, various nicotine replacement therapy options, bupropion hydrochloride (Zyban), varenidine (Chantix, a partial nicotine agonist), and alternative therapies such as hypnosis and acupuncture. Unfortunately, most patients are not successful in quitting and then maintaining abstinence for 2 to 3 months before a scheduled surgical procedure. Some physicians recommend no less than a full 2-month period of preoperative abstinence from cigarettes. This recommendation is supported by some observational studies in which discontinued cigarette use within several weeks of surgery actually increased the risk of perioperative pulmonary complications. Regardless, the quality of the evidence in the current medical literature is not sufficient to discourage any smoker from trying to cut down or quit before a scheduled procedure. If this is not possible, the patient should be advised at least to abstain from any cigarette use in the 12 hours before the surgical procedure. The rationale is to allow time for dissipation of systemic carbon monoxide before induction of anesthesia. **It is also suggested that the patient not resume smoking until 1 week after the surgical procedure, to improve postoperative wound healing outcomes** [● *Warner, 2005*].

Studies have shown that smoking cessation efforts in inpatients may be more effective than in outpatients. At home, the urge to smoke is commonly triggered by environmental cues that are strongly associated with cigarette use, and some patients have reported less intense withdrawal symptoms when they are hospitalized in a smoke-free environment. After experiencing a tobacco-related medical complication, a patient may be more receptive to learning about tobacco cessation programs. Abstinence rates have been shown to double for patients wearing a nicotine patch when compared with those receiving a placebo. Therefore, a nicotine patch should be considered for all smokers in the perioperative period, to reduce acute withdrawal symptoms and to help the motivated patient quit smoking. The dose may then be slowly tapered in the outpatient setting. Several studies have shown that nicotine replacement therapy is safe for use in patients with coronary artery disease, and **at least one RCT supports the idea that nicotine replacement therapy does not negate the beneficial effects of abstinence from cigarettes postoperatively** [❹ *Sorensen et al, 2003*].

PERIOPERATIVE MANAGEMENT OF THE PATIENT WHO ABUSES MARIJUANA

Marijuana, of the cannabis class, is the most commonly abused illicit drug in the United States. The fastest absorption occurs when it is smoked, but marijuana can be mixed into food and eaten as well. Peak intoxications occur within 10 to 30 minutes, and the effect lasts approximately 3 hours. The drug's plasma half-life is 20 to 30 hours, and the time course for urine drug screen detection varies greatly, depending on the individual extent of use. Manifestations range widely from euphoria to severe paranoia. Acute intoxication usually does not come to medical attention and does not warrant any specific pharmacologic treatment, but evidence of significant adverse events has been appearing in the medical literature.

Typical cardiovascular effects consist of a brief period of relative tachycardia and hypertension, followed by a longer period of relative bradycardia and hypotension. Patients may also present with nonspecific ECG changes, premature ventricular contractions, increased severity of anginal symptoms, myocardial infarctions, ischemic and thrombotic cerebrovascular accidents, and peripheral thromboembolic events.

Heavy marijuana users may complain of asthma-like symptoms, such as increased sputum production, wheezing, and bronchitis, as well as symptoms of exertional dyspnea that are equivalent to the effects of smoking one half-pack of cigarettes per day. There have been isolated case reports of spontaneous pneumothorax and lung bullae associated with marijuana abuse. Endocrinopathies and permanent neurologic changes have also been identified in some long-term users. Although it has not been proven in humans, teratogenicity has been reported in animals, and marijuana is known to impair the immune system's ability to recover from herpes-virus infections and genital warts.

In combination with other drugs, especially stimulants such as cocaine, marijuana can act synergistically to potentiate their toxic effects. Therefore, if a physician is evaluating an otherwise healthy, chronic user of marijuana for a surgical procedure and elicits unusual symptoms such as chest pain and episodes consistent with stroke or transient ischemic attacks, or notes physical findings suggestive of a hypercoagulable state, an elective procedure should be postponed until the patient can be further evaluated with appropriate diagnostic testing.

Selected Readings

Agency for Health Care Policy and Research: Smoking cessation clinical practice guideline. JAMA 275:1270-1280, 1996.

Al-Sanouri I, Dikin M, Soubani A: Critical care aspects of alcohol abuse. South Med J 98:372-381, 2005.

American Psychiatric Association: Practice Guidelines. Practice Guideline for the Treatment of Patients with Substance Abuse Disorders, 2nd ed, part A. Available at http://www.psychiatryonline.com

Busto U, Sellers EM, Naranjo CA, et al: Withdrawal reactions after long-term therapeutic use of benzodiazepines. N Engl J Med 315:854-859, 1986.

Ewing JA: Detecting alcoholism: The CAGE questionnaire. JAMA 252: 1905-1907, 1984. **Ⓐ**

Ferguson JA, Suelzer CJ, Eckert GJ, et al: Risk factors for delirium tremens development. J Gen Intern Med 11:410-414, 1996.

Ghuran A, Nolan J: Recreational drug misuse: Issues for the cardiologist. Heart 83:627-633, 2000.

Gordon R, Lowy F: Current concepts: Bacterial infections in drug users. N Engl J Med 353:1945-1954, 2005.

Hollander JE: The management of cocaine associated myocardial ischemia. N Engl J Med 333:1267-1272, 1995.

Hollander J, Henry T: Evaluation and management of the patient who has cocaine-associated chest pain. Cardiol Clin 24:103-114, 2006.

Kitchens JM: Does this patient have an alcohol problem? JAMA 272: 1782-1787, 1994.

Mayo-Smith MF, Beecher LH, Fischer TL, et al: Management of alcohol withdrawal delirium: An evidence based practice guideline [published correction appears in Arch Intern Med 164:2068, 2004]. Arch Intern Med 164:1405-1412, 2004. **Ⓒ**

Mendelson JH, Mello NK: Management of cocaine abuse and dependence. N Engl J Med 334:965-972, 1996.

Mouhaffel AH, Madu EC, Satmary WA, Fraker TD: Cardiovascular complications of cocaine. Chest 107:1426-1434, 1995.

Sorensen LT, Karlsmark T, Gottrup F: Abstinence from smoking reduces incisional wound infection: A randomized controlled trial. Ann Surg 238:1-5, 2003. **Ⓐ**

Sullivan JT, Sykora K, Schneiderman J, et al: Assessment of alcohol withdrawal: The revised Clinical Institute Withdrawal Assessment for Alcohol Scale (CIWA-Ar). Br J Addict 84:1353-1357, 1989.

Tonnesen H: Alcohol abuse and postoperative morbidity. Dan Med Bull 50:139-160, 2003. **Ⓑ**

Tonnesen H, Kehlet H: Preoperative alcoholism and postoperative morbidity. Br J Surg 86:869-874, 1999. **Ⓑ**

Tonnesen H, Peterson KR, Hojgaard L: Postoperative morbidity among symptom-free alcohol misusers. Lancet 340:334-337, 1992. **Ⓑ**

Warner D: Preoperative smoking cessation: The role of the primary care provider. Mayo Clin Proc 80:252-258, 2005. **Ⓒ**

Weber JE, Chudnofsky CR, Boczar M, et al: Cocaine-associated chest pain: How common is myocardial infarction? Acad Emerg Med 7:873-877, 2000.

West LJ, Maxwell DS, Nobel EP, et al: Alcoholism. Ann Intern Med 100: 445-446, 1984.

16 Perioperative Assessment and Management of the Surgical Patient with Neurologic Problems

RODNEY D. BELL, MD
GENO J. MERLI, MD

Patients with underlying neurologic disease who undergo surgical procedures present unique problems because all anesthetic agents affect neurologic function by altering muscle strength, ability to move, consciousness, or sensation. Because patients with neurologic disease already have at least one of these modalities affected, special understanding and optimization of medical parameters are necessary so that surgery may be carried out safely and with minimal complications.

NEUROMUSCULAR DISEASES

Myasthenia Gravis

Myasthenia gravis is an uncommon disorder; the estimated prevalence is 0.05 to 5 per 100,000 population, and the incidence is 0.4 per 100,000 population. Women are affected more frequently than men (2 to 3:1), and there are no racial or geographic predilections. The average age of onset is 26 years in women and 31 years in men. Two separate groups of patients are recognized, one with an early onset of disease and another with a peak incidence at 70 years. Myasthenia

Levels of Evidence:

Ⓐ—Randomized controlled trials (RCTs), meta-analyses, well-designed systematic reviews of RCTs. Ⓑ—Case-control or cohort studies, nonrandomized clinical trials, systematic reviews of studies other than RCTs, cross-sectional studies, retrospective studies. Ⓒ—Consensus statements, expert guidelines, usual practice, opinion.

gravis is an autoimmune disorder caused by antibodies directed against acetylcholine receptors.

Other autoimmune disorders have been associated with myasthenia gravis, such as pernicious anemia, rheumatoid arthritis, systemic lupus erythematosus, idiopathic thrombocytopenic purpura, pemphigus, autoimmune hemolytic anemia, and thyroid disease (hyperthyroid, hypothyroid, thyroiditis). Thyroid disease (most often hyperthyroidism) occurs in approximately 10% of patients. Thymomas occur in approximately 10% of patients and can usually be detected by chest computed tomography (CT) or magnetic resonance imaging (MRI). Although only 30% of patients with myasthenia gravis have antibodies to skeletal muscle, 90% of patients with thymoma and myasthenia have antiskeletal antibodies. Ten to 15% of patients with generalized myasthenia gravis do not have antibodies to the acetylcholine receptor.

The disease is characterized by fluctuating weakness and fatigue with exercise. The weakness generally is worse at the end of the day or after a period of exertion. However, strength may vary from hour to hour in the absence of any physical activity. Isolated ocular myasthenia occurs in 20% of patients. The most common presentations of generalized myasthenia gravis are fatigable weakness, eye movement abnormalities (40% to 50%), bulbar findings (e.g., difficulty swallowing, 20%), extremity weakness (30%), and neck flexion weakness.

The diagnosis of myasthenia gravis is made on the clinical history, the characteristic response of repetitive nerve stimulation at 3 to 5 Hz with a decremental pattern, the presence of acetylcholine receptor antibodies, and the characteristic response to acetylcholinesterase inhibitors, either edrophonium (Tensilon, 10 mg, with a 1- to 2-mg test dose intravenously) or neostigmine (Prostigmin, 0.04 mg/kg intramuscularly).

Myasthenic crisis develops when muscular weakness begins to worsen, leading to paralysis of respiratory muscles and respiratory failure. Systemic infection is a frequent cause of myasthenic crisis, but the condition can result from mal-absorption of the anticholinesterase medication or from progression of the disease. Cholinergic crisis occurs with an excess of anticholinesterase medication, which can occupy the same receptor as acetylcholine and thus reduces neuro-muscular transmission. Generally, other cholinergic effects are present, such as the following: nicotinic effects of muscle cramps; fasciculations; and increased weakness or musca-rinic effects, such as abdominal cramps, diarrhea, palpita-tions, sweating, increased secretions, salivation, tearing, bradycardia, and increased urination.

Thymectomy is now advocated for myasthenic patients less than 60 years of age who have generalized disease, be-cause of the greater 5- to 10-year survival, greater time in remission, and the 10% incidence of thymoma. Anticholin-esterases, steroids, immunosuppression, and plasmapheresis are all used to manage myasthenia gravis. The major respon-sibilities of the medical consultant are to be knowledgeable about treatment modalities and their adverse effects and to be able to recognize myasthenic and cholinergic crises.

Treatment

Despite the use of immunotherapy, anticholinesterase medi-cation is still the mainstay of therapy for many myasthenic patients. Pyridostigmine (Mestinon) is the most frequently used anticholinesterase for the management of myasthenia gravis. This medication is available in oral formulations (60-mg tablet and syrup, 12 mg/mL). Pyridostigmine is absorbed from the gut, although inactivation occurs, and the dosage required is greater than with other agents. The onset of action is 30 to 60 minutes, and the peak effect is at 2 hours. There is little effect after 4 hours. A sustained-action capsule is available, but release and absorption are erratic, and this mode of delivery is generally used only at bedtime. The usual starting dose of pyridostigmine is 15 to 60 mg every 4 to 6 hours and can be increased in 15- to 60-mg increments.

The side effects of the anticholinesterases can be divided into excess activity at nicotinic receptors (e.g., muscle cramps, fasciculations, and increased weakness) and muscarinic side effects (e.g., abdominal cramps, diarrhea, palpitations, sweating, increased nasal and bronchial secretions, increased urination, bradycardia, salivation, and tearing). The muscarinic side effects can frequently be controlled by oral atropine, 0.4 to 0.6 mg. The atropine is usually given with the pyridostigmine but can be given half an hour before pyridostigmine. Other medications used in the treatment of myasthenia gravis are listed in Table 16-1.

Corticosteroids are used extensively in the treatment of myasthenia gravis. Many patients experience complete reversal of their weakness with this treatment alone. Approximately 8% (44% of those patients treated with an initial high dose) of patients with myasthenia gravis who use steroids for the first time experience weakness. This effect can be reduced by initiating therapy with a low dose and gradually titrating the amount of steroid to achieve the desired effect on the patient's condition. An alternate-day dosing schedule is preferable to daily dosing. If patients are receiving long-term corticosteroids, appropriate preoperative and postoperative supplementation to avoid adrenal crisis will be necessary.

Azathioprine, at a dose of 2 to 3 mg/kg/day, has been used in the treatment of myasthenia gravis. Improvement in strength begins after 2 to 8 months, but the effect may not be maximal

TABLE 16-1	Anticholinesterase Drugs: Myasthenia Gravis	
Drug and Dose	**Route**	**Schedule**
Pyridostigmine (Mestinon)* 60 mg	PO, IV, IM	q4–6h
Pyridostigmine (Timespan), 180 mg	PO	q8–10h
Neostigmine (Prostigmin), 15 mg	PO, IV, IM	q4–6h
Ambenonium (Mytelase), 30 mg	PO	q4–6h

*IV dose 1/30 the total oral dose, q4–6h; IM dose 1/60 the total oral dose, q4–6h.
IM, intramuscularly; IV, intravenously; PO, by mouth; q, every.

until 12 to 24 months. The therapeutic effect is reported to occur only after the mean corpuscular volume increases by 10 U above the baseline value. Cyclophosphamide, at 3 to 5 mg/kg/day, preceded by 200 mg intravenously for 5 days, has been used in patients who are refractory to other forms of treatment. If cytotoxic agents are employed, patients should be assessed preoperatively for the known effects of these drugs (e.g., leukopenia, hemorrhagic cystitis, and hepatotoxicity). Cyclosporine and mycophenolate mofetil are immunosuppressants and steroid-sparing agents that have been shown to be beneficial in severe generalized, treatment-resistant myasthenia gravis.

Plasmapheresis is an effective short-term therapy for patients with severe weakness. It is particularly useful in the setting of recent exacerbation and in preparation for surgical procedures, and it can be used to offset the exacerbation of weakness seen with initiation of corticosteroid therapy. Plasmapheresis is believed to remove acetylcholine receptor antibodies and immune complexes. However, even patients who are seronegative for acetylcholine receptor antibodies may improve with plasmapheresis. The goal is removal of 2 to 4 L of plasma over 90 to 120 minutes three times a week, with 5% albumin replacement on alternate days. This should be completed until improvement in strength reaches a plateau. The onset of improvement is usually rapid, often beginning after the third exchange. Improvement usually lasts from 4 to 8 weeks. Plasmapheresis is being used increasingly with corticosteroids and azathioprine. The complications of plasmapheresis in the perioperative period are electrolyte imbalance, thrombosis, removal of clotting factors, and plasma-bound drugs.

Patients have been reported to improve with high doses of intravenous human immunoglobulin (Ig). The mechanism of action is poorly understood. Doses of 0.4g/kg/day over 2 to 5 days are associated with an improvement during the first week that lasts for weeks to months. Transient leukopenia is usually found in the first 24 to 48 hours. Aseptic meningitis and renal failure are seen uncommonly. Before administration of intravenous Ig, patients should be screened for selective IgA deficiency because an anaphylactic reaction to the IgA in IgG preparations can occur. The effect of intravenous Ig has a relatively short duration, and this agent can be used in the perioperative period in a manner similar to plasmapheresis.

Thymectomy is now widely used for myasthenic patients less than 60 years of age. The best results have been obtained with the transcervical-transsternal surgical approach. In a series of patients without thymoma, 96% benefited from the surgical procedure, 79% were symptom free, 46% were in remission, and 33% were symptom free when receiving minimal doses of pyridostigmine. No clear-cut relationship exists between the presence or titer of acetylcholine receptor antibodies and the patient's response to surgical procedures.

Perioperative Considerations

Numerous medications affect the myoneural junction and may exacerbate myasthenia gravis (Table 16-2). Local anesthetics of the ester group (cocaine, procaine, amethocaine) should be avoided because they are hydrolyzed by cholinesterase. Alternatively, anesthetics of the amide group (lignocaine, prilocaine, mepivacaine, bupivacaine) can be used because they are metabolized in the liver. Aminoglycoside antibiotics (gentamicin, tobramycin, neomycin, kanamycin, streptomycin) reduce the amount of acetylcholine released at the neuromuscular junction and can cause exacerbation of

TABLE 16-2	Perioperative Drugs That Exacerbate Myasthenia Gravis		
Local Anesthetics	**Antibiotics**	**Cardiac Medications**	**Analgesics**
Cocaine	Gentamicin	Quinidine	Morphine
Procaine	Tobramycin	Procainamide	Meperidine
Amethocaine	Neomycin	Propranolol	Barbiturates
Lidocaine	Kanamycin		
	Streptomycin		
	Polymixin		
	Ampicillin		

the patient's weakness and refractoriness to anticholinesterase medications. Other drugs such as morphine, quinidine, procainamide, and β-adrenergic blockers can worsen the neuromuscular transmission defect and exacerbate myasthenia gravis. If the preceding drugs are required in the perioperative period, they should be used with caution, with close monitoring of the patient's respiratory status.

Patients with myasthenia gravis can experience myasthenic crisis or cholinergic crisis with pulmonary impairment in the perioperative period. *Myasthenic crisis* is a worsening of the disease that may be a result of the surgery, an alteration of medication, postoperative infection, or part of the natural history of the disease. A *cholinergic crisis* may occur when the patient receives an excess of anticholinesterase medication. This excess leads to saturation of the same receptors as acetylcholine uses and decreases neuromuscular transmission. Both types of crisis may result in respiratory depression and failure. Crisis is treated by securing the airway and ventilating the patient [● *Younger et al, 1997*].

Postoperatively, the pulmonary care of the patient is most important. A prediction scale for the likelihood of need for mechanical ventilation has been shown to have a predictive accuracy of 91% (Table 16-3). Reinstitution of medication, incentive spirometry, and early mobilization

TABLE 16-3	Myasthenia Gravis: Risk Factors for Mechanical Ventilation	
Preoperative Factors		**Points**
Duration of myasthenia gravis >6 yr		12
History of chronic respiratory disease		10
Pyridostigmine dose >750 mg/day		8
Vital capacity <2.9 L		4
Risk Factor Prediction		
<10: Tracheal intubation		
10–34: Requires ventilator		

are all part of postoperative pulmonary care [● *Leventhal et al, 1980*].

Muscular Dystrophy

Muscular dystrophy refers to a group of genetically determined progressive myopathies. Each type of muscular dystrophy has specific genetic inheritance, medical problems, and long-term prognostic factors. The most frequently encountered myopathies are reviewed in this section.

Duchenne muscular dystrophy is inherited as an X-linked recessive trait and is the most common and severe of the myopathies. The onset is in early childhood, and the disease follows a progressive downhill course, with patients confined to a wheelchair at a mean age of 9.5 years. Survival after the age of 25 years is rare. Seventy percent of deaths among patients with Duchenne muscular dystrophy are from respiratory failure alone. Approximately 12% of deaths may be attributable to cardiac causes, but it is often difficult to distinguish between primary involvement of the cardiac muscle and cardiac decompensation caused by nocturnal hypoxemia and pulmonary hypertension.

Becker's dystrophy is a milder, less common allelic form of Duchenne muscular dystrophy. The muscle weakness is a slowly progressive process, with survival into the fourth and fifth decades of life. Pulmonary insufficiency is the major long-term problem.

Myotonic dystrophy is manifested as an autosomal dominant trait (chromosome 19) with variable expression, with an age of onset in the teens or 20s. It is probably the most frequently encountered muscular dystrophy in a general hospital. This disorder appears most commonly in the second and third decades of life, but a congenital form has been observed. The myopathy is slowly progressive, involving proximal and distal muscle groups; death occurs in the fifth and sixth decades of life. Myotonia is manifested clinically by an impaired ability to relax skeletal muscle. This can be seen by the inability to release a handshake or by percussion of the thenar muscles. Cardiac conduction abnormalities and respiratory insufficiency are the most frequent causes of death. Systemic weakness occurs with other associated findings, such as the following: frontal balding; high, arched palate; subcapsular cataracts; testicular atrophy; esophageal dysfunction; and glucose intolerance. The electromyogram has a characteristic spontaneous discharge that varies in amplitude and frequency and sounds like a "dive bomber."

The pulmonary deficit seen in chronic neuromuscular disease is somewhat different from that seen with acute neuromuscular diseases such as myasthenia gravis in which muscular weakness itself is the main problem. **In the chronic muscular dystrophies, the long-standing weakness produces other problems, including the following: scoliosis, which can compromise respiratory function; widespread microatelectasis with reduced lung compliance; recurrent sleep-related hypoxemia; thoracic mechanical abnormalities; a weak cough with retained secretions and repeated infections; and ventilation/perfusion imbalance. All these problems may be further complicated by a central disorder of ventilatory control [◉ Oliveira et al, 2004].**

The role of the consultant in preparing these patients for surgical procedures is to assess the degree of respiratory impairment and cardiac status with regard to myocardial function and arrhythmias and to assist with ventilatory management in the postoperative period.

Perioperative Considerations

Pulmonary assessment is directed to the degree of restrictive disease and the oxygenation status of the patient. Pulmonary function tests, with and without bronchodilators, and arterial blood gas determinations are performed preoperatively. The respiratory disability in patients with muscular dystrophy is a product of reduced muscle strength and decreased pulmonary and chest wall compliance. This is especially apparent when the respiratory system is stressed by ventilatory loading. The vital capacity closely reflects the degree of general disability from the time patients become confined to a wheelchair and appears to offer an accurate prognostic index. Patients with myotonic dystrophy may exhibit intercostal myotonia, which may interfere with regular breathing and result in respiratory complications. These patients also have oropharyngeal dysfunction and are at risk for aspiration pneumonia. The myotonia may be improved by use of the medications listed in Table 16-4.

Special attention should be given to the adverse affects of anesthetic agents used in patients with Duchenne muscular dystrophy. Acute hyperkalemia has been reported in these patients following administration of succinylcholine. Malignant hyperthermia (MH) has been reported following the administration of succinylcholine. These potential problems can be minimized by using narcotics instead of potent volatile anesthetics and nondepolarizing muscle relaxants instead of succinylcholine. Temperature should be monitored, and dantrolene should always be available for immediate use in case MH occurs. Local and regional anesthesia may be adequate for many of the surgical procedures these patients require.

Weaning from mechanical ventilation can be a problem in patients with chronic neuromuscular disease. In some cases, the imbalance between respiratory workload and respiratory muscle endurance is so severe and unremitting that standard weaning techniques are unsuccessful. Inspiratory muscle resistive training has been used successfully in some patients.

TABLE 16-4	Treatment of Myotonia	
Drug	**Route**	**Dose**
Phenytoin	PO, IV	5 mg/kg/day (q6h)
Procainamide	PO, IV	50 mg/kg/day (q6h)
Quinidine	PO	5–10 mg/kg/day (q6h)
IV, intravenously; PO, by mouth; q, every.		

The high frequency of cardiac abnormalities in myotonic muscular dystrophy results mainly from electrocardiographic conduction problems or atrial arrhythmias. **The most common electrocardiographic abnormalities are a prolonged P-R interval, QRS widening, and atrial arrhythmias. Cases of complete heart block have been reported. In Duchenne muscular dystrophy, cardiomyopathy with cardiac failure is common [● *Bertorini, 2004*].**

Preoperative assessment includes an electrocardiogram and an echocardiogram. Cardiac consultation may be required, depending on the degree of the patient's cardiac impairment and the need for intensive care unit management postoperatively.

Malignant Hyperthermia

MH is a rare, fatal complication of general anesthesia caused by an inherited myopathy. After exposure to inhaled anesthetics or depolarizing muscle relaxants, susceptible individuals experience a hypermetabolic state characterized by tachycardia, hyperpyrexia, fluctuation in blood pressure, metabolic and respiratory acidosis, cyanosis, and muscle rigidity. Multiple organ failure and death may result if the entity is not recognized and treated promptly.

The incidence of MH reactions in North America and Europe is approximately 1 in 15,000 anesthesia procedures in children and ranges from 1 in 50,000 to 1 in 150,000 anesthesia procedures in middle-aged adults. Clinical manifestations can occur with the presence of one autosomal dominant gene or two autosomal recessive genes.

The detection of susceptible individuals before anesthesia and surgery is of primary concern. Frequently, nothing in the clinical history or physical examination suggests that the patient may acquire MH. However, the following should alert the clinician to the possibility. Patients with a family history of unusual reactions or death from anesthesia are at risk for the development of MH. A history of unexplained muscle cramps or weakness, or both, with unexplained febrile responses or any difficulties in temperature control can mean potential susceptibility. The muscles in susceptible individuals are frequently round and bulky, with subclinical muscle weakness. Other associated clinical findings include strabismus, ptosis, kyphoscoliosis, hernia, club foot, and joint dislocations. Creatine kinase may be elevated in some, but not all, susceptible patients. The most definitive test is the in vitro contracture response of muscle to halothane and caffeine. This is an invasive test requiring a muscle biopsy and is not practical for general screening.

The pathophysiology of MH is not fully known. The most likely mechanism is a rise in concentration of myoplasmic calcium. Possible mechanisms that have been implicated include the following: excessive release of calcium from or decreased reuptake of calcium into the sarcoplasmic reticulum, or both; decreased reuptake by the mitochondria; excessively fragile sarcolemma with passive diffusion of calcium into the myoplasm from the extracellular fluid; and exaggeration of adrenergic innervation, with resulting multiple indirect effects.

Skeletal muscle rigidity and difficulty with endotracheal intubation, instead of the flaccid paralysis normally expected with anesthesia induction with succinylcholine, characterize an acute reaction. This reaction frequently begins in the masseter muscles. The most consistent early feature of an MH crisis is persistent sinus tachycardia. This occurs in 90% of patients within 30 minutes of anesthesia induction. Ventricular tachycardia may also occur. Instability of the systolic blood pressure secondary to increased cardiac output and arteriolar spasm results in hypertension. Hypotension occurs before cardiac arrest. The hypercatabolic state produces rapid, deep respirations (for the excretion of carbon dioxide) and excessive body temperature. A rise in the carbon dioxide tension is the first parameter that may be noticed. The patient has concomitant respiratory acidosis and metabolic acidosis (lactic acidosis). Frequently, there is a transient dilation of the vascular smooth muscle, resulting in a flush on the anterior chest. This is followed by vascular spasm and cyanosis. This process is not reversible with 100% oxygen. The rise in temperature is the result of both an increase in heat production and a decrease in heat loss from the peripheral vasospasm. Factors known to induce MH are shown in Table 16-5.

Management

The mainstay of treatment in MH is dantrolene sodium (Dantrium). Dantrolene is a phenytoin derivative that attenuates calcium release from the sarcoplasmic reticulum. An initial intravenous dose of 2.5 mg/kg is given and repeated every 5 to 10 minutes until a maximal dose of 10 mg/kg is given or until the episode is controlled. Control of MH is marked by decreasing temperature, decreasing muscle rigidity, and improving acid-base balance. Dantrolene has a half-life of 5 hours and should be continued for 24 hours at 1 to 2 mg/kg in four divided doses following control of the MH episode. Dantrolene should be reinstituted immediately if signs of increased metabolism or acidosis develop.

Symptomatic treatment of MH includes the administration of sodium bicarbonate at 1 to 4 mg/kg in accordance with blood gas pH measurements, maintenance of adequate urine output with intravenous fluids, and cooling of body temperature with a cooling blanket. The patient should be monitored in the intensive care unit with blood gas determinations, complete blood count, electrolyte determinations (especially potassium), and creatine kinase. **Patients thought to have MH can be pretreated with dantrolene, 2.5 mg/kg 1 hour preoperatively and then 4 to 7 mg/kg/day in divided intravenous doses** [● *Larach et al, 1987*].

Critical Care Neuropathy and Myopathy

Myoclonus is the most common movement disorder seen in the postoperative period, and myoclonic shivering is observed routinely as patients awaken from general anesthesia.

TABLE 16-5	Medications and Their Relationship to Malignant Hyperthermia	
Triggering Agents	**Potential Triggering Agents**	**Safe Agents**
Inhalational Anesthetics	Calcium, potassium salts	Nitrous oxide
Halothane	Ketamine	Barbiturates
Enflurane	Catecholamines	Local anesthetics
Isoflurane	Phenothiazines	Narcotics
Desflurane	Monoamine oxidase inhibitors	Nondepolarizing relaxants
Sevoflurane		Antibiotics
Depolarizing Blockers		Propranolol
Succinylcholine		Propofol
Decamethonium		Benzodiazepines
Suxamethonium		

From Kaus SJ, Rocko MA: Malignant hyperthermia. Pediatr Clin North Am 41:233, 1994.

Many drugs can induce myoclonus, some of which may be administered in the operating room or recovery room. The anesthetic agents etomidate and enflurane, penicillins, imipenem, quinolones, intravenous contrast media, dopamine-receptor blockers, and the opioids fentanyl and meperidine may cause myoclonus in the postoperative period.

Extensive evidence has accumulated that a type of axonal sensorimotor polyneuropathy, termed *critical illness polyneuropathy,* frequently occurs in patients who have multiorgan failure or who have received treatment, lasting a week or more, for sepsis. The acute myopathy of intensive care is associated with the use of intravenous corticosteroids and nondepolarizing neuromuscular junction blocking agents. Affected patients experience acute, diffuse, flaccid weakness often associated with failure to wean from mechanical ventilation. Creatine kinase elevations occur in many of these patients. With treatment of the underlying disorder and discontinuation of corticosteroids, the myopathy improves over weeks to months. Histopathologic evaluation shows predominantly a loss of thick (myosin) filaments. The medical consultant should recognize these entities so that appropriate supportive care can be given to the patient and should also be aware that it may take more time to wean the patient from the ventilator. Management consists of treating the underlying disease, discontinuing steroids, and adding physical therapy.

Parkinsonism

Parkinson's disease is one of the most common neurologic disorders the medical consultant will encounter in preoperative evaluation. This slowly progressive, degenerative disease is characterized pathophysiologically by a depletion of dopamine in the striatonigral pathways. Most cases are idiopathic, but atherosclerosis, infection, trauma, and medications can produce a parkinsonian syndrome. Tremor, rigidity, bradykinesia, and impaired postural reflexes are cardinal manifestations of the syndrome. Another important clinical manifestation is autonomic dysfunction manifested by orthostatic hypotension, inability to control temperature, abnormal sweating, and sialorrhea.

Several types of swallowing abnormalities have been identified in parkinsonian patients, such as the following: abnormal lingual control of swallowing; lingual festination, in which the elevated tongue prevents passage of the bolus of food into the pharynx; delayed swallowing reflex, with reduced pharyngeal peristalsis and aspiration; repetitive and involuntary reflux from the vallecula and piriform sinuses into the oral cavity; and difficulty in swallowing pills, with retention in the vallecula for long periods. Most patients with moderate to severe Parkinson's disease have one or more of these abnormalities. These abnormalities may or may not respond to antiparkinsonian medication. Patients with moderate to severe Parkinson's disease and patients who complain of swallowing difficulties should have their swallowing evaluated by a video barium swallow preoperatively. If an abnormality exists, patients can be taught preoperatively the voluntary airway protection technique, in which they are instructed to hold the breath, tilt the chin to the chest, swallow, cough, and then swallow again.

The medical consultant's major concern is the perioperative effect of impaired motor dysfunction resulting from withdrawal of parkinsonian medication [⊙ *Galvez-Jimenez and Lang, 2004*]. The expected worsening of parkinsonian rigidity and bradykinesia coupled with swallowing difficulties and the inability to clear oral and pulmonary secretions make these patients prone to postoperative complications such as aspiration pneumonia and deep vein thrombosis.

Parkinsonian Medications

The cardiovascular system is affected by antiparkinsonian therapy. The metabolite of levodopa and levodopa-carbidopa therapy, dopamine, acts on three receptors in the cardiovascular system. Dopamine acts directly on myocardial β-adrenergic receptors, and the result is release of norepine-phrine, which can be arrhythmogenic. To avoid this complication, at least 100 mg of carbidopa, the peripheral decarboxylase inhibitor, is recommended. Dopamine affects β-adrenergic receptors and thus causes vasoconstriction and elevation in blood pressure. Vasodilation of renal and mesenteric vessels results from stimulation of the dopaminergic receptor, which can cause hypotension. Levodopa-carbidopa has a duration of action of 3 to 4 hours. Because of the short duration of action, these drugs can be given the night before the surgical procedure, to avoid arrhythmias in the perioperative period.

Bromocriptine and pergolide are dopamine agonists that are classified as ergots. These agents have been linked to cases of valvulopathy and pulmonary fibrosis. Because of these risks, these drugs are no longer used for the management of Parkinson's disease. Nonergot drugs, which include ropinirole and pramipexole, are currently used for treatment.

Amantadine hydrochloride (Symmetrel) is an anti-influenza drug. It acts in Parkinson's disease by releasing endogenous dopamine. It is generally used as adjunct therapy.

Selegiline hydrochloride (Eldepryl) is a monoamine oxidase (MAO) inhibitor. One of the pathways of metabolism of dopamine is through the MAO system. Inhibition of this system decreases the amount of dopamine broken down and increases the amount of dopamine in the nigrostriatal pathways. Selegiline is used as an adjunct with levodopa-carbidopa in the treatment of Parkinson's disease. The most common side effects are dizziness, nausea, and fainting. Antiparkinsonian medications are shown in Tables 16-6 and 16-7. Rasagiline (Azilect) is a second-generation MAO-B inhibitor structurally related to selegiline, but it is more potent and more selective for MAO-B, and it does not have the amphetamine metabolite that selegiline possesses. This newer agent can be used in monotherapy or adjunct therapy. Its main side effects are nausea, hypotension, dizziness, abdominal pain, and confusion.

TABLE 16-6	Antiparkinsonian Medications (Dopaminergic Action)*	

Drug	Dose	Schedule
Carbidopa/L-dopa		
Carbidopa/levodopa (Parcopa)	10 mg/100 mg, 25 mg/100 mg, 25 mg/250 mg	0.5–1 g/day up to 8 g/day
		Tablets/capsules
Carbidopa/levodopa (Sinemet)†	10/100 mg, 25/100 mg, 25/250 mg	1 tablet, tid; titrate upward based on clinical response
Monoamine Oxidase-B Inhibitors		
Selegiline (Eldepryl)	5 mg	5–10 mg bid
Rasagiline (Azilect)	0.5 mg, 1 mg	0.5 mg adjunct therapy
Dopamine Agonists (Nonergot)		
Ropinirole (Requip)	0.25 mg, 0.5 mg, 1 mg, 2 mg, 3 mg, 4 mg, 5 mg	Titrate to maximum dose 3 mg tid
Pramipexole (Mirapex)	0.125 mg, 0.25 mg, 0.5 mg, 1 mg, 1.5 mg	Titrate to maximum dose 1.5 mg tid
Catechol-O-Methyltransferase		
Entacapone (Comtan)	200 mg	200 mg tid
Entacapone + carbidopa/ levodopa (Stalevo)	12.5 mg/50 mg/200 mg 25 mg/100 mg/200 mg 37.5 mg/150 mg/200 mg	tid dosing tid dosing tid dosing

*Bromocriptine and pergolide no longer used because of valvulopathy and pulmonary fibrosis. Individual patients may require more than one medication and more than one dosage regimen in any 24-hour period.
†Sinemet CR no longer used because of erratic absorption.
bid, twice daily; tid, three times daily.

Perioperative Considerations

Pulmonary care in the perioperative period is directed toward the restrictive lung impairment secondary to the rigidity and bradykinesia of the respiratory muscles. This problem is exacerbated by the postoperative withdrawal of antiparkinsonian medication. In addition, kyphosis, pharyngeal dysfunction, and sialorrhea compound the restrictive dysfunction [● *Frucht, 2004*].

TABLE 16-7	Antiparkinsonian Medications (Anticholinergic Action)	
Drug	**Dose**	**Schedule**
Trihexyphenidyl (Artane)	2 mg	≤5 mg tid
Benztropine (Cogentin)	2 mg; 1-mg ampule	≤2 mg tid or 0.5–1 mg IM, up to 1–7 mg/day
Procyclidine (Kemadrin)	10 mg	≤10 mg qid
Diphenhydramine (Benadryl)	50-mg ampule	10–50 mg IM/IV, up to 150 mg/day

IM, intramuscularly; IV, intravenously; qid, four times daily; tid, three times daily.

These mechanisms collectively result in respiratory compromise. Preoperatively, pulmonary function tests and arterial blood gas determinations are obtained to assess the degree of impairment. Postoperatively, management includes incentive spirometry, postural drainage, percussion, and reinstitution of antiparkinsonian medications. In an uncontrolled trial, levodopa was shown to improve minute ventilation and vital capacity in patients with parkinsonism.

If the patient is unable to take oral medication, parenteral anticholinergic drugs (e.g., biperiden, benztropine, or diphenhydramine) can be used (see Table 16-7). These drugs can be given parenterally (intravenously or intramuscularly) for the management of rigidity and bradykinesia. They should be used in as low a dose as possible because they may precipitate an acute confusional state in the postoperative period. Diphenhydramine, an H_1-receptor blocking antihistamine that has central anticholinergic activity, has been used as the sole agent in ophthalmic surgery. Diphenhydramine administered in 25-mg increments produces a well-sedated patient with minimal tremor. With this regimen, oversedation or delirium is rare.

The need for postoperative intensive care depends on the degree of pulmonary disease, hypotension necessitating volume replacement, and concomitant medical problems. The major perioperative management of a patient with Parkinson's disease involves assessment of pulmonary function, correct application of antiparkinsonian medications, and maintenance of volume status.

All antiparkinsonian medications are active in the central nervous system and can cause an alteration in mental status. Carbidopa-levodopa, amantadine, and anticholinergic agents can produce side effects such as dyskinesias, dizziness, hallucinations, dystonia, confusion, somnolence, and insomnia. It is important to recognize this possibility in the postoperative elderly patient, in whom reinstituting medication or altering the dosage can produce significant neurologic side effects.

EPILEPSY

Epilepsy is one of the most common neurologic disorders encountered in clinical practice, affecting an estimated 2 to 4 million people in the United States, approximately 1 in 50 children and 1 in 100 adults. Seizures are classified into (1) partial seizures with elementary symptoms (these may occur without an alteration in consciousness, e.g., focal motor seizures), (2) partial seizures with complex symptoms (temporal lobe or psychomotor seizures), and (3) generalized seizures (petit mal, grand mal, tonic-clonic seizures). The complete classification of seizures is complex and is not discussed here; however, the problem facing the consultant is not the diagnosis or classification of the seizure disorder but management of the antiepileptic drugs and prevention of recurrent seizure activity preoperatively and postoperatively.

Stage I (excitation) and stage II (delirium) of anesthesia are the periods of risk for seizure activity. Knowledge of the pharmacokinetics and toxicity of antiepileptic drugs is important for the prevention of seizures and for understanding the possible adverse reactions in the patient undergoing surgery.

Categorization of Patients

Preoperative patients with seizure disorders who are to undergo elective or emergency surgical procedures can be classified as having well-controlled or poorly controlled disorders. Contributing factors are sought for the patient with a poorly controlled seizure disorder such as noncompliance, alcohol ingestion, or concurrent illness.

Treatment Modalities

Phenytoin is the most frequently used parenteral antiepileptic drug. To avoid the risks of hypotension and asystole, this drug must be administered in saline solution or lactated Ringer's solution at a rate no faster than 50 mg/minute. An oral loading schedule of an initial 400 mg, followed by 300 mg every 2 hours for a total of 1 g, will achieve a therapeutic range of phenytoin. Phenytoin should not be given intramuscularly or rectally because of erratic absorption. Phenytoin is given in an intravenous loading dose of 15 to 18 mg/kg and a maintenance dose of 4 to 8 mg/kg/day. When given intravenously, phenytoin should be given in divided doses.

Fosphenytoin sodium is a water-soluble prodrug of phenytoin that can be administered intravenously and intramuscularly. It has the advantages of being better tolerated at the injection site, and a loading dose of 15 to 20 mg/kg can be given at a rate of 150 mg/minute. Fosphenytoin may be given intramuscularly when intravenous access is not available.

Phenobarbital is the second most frequently used parenteral antiepileptic medication. It is given in a loading dose of 2 to 6 mg/kg and a maintenance dose of 1 to 5 mg/kg/day. It can be given intramuscularly or intravenously if the oral route is not available. If administered parenterally, phenobarbital should be given in divided doses.

Many newer antiepileptic drugs are available (Table 16-8). These agents are all formulated as oral preparations, except for valproate sodium and levetiracetam, which are available in parenteral form. Valproate sodium is given at 10 to 15 mg/kg/

TABLE 16-8   Anticonvulsant Medication (Adult Dosing)

Drug	Route	Half Life	Therapeutic Range (mg/L)	Dose
Phenytoin (Dilantin)	PO, IV	24±12	10–20 mg/L	200–600 mg/day
Carbamazepine (Tegretol)	PO	9–15	8–12 mg/mL	400–2000 mg/day divided dose
Oxcarbazepine (Trileptal)	PO	9	10–35 mg/mL	300–2400 mg/day divided dose
Valproic acid (Depakene)	PO	5–20	50–100 mg/L	1000–3000 mg/day divided dose
Valproate sodium	IV	5–20	50–100 mg/L	10–15 mg/kg/day administered over 1 hr (>20 mg/min)
Divalproex sodium (Depakote)	PO	6–16 hr	50–100 mg/L	750–3000 mg
Phenobarbital (Luminal)	PO, IV, IM	24–110 hr	10–40 mg/L	60–240 mg/day
Primidone	PO	12–36 hr	6–12 mg/L	500–2000 mg/day
Clonazepam (Klonopin)	PO	18–50 hr	20–80 μg/mL	0.5–20 mg/kg; divided doses
Diazepam	IV, PO, IM, IV, PO 24	0.5–4	100–1000 mg/L	0.3 mg/kg, maximum 20 mg
Lorazepam	IV, PO, IM, IV	1–4	10–30 mg/L	2 mg IV followed by another 2 mg; can repeat up to 6-8 mg
Ethosuximide (Zarontin)	PO	30–60 hr	40–80 mg/L	20–40 mg/kg/day divided dose
Topiramate (Topamax)	PO	20 hr	15 mg	200–400 mg/day
Levetiracetam (Keppra)	PO	6–8 hr	N/A	1000–3000 mg/day
Felbamate (Felbatol)	PO	14–20 hr	N/A	1200–3600 mg/day
Lamotrigine (Lamictal)	PO	11–60 hr	N/A	300–500 mg/day; 100–150 mg/day with other medications
Zonisamide (Zonegran)	PO	60 hr	N/A	400–600 mg/day
Gabapentin (Neurontin)	PO	5–7 hr	N/A	900–1800 mg/day

day in divided doses. It should be administered over 1 hour at faster than 20 mg/minute. In patients who develop multifocal myoclonus secondary to a hypoxic event (e.g., following cardiac arrest), benzodiazepines and valproic acid are the drugs of choice.

Perioperative Considerations

Seizures can occur following withdrawal from any sedative-hypnotic medication, but patients in withdrawal from alcohol or barbiturates are particularly prone to generalized convulsions. Acute ingestion of alcohol can also cause alcoholic ketoacidosis and hypoglycemia. If the patient has no history of a previous seizure disorder, a toxicology screen should be obtained. Seizures associated with enflurane administration may occur during inhalation induction, on emergence, or during the postoperative period. Local anesthetic overdose (excessive dose of local anesthetic, intravascular injection, or rapid uptake) can cause generalized convulsions. Meperidine in large doses, or administered to patients receiving MAO inhibitors, may cause seizures. Seizures may also be seen after injection of retrobulbar block for ophthalmic surgery.

Most nonepileptic patients with perioperative seizures have a metabolic derangement. Hyponatremia is common after subarachnoid hemorrhage, and hypercalcemia may be seen after thyroid or parathyroid surgical procedures. Patients with seizures postoperatively should be screened for electrolyte abnormalities guided by the operative procedure and the preoperative electrolyte balance. Acute organ failure from any cause may produce seizures. Sepsis can cause seizures and should be considered in any trauma patient with an obvious source of infection or with spillage of bowel contents. Rapidly developing MH may manifest with seizures. Although alcohol withdrawal may cause generalized seizures, many alcoholic patients have a predisposing cause for the development of a chronic seizure disorder, such as head trauma. If the seizure is clearly a generalized withdrawal seizure, no chronic anticonvulsant medication is generally required. The convulsion can be aborted with either diazepam or lorazepam. If the seizure is focal, it generally implies an underlying structural brain pathologic condition, and the patient should receive long-term anticonvulsant medication. In situations that are not clearly withdrawal seizures, an electroencephalogram (EEG) can be helpful. In withdrawal seizures, the EEG is normal. If the EEG shows a potential epileptic focus, the patient should receive long-term anticonvulsant therapy. Commonly used anticonvulsants are shown in Table 16-8.

The use of prophylactic anticonvulsants in neurologically injured patients is controversial. Patients with head injuries have a 5% risk of having a seizure in the first week, and another 5% of patients will have a seizure some time after the first week. In patients with trauma, risk factors known to predispose to epilepsy are linear skull fracture (6%), age less than 5 years (9%), depressed skull fracture (10%), posttraumatic amnesia exceeding 24 hours (12%), focal neurologic deficit (13%), and intracranial hematoma (27%). Twenty-five percent of early epilepsy occurs within 1 hour of the injury, and 25% occurs within 24 hours of the injury. Approximately two thirds of patients who have a single seizure will have a second episode, and 25% will have late seizures. Late epilepsy is more likely to develop in patients with an acute hematoma (31%), early epilepsy (25%), or depressed skull fractures (15%). Fifty percent of late seizures occur within the first year, with a progressive decrease in each subsequent year. The risk after 5 years is equal to that of the general population. Fifty percent of late seizures are focal, 35% of patients have frequent seizures, and 25% have long-term remissions.

The incidence of seizures following intracranial surgery depends on the underlying pathologic condition, the location, and the degree of brain retraction required to perform the procedure. In surgical procedures requiring extensive retraction, the incidence of postoperative seizures is approximately 25% (e.g., intracranial versus carotid ligation for aneurysmal surgery). In patients with subarachnoid hemorrhage, seizures occur with the initial bleeding and at the time of rebleeding. Late seizures occur in approximately 10% of survivors. The incidence seems to be highest with middle cerebral artery aneurysms.

Patients with brain tumors are at risk for the development of seizures inversely related to the malignancy of the tumor, that is, oligodendroglioma (81%), astrocytoma (66%), ependymoma (50%), glioblastoma (42%), meningioma (40%), and metastases (19%). The location of the tumor is also important; seizures are more frequent in tumors around the motor cortex and are less common in tumors involving the occipital cortex. Approximately 50% of patients with subdural empyema and 36% to 79% of patients with intracerebral abscesses experience seizures.

Phenytoin and phenobarbital are the most common anticonvulsants used for seizure prophylaxis. Approximately 10% of patients have toxic side effects that cause the medication to be changed or altered. Based on this information, many consultants recommend prophylaxis in those patients who are at a 15% risk of development of seizures. Included in this risk category are the following: patients with intracranial abscess or subdural empyema; postoperative trauma in patients with intracranial hematoma, early posttraumatic seizures, penetrating head wounds, and depressed skull fractures; patients with tumors located near the motor strip; and surgical procedures in which a seizure would produce catastrophic results, for example, a rapid rise in intracranial pressure. The length of time that patients should receive prophylaxis is unknown, but most continue for 1 to 3 years.

CEREBROVASCULAR DISEASE

Stroke

Stroke is the third leading cause of death in the United States, after myocardial infarction and cancer. Stroke also accounts for half of all patients hospitalized for acute neurologic disease.

The major risk factors for stroke are age, hypertension, coincident coronary heart disease, diabetes, and smoking. Stroke is a syndrome and includes hemodynamic obstruction, artery-to-artery emboli, occlusion of small penetrating arteries producing a lacunar infarction, cardiogenic emboli, ruptured intracranial aneurysms, and intracranial hemorrhages.

Large multicenter clinical trials have provided the clinician with information regarding the management of the patient with cerebrovascular disease:

1. Prevention of Cerebral Ischemic Events in Patients with Noncardioembolic Transient Ischemic Attack (TIA) or Stroke: Acceptable options for initial therapy are as follows: aspirin, at a dose of 50 to 325 mg once daily; or the combination of aspirin, 25 mg, and extended-release dipyridamole, 200 mg, twice daily; or clopidogrel, 75 mg, once daily.

2. Prevention of Cardioembolic Cerebral Ischemic Events: Atrial fibrillation is a risk factor for stroke, and that risk can be reduced by anticoagulation with warfarin with an international normalized ratio (INR) of 2 to 3. Patients may receive aspirin for management if warfarin is contraindicated.

3. In patients with recent TIA or ischemic stroke within the last 6 months and ipsilateral severe carotid artery stenosis (70% to 99%), carotid endarterectomy by a surgeon with a record of perioperative morbidity and mortality of less than 6% is recommended. When the degree of stenosis is less than 50%, there is no indication for carotid endarterectomy.

4. Among patients with symptomatic severe stenosis (>70%) in whom the stenosis is difficult to access surgically, who have medical conditions that greatly increase the risk of surgery, or when other specific circumstances exist such as radiation-induced stenosis or restenosis after carotid endarterectomy, carotid artery stenting is not inferior to endarterectomy and may be considered.

5. Acute ischemic stroke: For eligible patients, tissue plasminogen activator is given within 3 hours of the clearly defined symptom onset at a dose of 0.9 mg/kg (maximum,

90 mg), with 10% of the total dose administered as an initial bolus and the remainder infused over 60 minutes.

Asymptomatic Carotid Bruit

A relatively common problem for the medical consultant is the discovery of an asymptomatic carotid bruit on a preoperative physical examination. Asymptomatic carotid bruits occur in approximately 4% of patients who are more than 40 years old. Ropper and associates found that 14% of all surgical patients who were more than 55 years old had carotid bruits. The correlation between the presence of a bruit and significant carotid disease was found to be 21% by oculoplethysmography. In contrast, 47% of the patients with cervical bruits had hemodynamically significant stenosis by arteriography [Ropper et al, 1982]. One can conclude from these data that anywhere between 40% and 60% of asymptomatic patients with audible cervical bruits will not have hemodynamically significant internal carotid lesions by noninvasive studies or arteriography.

The cervical bruit is more highly correlated with diffuse arteriosclerosis and coronary artery disease than it is with hemodynamically significant carotid disease. The annual risk for stroke with an asymptomatic carotid bruit is approximately 2%. Longitudinal studies in patients with asymptomatic carotid bruits have shown a higher incidence of cerebral ischemic events when correlated with the degree and progression of the stenosis. An increase in preoperative stroke has not been demonstrated in patients with asymptomatic carotid bruits who are undergoing general or vascular surgical procedures. In contrast, the risk of stroke or TIA is increased 3.9-fold in the patient with a carotid bruit who undergoes coronary artery bypass surgery. This risk approaches the risk of stroke from carotid endarterectomies of approximately 2.9% (Table 16-9).

Perioperative Considerations

Perioperative stroke is uncommon, occurring in 0.2% to 0.5% of patients undergoing general surgical procedures. Patients undergoing aortoiliac surgery who are at additional risk because of generalized atherosclerosis and intraoperative

TABLE 16-9	Suggested Limits of Surgical Morbidity and Mortality for Carotid Endarterectomy	
Indication		**Limit**
Absence of symptoms		<3%
Transient ischemic attacks		<5%
Ischemic strokes		<7%
Recurrent carotid disease in same artery postendarterectomy		<10%

hypotension have a perioperative stroke rate of 1%. Strokes, if they occur, tend to take place in the postoperative period. Hart found that 83% of strokes occurred postoperatively, and 17% occurred during the operative period. Presumed cardiogenic embolism with atrial fibrillation is a common finding (33%).

The presence of a carotid bruit without symptoms may raise the risk of postoperative stroke 1%. Patients with ultrasound-documented carotid stenosis have a perioperative stroke risk of 3.6%. Patients with a prior history of stroke have a 2.9% incidence of postoperative stroke. One case-controlled study defined adjusted odds ratios (AORs) for increasing the risk of perioperative stroke as follows: prior stroke (AOR, 12.51), chronic obstructive pulmonary disease (AOR, 7.51), and peripheral artery disease (AOR, 5.35).

A strong association exists between carotid artery disease and coronary artery disease. Aggregate data show a consistently higher percentage of cardiac deaths than stroke deaths following TIA. Approximately 70% of all late deaths following carotid endarterectomy have a cardiac cause.

Perioperative Considerations

In patients with a recent stroke or TIA who need surgery, the following question arises: At what time is it appropriate to proceed with a surgical procedure? **Because it can take up to 2 weeks for cerebral autoregulation to return to baseline after an ischemic stroke, deferring elective surgical procedures for 2 weeks at minimum after a moderate or large** stroke seems reasonable to prevent hypotension-induced enlargement of the ischemic penumbra [● Whisnant et al, 1983]. If the patient is having recurrent TIAs with an appropriate carotid lesion, we recommend evaluation of the carotid disease and urgent surgical repair.

A combined procedure is used only in patients with neurologic symptoms in conjunction with unstable coronary artery disease and who have a high-grade (>80%) carotid stenosis. Patients with embolic strokes related to valvular heart disease, prosthetic valves, or dysrhythmia are frequently maintained on long-term warfarin.

Subarachnoid Hemorrhage

Rupture of an intracranial aneurysm is a catastrophic event. Approximately 27,000 patients in the United States and Canada suffer from a ruptured intracranial aneurysm every year. Subarachnoid hemorrhage is more common in women than in men (2:1). Of those 27,000 patients, approximately 10,000 die of the initial insult, 3000 die of a massive hemorrhage, and 7000 die as a result of misdiagnosis or a delay in surgery. Of the 17,000 patients who reach neurosurgical care, approximately 50% of them die or become disabled.

Rebleeding is one of the major causes of death and disability after subarachnoid hemorrhage. Two to 4% of patients hemorrhage again within the first 24 hours after the initial episode, and approximately 15% to 20% bleed a second time within the first 2 weeks. The recent emphasis has been on early clipping or coiling of the aneurysm to prevent the bleeding. Patients who have grade III or greater in the Hunt modified system (Table 16-10) are generally submitted to early angiography and immediate surgical clipping or coiling of the aneurysm. This approach prevents recurrent bleeding and allows for the treatment of vasospasm.

Angiographic evidence of vasospasm following subarachnoid hemorrhage occurs in approximately 60% of patients. The angiographic appearance of vasospasm is correlated with

TABLE 16-10	Hunt and Hess Classification of Subarachnoid Hemorrhage
Grade	**Clinical Symptoms**
I	Asymptomatic bleeding or minimal headache and slight nuchal rigidity
Ia	Fixed neurologic deficit with no acute meningeal or brain reaction
II	Moderate to severe headache and nuchal rigidity; no neurologic deficit other than cranial nerve palsy
III	Drowsiness, confusion, or mild focal deficit
IV	Stupor, moderate to severe hemiparesis, possibly early decerebrate rigidity or vegetative disturbances
V	Deep coma, decerebrate rigidity, moribund status

the appearance of delayed cerebral ischemia, which is sometimes referred to as vasospasm. Nimodipine, a calcium channel blocker, is indicated for the improvement of neurologic outcome by reducing the incidence and severity of ischemic deficits in patients with subarachnoid hemorrhage. The dose of nimodipine is 60 mg every 4 hours for 21 days. If hypotension occurs, 30 mg of nimodepine is given every 2 hours. Clinical signs of vasospasm occur in approximately 30% of patients, with the peak of spasm beginning 7 days after the subarachnoid hemorrhage. This may last for 2 to 3 weeks.

The principal options for treating delayed cerebral ischemia are hemodynamic augmentation and endovascular therapy. **The concept of hemodynamic augmentation consists of hypertension, hypervolemia, and hemodilution, known as *triple-H therapy*. The fundamental idea is to expand the blood volume and to raise the blood pressure to open arteries that are in spasm while improving the rheologic characteristics of the blood cells with hyperosmolar therapy** [● *Naval et al, 2006*]. These patients should be cared for in the intensive care unit with hemodynamic monitoring. The hematocrit is maintained between 35% and 40% by transfusion of packed red blood cells. Mannitol and albumin may be given to improve red blood cell rheologic characteristics. Pulmonary capillary wedge pressure is maintained between 15 and 18 mm Hg by administering fluids, either normal saline or colloid. The usual requirement for individuals with normal cardiac function is from 150 to 400 mL/hour. In a patient whose condition continues to deteriorate or is rapidly deteriorating, the mean arterial pressure (MAP) can be elevated. The choice of pressors varies. Frequently, phenylephrine, in a concentration of 10 to 40 μg/minute, is administered to elevate the MAP to 125±10 mm Hg. This drug can be rapidly titrated under constant observation. Bradycardia often follows administration of phenylephrine, with the consequent buffering of the initial rise in MAP. This is best treated by increasing the heart rate and cardiac contractility simultaneously with dopamine in concentrations that provide between 5 and 15 μg/kg/minute.

The combination of phenylephrine and dopamine allows rapid MAP elevation without excessive reliance on elevating cardiac output or altering systemic vascular resistance. The cardiac output is generally kept in the range of 5 to 10 L/minute, and systemic vascular resistance is maintained at 1200 to 1700 resistance units. If the neurologic deficits do not reverse in the first 30 minutes, the MAP and pulmonary wedge pressure can be elevated to a pulmonary wedge pressure of 18±2 mm Hg and an MAP of 135±10 mm Hg. If no improvement of neurologic status occurs, these parameters are generally maintained for at least 24 hours. This situation is maintained until the patient is stable for 12 to 24 hours before the pressors and volume expanders are tapered.

Stable neurologic function is defined as the patient's performance capabilities before aneurysm rupture. Tapering of hypervolemic hypertensive therapy can usually be accomplished within 3 to 4 days after the initiation of treatment. Treatment is not continued if the patient's deficits do not respond within 24 hours or a completed cerebral infarction can be demonstrated by CT. For patients showing improvement, dopamine or phenylephrine is tapered to decrease the MAP 5 mm Hg in 4- to 5-hour increments. Patients may require 7 to 10 days of hypervolemic hypertensive therapy.

They may require support of intravascular volume for an additional 4 to 7 days after discontinuation of pressor therapy.

Endovascular treatments of cerebral vasospasm include transluminal balloon angioplasty and the intra-arterial delivery of vasodilating compounds. These techniques are most commonly used in patients with symptomatic vasospasm that has been resistant to triple-H therapy. Complications of transluminal balloon angioplasty include trauma to the arterial wall leading to dissection, rupture, and thrombosis, with consequent cerebral infarction or hemorrhage. Verapamil and nicardipine have been used as vasodilator agents, but their safety and efficacy are largely anecdotal.

CHANGE IN MENTAL STATUS

The medical consultant is frequently asked to see a postoperative patient for a change in mental status. The two major considerations are the presence of structural central nervous system disease and metabolic derangement causing the alteration of mental status.

Assessment

The neurologic examination generally can demonstrate focal structural disease. This disorder may be manifested by cranial nerve findings, subtle motor weakness, or even abnormal postures. Ancillary evidence from imaging techniques, such as CT or MRI, is helpful in the diagnosis of structural disease, especially in the frontal and temporal lobes, which may be relatively silent areas on physical examination. Perioperative stroke is an infrequent complication in general surgical patients and occurs at a rate of 0.3% to 3.5%, depending on the age of the patient and other complicating factors, such as the possibility of cardiogenic emboli during cardiovascular surgery. These strokes generally produce a focal examination, but there are silent areas in which a confused patient's focalization may not be easily discernible.

More difficult to address are the metabolic derangements that can produce a change in mental state or a confusional state. The term *confusional state* implies an alteration in attentiveness in which the patient is unable to maintain a cohesive train of thought. This is part of a broader clinical spectrum that ranges from lack of attention, to agitation, to lethargy proceeding to coma. These patients are frequently disoriented about person, place, date, and time. Confused patients are also unable to remember four objects in 3 minutes and are unable to perform serial subtractions. Perceptual changes with illusions and visual hallucinations can also occur, particularly with the toxic metabolic encephalopathies or encephalopathies related to drug intoxication or drug withdrawal.

Toxic metabolic encephalopathy has several signatures, including tremors, asterixis, and multifocal myoclonus. The characteristic tremor and asterixis seen in metabolic encephalopathies occur after a latent period of 20 to 36 seconds after postural fixation, with the tremor appearing first. The tremor has two separate components. The first component is a varying oscillation of the fingers, usually in the anteroposterior direction, but with a rotary component at the wrist. The second component is a tiny, but clearly defined, random motion of the fingers at the metacarpophalangeal joint once or twice per second. Usually, the tremor increases in amplitude while the hands remain dorsiflexed. The oscillation becomes wider and more variable, and the tiny finger motions become more rapid than propulsive, followed by the hand with the fingers leading, last being forward 2 to 5 cm, only to be jerked to the hands' original position. This situation produces the characteristic asterixis (flap). Patients have no control over these movements and have no warning of their occurrence. The flaps may be either synchronous or asynchronous. Commonly, one flap of asterixis is followed in quick succession by two to three others, with a return to the original fixed posture on amelioration of the tremor. This pattern then repeats over and over. Asterixis with tremor is seen in a variety of metabolic encephalopathies, including uremia, hypokalemia, polycythemia, congestive heart failure, chronic obstructive pulmonary disease with carbon dioxide narcosis, hepatic failure, idiopathic steatorrhea, Whipple's disease and other malabsorption syndromes, magnesium deficiency, and intoxication with bromide and other potentially toxic compounds, including acetazolamide, chlorothiazide, and methionine. Rarely, asterixis can be seen in structural nervous system disease involving the thalamus or parietal lobe. In these patients, asterixis is associated with a severe loss of position sense.

Multifocal myoclonus is a sudden nonrhythmic, nonpatterned, and gross twitching of various muscle groups in the body. Myoclonus may occur in a single fascicle of muscle without displacement of a joint, in a muscle in its entirety, or in a group of muscles with gross movement of the attached structures or limb. It may be either a single muscle contraction or a series of contractions, the latter being an irregular pattern of movement in a rhythmic sequence or a rhythmic unpatterned succession of contractions with each muscle acting in disorderly relation to the others. Multifocal myoclonus can be prominent in uremic and hypoxic encephalopathies and is frequently more pronounced in the face muscles and the tongue. Myoclonus indicates a severe metabolic disturbance that may or may not be reflected in the EEG. Occasionally, the myoclonus can be brought on by a startle response such as is elicited with a sudden clap or loud noise. The myoclonus frequently disappears with appropriate treatment of the encephalopathy.

The pupillary light response to bright light is generally preserved in metabolic encephalopathies, even in patients in profound coma, with certain exceptions. Glutethimide, methaqualone, and atropine poisoning and amphetamine overdoses are notorious for producing large pupils. Large, fixed pupils can also occur with high doses of dopamine. Opiates and pilocarpine drops produce a constricted or pinpoint pupil. Preserved pupillary responsiveness to bright lights despite respiratory depression, caloric unresponsiveness, and decerebrate posture still points to a metabolic cause for the altered state of consciousness.

Almost all types of eye positioning or movement can be observed in metabolic encephalopathy. Downward conjugate gaze and random roving eye movements are frequently seen. Persistent conjugate lateral deviation suggests structural brain or brainstem disease. Ice water calorics (oculovestibular reflex) are of value in the evaluation of the comatose or obtunded patient. Ice water placed in the ear after examination, to ensure the absence of structural abnormalities in the ear canal, produces tonic conjugate deviation toward the ear containing the ice water in patients with an intact brainstem. The oculovestibular reflex can be lost in hypothermia and as a result of massive sedative hypnotic overdoses.

Changes in tone, focal weakness, and decerebrate and decorticate posturing can all occur with diffuse toxic metabolic encephalopathy. Frequently, one can elicit frontal release signs: paratonia, grasp, rooting, suck.

Focal or generalized convulsions can result from all metabolic derangements. Although the convulsions are most often generalized, focal seizures do occur and may appear to be migratory. These seizures may be extremely difficult to control, particularly until the metabolic derangement is corrected, or if the patient has underlying hypoxia.

Perioperative Considerations

Delirium or a confusional state may develop in the immediate postoperative period as the patient emerges from anesthesia, or it may follow lucid intervals for several days. Although the typical course runs 1 or 2 days, it may be longer, especially in patients with underlying structural brain disease, and occasionally it lasts for weeks. The three possible outcomes in a delirious patient are recovery, progression to dementia, or progression to death.

Caring for these types of patients is extremely difficult. Patients may have difficulty communicating their symptoms and may have totally unpredictable behavior. They may be agitated, hypervigilant, fearful, and paranoid, or alternatively sluggish, lethargic, and obtunded. Alterations between these two extremes are common. Night is the most common time for the symptoms to worsen, hence the common reference to "sundowning." The incidence of an agitative delirium varies with the surgical procedure but is said to approach 100% after cardiotomy.

Patients with organic brain disease are known to become more confused postoperatively because of their baseline limitations in coping mechanisms. They already have deficits in perception and processing of information; therefore, it is common for these patients to have delusions, hallucinations, and paranoia after a surgical procedure.

Patients with seizure disorders whose anticonvulsants have been withdrawn may become confused, particularly if they are having nonconvulsive seizures. Patients who have an addiction to drugs or alcohol are also at risk. It is not uncommon to see delirium tremens precipitated by a cessation of alcohol during or following the surgical procedure. Certain diseases can result in postoperative deterioration, particularly porphyria, hypothyroidism, and cancer.

The type of operation, in some instances, must be considered a risk factor for confusion. The most widely recognized example is *postcardiotomy delirium*. *Black patch delirium* following ophthalmologic surgery has been recognized since the 19th century. The incidence of delirium when the eye is patched approaches 16%. The figure rises in patients with preexisting organic brain syndrome. In a group of 100 elderly patients who were more than 80 years old and who were undergoing total hip replacement, infection was the most common postoperative complication, followed in frequency by confusional states and adverse drug reactions. Burn victims, women having abortion or hysterectomy, transplant recipients, and patients with chronic pain are also at high risk for delirium.

Numerous metabolic derangements are associated with sepsis, including hyperdynamic circulation, hypercatabolic states, and altered hormonal patterns with elevated catecholamine levels. When sepsis is associated with multiorgan system failure, the mortality is 95%. The encephalopathy of sepsis may include hyperventilation, fever, seizures, focal or nonfocal examination, and a diffusely slow EEG. Nonconvulsive status epilepticus may occur in an intensive care setting. If the patient is unresponsive without an explanation, continuous EEG monitoring is warranted.

Approach to the Patient

The approach to the patient with a postoperative change in mental status is based on the knowledge of the patient's preoperative baseline. If the patient has an underlying organic or psychiatric disease, confusion and disorientation postoperatively can be anticipated, and the patient can be supported appropriately.

More commonly, the change in mental status is an acute event in the postoperative period. The basic approach to the patient is with physical examination, imaging techniques, and metabolic screening. The physical examination can help one to assess ongoing underlying changes. Changes in vital signs and asterixis, tremor, and myoclonus are all physical signs of underlying metabolic problems. Arterial blood gas, electrolyte, blood urea nitrogen and creatinine determinations, a complete blood count, and liver function tests are valuable in defining the cause of the change in mental status. In addition, attention should be given to the patient's calcium, phosphorus, and magnesium levels, abnormalities of which can alter mental status and produce a confusional state.

One of the first tasks in evaluating these patients is the assessment of concurrent medications. Probably the most common cause of a change in mental status, other than sepsis and electrolyte abnormalities, is the medication given for sedation.

Anticholinergic medications have long been implicated as causes of confusional states. Not only atropine but also phenothiazines, antihistamines, hypnotics, barbiturates, and analgesics may induce anticholinergic effects. Other examples of drugs that can cause confusional states include corticosteroids and cimetidine. They do so either by a direct central nervous system effect or by impairing the metabolism of other medications by inhibiting the hepatic microsomal system. Ketamine can produce hallucinations, particularly in younger patients. Narcotics, particularly meperidine (Demerol), can induce seizures and changes in mental status. The first approach to these patients is to stop all the sedative hypnotics and analgesics, at least to the point of pain tolerance. The suggested approach to these patients is given in Table 16-11.

PERIOPERATIVE PERIPHERAL NERVE LESIONS

Peripheral nerve injuries associated with surgery may be caused by a variety of factors, including improper operative positioning, regional anesthesia, and surgical misadventures. These injuries may be either permanent or temporary. External pressure may cause an interruption of the blood supply to a peripheral nerve that results in the sensation of numbness or tingling, or both. This is termed *neurapraxia* and is a transient phenomenon. During surgical procedures, patients are not able to move, and prolonged pressure on a nerve may result in ischemia and axonal damage. This condition is called *axonotmesis*. Recovery after both of these types of injuries is usually complete.

Neurapraxia is a transient phenomenon, and recovery occurs in a space of hours. With axonotmesis, recovery is also complete, but axonal regeneration progresses at a slower rate. The most severe injuries involve cutting or stretching a nerve.

TABLE 16-11	Change in Mental Status: What Is the Patient's Baseline?	

Focal Examination	**Nonfocal Examination**
Hemiparesis	Confusion-delirium tremor
Abnormal posture	Asterixis
Cranial nerve abnormalities	Myoclonus
Seizures	
Imaging	**Laboratory Examination**
Computed tomography	Arterial blood gas determinations
Magnetic resonance imaging	SMA7–SMA12
Electroencephalography	
Blood cultures	
Cortisol, phosphorus levels; hemo-	
globin, hematocrit, platelet	
count, partial thromboplastin	
time, prothrombin time	
Lumbar puncture	
STOP	
S	Stop all sedative hypnotics or central nervous system–active drugs
T	Treat sepsis if present
O	Optimize metabolic status
P	Patience: Patients with altered mental status at baseline are going to take longer to return to baseline

SMA7–SMA12, chemistry screens including electrolytes, renal function, liver function.

This is called *neurotmesis* and implies that both the axon and the Schwann cells are interrupted. The prognosis for this type of injury is poor despite surgical intervention. The patient may have only a partial return of nerve function.

Specific Nerve Injuries

Optic Nerve

The retina is supplied by the central retinal artery that enters the optic nerve just distal to the point at which the artery branches from the ophthalmic artery. If external pressure is applied to the eye, the intraocular pressure can be increased to the point at which it exceeds the pressure in the central retinal artery. Blood flow through the artery then ceases, and retinal ischemia results. Approximately 4 minutes of ischemia to the retina can result in retinal blindness from ischemic necrosis of the light-sensing cells.

Branches of the Trigeminal Nerve (Cranial Nerve V)

The supraorbital, infraorbital, and supratrochlear and infratrochlear nerves supply sensory fibers to the face and the vicinity of the eyes and nose. Pressure from the anesthesia mask can produce neurapraxia or even axonotmesis in one or more of these nerves. This may result in loss of sensation in selected areas of the face.

Facial Nerve

Peripheral branches of the facial nerve pass beneath the lower ramus of the mandible to the muscles of the face. When a face mask is used for the administration of anesthesia, a retainer is also frequently employed to assist in holding the mask in place. If pressure is placed on the facial nerve at this point, facial nerve palsy may result. This condition is usually transient.

Brachial Plexus

The brachial plexus involves nerve roots C5 to T1. The plexus usually also receives small branches from the four cervical and second thoracic spinal nerves. The plexus passes from the inferolateral aspect of the neck behind the cervical triangle and enters the axilla. In the axilla, the plexus is initially located on the lateral aspect of the axillary artery. It then completely surrounds the artery with one cord laterally, one medially, and one posteriorly. In the inferior axillary space, the plexus breaks into three terminal branches, forming the radial, median, and ulnar nerves supplying the upper extremity. The plexus may be injured by the placement of a brace or other devices in the back of the neck before the plexus descends behind and beneath the clavicle. If the braces are in the posterior triangle, the roots of the plexus may be injured by exerting pressure directly on them.

The plexus may also be injured by excessive depression of the shoulder girdle during anesthesia with the patient in the Trendelenburg position. This occurs if the patient is supported solely by wrist straps or shoulder braces during steep Trendelenburg positioning. The upper roots of the brachial plexus may be stretched in such a situation.

The brachial plexus may also be injured if the arm is abducted 90 degrees or more from the body and allowed to remain in that position for some time. As the arm is abducted, the head of the humerus tends to descend into the axilla. The brachial plexus, in passing from the supraclavicular area into the axilla, goes caudad to the head of the humerus. Stretch and compression may occur in this location.

The lower brachial plexus may also be injured in patients undergoing open heart surgery. This usually involves the lower roots of C8 and T1. The brachial plexus may also be injured during thoracic outlet surgery with transaxillary rib resection. The radial, median, and ulnar nerves are all derived from the brachial plexus. These nerves can be injured anywhere along their course.

The median nerve is not subject to positional injury. It can be injured during a venipuncture attempt in the antecubital space. This can occur particularly when the patient is receiving general anesthesia.

Radial Nerve

The radial nerve spirals around the lateral aspect of the humerus about the midposition of the forearm. Perioperative compression from a tourniquet or improper padding of the dependent arm of the patient placed in the lateral decubitus position can produce radial nerve palsy. This disorder is manifested by a wrist drop and sensory anesthesia of the skin of the dorsum of the radial two thirds of the hand.

Ulnar Nerve

The ulnar nerve is supplied by the C8 and T1 nerves. It passes across the elbow in the olecranon groove, between the medial condyle of the humerus and the olecranon process of the ulna. It then passes into the forearm between the heads of the flexor carpi ulnaris and extends onto the posteromedial aspect of the arm. This nerve may be injured anywhere along its course. The ulnar groove injury usually occurs when the arm is adducted along the side of the body and the hand is supinated. In this position, the elbow may gravitate downward to the edge of the operating table, coming into contact with the ulnar groove. This situation may be avoided by pronating the patient's hand before placing the forearm within draw sheets. The ulnar nerve may also be injured at the point just below the elbow. This generally occurs with the hand abducted and pronated, a position that subjects the ulnar nerve to external pressure.

When the ulnar nerve is injured, paresthesias of the fifth finger, the ulnar half of the ring finger, and the ulnar third of the hand occur. A claw hand may develop. Because the proximal phalanges cannot be flexed, they are hyperextended by the unopposed long extensors. The middle and distal phalanges cannot be extended, and those of the index and middle finger are hyperflexed by the unopposed long flexors. Atrophy of the interosseous muscles can also occur.

Sciatic Nerve

Injuries to the sciatic nerve have resulted from injections to the buttocks, secondary to failure to give the injection appropriately in the upper outer quadrant of the patient's buttock. This can cause foot drop, impaired extension at the hip, flexion of the knee, and anesthesia of the skin, leg, and foot.

Lateral Femoral Cutaneous Nerve of the Thigh

The lateral femoral cutaneous nerve of the thigh may receive excessive pressure if the patient is placed in a prone jackknife position during surgical procedures. The nerve enters the thigh beneath the inguinal ligament near the anterosuperior iliac spine. Inadequate padding between the operating table and the anterior thigh, just distal to the inguinal ligament, can result in compression of the nerve. Alternatively, excessive flexion of the leg at the hip may compress the nerve. Sensory loss with paresthesias over the anterolateral portion of the thigh may result. This condition is also sometimes referred to as *meralgia paresthetica*. It has been reported with groin flap procedures.

Common Peroneal Nerve

The common peroneal nerve, which is a branch of the sciatic nerve, passes across the lateral aspect of the popliteal fossa to the head of the fibula close to the medial margin of the tendon of the biceps femoris muscle. It then passes in close proximity to the neck of the fibula. At this point, the nerve may be injured by excessive external pressure. Improper padding along the lateral aspect of the knee with the patient in the lateral decubitus position, or in stirrups, may result in injury to this nerve. This injury causes a sensory loss over the lateral aspect of the leg distal to the knee and dorsum of the foot. Foot drop is a common finding.

Special Considerations

Total hip arthroplasty can result in injury to the sciatic femoral nerve or obturator nerve. This can occur with direct surgical trauma, bleeding, or stretching of the nerve itself.

The femoral nerve may be damaged during renal transplantation. This injury is frequently caused by a hematoma. This nerve may also be injured during delivery of a baby and may be unilateral or bilateral. A good outcome is generally expected. Meralgia paresthetica can also occur from injury to the lateral femoral cutaneous nerve during bone procurement from the iliac crest for purposes of grafting.

Lower abdominal surgery for hernia repair or gynecologic surgery may cause damage to local nerves traversing the abdominal wall. The ilioinguinal nerve may be damaged during surgical hernia repair. This nerve originates from T12 to L1 nerve roots, crosses retroperineally, and becomes extraperitoneal just after passing the medial to the anterior iliac crest. It then runs along the inguinal canal with its spermatic cord. When this nerve is damaged during surgery, the patient complains of pain and may have sensory loss in a strip of skin extending along the inguinal canal to the base of the penis and scrotum or to the labia. The iliohypogastric nerve is slightly caudal to the ilioinguinal nerve. Damage to this nerve causes sensory loss to the region of the skin over the greater trochanter into the lower abdominal wall just above the pubis. The genital femoral nerve supplies the femoral triangle and a small area of skin on the medial thigh with most of the scrotum, penis, or labia. Damage to this nerve in the retroperitoneal area can produce loss of sensation in those areas.

Selected Readings

Albers GW, Amarenco P, Easton JD, et al: Antithrombotic and thrombolytic therapy for ischemic stroke. Chest 126:483S-512S, 2004.

Aldrieh TK, Uhrlass RM: Weaning from mechanical ventilation: Successful use of modified inspiratory resistive training in muscular dystrophy. Crit Care Med 15:247-249, 1987.

Alvine FG, Schurrer ME: Postoperative ulnar nerve palsy: Are there predisposing factors? J Bone Joint Surg Am 69:255-259, 1987.

Albin RL: Parkinson's disease: Background, diagnosis, and initial management. Clin Geriatr Med 22:735-751, 2006.

Bell RD: Perioperative seizures in decision making. In Bready LL, Smith RB (eds): Anesthesiology. Toronto, BC Decker, 1987, pp 224-225.

Bell RD, Lastimosa AC: Metabolic encephalopathies. In Rosenberg RN (ed): Neurology. New York, Grune & Stratton, 1980, pp 115-164.

Bernstein RA: Risks of stroke from general surgical procedures in stroke patients. Neurol Clin 24:777-782, 2006.

Bertorini TE: Perisurgical management of patients with neuromuscular disorders. Neurol Clin 22:293-313, 2004. ⊕

Blacker DJ, Flemming KD, Wijdicks EF: Risk of ischemic stroke in patients with symptomatic vertebrobasilar stenosis undergoing surgical procedures. Stroke 34:2659-2663, 2003.

Brisman JL, Song JK, Newell DW: Medical progress: Cerebral aneurysms. N Engl J Med 355:928-939, 2006.

Cooper DE, Jenkins RS, Bready L, Rockwood CA: The prevention of injuries of the brachial plexus secondary to malposition of the patient during surgery. Clin Orthop 228:33-41, 1988.

Dawson DM, Krarup C: Perioperative nerve lesions. Arch Neurol 46:1355-1360, 1989.

Deutschman CS, Haines SJ: Anticonvulsant prophylaxis in neurologic surgery. Neurosurgery 17:510-517, 1985.

Dorenette WH: Compression neuropathies: Medical aspects and legal implications. Int Anesth Clin 24:201-229, 1986.

Frucht SJ: Movement disorder emergencies in the perioperative period. Neurol Clin 22:379-387, 2004. **ⓒ**

Galvez-Jimenez N, Lang AE: The perioperative management of Parkinson's disease revisited. Neurol Clin 22:367-377, 2004. **ⓒ**

Goudreau JL: Medical management of advanced Parkinson's disease. Clin Geriatr Med 22:753-772, 2006.

Hasselgreen PO, Fischer JE: Septic encephalopathy. Intensive Care Med 12:13-16, 1986.

Jackson AC, Gilbert JJ, Young GB, Bolton CF: The encephalopathy of sepsis. Can J Neurol Sci 12:303-307, 1985.

Larach MG, Rosenberg H, Broennle AM: Prediction of malignant hyperthermia susceptibility by clinical signs. Anesthesiology 66:547-550, 1987. **ⓒ**

Leventhal SR, Orkin FK, Hirsch RA: Prediction of the need for postoperative mechanical ventilation in myasthenia gravis. Anesthesiology 53:26-30, 1980. **ⓒ**

Limburg M, Wijdicks EF, Li H: Ischemic stroke after surgical procedures: Clinical features, neuroimaging, and risk factors. Neurology 50:895-901, 1998.

Naval NS, Stevens RD, Mirski MA, Bhardwaj A: Controversies in the management of aneurysmal subarachnoid hemorrhage. Crit Care Med 34:511-524, 2006. **ⓒ**

Oliveira E, Michel A, Smolley L: The pulmonary consultation in the perioperative management of patients with neurologic diseases. Neurol Clin 22:277-291, 2004. **ⓒ**

Ropper AH, Wechsler LR, Wilson LS: Carotid bruit and risk of stroke in elective surgery. N Engl J Med 307:1388-1390, 1982.

Wackym PA, Dabrow TJ, Abdul-Rasool IH, Peacock WJ: Neurosurgery in the malignant hyperthermia-susceptible patient. Neurosurgery 22:1032-1036, 1988.

Whisnant JP, Sandok PA, Sundt TM: Carotid endarterectomy for unilateral carotid system transient cerebral ischemia. Mayo Clin Proc 58:171-175, 1983. **ⓒ**

Younger D, Worral B, Pen A: Myasthenia gravis: Historical perspectives and overview. Neurology 48(Suppl 5):1-7, 1997. **ⓒ**

17 Perioperative Care of the Elderly Patient

MICHAEL F. LUBIN, MD

Currently, approximately one third of the surgical procedures in the United States are performed on patients more than 65 years old. This percentage will certainly increase over the next decades because elderly persons will make up more than 20% of the population by early in the next century. The group of patients older than 85 years of age constitutes the fastest growing segment of the U.S. population.

Elderly patients, as a whole, are at greater surgical risk than their younger counterparts, for two reasons: (1) elderly patients have an increased likelihood of underlying chronic disease (e.g., heart or lung disease), which increases surgical risk; and (2) elderly persons have decreased physiologic reserve; these make them less able to withstand the stress of surgery and the perioperative period. Despite these challenges, healthy elderly patients often tolerate surgery well, with resultant improvement in quality and length of life.

This chapter reviews the following:
- The physiologic changes associated with aging that affect the patient's ability to undergo surgery successfully
- The preoperative assessment and perioperative management of elderly patients
- Common postoperative problems and their management
- Special surgical issues in the geriatric age group

Levels of Evidence:

Ⓐ—Randomized controlled trials (RCTs), meta-analyses, well-designed systematic reviews of RCTs. Ⓑ—Case-control or cohort studies, nonrandomized controlled trials, systematic reviews of studies other than RCTs, cross-sectional studies, retrospective studies. Ⓒ—Consensus statements, expert guidelines, usual practice, opinion.

PHYSIOLOGIC EFFECTS OF AGING

It has not always been possible to separate clearly the effects of aging from the effects of diseases, such as atherosclerosis, which are more common in older patients. Many elderly patients have decrements in physiologic function that are caused by both aging and the added effects of chronic disease. Even in the healthy elderly patient, however, age-related changes affect vital organs and decrease the ability of the patient to respond to stresses such as surgery or infection.

The following sections summarize the overall effects of aging. There is great heterogeneity within the geriatric age group, however, so each patient must be assessed individually.

Cardiovascular Effects

Cardiac output at rest may not decrease with age, but the maximal heart rate and maximal cardiac output decline. The ventricular filling rate decreases, ventricular compliance decreases, and atrial contraction becomes more important in maintaining cardiac output. Peripheral resistance increases as aortic stiffness increases, and the vascular bed cross-sectional area decreases. Responsiveness to catecholamine stimulation decreases. The net result is that the elderly heart is likely to be less able to withstand severe stress such as volume overload or hypotension.

In addition to changes related to aging, underlying cardiovascular disease becomes more prevalent; up to 50% of patients who are more than 65 years old have some sort of heart disease. Up to 50% of patients more than 70 years old have hypertension, and up to 20% have coronary artery disease. More than half of elderly patients have systolic murmurs, which usually represent valvular sclerosis rather than stenosis. The identification of aortic stenosis is important, however, because this condition increases the surgical risk.

Pulmonary Effects

Physiologic changes in lung function begin at the age of 30 years and accelerate with advancing age. Lung elasticity decreases, the chest wall becomes stiffer, and the respiratory muscles weaken. The consequences of these changes are decreased vital capacity and increased residual volume. Expiratory flow rates and maximal minute ventilation decrease, as does closing volume. In elderly persons, closing capacity may exceed residual functional capacity. Thus, closure of small airways occurs during normal breathing. This predisposes the individual to lower lobe atelectasis postoperatively. Ventilation/perfusion mismatches occur with resultant decreases in oxygen tension. Many of these changes are exacerbated by smoking, a history of which is quite common in older patients.

Renal Effects

Renal mass decreases by 25% to 30% between the ages of 30 and 90 years. Creatinine clearance and renal blood flow diminish with age in most individuals. By 80 years of age, the glomerular filtration rate is only one half to two thirds of what it was at 30 years of age. However, serum creatinine levels may remain normal, because lean body mass also decreases. Thus, a normal serum creatinine level may mask significant renal dysfunction. Creatinine clearance in men may be estimated by the Cockroft-Gault equation:

$$\text{Creatinine clearance} = (140 - \text{age}) \times \text{weight (kg)} / (72 \times \text{serum creatinine})$$

For an estimate in women, 0.85 of this value is used.

Tubular function is also affected by age. Changes include an impaired ability to concentrate and dilute urine maximally. Because thirst in response to volume depletion is decreased, elderly persons are more prone to dehydration. Elderly persons also show decreased excretion of sodium, potassium, and acid loads.

Drug Metabolism

An understanding of how drug metabolism differs in the elderly is important, because these patients frequently have adverse drug reactions. Some of these reactions may be prevented with a good understanding of the changes that commonly occur in aging (Box 17-1 and Table 17-1).

Drug Distribution

Lean body mass and total body water decrease with age, whereas total body fat increases. Thus, drugs that are water soluble may have higher concentrations in elderly patients than in young patients. Drugs that are fat soluble may have prolonged half-lives.

Renal Excretion

Creatinine clearance declines with age, and drugs excreted by the kidney must be given in decreased doses based on measured drug levels or measured or estimated creatinine clearance.

Box 17-1	IMPORTANT CONSIDERATIONS IN GERIATRIC DRUG THERAPY

1. Pharmacokinetics are often different (e.g., decreased renal clearance and decreased distribution secondary to lower lean body mass).
2. Homeostatic functions are impaired and susceptible to effects of drugs (e.g., orthostatic hypotension is more common).
3. Certain conditions that increase the likelihood of adverse drug reactions are more prevalent (e.g., renal impairment and prostatic hypertrophy).
4. Some conditions are caused or exacerbated by drug therapy.
5. Polypharmacy is common and may increase the likelihood of adverse drug reactions.

TABLE 17-1	Examples of Common Drugs Used Perioperatively with Pharmacokinetic Changes in the Elderly	
Drug	**Change**	**Cause**
Benzodiazepines (long acting)	Increased half-life	Higher body fat
		Lower hepatic metabolism
Nonsteroidal anti-inflammatory drugs	More frequent renal toxicity	Lower renal blood flow (?)
Aminoglycosides	Decreased maintenance dose	Lower renal excretion
β-blockers	Diminished responsiveness	Lower β-adrenergic receptor responsiveness

Hepatic Excretion

Although some decrease in oxidative metabolism occurs, overall hepatic metabolism and excretion are less affected by age than is renal excretion. These changes vary considerably among elderly persons.

Absorption

Drug absorption changes little with age.

Other Considerations

Elderly persons, especially those with dementia, often suffer further cognitive decline as a result of drugs. Sedatives, anti-hypertensive agents, and analgesic agents can all lead directly or indirectly to cognitive decline. This age group is also more subject to drug-induced delirium.

PREOPERATIVE ASSESSMENT

General Principles

There is a modest increase in surgical risk associated with age, but age alone should not be a reason to forgo necessary surgery if the benefit outweighs the risk. The life expectancy of the average 75-year-old man is approximately 9 years; for a woman, it is 11 years. **Population studies of patients undergoing surgical procedures in their 90s demonstrated that** the long-term age-matched survival of these patients was similar to that of controls [● *Hosking et al, 1989*]. Reports on surgery in the elderly have demonstrated that the overall perioperative mortality rates for major elective surgery are in the 5% to 10% range, whereas many procedures performed on elderly patients have mortality rates lower than 5%. The 2007 revision of the American College of Cardiology/American Heart Association Guidelines on Perioperative Cardiovascular Evaluation and Care for Noncardiac Surgery no longer considers advanced age (older than 70 years) to be an independent risk factor for cardiac complications in noncardiac surgery.

Emergency surgery, in contrast, is poorly tolerated by elderly patients and is associated with a much higher morbidity and mortality, usually three or more times higher. Thus, earlier identification of surgically correctable problems may decrease mortality.

The goals of preoperative assessment are no different in elderly patients than in the young. They include the following:

• Identification of all medical conditions that affect surgical risk
• Management of medical problems perioperatively to reduce risk, if possible
• Identification of patients in whom surgical risk is excessive

History

The history should address all medical problems, especially those concerning the heart and lungs. Most elderly patients undergoing surgical procedures have underlying medical problems in addition to the surgical indication. For example, Vaz and Seymour found that only 20% of general surgical patients who were more than 65 years old had no preoperative medical problems [● *Vaz and Seymour, 1989*]. Each of those underlying medical problems must be identified so that its impact on surgical risk can be assessed and managed perioperatively.

History taking may be difficult in this population. Elderly patients often have poor recollection of their medical history and may have impaired memory, factors that often make the information they give inaccurate. These patients frequently minimize symptoms because they believe the symptoms to be part of the aging process.

A careful cardiac history is necessary. As in all patients, a history of recent myocardial infarction or angina should be sought. The degree of exercise tolerance is exceedingly important; many studies have shown a clear correlation between an ability to exercise and a decrease in mortality. If a patient has a history of ischemic heart disease and no recent chest pain, this may indicate either a good prognosis (i.e., no angina) or lack of enough exertion to induce angina. The clinician should ask specifically about the patient's activity level. Can the patient climb stairs without stopping? Can he or she go to the grocery store and carry groceries home? In a younger individual, one may take these things for granted, but many elderly patients have significant limitations in their exercise tolerance.

The elderly patient with ischemic heart disease and poor exercise tolerance of noncardiac origin (e.g., arthritis) poses a problem for the consultant, because the degree of angina is not ascertainable. Poor functional capacity, even if it does not have a cardiac cause, is a risk factor for cardiac complication associated with noncardiac surgical procedures. Gerson and associates demonstrated that these patients are at higher risk overall [❾ *Gerson et al, 1990*]. The physician should ask about exertional shortness of breath, because this sign may be an anginal equivalent or may represent underlying lung disease. Elderly patients are somewhat less likely to have typical anginal chest pain, so exertional dyspnea may be the only clue to underlying coronary artery disease. A history of smoking, chronic cough, and dyspnea are all important in identifying the patient with lung disease.

A formal evaluation for dementia should be performed, especially in patients more than 75 years of age. Dementia increases surgical risk, affects the ability of the patient to cooperate postoperatively, and lowers the likelihood that the

patient will be able to return home after the surgical procedure. In addition, dementia is a clear risk factor for postoperative delirium, which also increases morbidity and mortality. A short mental status assessment such as the Mini-Mental
Status Examination (Table 17-2) should be routine. A low

TABLE 17-2   Mini-Mental State Examination

Maximum Score	Patient Score
Orientation	
5	_____ What is the (year) (season) (date) (day) (month)?
5	_____ Where are we (state) (county) (town) (hospital) (floor)?
Registration	
3	_____ Name three objects—one second to say each—then ask the patient all three after you have said them. Give one point for each correct answer. Then repeat them until patient learns all three. Count trials and record. Number of trials _____
Attention and Calculation	
5	_____ Serial sevens. One point for each correct answer. Stop after five answers. If subject refuses, ask to spell "World" backwards.
Recall	
3	_____ Ask for three objects repeated above. Give one point for each correct.
Language	
9	_____ Name a pencil and watch (2 points). Repeat the following: "No ifs, ands, or buts" (1 point). Follow a three-stage command: "Take a paper in your right hand, fold it in half, and put it on the floor" (3 points). Read and obey the following: "Close your eyes" (1 point). Write a sentence (1 point). Copy a design (1 point).
30	_____
Maximum_____	Patient Score_____ Total___

Assess Level of Consciousness Along a Continuum
Alert—Drowsy   Stupor—Coma
A score <24 is considered abnormal.

score does not distinguish among dementia, delirium, and low education, but it is useful as a baseline. Significant numbers of elderly patients, even in the absence of dementia, suffer postoperative delirium.

It is important to identify all drugs taken by the patient, because their use must be managed in the perioperative period. Many elderly patients receive medications from multiple doctors, use many over-the-counter drugs, and often take alternative herbs and supplements that can interact with standard medications. Drugs with anticholinergic effects may increase the chance of postoperative delirium.

Physical Examination

A standard physical examination should be performed, with particular attention to the presence of heart or lung disease. A baseline weight should be obtained. The state of hydration in elderly patients may be difficult to assess occasionally. Neck vein distention and skin turgor over the forehead (not on arms or other areas of decreased subcutaneous support) are helpful indications of the state of hydration.

Although an asymptomatic carotid bruit is a marker for underlying vascular disease, it is not associated with an increased risk of perioperative stroke [● *Ropper et al, 1982*]. Evidence of active congestive heart failure, especially an S_3 gallop, is important to identify because it is an important risk factor in perioperative morbidity and mortality.

Many elderly patients have systolic murmurs, which may suggest aortic stenosis, a well-documented risk factor for cardiac complications. Physical examination may be misleading in elderly patients. In the elderly patient with significant aortic stenosis, the typical signs may be absent. Hypertension may be present (rather than hypotension), and the slowed and delayed carotid upstroke may be absent. In a patient whose history and physical examination suggest aortic stenosis, an echocardiogram with Doppler imaging should be performed, because it is important to identify significant aortic stenosis preoperatively given that it increases surgical risk. I also consider echocardiography for the patient whose preoperative physical examination suggests the presence of previously unidentified significant valvular heart disease.

Laboratory Studies

Currently, no uniform standardized approach to preoperative laboratory testing in the elderly patient exists. A complete blood count, serum electrolytes, and creatinine determinations are usually performed. Age alone does not cause anemia, but significant numbers of older patients are found to have anemia, the cause of which should be investigated (although this may not be necessary in all cases before important surgical procedures). As noted previously, a normal creatinine level in an elderly person is often not indicative of normal creatinine clearance. Lean body mass decreases with age, and body fat increases. The Cockcroft-Gault equation mentioned earlier should be used to estimate clearance so that this can be taken into account for drug dosing and other uses. Even if only minimally elevated, a raised creatinine level indicates significant renal impairment in the geriatric age group. An electrocardiogram and chest radiograph should be obtained as baseline studies; many older people have abnormalities on their electrocardiographic tracings and chest films that would not be expected from the history. The presence of abnormalities on these tests may be needed postoperatively for accurate evaluation of complications or symptoms.

Beyond these basic tests, the necessity of routinely ordering more involved and invasive tests is controversial. Pulmonary function tests have been recommended by some authors for all elderly patients. No good evidence indicates that these tests are useful for surgical decision making for most patients. This patient population undergoes few minor elective surgical procedures; thus, most surgery is necessary and important. As in younger patients, pulmonary function tests should generally be limited to patients who are having lung resection procedures.

ANESTHESIA

Local anesthesia is associated with low risk in elderly patients. If local anesthesia is not feasible, the choice between spinal and general anesthesia is the surgeon's and anesthesiologist's, based on the patient's medical condition and preference. There is no significant difference in mortality between the two routes. Although general anesthesia is often followed by a short-term cognitive decline, in some studies spinal anesthesia had a similar effect.

POSTOPERATIVE COMPLICATIONS

General Complications

Older patients face the same postoperative complications as younger patients. However, older patients have less physiologic reserve. There are significant decreases in function of important physiologic systems, as discussed earlier; the older patient is less able to compensate for these changes, and complications are more likely to ensue. The older patient is also more likely to have underlying chronic disease that predisposes to complications. The most serious complications in elderly patients, as in younger patients, are cardiac and pulmonary problems; in addition, neurologic complications such as delirium are more likely to occur in this patient population.

Cardiac Complications

Congestive heart failure may manifest postoperatively even in patients who never had a history of heart disease. This finding was noted in Goldman's initial study in which many of the cases of congestive heart failure were found in patients older than 60 years and without a history of heart disease. It is important to ask about shortness of breath, orthopnea, and paroxysmal dyspnea. Physical findings of elevated neck veins or S_3 gallop are useful, whereas rales are a nonspecific finding with a variety of causes. If congestive heart failure occurs, a cause should be sought. Postoperative myocardial infarction is not accompanied by chest pain in more than half of patients and may manifest as congestive heart failure, hypotension, arrhythmias, or, especially in the elderly, as a change in mental status.

Pulmonary Complications

Pulmonary complications are probably the most common postoperative problems. As many as 40% of elderly patients suffer postoperative pulmonary problems, which often contribute to the cause of death. Atelectasis is extremely common and, if allowed to go unchecked, may lead to collapse of major lung segments or pneumonia.

The prevention of these complications is possible with good preoperative planning. Ideally, patients should stop smoking at least 6 weeks preoperatively. Inspiratory maneuvers such as inspiratory incentive spirometry appear to be effective deterrents to atelectasis and pneumonia, and these techniques should be taught preoperatively. In patients with known chronic obstructive pulmonary disease or asthma, maximization of preoperative pulmonary status with bronchodilators should be considered. The use of chest physiotherapy has not been well studied, but it should probably be used in patients at high risk of pulmonary complications.

Deep Venous Thrombosis

Deep venous thrombosis and pulmonary embolism are important causes of postoperative complications. Despite concerns about using anticoagulation in elderly patients, the benefit clearly outweighs the risk.

Delirium

Delirium, also known as acute confusional state, is often seen postoperatively in elderly patients. It is associated with increased hospital morbidity, mortality, and a longer length of stay. Although delirium is more common in demented patients, it can be seen in elderly patients with no prior dementia and must be distinguished from dementia by the examining physician. Box 17-2 shows the DSM-IV criteria for delirium established in the fourth edition of the *Diagnostic and Statistical Manual of Mental Disorders*.

Like dementia, delirium is associated with a decrease in cognition, which may include disorientation about time. Unlike in dementia, however, the patient's level of consciousness is sometimes reduced, and the patient frequently has difficulty attending to stimuli. The delirious patient may have an increased or reduced activity level. Delirium, in

Box 17-2	**DSM-IV DIAGNOSTIC CRITERIA FOR DELIRIUM**

1. Disturbance of consciousness (e.g., reduced clarity of awareness of the environment) in conjunction with reduced ability to focus, sustain, or shift attention
2. A change in cognition (such as memory deficit, disorientation, or language disturbance) or the development of a perceptual disturbance that is not better accounted for by a preexisting, established, or evolving dementia
3. Development of the disturbance during a brief period (usually hours to days) and a tendency for fluctuation during the course of the day
4. Evidence from the history, physical examination, or laboratory findings that the disturbance is caused by
   a. A general medical condition
   b. A substance intoxication or side effect
   c. Substance withdrawal
   d. Multiple factors

Based on Diagnostic and Statistical Manual of Mental Disorders, 4th ed (DSM-IV). Modified from the American Psychiatric Association. Copyright 1994 American Psychiatric Association. Reprinted with permission from the Diagnostic and Statistical Manual of Mental Disorders, copyright 2000. American Psychiatric Association.

contrast to dementia, is usually of acute onset and commonly fluctuates during the day, often worsening at night ("sundowning"). Table 17-3 contrasts dementia with delirium. The significance of postoperative delirium is its frequent association with either worsening medical illness or drug toxicity, the latter of which is preventable and both are reversible. These causes must be carefully sought. Infections, acute myocardial infarction, congestive heart failure, metabolic disturbances, and dehydration and many other medical complications can all manifest with prominent delirium in elderly patients. Similarly, alcohol and sedative-hypnotic withdrawal can appear postoperatively. Drugs, especially those agents with anticholinergic effects, are often implicated in delirium in elderly patients. Box 17-3 lists some of the drugs associated with delirium.

Thus, in an elderly patient with postoperative delirium, a thorough medical evaluation should be performed. Several conditions may precipitate delirium: infections, especially

TABLE 17-3	Clinical Features of Delirium and Dementia	
Characteristic	**Delirium**	**Dementia**
Onset	Acute	Insidious
Course over 24 hours	Fluctuating, often worse at night	Stable
Consciousness	May be reduced	Clear
Attention	Globally disordered	Normal, except in severe cases
Cognition	Globally disordered	Globally impaired
Hallucinations	Usually visual or visual and auditory	Usually absent
Delusions	Fleeting, poorly systematized	Often absent
Orientation	Usually impaired at least for a time	Often impaired
Psychomotor activity	Increased, reduced, or shifting unpredictably	Often normal
Speech	Often incoherent, slow, or rapid	Difficulty finding words
Involuntary movements	Often asterixis or coarse tremor	Often absent

From Lipowski ZJ: Delirium in the elderly patient. N Engl J Med 320:578-582, 1989.

Box 17-3	DRUGS THAT CAUSE DELIRIUM OR COGNITIVE IMPAIRMENT

DRUGS THAT PRODUCE CENTRAL ANTICHOLINERGIC EFFECTS

- Anticholinergic drugs
- Tricyclic antidepressants or trazodone
- Phenothiazines
- Antipsychotic drugs
- Antihistamine agents
- Benzodiazepines
- Opiate analgesics
- Disopyramide
- Phenobarbital

OTHER DRUGS THAT CAN ALSO CAUSE CONFUSION

- Alcohol
- Amantadine
- β-Blockers
- Bromocriptine
- Cimetidine
- Corticosteroids
- Digoxin
- Diuretics
- Levodopa
- Nonsteroidal anti-inflammatory drugs
- Penicillin
- Phenytoin, primidone
- Quinidine

those of the respiratory tract; acute myocardial infarction or congestive heart failure; electrolyte abnormalities or metabolic problems, such as hyperglycemia or hypoglycemia or hypernatremia or hyponatremia; renal or liver failure; and hypoxia. A central nervous system cause such as stroke is possible but uncommon in the absence of localizing signs. All nonessential drugs should be stopped, especially those listed in Box 17-3. In elderly patients, the cause often turns out to be multifactorial, and it may be impossible to pinpoint only one or two etiologic factors.

Management should be directed at identifying the underlying causes and correcting them, if possible. General supportive measures, including good nursing care with a quiet and well-lit room, and reassurance, and reorientation of the patient, are recommended.

If restlessness is severe, pharmacologic intervention may be required. The newer atypical antipsychotic drugs such as risperidone and quetiapine have been used effectively. Doses should start at low levels and be increased if needed. Haloperidol was used in the recent past because of its sedating potential and relatively limited anticholinergic effects; although this drug is effective, its side effects are more common than those of the newer medications. If alcohol or sedative-hypnotic withdrawal is suspected, benzodiazepines are the drugs of choice. Sedation, however, should not be a substitute for careful evaluation of the delirious patient. If true sedation is needed, low doses of short-acting benzodiazepines are used by some experts.

Studies have shown that delirium is preventable with careful preoperative assessment and planning. Attention to a variety of precipitating causes before the surgical procedure can prevent many cases. Marcantonio and colleagues showed that attention to 10 major areas, including multiple metabolic factors, treatment of pain, medications, and mobilization, for example, decreased the incidence significantly [◉ *Marcantonio et al, 2001*].

Hypothermia

Another important but lesser known problem is postoperative hypothermia. Most operating rooms and recovery suites are kept at low ambient temperatures, and many patients have been found to have temperatures lower than 36°C. Although this temperature does not cause problems for most patients, in some it may contribute to hypoxia, hypotension, and altered mental status.

SPECIAL ISSUES IN GERIATRIC SURGERY

Nonspecific Presentations

Illness in elderly patients, especially the frail elderly, often presents atypically. Nonspecific presentations include weakness, falling, incontinence, failure to eat, and change in mental status (i.e., delirium). These symptoms and signs may be the earliest presentations of serious problems such as respiratory or urinary tract infections, congestive heart failure, or metabolic derangements. The elderly patient may have little or no fever despite serious infection. Thus, in evaluating the perioperative elderly patient who has a change in status, the clinician must keep in mind that these nonspecific presentations may be the only clues to many serious underlying illnesses, and a thorough evaluation must be performed to identify and treat these disorders.

Different Presentations

Certain surgical diseases may manifest differently in elderly patients. Appendicitis, although more common in younger age groups, has a higher mortality in elderly patients (6% to 10%). Two reasons are generally cited for this phenomenon: (1) delay in diagnosis and (2) increased rate of perforation.

The delay in diagnosis is attributed to both a delay on the part of the elderly person in seeking medical attention and a failure by the physician to make the correct diagnosis preoperatively. Symptoms in elderly patients may be less severe, because fever is less common and abdominal pain is usually milder. Right lower quadrant tenderness is present in 80% to 90% of patients, however. Rebound tenderness is less common in elderly patients. Abscess formation may result in a right lower quadrant mass that may be mistakenly diagnosed as cecal carcinoma. Perforation is common, occurring in up to 70% in elderly individuals versus 20% in young patients, probably because the appendix atrophies with age and the blood supply may be compromised by atherosclerosis. Thus, with infection and increased pressure in the appendix, the blood supply is quickly impeded, and the thinned wall easily perforates.

Cholecystitis may likewise present in a different fashion in elderly patients. Peritoneal signs are seen in only one half of cases, fever is frequently low grade, and up to one fourth of patients may have no abdominal tenderness. Nonetheless, elderly patients are more likely to have gangrene and empyema by the time they present for treatment. Acute cholecystitis, which requires emergency surgery, thus has a high mortality rate in this age group (8% to 17%).

Finally, peptic ulcer disease more often manifests without pain in elderly patients. Occult gastrointestinal bleeding occurs frequently, whereas perforation may be manifested by shock, hemorrhage, or abdominal distention rather than by pain.

Cardiac Surgery

Coronary artery bypass grafting (CABG) is routinely performed in elderly patients. Many studies have been conducted and have shown good results with low mortality. One study demonstrated a mortality rate of 2.6% in patients who were more than 75 years old; good results were assessed by angina relief and quality of life improvement. Off-pump coronary artery surgery has been suggested to be associated with lower morbidity and mortality in elderly patients.

Surgery for valvular disease, however, has higher mortality in the elderly. One study of patients who were more than 80 years old showed a mortality rate of 2.9% for CABG but a rate of 16% for those having valve replacement surgery or CABG with valve surgery. Studies have shown that minimally invasive aortic valve surgery can be done in elderly patients with good results.

Vascular Surgery

Abdominal aortic aneurysm repair can be performed electively in elderly patients with reasonable morbidity and mortality rates. Investigators have shown that endovascular procedures can also be performed in patients who are more than 80 years old, with good results. One study showed mortality rates of 2.2% in endovascular elective surgery and 3.3% in open elective surgery. Mortality rates for ruptured or symptomatic aneurysms were substantially higher.

Carotid endarterectomy is a common operation in elderly patients. One study of octogenarians demonstrated a mortality rate of 1.4% and an ipsilateral stroke rate of 1.7%. Overall survival was 86% at 6 years, with a stroke-free survival of 76%.

Abdominal Surgery

Abdominal surgery in elderly patients is not benign; however, results of elective abdominal surgery are rather good. In a study of major abdominal surgery in patients who were more than 80 years old, the mortality rate for elective surgery was 7.5%; results for emergency surgery were much worse, with a mortality rate of 29%. Numerous studies have investigated laparoscopic procedures. Elderly patients can undergo these types of procedures with good results and very favorable morbidity and mortality rates. Excellent results have been shown for cholecystectomy and colonic surgery.

Cancer

General Considerations

Because the risk of most cancers increases with age, elderly patients have a disproportionate number of malignant tumors, and surgery is the primary treatment for many of them. The decision to perform cancer surgery in the elderly patient, however, rests on certain factors. The first is the combination of the life expectancy of the patient without surgical intervention and the natural history of the underlying cancer. Radical surgery for prostate cancer in an ill 90-year-old man is not indicated, whereas resection of bowel carcinoma in a vigorous 70-year-old patient certainly is. The second factor is the availability of nonsurgical therapy and its relative toxicity. The final factor is the risk of the proposed surgical procedure in relation to the chance of cure or prolongation of life.

Lung Cancer

Half of all lung cancer occurs in patients older than 65 years of age. Surgical resection is a potentially curative form of treatment. One study retrospectively reviewed morbidity and mortality following thoracotomy in a group of patients who were more than 70 years old. The elderly group had a mortality of 12.8% versus 4.7% for a group of controls younger than 70 years of age. Complication rates and actuarial survival were similar between the two groups, with a 5-year survival of 29.8% in the group older than 70 years of age versus 33% in the younger group [Thomas et al, 1993]. Other studies have shown similar results, with a small increase in short-term mortality in elderly patients reported as 3% to 14%. A more recent study of patients more than 80 years old showed a perioperative death rate of only 1.6% and a rate of major complications of 13%. Overall 5-year survival was 38%, and it was 82% for patients with stage IA disease. In addition, studies have shown that video-assisted thoracic surgery is feasible for lung cancer treatment in elderly patients. Age alone therefore should not be a contraindication to potentially curative therapy if the patient has reasonable cardiopulmonary function.

Colon Cancer

Two thirds of colon cancer cases present in persons older than 65 years of age. There is no nonsurgical therapy. Some studies have looked at morbidity, mortality, and long-term survival in elderly patients undergoing colon resection. For elective surgery with curative intent, mortality rates have been reported to be between 3% and 11%. One study of hospitals found a mortality rate of only 2.9% in patients who were more than 65 years old and 6.9% in those older than 80 years [Dimick et al, 2003]. Studies of laparoscopic procedures for bowel cancer have demonstrated good results with lower morbidity and mortality rates.

In one study, emergency surgery carried a much higher mortality rate (38%) in patients who were more than 80 years of age. Operations for palliation rather than for cure also had a higher surgical mortality. Thus, elective surgery carries a reasonable prognosis, even in those older than 80 years of age, but emergency surgery is poorly tolerated, especially in very old patients.

Gastric Carcinoma

Similar results have been found in gastric cancer. In one report of a small number of patients but with young controls, the mortality rate was slightly higher in the elderly patients than in the younger control patients (8% versus 4%) but with similar 5-year survival rates (16% versus 20%).

Conclusions

Overall, the results of these and other studies suggest that elective surgery can be performed with acceptable mortality rates, especially in younger elderly patients (<80 years of age) and in older patients without multiple medical problems. Emergency surgery is poorly tolerated, especially in patients who are more than 80 years old. Newer, less invasive procedures such as laparoscopic surgery, video-assisted thoracic surgery, and other minimally invasive surgical procedures have shown excellent results with lower morbidity and mortality rates that have rendered even more patients eligible for surgery and have given them a chance for longer lives with better quality of life.

Key Points

- Surgical procedures in elderly patients, in appropriately selected cases, can be performed with reasonable morbidity and mortality rates.
- Many elderly patients can enjoy longer lives with improved quality and more productivity after appropriate surgical procedures.
- Emergency surgery has very much higher morbidity and mortality than elective surgery. Elective surgery should be performed before an emergency procedure must be done.
- Elderly patients have less physiologic reserve than younger patients and should be in optimal condition before surgical procedures are undertaken, if possible.
- Older patients often have significant numbers of underlying disease processes that put them at additional risk for surgery.
- Many older patients are taking many medications that put them at risk for surgical complications.
- Elderly patients are at much higher risk for postoperative delirium because of age and medications; delirium increases the risk of postoperative morbidity and mortality.
- Improvements in surgical techniques such as endoscopic procedures make many operations available to older patients, with much improved outcomes (e.g., laparoscopic cholecystectomy).

Selected Readings

Abbas S, Booth M: Major abdominal surgery in octogenarians. N Z Med J 116:1-8, 2003.

Beck LH: Perioperative renal fluid, and electrolyte management. Clin Geriatr Med 6:557-569, 1990.

Berggren D, Gustafson Y, Eriksson B, et al: Postoperative confusion after anesthesia in elderly patients with femoral neck fractures. Anesth Analg 66:497-504, 1987.

Bridget P, Bellows W, Leung JM: The prevalence of preoperative diastolic filling abnormalities in geriatric surgical patients. Anesth Analg 97: 1214-1221, 2003.

Conaway DG, House J, Bandt K et al: The elderly: Health status benefits and recovery of function one year after coronary artery bypass surgery. J Am Coll Cardiol 42:1421-1426, 2003.

Dimick JB, Cowan KA, Upchurch GR, et al: Hospital volume and surgical outcomes for elderly patients with colorectal cancer in the United States. J Surg Res 114:50-56, 2003.

Gerrah R, Izhar U, Elami A, et al: Cardiac surgery in octogenarians: A better prognosis in coronary artery disease. Isr Med Assoc J 5:713-716, 2003.

Gerson MC, Hurst JM, Hertzberg VS, et al: Prediction of cardiac and pulmonary complications related to elective abdominal and noncardiac thoracic surgery in geriatric patients. Ann Intern Med 88:101-107, 1990. **Ⓑ**

Hamel MB, Henderson WG, Khuri SF, et al: Surgical outcomes for patients aged 89 and older: Morbidity and mortality from major noncardiac surgery. J Am Geriatr Soc 53:424-429, 2005.

Hosking MP, Warner MA, Lobdell CM, et al: Outcomes of surgery in patients 90 years of age and older. JAMA 161:1909-1915, 1989. **Ⓒ**

Lewis AAM, Khourg GA: Resection for colorectal cancer in the very old: Are the risks too high? BMJ 296:459-461, 1988.

Lien CA: Regional versus general anesthesia for hip surgery in older patients: Does the choice affect patient outcome? J Am Geriatr Soc 50:191-194, 2002.

Lipowski ZJ: Delirium in the elderly patient. N Engl J Med 320:578-582, 1989.

Marcantonio ER, Flacker JM, Wright RJ, et al: Reducing delirium after hip fracture: A randomized trial. J Am Geriatr Soc 49:516-522, 2001. **Ⓒ**

McCallion J, Canning GP, Knight PV, et al: Acute appendicitis in the elderly: A 5-year retrospective study. Age Ageing 16:256-260, 1987.

Morrow DJ, Thompson J, Wilson SE: Acute cholecystitis in the elderly: A surgical emergency. Arch Surg 113:1149-1152, 1978.

Patel AP, Langan EM, Taylor SM, et al: An analysis of standard open and endovascular surgical repair of abdominal aortic aneurysms in octogenarians. Am Surg 69:744-748, 2003.

Port JL, Kent M, Korst RJ, et al: Surgical resection for lung cancer in the octogenarian. Chest 126:733-738, 2004.

Pruner G, Castellano R, Jannello AM, et al: Carotid endarterectomy in the octogenarian: Outcomes of 345 procedures performed from 1995-2000. Cardiovasc Surg 11:105-112, 2003.

Ropper AH, Wechsler LR, Wilson LS: Carotid bruit and the risk of stroke in elective surgery. N Engl J Med 307:1388-1390, 1982. **Ⓒ**

Saidi RF, Bell JL, Cucrick PS: Surgical resection for gastric cancer in elderly patients: Is there a difference in outcome? J Surg Res 118:15-20, 2004.

Seymour DG, Vaz FG: Prospective study of elderly general surgical patients. II. Postoperative complications. Age Ageing 18:316-326, 1989.

Sherman S, Guidot CE: The feasibility of thoracotomy for lung cancer in the elderly. JAMA 258:927-930, 1987.

Thomas P, Sielezneff I, Ragni J, et al: Is lung cancer resection justified in patients aged over 70 years? Eur J Cardiothorac Surg 7:246-251, 1993.

Vaz FG, Seymour DG: A prospective study of elderly general surgical patients. I. Preoperative medical problems. Age Ageing 18:309-315, 1989. ⓒ

Weber DM: Laparoscopic surgery: An excellent approach in elderly patients. Arch Surg 138:1083-1088, 2003.

Weitz HH: Noncardiac surgery in the elderly patient with cardiovascular disease. Clin Geriatr Med 6:511-529, 1990.

18 Surgery in the Patient with Kidney Disease

BRENDA HOFFMAN, MD
TRACY McGOWAN, MD

- An estimation of glomerular filtration rate (GFR) in the surgical patient with an elevated serum creatinine concentration will provide the practitioner with an accurate assessment of the stage of renal failure and will facilitate the appropriate perioperative medical management of that patient.
- Cardiovascular disease is the most common cause of mortality in patients with chronic kidney disease (CKD). Dipyridamole thallium scanning and dobutamine echocardiography are the preferred noninvasive tests for preoperative cardiac risk assessment in the patient population with CKD.
- Poorly controlled hypertension is prevalent in patients with CKD and is usually aggravated by hypervolemia. Patients undergoing dialysis should be well dialyzed and near their dry weight at the time of surgery.
- Hyperkalemia and acidemia should be corrected medically or with dialysis before proceeding with surgery.
- Bleeding times are not helpful in identifying patients with CKD who are at risk for uremic bleeding, and these tests should not be routinely ordered preoperatively. Bleeding risk can be decreased with correction of anemia and adequate dialysis. Active bleeding can be treated specifically with desmopressin acetate (DDAVP), cryoprecipitate, and conjugated estrogens.

- Care must be taken to administer all drugs at doses appropriate to the level of GFR in patients with CKD in the perioperative period.
- Postoperative renal failure is associated with high mortality and is usually caused by prerenal failure or acute tubular necrosis (ATN).
- The treatment of postoperative renal failure is largely supportive and should focus on normalization of volume status, optimization of hemodynamics, avoidance of nephrotoxins, and the timely provision of renal replacement therapy (RRT) if necessary.

The need for both elective and emergency surgery in patients with acute renal failure (ARF) and CKD is not uncommon and has resulted in the development of a specialized surgical approach to their care. These patients undergo operations for surgical problems, such as those encountered in the general population, as well as for problems that arise specifically as a result of renal failure, such as vascular access surgery. Regardless of the surgical procedure, these patients present unique management challenges. Recognition of the potential sequelae of kidney disease and their appropriate management by the medical consultant will result in optimal perioperative care of these patients.

ASSESSING RENAL FUNCTION

The most frequently used screening tool for identifying a patient with impaired renal function is the serum creatinine concentration. In the hospitalized patient, an elevated serum creatinine may represent either acute kidney disease or CKD. Therefore, when evaluating a patient with an elevated serum creatinine for a possible surgical procedure, it is first important to determine whether this condition is acute or chronic. A careful history and review of the patient's records should provide insight into whether the current elevation in creatinine is new or old.

ACUTE RENAL FAILURE

ARF, as indicated by a sudden rise in creatinine, is common in the hospitalized patient. The causes are grouped into three categories: prerenal (hypoperfusion of the kidneys), intrinsic renal damage, and postrenal (obstruction). If ARF is suspected in a patient who needs a surgical procedure, prompt consultation with a nephrologist is recommended to determine what interventions are available to restore the patient's renal function to baseline. In general, it is best to wait for the resolution of ARF before proceeding to surgery, if at all possible, both to minimize surgical risk and to promote full renal recovery. If it is necessary for a patient with ARF to have an operation, care should be taken to prevent intraoperative hypotension because any decrease in renal blood flow could prolong the duration of the renal failure and perhaps aggravate the extent of irreversible kidney damage.

CHRONIC KIDNEY DISEASE

In contrast to ARF, CKD is reflected by a stable elevation in serum creatinine. Serum creatinine is merely a screening test to identify patients who may have impaired renal function. To characterize true renal filtration function accurately, one needs to measure GFR. This measurement requires injection of inulin or a radiolabeled substance such as iothalamate and the collection of both timed blood and urine samples to calculate clearance. This approach provides an accurate assessment of the GFR, but it is time consuming, costly, and inconvenient for the patient. Measurement of a 24-hour creatinine clearance (ClCr) is a good estimate of GFR but still requires both a blood sample and a timed urine collection. To estimate GFR quickly from an easily obtained serum creatinine measurement simply requires employing any of several equations that have been validated to estimate GFR. **Two frequently used equations are the simplified Modification of Diet in Renal Disease Study Group (MDRD) formula:**

GFR, in mL/minute/1.73 m^2 =186.3 $\times$
Serum creatinine$^{[-1.154]}$ $\times$ Age$^{[-0.203]}$ $\times$(0.742 if female) $\times$
(1.21 if African American) [Stevens et al, 2006]

and the simpler formula of Cockcroft and Gault:

ClCr, in mL/minute = (140−age) $\times$ Lean body weight [kg] $\div$
(PCr [mg/dL] $\times$ 72) $\times$ (0.85 if female)

Where PCr is plasma creatine [❂ *Stevens et al, 2006*].

By applying one of these equations, the clinician may estimate the patient's true level of filtration function. To understand the implications of different levels of GFR more clearly, the National Kidney Foundation established a classification of the stages of CKD [National Kidney Foundation, 2002] (Table 18-1). Patients in stages 1 and 2 CKD have fairly well-preserved GFR and typically have no special perioperative considerations based on their renal function. Patients in stages 3, 4, and 5 need special consideration in the preoperative and postoperative period.

General Considerations

Diabetes mellitus (50%) and hypertension (33%) are the two primary causes of end-stage renal disease (ESRD) in the United States; the remaining cases result from glomerulonephritides and a variety of other causes. However, although only one third of patients have hypertension as the cause of

TABLE 18-1	Stages of Chronic Kidney Disease by Glomerular Filtration Rate	
Stage	**Description**	**GFR (mL/min)**
1	CKD with normal or ↑ GFR	>90
2	Mild ↓ GFR	60–89
3	Moderate ↓ GFR	30–59
4	Severe ↓ GFR	15–29
5	Kidney failure, ESRD	<15 or dialysis

CKD, chronic kidney disease; GFR, glomerular filtration rate.

their CKD, almost 100% of patients develop hypertension as a result of CKD by the time they need RRT (either dialysis or kidney transplantation). Moreover, these patients often require two or more drugs to achieve adequate blood pressure control. Uncontrolled blood glucose levels and blood pressure must be managed before these patients can safely proceed to surgery.

Regardless of the cause, patients with advanced stages of CKD have impairment of the kidneys' excretory function, as evidenced by the accumulation of urea nitrogen and creatinine. Similarly, drug excretion is impaired for drugs that depend on the kidney as their route of elimination. Therefore, dose adjustment of renally eliminated drugs based on the patient's GFR is imperative to avoid toxicity. Other compounds that can accumulate in patients with CKD include the following: potassium, which leads to hyperkalemia and possible cardiac arrhythmias; phosphorus, which contributes to hyperparathyroidism; acids leading to metabolic acidosis, which weakens bones and muscles; and sodium and water, which result in edema and possibly congestive heart failure. Uremia may lead to malnutrition that can affect wound healing, to pericarditis, and possibly to pericardial tamponade, as well as predisposing patients to increased bleeding by inhibiting normal platelet aggregation.

In CKD, the kidneys' synthetic function is also impaired, resulting in decreased production of erythropoietin with consequent anemia, as well as decreased conversion of vitamin D to its active form, a process that causes hypocalcemia, secondary hyperparathyroidism, and renal osteodystrophy. Impaired kidney function can lead to decreased metabolism of substances such as insulin; the results are an increased sensitivity to the effects of endogenous insulin and a decreased need for both exogenous insulin and oral hypoglycemic agents as renal failure progresses. Profound hypoglycemia may therefore occur in the diabetic patient with CKD in whom food is withheld preoperatively.

All the foregoing conditions associated with CKD must be considered when evaluating and managing patients with impaired renal function in the perioperative period. ***Renal insufficiency* (creatinine ≥2.0) is an independent risk factor for cardiac complications in the patient who undergoes noncardiac surgical procedures** [● *Eagle et al, 2002*]. Patients with CKD have a higher incidence of vascular disease, coronary artery disease, and peripheral vascular disease, as well as greater myocardial dysfunction, than the general population. In addition to an increased prevalence of traditional risk factors for coronary artery disease such as diabetes, hyperlipidemia, and hypertension, these patients have other, less traditional risk factors such as abnormal calcium and phosphorus balance and uremia itself.

History and Physical Examination

The history of the patient with CKD should focus on prior surgical procedures, bleeding tendencies, and cardiac history, including a thorough review of systems with attention to a history of angina, pulmonary symptoms, and arrhythmias. A complete list of medications needs to be ascertained, especially potentially nephrotoxic drugs, medications that need therapeutic drug monitoring, and medications whose abrupt withdrawal can lead to rebound hypertension (i.e., β-blockers and clonidine). The physical examination should emphasize evidence of volume overload (i.e. signs of peripheral or pulmonary edema or elevated jugular venous pressure) and evidence of both cardiac disease (e.g., murmurs, rubs, or gallops) and peripheral vascular disease, (i.e., bruits or decreased or absent peripheral pulses).

Laboratory Tests and Other Diagnostic Studies

Appropriate laboratory tests and other studies include a chemistry panel to look for abnormalities in electrolytes, including sodium, potassium, calcium, and phosphorus. A complete blood count should be ordered to assess for anemia. If anemia is present, iron studies should be checked. A baseline electrocardiogram (ECG) should be performed and compared with previous ECGs if available. Drug levels should be measured for appropriate medications such as digoxin and calcineurin inhibitors (CNIs) in patients with renal transplants. If there is any question of pulmonary compromise from either the history or physical examination, a chest radiograph should be obtained. Finally, as part of the preoperative evaluation, one must pay special attention to cardiovascular risk assessment, blood pressure control and volume status, electrolyte and acid-base balance, and optimization of hematologic parameters.

Assessment of Cardiovascular Risk

Cardiovascular disease is extremely common in patients with CKD stages 3 to 5 and is the primary cause of death in this population. In ESRD, mortality from cardiovascular disease is reported to be at least 10 times higher than in the general population and is even greater when the underlying cause of renal failure is diabetes. Overall risk assessment must take into account both the patient's clinical risk profile and the specific risk of the surgical procedure itself. The American College of Cardiology/American Heart Association preoperative evaluation guideline should be utilized to estimate perioperative risk (see Chapter 7).

For the patient with CKD in whom evaluation suggests that cardiac stress testing should be performed, it is important to consider the patient's functional and exercise capacity. Patients with CKD have been shown to have a lower functional capacity and may be less likely to achieve a target heart rate on a conventional treadmill stress test. This situation limits the sensitivity of treadmill stress testing. Although stress testing in conjunction with nuclear perfusion imaging is more applicable in patients with known coronary disease or baseline abnormalities on the ECG, these tests are similarly limited in patients who are unable to achieve target heart rates and have been shown to have a poorer positive predictive value in patients undergoing dialysis. Therefore, studies of dialyzed patients lead us to suggest that patients undergoing high-risk procedures and those who are unable to exercise should undergo either dipyridamole thallium-201 imaging or dobutamine stress echocardiography. In the foregoing studies, the dipyridamole thallium and dobutamine echocardiographic tests had sensitivities, at best, of 92% and 95% and specificities of 89% and 86%, respectively.

Patients with CKD not only have an increased incidence of coronary artery disease but also have a very high incidence of left ventricular wall motion abnormalities. The incidence of left ventricular hypertrophy is approximately 30% when the GFR is in the range of 50 to 75 mL/minute and increases to almost 80% by the time the patient is in need of RRT.

Management of Blood Pressure and Volume Status

Volume overload in the patient with CKD is a common cause of hypertension that is difficult to control. A careful physical examination for signs of intravascular or peripheral volume excess is critical. In dialysis-dependent patients, volume control is achieved by ultrafiltrating fluid to take the patient to his or her appropriate dry weight. Overly aggressive fluid removal must be avoided because patients below their dry weight can develop profound hypotension during the induction of anesthesia that can lead to complications such as thrombosis of the dialysis access site.

Most patients have hemodialysis with ultrafiltration performed the day before the surgical procedure to ensure that they are as near to their dry weight as possible for the operating room. Patients undergoing peritoneal dialysis should continue exchanges until the time of surgery, at which point their peritoneal cavity should be drained. For patients not receiving RRT who have signs of volume overload, diuretics should be used to achieve euvolemia. Typically, loop diuretics are used for this purpose. However, if a patient develops diuretic resistance, a combination of diuretics may be necessary.

In cases of severe volume overload, especially when pulmonary edema is present in a patient who needs to go to the operating room and there is not sufficient time to optimize volume status with medical therapy, a temporary dialysis catheter should be placed, and the patient should be ultrafiltrated. This catheter can be removed postoperatively if the patient's renal function is sufficient to maintain the volume status or changed to a more permanent access if prolonged dialysis is anticipated.

In the patient with CKD and hypertension in the absence of volume overload, parenteral antihypertensive medications should be used in the perioperative period while the patient is unable to take oral medications. Parenteral antihypertensive agents that may be used include labetalol (a combined α-and β-adrenergic blocker), α-methyldopa (a centrally acting agent), and hydralazine (a direct arteriolar vasodilator that should be given with a β-blocker to minimize reflex sympathetic stimulation). Nicardipine is a dihydropyridine calcium channel blocker that can be given as an intravenous infusion. Its major limitation is a long half-life, which limits the ability for rapid titration. Fenoldopam is a peripheral dopamine-1 receptor agonist, which has the added advantage of maintaining or increasing renal perfusion while it lowers blood pressure, thus making it an attractive choice for patients with CKD. Unlike many other parenteral antihypertensives, fenoldopam does not lead to rebound hypertension when it is discontinued. Finally, enalaprilat is an intravenous form of the angiotensin-converting enzyme inhibitor enalapril. The response to enalaprilat depends heavily on the plasma volume and plasma renin activity. This drug should be used with caution in patients with advanced CKD and should be avoided in new kidney transplant recipients and in patients with ARF. Nitroglycerin can be administered intravenously, but the more potent nitroprusside should be avoided in patients with renal insufficiency because it is metabolized to cyanide, and accumulation can be toxic.

Hypotension, albeit less common, can occur in patients with CKD. In dialyzed patients, low blood pressure is usually the result of too much volume removal. In this case, fluid replacement with isotonic saline is appropriate. Once oral intake is stopped preoperatively (NPO status), it is appropriate to give 500 mL/day of maintenance fluids in addition to replacing any ongoing fluid losses, which include increased insensible losses from factors such as mechanical ventilation and fever. In the euvolemic patient, hypotension can be caused by autonomic neuropathy, particularly in patients with diabetes, severe left ventricular dysfunction, pericardial tamponade (possibly from uremia), oversedation, or adrenal insufficiency (in patients who received kidney transplants in the days before steroid-sparing regimens were routinely employed). In patients with an abnormal response to cosyntropin stimulation testing, stress-dose steroids should be considered in the perioperative period.

Hyperkalemia

Hyperkalemia is common as the GFR falls and is secondary to impaired renal excretion of hydrogen and potassium. Ordinarily, hyperkalemia in patients with CKD but with some residual renal function is managed by dietary potassium restriction and diuretics. However, even in these patients, dialysis may be necessary in catabolic states, during which potassium release can be immense. Blood in the gastrointestinal tract or the administration of units of packed red blood cells, especially cells with an older shelf life, can also result in a heavy potassium load caused by the lysis of red blood cells.

Hyperkalemia in CKD can be treated in several ways, depending on its severity. As a general rule, potassium levels less than 6 mEq/L rarely result in changes in the ECG and do not require emergency therapy. Potassium levels greater than 6 mEq/L require an ECG to interpret the effects of hyperkalemia on the cardiac conduction system. Tall, peaked T waves are an early sign of hyperkalemia. As potassium levels increase in the toxic range, the cardiac conduction system is further depressed and exhibits loss of P waves and widening of the QRS complex. Ultimately, ventricular fibrillation with cardiac arrest may occur.

Ion-exchange resins, such as sodium polystyrene sulfonate (Kayexalate, 15 to 60 g), lower serum potassium levels by causing potassium losses in the gut. Both glucose-insulin therapy, (10 U of insulin in addition to 50 mL of a 50% glucose solution, followed by continuous infusions of both glucose and insulin titrated to maintain normal blood glucose values) and sodium bicarbonate (50 to 100 mEq) lower serum levels by shifting potassium intracellularly. Their effect is only temporary. Intravenous calcium infusions do not lower potassium levels but directly antagonize the effects of potassium on the cell membrane. Mild hyperkalemia (<6 mEq/L) can be treated with sodium polystyrene sulfonate alone (by enema or orally). More severe cases are treated with glucose and insulin or intravenous bicarbonate therapy, to lower serum potassium levels acutely, coupled with sodium polystyrene sulfonate to lower potassium stores.

The infusion of calcium salts is reserved for patients who have severe changes on the ECG related to hyperkalemia, such as widening of the QRS complex or cardiac arrest. Calcium therapy must be combined with glucose-insulin or bicarbonate therapy, which lowers potassium levels acutely, followed by either sodium polystyrene sulfonate or dialysis to lower potassium stores. β-agonists, such as inhaled albuterol, can be useful in lowering serum potassium levels. These agents are best used in conjunction with glucose and insulin. Care must be taken, however, because the doses are higher than in conventional use, and cardiovascular complications can occur, especially arrhythmias in conjunction with anesthesia.

Dialysis-dependent patients should be routinely dialyzed 24 hours before a surgical procedure. If necessary, patients can undergo urgent dialysis to treat hyperkalemia acutely. With the removal of approximately 25 to 50 mEq/hour of potassium, most patients can be stabilized for surgery with a 2-hour dialysis treatment. Immediate postdialysis potassium levels may not reflect the true equilibrium potassium level reached several hours later.

Acidemia

Patients with renal failure can have either normal anion gap or elevated anion gap acidosis. The former occurs when renal failure is mild to moderate (ClCr >20 mL/minute), and the latter occurs in more severe renal dysfunction. When a patient with CKD is acidemic and dialysis is not feasible or indicated, correction to a minimum pH of 7.25 is indicated preoperatively. Bicarbonate deficit can be calculated by the following formula:

$$(\text{Desired } HCO_3 - \text{observed } HCO_3) \times 50\% \text{ body weight (kg)}$$

where HCO_3 is bicarbonate.

The patient with CKD may have acidemia for reasons other than CKD alone, especially when it is high anion gap metabolic acidosis. High anion gap can be caused by ketoacids, lactic acid, and poisoning with ethylene glycol, aspirin, or methanol.

Hematologic Considerations

Progressive anemia is common as the GFR falls to less than 60 mL/minute. Moreover, as renal function declines, the degree of anemia worsens. Anemia of CKD is normochromic and normocytic. The principal cause of the anemia relates to relative underproduction of erythropoietin, although the uremic milieu causes suppression of erythroid progenitor cells. **Recombinant human erythropoietin is the mainstay of treatment for uremic anemia in all stages of CKD** [Ⓐ *Eschbach et al, 1987*]. In dialysis for ESRD, the removal of uremic toxins may also help to stimulate erythropoiesis. However, both dialysis and erythropoietin therapy are slow to correct anemia and thus are of little practical benefit in the perioperative period. Although younger patients without coronary disease may tolerate major surgical procedures with hemoglobin levels of 6 to 7 g/dL, **it is prudent to transfuse packed red blood cells in an amount sufficient to provide a hemoglobin of approximately 9 to 10 g/dL in older patients with concomitant cardiac or pulmonary disease** [*Livio et al, 1982*].

Correction of anemia to a hematocrit of 26% to 30% is a mainstay of treatment for the increased bleeding tendency experienced by some patients with CKD. Uremic bleeding relates to disorders of platelet function because most patients have normal platelet counts as well as normal coagulation studies. In addition, not all uremic patients have bleeding diatheses. Conversely, some patients are hypercoagulable. The pathophysiology underlying uremic platelet disorders is incompletely understood. Anemia can contribute to prolonged bleeding times through rheologic mechanisms. Other abnormalities that may affect bleeding time include abnormal arachidonate metabolism, acquired platelet storage pool deficiency, disturbed regulation of platelet calcium content, and qualitative or quantitative abnormalities of von Willebrand factor.

There are several approaches to correcting the bleeding time of a uremic patient. Dialysis alone improves bleeding time in about half the patients and can be instituted if other indicators for its use are present. Specific therapy is indicated for bleeding time abnormalities in the uremic patient who is actively bleeding, either postoperatively or, for example, from the gastrointestinal tract. The indication for attempting to correct bleeding time before an elective procedure, however, is less clear. Although it is true that uremic patients are more prone to bleeding and that some patients have a demonstrably abnormal bleeding time, the correlation between which patients will bleed and the actual bleeding time is poor. For this reason, we no longer measure bleeding time routinely before procedures such as percutaneous renal biopsy or surgery. Patients with a bleeding diathesis are treated as outlined later.

Cryoprecipitate (10 U intravenously every 12 to 24 hours) can correct bleeding time, likely by providing von Willebrand factor. Its onset of action is rapid, and thus it is useful when immediate correction of bleeding time is desired. The principal risk of cryoprecipitate use is infection, similar to other blood products. Arginine vasopressin, or DDAVP (0.3 μg/kg intravenously), also has a rapid effect on bleeding time and is well tolerated. The effect may relate to release of stored von Willebrand factor. Its principal drawback relates to a relatively short duration of effect; tachyphylaxis tends to develop after only two doses, probably resulting from depletion of factor VIII-von Willebrand factor stores.

Conjugated estrogens can also shorten bleeding time. The onset of action is relatively slow. Some effect occurs in 6 hours, but the peak effect occurs between 5 and 7 days. However, the duration of effect of conjugated estrogens may be as long as 14 days, thus making estrogen therapy a promising approach when a prolonged effect on bleeding time may be desirable (e.g., in difficult to control gastrointestinal bleeding).

Finally, it is important to avoid the use of heparin during dialysis if the patient is to undergo a surgical procedure immediately after treatment. Typically, the coagulation profile returns to normal within 4 hours after hemodialysis. If surgery is urgent, the effects of heparin can be reversed by the administration of protamine.

Intraoperative Considerations

Anesthesia

CKD can affect the disposition of commonly used anesthetic drugs by changes in the renal excretion of drug and active metabolites and by changes in protein binding. The benzodiazepines diazepam, lorazepam, and midazolam are highly protein bound agents. In renal failure, displacement of benzodiazepines from protein by other molecules results in an increased free fraction of these agents. This process, in addition to the accumulation of active metabolites with repetitive administration, makes renal patients very sensitive to the sedative effects of these agents.

Propofol, which is primarily metabolized by the liver, is usually well tolerated in patients with renal disease. The depolarizing neuromuscular blocker succinylcholine may cause an increase in serum potassium level of approximately 0.5 to 1.0 mEq/L and should not be used in patients with CKD unless serum potassium is normal. The long-acting muscle relaxant pancuronium is excreted primarily by the kidneys and can result in prolonged paralysis after a single dose in patients with CKD. Atracurium undergoes spontaneous Hofmann elimination in the plasma and tissues and can be safely used in patients with CKD. In general, recovery from neuromuscular blockade is variable in patients with CKD and needs to be monitored carefully. Fluoride ions can accumulate with the use of the inhalational agents enflurane, sevoflurane, and methoxyflurane and can lead to renal toxicity. The use of these agents should be avoided in patients with preexisting renal failure.

Perioperative pain relief may be provided by a variety of agents. Fentanyl may be used safely in patients with CKD, but large or prolonged doses of meperidine should be avoided. Normeperidine is an active metabolite of meperidine that accumulates in kidney failure and can cause myoclonic jerks, seizures, and respiratory depression. Morphine-6-glucuronide, the active metabolite of morphine, can also accumulate in CKD and cause prolonged opioid effects when morphine is given in repeated doses or infusion.

Antibiotic Prophylaxis

Many patients with CKD receive prophylactic antibiotics for surgical procedures. In general, perioperative antibiotics should be administered in accordance with general surgical principles as long as appropriate dose adjustments are made for the level of renal function. Empirical vancomycin should be avoided, if possible, because of the increased incidence of resistant bacteria. Antibiotic prophylaxis using standard bacterial endocarditis regimens is recommended for dialyzed patients with synthetic vascular access grafts or catheters.

Hemodynamic Monitoring and Fluid and Electrolyte Management

Special care must be taken to avoid intraoperative hypotension, decreased renal perfusion, and further worsening renal function. Adequate venous access should be established. Arterial and central venous lines may aid in the assessment of volume status. The use of pulmonary artery catheters may be required in patients with CKD who have severe coronary artery disease, valvular heart disease, or decreased systolic function. Volume replacement fluids should be given in the form of isotonic saline or blood products. The intraoperative infusion of potassium-containing (4 mEq/L) lactated Ringer's solution should be avoided.

As previously mentioned, patients undergoing dialysis should ideally be dialyzed within 24 hours before going for elective surgical procedures, to prevent volume overload, hyperkalemia, and metabolic acidosis. Aggressive volume replacement intraoperatively may result in pulmonary edema and the need for emergency dialysis in the postoperative period. A small study conducted in dialyzed patients undergoing cardiac surgery suggested that intraoperative hemodialysis may allow a delay in performing postoperative dialysis, but no data suggest that overall outcome is improved with the performance of intraoperative dialysis. In general, intraoperative hemodialysis can be logistically difficult and can lead to further hemodynamic instability. In certain circumstances, such as during liver transplantation, continuous dialysis (continuous arteriovenous hemofiltration or continuous venovenous hemofiltration) may be performed in the operating room to prevent massive fluid overload.

Serum potassium should be closely monitored by the anesthesia team during long procedures, especially in the event of tissue ischemia and necrosis or the transfusion of blood. Severe hyperkalemia that occurs intraoperatively can best be treated with intravenous calcium to stabilize membranes and with glucose and insulin to drive potassium intracellularly. Worsening acidosis may be treated with sodium bicarbonate, but this can lead to volume overload. The hyperkalemic or acidemic patient will most likely need to be dialyzed soon after the surgical procedure.

Vascular Access

During surgical procedures, the anesthesia team must take special measures to protect the dialyzed patient's vascular access. The limb should be properly positioned without restraints to prevent prolonged occlusive pressure and possible thrombosis of the access site. Needle sticks and blood pressure measurements should also be avoided in the access-related limb. Central lines should be avoided on the same side as the vascular access if at all possible. Internal jugular lines are preferred over subclavian lines to prevent venous stenosis and loss of potential access sites. Intraoperative hypotension can also lead to thrombosis of the access. The anesthesiologist should auscultate the access frequently during the surgical procedure to verify patency. In the event of thrombosis, prompt thrombectomy should be arranged. Special care must be taken in patients with CKD who are not yet receiving dialysis to protect potential vascular access sites. The forearm and upper arm veins of the nondominant arm should be protected from needle sticks. Displaying a sign at the patient's bedside to save the designated arm may be helpful.

In kidney transplant recipients, femoral access, such as arterial or venous catheters or intra-aortic balloon pumps, should generally be avoided on the side ipsilateral to the renal allograft. In the event of cross-clamping of the abdominal aorta, a temporary bypass, usually from the ipsilateral axillary artery to the femoral artery, must be performed to maintain the arterial blood supply to the transplanted kidney.

Patients undergoing peritoneal dialysis should have their peritoneal cavity drained of dialysate preoperatively. The peritoneal catheter can remain in place unless the peritoneal cavity becomes contaminated intraoperatively with intestinal contents. In the event of abdominal surgical procedures, a central venous hemodialysis catheter will need to be placed for performance of temporary hemodialysis until the incision is adequately healed to permit resumption of peritoneal dialysis (usually 2 to 3 weeks).

Postoperative Management

Pharmacotherapy

Care must be taken to administer all postoperative medications at doses appropriate to the patient's level of renal function. The use of prewritten postoperative order templates can create increased potential for inappropriate dosing of medications in patients with CKD and should be avoided. ClCr should be calculated or estimated for all patients, and doses of medications should be adjusted accordingly. Special care must be taken with those drugs that are excreted primarily by the kidney and that have narrow toxic-therapeutic windows such as digoxin and aminoglycoside antibiotics. In these situations, drug levels must be monitored frequently. The use of magnesium- or phosphate-containing antacids and cathartics in the postoperative setting can lead to dangerous hypermagnesemia and hyperphosphatemia in patients with advanced CKD and should generally be avoided.

Options for postoperative analgesia include acetaminophen, fentanyl, and oxycodone. As mentioned earlier, meperidine should not be used in patients with CKD because of the accumulation of its neurotoxic metabolite, and morphine should be used cautiously because of prolongation of its sedative effects. Other drugs that should be used with caution include angiotensin-converting enzyme inhibitors, angiotensin II receptor blockers, and nonsteroidal anti-inflammatory agents (NSAIDs). These agents can decrease renal blood flow and GFR and can lead to further decrement in kidney function, especially during periods of effective circulating volume depletion that can occur postoperatively. The low-molecular-weight heparin enoxaparin is eliminated primarily by the kidney, and administration at fixed doses without monitoring has an unpredictable anticoagulant effect in patients with CKD. If this agent is used, doses should be reduced and anti–factor Xa activity frequently monitored. To date, enoxaparin has not been approved by the U.S. Food and Drug Administration for use in dialyzed patients.

Drug dosing in the renal transplant recipient can create unique challenges in the perioperative setting. Immunosuppressant medications must be continued in renal transplant recipients perioperatively to prevent organ rejection. The use of stress-dose steroids is not indicated for routine, elective surgical procedures unless the patient has documented adrenal insufficiency. The CNIs cyclosporine and tacrolimus can be given intravenously at one third the usual dose for those patients who cannot yet take oral medications. Trough drug levels must be monitored very closely to verify appropriate perioperative dosing. Moreover, CNIs are metabolized by the cytochrome P-450 system, and numerous drug interactions can occur. Some of the more frequently prescribed drugs metabolized by this system include diltiazem, verapamil, fluconazole, ketoconazole, and erythromycin, which increase CNI levels, as well as rifampin, barbiturates, phenytoin, and carbamazepine, which decrease CNI levels. The immunosuppressant agent sirolimus may have a negative effect on fibrosis, and some evidence suggests a higher incidence of surgical wound complications, such as infection and hernia, with this agent.

Nutrition

Careful attention must be paid to the postoperative nutritional needs of patients with CKD. There is an overall high prevalence of protein-calorie malnutrition in these patients that must be taken into account when prescribing postoperative nutritional support. Caloric intake should be high, and protein intake should be adequate to minimize tissue catabolism and to promote wound healing. A caloric intake of 30 to 35 kcal/kg with a protein intake of 1.2 to 1.5 g/kg is usually optimal for patients with CKD. Formulas with high caloric density may be needed in dialyzed patients to limit the amount of fluid administered. Electrolyte-free formulas of parenteral nutritional solutions may need to be used to prevent hyperkalemia, hyperphosphatemia, and hypermagnesemia. If enteral supplements can be used, then renal specific formulas that are lower in potassium should be used.

Fluid-Electrolyte Management

Patients with renal failure are prone to electrolyte abnormalities in the postoperative period. Hyperkalemia should be treated as outlined earlier. Enemas containing the cation-exchange resin Kayexalate and sorbitol should be used with extreme caution to treat hyperkalemia in patients after surgical procedures because of the increased incidence of intestinal necrosis. This usually occurs in the setting of decreased colonic motility and may be precipitated by hyperosmotic sorbitol-induced tissue damage. Dialysis should be performed in patients with CKD who have persistent hyperkalemia despite medical therapy. Dialysis treatments performed in the first 24 to 48 postoperative hours should be done without the use of heparin to prevent bleeding. Care must be taken not to administer large amounts of hypotonic fluids to patients with advanced renal failure because this may lead to severe hyponatremia. Fluid replacement should generally be given with isotonic saline. Hypotonic saline should be reserved for those patients who have increased free water losses, such as patients with osmotic diarrhea or diuresis or patients who are already hypernatremic.

POSTOPERATIVE ACUTE RENAL FAILURE

Incidence and Impact

Postoperative ARF (acute or acute superimposed on chronic) is a common complication of major vascular, cardiac, and abdominal surgical procedures. Identifying the exact incidence is made difficult mainly because of the lack of a consistent definition of ARF and the lack of uniformity in the surgical populations studied. The best-studied population represents patients undergoing cardiac surgery. Estimates of postoperative ARF in this population range from 1% to 15%. Despite the many advances in the care of surgical patients, ARF that develops postoperatively remains a serious complication that is associated with high mortality and resource utilization. Over the last decade, mortality has been shown to still be as high as 50% in some series of patients who have developed ARF postoperatively. One study performed in cardiac surgical patients showed that in-hospital mortality was 14.5% in those patients who developed postoperative ARF compared with 1.1% in those patients without ARF [Loef et al, 2005]. Long-term (>5-year) mortality risk remained elevated in these patients even when renal function had recovered at the time of discharge. Patient-specific risk factors shown to be predictive of developing postoperative renal failure include preoperative renal dysfunction, perioperative cardiac dysfunction, sepsis, hepatic failure, obstructive jaundice, hypovolemia, and advanced age. **Higher-risk surgical procedures include cardiac surgery requiring cardiopulmonary bypass, vascular procedures requiring aortic cross-clamping, liver transplantation, and, for obvious reasons, renal transplantation** [Ⓒ *Sadovnikoff, 2001*].

Differential Diagnosis

Although the surgical setting creates unique conditions that can lead to ARF, the general approach to the patient and the generation of the differential diagnosis are the same in all patients with ARF. In the postoperative setting, ARF may have prerenal, intrinsic renal, or postrenal (obstructive) causes.

Prerenal failure results from decreased renal perfusion and is very common in the postoperative setting, in which hypovolemia from blood loss, third spacing of fluid, and gastrointestinal fluid loss is common. Decreased renal perfusion resulting from impaired cardiac contractility occurs frequently in the cardiac surgical patient. Cross-clamping of the abdominal aorta during aneurysm repair also results in decreased renal perfusion and can lead to ARF. The *abdominal compartment syndrome* is an unusual cause of decreased renal perfusion associated with increased intra-abdominal pressure. This syndrome is most commonly seen in trauma patients who require massive volume resuscitation, but it also can be seen with tight surgical closures and scarring after burn injuries.

Potential *intrinsic renal causes* of postoperative ARF are many. The most common cause of renal failure in this category is ATN. Because ATN can be seen with severe renal ischemia, any prerenal insult discussed earlier may lead to ATN if it is severe or prolonged or both. ATN may also be seen with exposure to various toxins. Common toxins encountered in the perioperative setting include aminoglycoside antibiotics, amphotericin, and intravenous contrast agents. Myoglobin, an endogenous toxin, can lead to ATN during rhabdomyolysis that occurs with muscle trauma or ischemia. Rhabdomyolysis can also be seen with prolonged perioperative immobilization of morbidly obese patients. Other common intrinsic causes of ARF include release of atheroemboli during vascular manipulation and acute interstitial nephritis resulting from a hypersensitivity response to various medications such as NSAIDs.

Postrenal failure can occur anytime there is obstruction to urinary flow, and potential causes in the surgical setting are many. An important cause is bladder outlet obstruction resulting from prostatic hypertrophy that is often aggravated by impaired bladder motility in the postanesthesia setting.

Other causes include obstruction related to gross hematuria and blood clots, formation of retroperitoneal hematoma, and actual damage to the ureters during surgical procedures.

Diagnosis

Most cases of postoperative ARF are the result of prerenal failure or ATN usually related to prolonged renal ischemia. Differentiating between these two disorders can sometimes be difficult, because they often exist on a continuum. Proper diagnosis is important, however, in that management of the patient differs depending on the cause.

A thorough history should focus on episodes of volume loss such as vomiting, diarrhea, hemorrhage, and aggressive diuresis. Third spacing of fluid can be tremendous in pancreatitis, and insensible losses of fluid can be high with fever, mechanical ventilation, and severe burns. The intraoperative flow sheets must be reviewed for episodes of hypotension. The medical record must be thoroughly reviewed to ascertain any exposure of the patient to nephrotoxins such as intravenous contrast agents, aminoglycosides, NSAIDs, or myoglobin.

The physical examination should focus on accurate assessment of volume status and cardiac function and the presence of rash, livedo reticularis, or embolic stigmata. Diagnostic studies that can assist in making the proper diagnosis include urine electrolytes and urinalysis with examination of spun urinary sediment. **Low urine sodium (<10 mEq/L) with a fractional excretion of sodium less than 1% and a bland urinary sediment suggests a diagnosis of prerenal failure. In an oliguric patient, high urine sodium (>20 mEq/L) with fractional excretion of sodium greater than 1% and the presence of renal tubular epithelial cells and granular casts in the urine is indicative of ATN** [⦿ *Miller et al, 1978*]. A renal ultrasound scan should always be performed in postoperative ARF to rule out hydronephrosis and urinary obstruction quickly. Urine eosinophils may be present in interstitial nephritis and atheroemboli syndrome. The serum creatine phosphokinase level should be checked, and it usually exceeds 10,000 mg/dL when associated with ATN resulting from rhabdomyolysis.

Management

The management of postoperative ARF is mainly supportive and initially involves the treatment of intravascular volume depletion with isotonic fluids or blood products. Renal blood flow should be maximized by optimizing cardiac output. This may require controlling rhythm disturbances if present, reducing afterload, and possibly using inotropic agents. The use of diuretic therapy may be necessary for oliguria that persists despite the repletion of intravascular volume and the optimization of hemodynamic status. Emphasis and energy are often placed on the conversion of oliguric to nonoliguric renal failure. Although the ability of a patient to respond to diuretics does generally imply less severe disease and can facilitate management, the successful ability to convert a patient from oliguric to nonoliguric renal failure has not been shown to improve the clinical outcome. In fact, **some evidence suggests that the use of diuretics in ARF may be associated with poorer renal functional outcome** [● *Mehta et al, 2002*]. High doses of loop diuretics are needed to induce natriuresis in patients with renal failure. Continuous infusion of loop diuretics may produce a greater percentage of increase in sodium excretion compared with large-bolus dosing. RRT is indicated for patients with hypervolemia resistant to diuretics, hyperkalemia or metabolic acidosis that does not respond to medical therapy, and uremic manifestations such as pericarditis, increased bleeding, or decreased mental status.

The use of agents to reverse renal failure or potentially to hasten the recovery of renal function has generated much interest. Dopamine, at "renal doses," has been one such agent that continues to be used frequently in the surgical setting. The theoretical benefit of lower-dose dopamine is based on the ability of this agent to increase renal blood flow, increase

GFR, and induce natriuresis in experimental situations. However, **no convincing evidence has been provided that dopamine prevents postoperative renal failure, decreases the need for RRT, or changes clinical outcomes** [● *Holmes and Walley, 2003*]. This lack of evidence, along with the potential risks of therapy such as increased myocardial oxygen demand, increased frequency of arrhythmias, decreased splanchnic circulation, and blunted immune response, should argue against the routine use of renal-dose dopamine in patients with postoperative renal failure.

Mannitol is another agent that has been used to treat postoperative renal failure. Mannitol has been proven to be of benefit in the prevention of ATN in renal transplant recipients if the drug is administered before the release of the renal artery cross-clamp, and it is also still frequently used in the prime solution during cardiopulmonary bypass. However, no controlled trails have been conducted to show the benefit of mannitol in established renal failure.

Prevention

Given the lack of current therapy to treat postoperative renal failure, emphasis should focus on its prevention. Strategies to prevent postoperative renal failure include the early identification of at-risk surgical patients, the maintenance of effective intravascular volume status and the optimization of cardiovascular performance, the avoidance of nephrotoxins, and the proper spacing of procedures. Many pharmacologic agents have been investigated for benefit in preventing ARF. Agents that have been studied but so far have not shown to be of benefit include renal-dose dopamine, loop diuretics, calcium channel blockers, atrial natriuretic peptide, and various growth factors such as insulin-like growth factor and fibroblast growth factor.

Two agents that have shown some promise in the prevention of ARF resulting from intravenous contrast agents are N-acetylcysteine and the dopamine analogue fenoldopam.

Whether there is some benefit in the use of these agents for the prevention of postoperative renal failure remains to be elucidated. One review of evidence-based strategies to lower the risk of contrast-induced nephropathy suggested that patients at increased risk for contrast-induced nephropathy be considered to receive N-acetylcysteine, 600 to 1200 mg orally twice daily for two doses before the contrast-related procedure and two doses after the procedure, OR ascorbic acid, 3 g orally 2 hours before the procedure and 2 g orally twice daily after the procedure. These patients should also receive intravenous hydration before the procedure (intravenous normal saline, 1 mL/kg/hour for 6 to 12 before the procedure, OR intravenous 5% dextrose and water AND sodium bicarbonate, 3 mL/kg for 1 hour before the procedure, with monitoring for metabolic alkalosis) and intravenous hydration following the procedure (intravenous normal saline, 1 mL/kg/hour for 6 to 12 hours, OR intravenous 5% dextrose and water AND sodium bicarbonate, 154 mEq/L, 1 mL/kg for 6 hours, with monitoring for metabolic alkalosis). Because these preprocedure and postprocedure hydration regimens use a significant volume load, it is essential to monitor the patient carefully for volume overload. It is also recommended that the minimum possible volume of iso-osmolar or low-osmolar contrast agent be used [● Pannu et al, 2006].

Selected Readings

Brown K, Rimmer J, Haisch C: Non-invasive cardiac risk stratification of diabetic and non-diabetic uremic renal allograft candidates using dipyridamole-thallium-201 imaging and radionuclide ventriculography. Am J Cardiol 64:1017-1021, 1989.

Burke JF, Francos GC: Surgery in the patient with acute or chronic renal failure. In Merli GJ, Weitz HH (eds): Medical Management of the Surgical Patient, 2nd ed. Philadelphia, WB Saunders, 1998, pp 326-337.

Camp A, Garvin P, Hoff J: Prognostic valve of intravenous dipyridamole thallium imaging in patients with diabetes mellitus considered for renal transplantation. Am J Cardiol 65:1459-1463, 1990.

Chobanian AV, Bakris GL, Black HR, et al: The seventh report of the Joint National Committee on Prevention, Detection, Evaluation and Treatment of High Blood Pressure. JAMA 289:2560-2572, 2003.

Cockcroft D, Gault M: Prediction of creatinine clearance from serum creatinine. Nephron 16:31-41, 1976.

Conger J: Interventions in clinical acute renal failure: What are the data? Am J Kidney Dis 26:565-576, 1995.

Dahan M, Viron B, Faraggi M, et al: Diagnostic accuracy and prognostic value of combined dipyridamole-exercise thallium imaging in hemodialysis patients. Kid Int 54:255-262, 1998.

Dean M: Opioids in renal failure and dialysis patients. J Pain Symptom Manage 28:497-504, 2004.

Eagle K, Berger P, Calkins H: ACC/AHA guideline update for perioperative cardiovascular evaluation for noncardiac surgery—executive summary: A report of the American College of Cardiology/American Heart Association Task Force on Practice Guidelines. J Am Coll Cardiol 39:542-553, 2002. **C**

Eschbach J, Egrie J, Downing M: Correction of the anemia of end-stage renal disease with recombinant human erythropoietin: Results of a combined phase I and phase II clinical trial. N Engl J Med 316:73-78, 1987. **A**

Holley J, Fenton R, Arthur R: Thallium stress testing does not predict cardiovascular risk in diabetic patients with end-stage renal disease undergoing cadaveric renal transplantation. Am J Med 90:563-570, 1991.

Holmes C, Walley K: Bad medicine: Low-dose dopamine in the ICU. Chest 123:1266-1275, 2003. **C**

Kidney Disease Outcomes Quality Initiative (K/DOQI): K/DOQI clinical practice guidelines on hypertension and antihypertensive agents in chronic kidney disease. Am J Kidney Dis 43(Suppl):S1-S290, 2004.

Lemmens H: Kidney transplantation: Recent developments and recommendations for anesthetic management. Anesthesiol Clin North Am 22: 651-662, 2004.

Lind S: The bleeding time does not predict surgical bleeding. Blood 77:2547-2552, 1991.

Livio M, Gotti E, Marchesi D: Uraemic bleeding: Role of anaemia and beneficial effect of red cell transfusions. Lancet 2:1013-1015, 1982. **B**

Loef BG, Epema AH, Smilde TD, et al: Immediate postoperative renal function deterioration in cardiac surgical patients predicts in-hospital mortality and long-term survival. J Am Soc Nephrol 16:195-200, 2005.

Mazze R: Anesthesia for patients with abnormal renal function and genitourinary problems. In Miller RD (ed): Anesthesia, 2nd ed. Philadelphia, JB Lippincott, 1986.

Mehta RL, Pascual MT, Soroko S, et al: Diuretics, mortality, and nonrecovery of renal function in acute renal failure. JAMA 288:2547-2553, 2002. **C**

Miller TR, Anderson RJ, Linas SL, et al: Urinary diagnostic indices in acute renal failure: A prospective study. Ann Intern Med 89:47-50, 1978. **Ⓐ**

National Kidney Foundation: K/DOQI clinical practice guidelines for chronic kidney disease: Evaluation, classification and stratification. Am J Kidney Dis 39(Suppl):S1-S266, 2002.

Pannu N, Wiebe N, Tonelli M: Prophylaxis strategies for contrast-induced nephropathy. JAMA 295:2765-2779, 2006. **Ⓒ**

Pannu N, Manns B, Lee H, Tonelli M: Systematic review of the impact of N-acetylcysteine on contrast nephropathy. Kidney Int 65:1366-1374, 2004.

Reddy V: Prevention of postoperative acute renal failure. J Postgrad Med 48:64-70, 2002.

Remuzzi G: Bleeding disorders in uremia: Pathophysiology and treatment. Adv Nephrol Necker Hosp 19:171-186, 1989.

Sadovnikoff N: Perioperative acute renal failure. Int Anesthesiol Clin 39:95-109, 2001. **Ⓒ**

Schillaci G, Reboldi G, Verdecchia P: High-normal serum creatinine concentration is a predictor of cardiovascular risk in essential hypertension. Arch Intern Med 161:886-891, 2001.

Singri N, Ahya S, Levin M: Acute renal failure. JAMA 289:747-751, 2003.

Stevens LA, Coresh J, Greene T, Levey AS: Assessing kidney function: Measured and estimated glomerular filtration rate. N Engl J Med 354:2473-2483, 2006. **Ⓒ**

Stone G, McCullough PA, Tumlin JA, et al: Fenoldopam mesylate for the prevention of contrast-induced nephropathy: A randomized controlled trial. JAMA 290:2284-2291, 2003.

Tepel M, van der Giet M, Schwarzfeld C, et al: Prevention of radiographic-contrast-agent–induced reductions in renal function by acetylcysteine. N Engl J Med 343:180-184, 2000.

19 | Perioperative Management of the Patient with Arthritis or Systemic Autoimmune Disease

BRIAN F. MANDELL, MD, PhD

The systemic autoimmune diseases encompass a heterogeneous group of disorders that provide the patient, surgeon, and medical consultant with unique concerns in the perioperative setting. Because perioperative assessment and management depend on the specific disorder, the medical consultant should try to confirm the diagnosis by discussion with the patient's rheumatologist or review of prior records. Details regarding rheumatologist-prescribed medications (e.g., cyclophosphamide, intravenous immune globulin, azathioprine, anti-tumor necrosis factor [anti-TNF] therapy) may give insight into the severity and course of the disease. An assessment of current disease activity that includes the degree of end-organ damage and could influence the patient's perioperative course should be a component of the preoperative evaluation. The consultant should not assume that baseline laboratory tests will be normal, even in young, apparently healthy patients with systemic autoimmune disease.

Patients with these disorders are frequently ingesting many prescribed and alternative medications. The patient should be particularly asked regarding the use of nonprescription medications taken for pain relief, to "boost their immune system," or to increase energy.

Levels of Evidence:

A—Randomized controlled trials (RCTs), meta-analyses, well-designed systematic reviews of RCTs. **B**—Case-control or cohort studies, nonrandomized controlled trials, systematic reviews of studies other than RCTs, cross-sectional studies, retrospective studies. **C**—Consensus statements, expert guidelines, usual practice, opinion.

Issues that may affect successful postoperative rehabilitation should be considered preoperatively. Recommendations regarding pain and anti-inflammatory medications are likely to affect the postoperative course. This is particularly important in patients with inflammatory arthritis. Preoperative withdrawal of nonsteroidal anti-inflammatory drugs (NSAIDs) and withholding of methotrexate in the perioperative period may result in significant exacerbation of inflammatory joint pain postoperatively. This complication may be blunted or prevented if perioperative "stress-dose" corticosteroids are required or by the judicious use of low-dose postoperative prednisone. Narcotics are often surprisingly ineffective at relieving the pain and stiffness of active inflammatory joint disease.

SYSTEMIC AUTOIMMUNE ARTHRITIS

Rheumatoid Arthritis

Disease Characteristics

Rheumatoid arthritis (RA) is the most common inflammatory arthritis affecting women. More than 1% of the population may have the disease. RA is characterized by chronic symmetrical, often destructive, polyarticular synovitis. RA involves the small and large joints while sparing the distal finger joints and noncervical spine. It is a systemic disease, frequently with extra–articular manifestations (Table 19-1). The advent of more effective therapies, employed in a more aggressive fashion, has probably made these complications less common.

RA-associated surgery includes arthroplasty, tendon reconstruction, carpal tunnel decompression, subcutaneous nodule removal, and intrathoracic nodule biopsy. Carpal tunnel surgery in RA is often more extensive than idiopathic or diabetes-associated carpal tunnel decompression. In RA, the surgical procedure often requires exploration and synovectomy. For the patient with RA who requires joint replacement, the risk of prosthetic joint infection is slightly higher

TABLE 19-1	Complications of Rheumatoid Arthritis
Complication	**Comments**
Fatigue	Multifactorial, associated with inflammation, disordered sleep, anemia
Anemia	Usually mild, not iron responsive; ferritin level >60 suggests anemia of inflammatory disease, not iron deficiency
Felty's syndrome	Splenomegaly and neutropenia, often with leg ulcers; thrombocytopenia can occur
Interstitial lung disease; pleural effusions	
Neuropathies	Compressive (median nerve at wrist; ulnar at elbow); cervical myelopathy; mononeuritis multiplex (vasculitic), polyneuropathy (vasculitic, amyloidosis)
Coronary artery disease	Independent of usual risk factors
Pericarditis	Usually mild and asymptomatic
Adenopathy	Common, but risk of lymphoma is also higher than normal population
Scleritis	
Sjögren's syndrome	
Cricoarytenoid arthritis	Hoarseness; ear, nose, and throat evaluation before intubation

than in the patient whose joint replacement is necessitated by osteoarthritis (OA). The question whether a lung nodule in a patient with severe RA is a rheumatoid nodule can be answered only by tissue biopsy. In a series of 64 pulmonary nodules, only 6% were rheumatoid nodules, and 38% were malignant. This finding should be considered if a lung lesion is discovered on a preoperative chest radiograph.

Rheumatoid involvement of the cervical spine affects the ease and safety of endotracheal intubation [● *Nguyen et al, 2004*]. Preoperative assessment includes evaluation of articular structures that may influence the outcome of intubation, as well as a focused baseline neurologic examination. Involvement of the temporomandibular joint affects the ease of endotracheal intubation, and this joint should be assessed. Hoarseness or any history of voice change, odynophagia, or stridor should raise concern regarding cricoarytenoid arthritis. **The possibility of cricoarytenoid joint**

dysfunction should prompt preoperative ear, nose, and throat evaluation, to avoid a potential postextubation airway catastrophe resulting from vocal cord closure caused by joint dysfunction [ⓒ *Kolman and Morris, 2002*]. An otolaryngologist can inject the inflamed joints with corticosteroids preoperatively if necessary. RA does not affect the lower spine; hence epidural catheter insertion is not usually problematic.

The patient with severe RA is more likely to require arthroplasty subsequently. In this patient group, radiographic cervical instability has been demonstrated in approximately 60%. Up to 80% of patients with radiologic changes of cervical instability have no clinical symptoms (jumping legs, Lhermitte's sign, clumsiness, incontinence) or findings (hyperreflexia) of spinal cord compression. The neurologic examination in patients with RA may be difficult because of peripheral joint destruction or peripheral compressive neuropathies. Nonetheless, a focused baseline neurologic examination should be performed and recorded. Patients with recent-onset disease are less likely to have significant cervical spine instability, which results from ligamentous laxity usually subsequent to more than 3 years of inflammatory disease. Cervical instability is most common at the atlantoaxial level. Subaxial instability is less frequent, and cranial settling is least common. Pannus extending from the articular joints of the spine may also compress the spinal cord. Pannus can be documented only by magnetic resonance imaging or computed tomography.

Postoperative neurologic complications are rare, even in patients with cervical involvement. To assess the risk of perioperative cervical spinal cord compression, preoperative lateral cervical spine radiographs should be obtained in the neutral position as well as with flexion and extension views. Several methods are used to analyze the extent of radiographic instability and canal narrowing, but none is ideal at predicting complications. Radiographic findings suggestive of spinal cord impingement are much less common than demonstration of laxity. If the patient has any neurologic symptoms or findings suggestive of myelopathy, neurosurgical consultation should be obtained before elective surgery. Cervical stabilization procedures have associated morbidity and mortality and are not routinely considered prophylactically before other surgical procedures. The indications for surgery, outside of overt myelopathy in the setting of spinal cord compression, are controversial. For patients with severe RA, wearing a soft cervical collar encourages more gentle transfers during movement around the hospital, but it does not afford complete protection of the cervical spinal cord.

Patients with RA have an increased burden of cardiovascular disease compared with their age- and risk-matched counterparts without RA [● *Maradit-Kremers et al, 2005*]. The reason for the increased cardiovascular morbidity in RA is not known. In addition, because of deconditioning or the direct effects of RA, patients may be unable to exert themselves sufficiently to note symptoms of physiologically significant coronary artery disease, thereby masking the presence of coronary artery disease. Patients with severe articular involvement are also likely to be deconditioned. Sjögren's syndrome is common in patients with RA. Before extensive surgical procedures, long-acting lubricating eye ointment (not drops) should be applied. Patients with severe RA may have unrecognized interstitial lung disease or pleural effusions.

Spondylitis, Including Ankylosing Spondylitis

Disease Characteristics

Ankylosing spondylitis (AS) is the prototypic human leukocyte antigen (HLA)-B27-associated spondyloarthropathy. Spinal involvement tends to be symmetrical, whereas it is more asymmetrical in other seronegative spondyloarthropathies (psoriatic, enteropathic). The arthritis may involve all levels of the spine from the sacrum through neck, as well as the peripheral joints. Unlike in RA, spinal involvement in AS is characterized more by fusion and reduced mobility than by instability. This reduced mobility may compromise the patient's ability to be intubated or positioned. This involvement should be evaluated by physical examination preoperatively. The peripheral arthritis is also asymmetrical. Enthesitis and dactylitis are common. This situation may be relevant in the case of a postoperative flare, when the extremely inflammatory, asymmetrical synovitis may resemble joint space infection.

Patients with spondylitis, or with the HLAB27 gene without recognized spine disease, are at risk for aortitis. This disorder may be accompanied by aortic valve insufficiency, conduction disease, and atrial fibrillation. The valvular disease is rarely acute, but it may predispose the patient to bacterial endocarditis.

Heterotopic ossification (HO) complicates total hip replacement in up to 50% of cases (all diagnoses), and it is severe in up to 19%. Male patients with spondylitis are especially predisposed to develop HO around the prosthetic joint. The highest risk is in those patients who had HO associated with a prior joint operation. HO may be prevented with the preoperative use of single-dose radiation or postoperative NSAIDs (selective or nonselective). Thus, recognition of the diagnosis of spondylitis warrants review of the patient's tissue response to prior orthopedic surgery and discussion with the surgeon.

Medication Management in Systemic Autoimmune Arthritis

Medications used in systemic arthritis in the perioperative period are shown in Table 19-1.

Nonsteroidal Anti-inflammatory Drugs

The traditional nonselective NSAIDs inhibit platelet function, and preoperative use of NSAIDs has been associated with increased surgical bleeding. Thus, NSAIDs are generally discontinued preoperatively. Because platelet function is reversibly inhibited, stopping the drug four to five half-lives before a surgical procedure should be sufficient to permit return of adequate platelet function and hemostasis. Rather than looking up the individual NSAID's half-life, discontinuing any NSAID 5 days preoperatively is a reasonable guideline. The exception is a drug with a longer half-life, such as piroxicam, which should be stopped 10 days preoperatively. Aspirin, unlike other NSAIDs, is an irreversible inhibitor of platelet cyclooxygenase; it, too, should be stopped 10 days or more before surgical procedures. The nonacetylated salicylates do not affect platelet function. Although NSAIDs have been associated with increased surgical bleeding, they are ineffective agents for the prevention of perioperative deep venous thrombosis.

The cyclooxygenase-2 (COX-2) selective NSAIDs (e.g., celecoxib) do not affect platelet function. In short-term, small trials, they have not adversely affected wound healing or bleeding. They can provide sufficient analgesia when given preoperatively to reduce the need for postoperative narcotics.

All NSAIDs are associated with increased risk for (usually reversible) acute renal insufficiency, particularly in the setting of decreased renal blood flow. Parenteral administration of NSAIDs offers no gastric or renal safety advantage over orally administered drugs. All NSAIDs may increase the risk of gastrointestinal hemorrhage.

Methotrexate

Methotrexate (MTX) is usually prescribed once weekly, along with daily folic acid (1 mg) to reduce side effects. MTX is normally cleared very rapidly from the circulation following each administration; but because the kidney excretes methotrexate, the drug should not be given immediately before any procedure likely to be associated with significant renal insufficiency. No data have strongly shown that the use of methotrexate within the week before surgery adversely affects surgical outcome. Several small, controlled studies demonstrated the safety of providing the drug a week before a surgical procedure. Preoperative withdrawal of the drug has been associated with flare of the underlying disease that adversely affects rehabilitation. Thus, there is no demonstrated need to withhold the drug for 1 week or longer before a procedure.

Leflunomide

Leflunomide is an antimetabolite used in the treatment of RA and occasionally other inflammatory disorders. It has an extremely prolonged tissue half-life. Preoperative withdrawal of the drug is not likely to affect tissue or plasma levels significantly. Although data are insufficient to make strong recommendations, it is reasonable to withhold the drug several days before and after the surgical procedure to avoid the possibility of acutely elevated serum drug levels should acute renal failure complicate surgery. Missing a few doses is not likely to provoke a flare in arthritis.

Corticosteroids

Patients with RA or spondyloarthropathy may be taking daily low-dose or intermittent prednisone as therapy for their arthritis. Physiologic studies have repeatedly shown that patients taking supraphysiologic doses of prednisone for more than 2 weeks have a submaximal cortisol release response to challenge with adrenocorticotropic hormone (ACTH). However, this blunting of the stress response has not been shown to have any clinically significant effect on the outcome of surgery.

For the patient who has been receiving supraphysiologic doses of corticosteroids for more than 2 weeks during the year before a surgical procedure, it has become routine practice to administer 50 to 100 mg of intravenous hydrocortisone before induction of anesthesia and every 8 hours until the patient is stable. In many hospitals, all patients with demonstrably or assumed blunted adrenal responses receive this regimen. Nonetheless, several small studies demonstrated that steroid-treated patients who receive only their baseline corticosteroid dose, without supplementation, do not suffer adverse effects. **Evidence does not mandate the prolonged use of stress-dose corticosteroids during the**

perioperative period in patients receiving long-term corticosteroid therapy [● *Salem et al, 1994*].

If perioperative stress-dose corticosteroids are provided, a return to the patient's baseline dosing (even if zero) should be anticipated as soon as the patient is stable. Investigators have proposed that the perioperative intravenous coverage should be linked to the severity of the surgical procedure: minor procedures warrant 25 mg every 8 hours until the patient is stable, and patients undergoing procedures with greater hemodynamic stress should receive 50 mg intravenously every 8 hours until they are stable. There is no need for prolonged (days) tapering regimens. Long-term corticosteroid therapy may adversely affect wound healing, although supportive data from controlled studies are limited. Administration of corticosteroids elicits neutrophilia by increasing the demargination of neutrophils and slightly accelerating release of young neutrophils from the bone marrow. This situation may cause diagnostic confusion because the elevated white blood cell count may suggest the presence of infection. Corticosteroids may mask the presence of infection by blunting the fever response and reducing inflammatory pain. They may also cause hyperglycemia. The recommendations listed above do not relate to the patient with adrenal insufficiency for reasons other than suppression by exogenous long-term corticosteroid administration.

Anti–Tumor Necrosis Therapies

Limited data exist regarding anti-TNF agents (adalimumab, etanercept, infliximab) and the risk of postoperative infection. In patients with inflammatory bowel disease, there is no suggestion of an increased wound infection rate from retrospective studies. However, these studies suffered from heterogeneity in timing between the last dose of medication and the surgical procedure. Many rheumatologists suggest holding these therapies for several half-lives of the drug before significant surgical procedures and restarting them when the patient's wound is healing satisfactorily. A single retrospective review of 91 patients with RA who underwent orthopedic procedures demonstrated a greater risk of postoperative infections (adjusted odds ratio, 5.3) in patients taking anti-TNF therapy [Giles et al, 2006], although smaller studies did not demonstrate a similar risk. Other recent studies, presented in abstract form, also suggest that the agents should be "held" for at least several weeks before surgery.

Postoperative Complications

Postoperative flares of disease are usually the result of withholding medications. Anti-inflammatory medications should be reinstituted as soon as possible. Low-dose corticosteroids ($\leq$7.5 mg prednisone daily) may be helpful, as may NSAIDs. Postoperative fever is not likely the result of a flare in RA or spondylitis. A monoarticular "flare" should be assumed to be an infection until proven otherwise by arthrocentesis, even in the absence of leukocytosis or fever. Postoperative neurologic complications can be caused by myelopathy, but they are more commonly the result of compressive neuropathies.

CRYSTALLINE ARTHRITIS

Disease Characteristics

It is useful to try to document the validity of the prior diagnosis of gout or pseudogout. Frequently, the diagnosis of gout has been unreliably based solely on the presence of hyperuricemia or an episode of foot pain. The frequency of attacks and the need for aggressive prophylaxis should be ascertained from the patient and prior medical records. Previous episodes of postoperative attacks of arthritis are noteworthy. Hyperuricemia is strongly associated with coronary artery disease and the metabolic syndrome; thus, an especially careful cardiac risk assessment should be obtained.

Medications

Postoperative flares are particularly common and may prolong hospitalization. It is therefore important to consider perioperative prophylaxis. For the patient who takes allopurinol or colchicine on a long-term basis, we recommend that these medications be continued up to the time of surgery and restarted immediately thereafter. Given orally, colchicine can cause dose-related diarrhea or nausea, but it is not ulcerogenic. We generally avoid low-dose intravenous prophylaxis or treatment with intravenous colchicine because of the reported fatal complications with the intravenous form of this medication. For the patient who has a history of frequent or recent attacks of gout but who comes to surgery not taking allopurinol or colchicine, prophylactic oral low-dose (0.6 mg once to twice daily) colchicine can be considered if renal function and biliary function are normal. However, the possibility of diarrhea exists, even with low doses. NSAIDs or corticosteroids can be used as prophylactic therapy, but because of their myriad of side effects in this setting, these drugs are generally used as therapy if an attack should occur.

Postoperative Flares

Flares (attacks) of gout are common and are frequently associated with fever. Patients have usually experienced previous gout attacks, although that history may not have been elicited at the time of surgical admission. Acute arthritis in the postoperative setting warrants arthrocentesis not only to diagnose crystalline arthritis definitively, but also to exclude infection. Indirect evaluation (presence or absence of fever, leukocytosis, or erythrocyte sedimentation rate elevation) is inadequate to distinguish infection from crystalline arthritis. There is no diagnostic value in obtaining radiographs or nuclear imaging studies to distinguish between acute septic and crystalline arthritis. Unrecognized crystal-induced arthritis is a cause of unexplained fever, particularly in intubated or uncommunicative patients.

Treatment options for acute crystalline arthritis include NSAIDs, selective or nonselective, based on the clinical concern for suppression of platelet function (nonselective), cardiovascular risk (especially with the COX-2-selective NSAIDs), and induction of gastric injury (nonselective). All NSAIDs can adversely affect renal function. Corticosteroids and ACTH in high doses are also effective therapies for acute gout. Oral or intravenous colchicine is effective, but the intravenous route is fraught with potentially life-threatening complications, especially if an inappropriate dose is used. Hence many clinicians avoid this route of administration other than in unusual circumstances. Oral colchicine regimens (i.e., 0.6 mg orally every hour until resolution of pain or onset of diarrhea) are often inadvisable perioperatively because diarrhea is almost inevitable, and it usually occurs before resolution of the gouty attack.

Hypouricemic therapy should generally not be initiated or significantly altered in the setting of an acute flare of gout. This recommendation is based on the observation that acute hypouricemia can provoke an attack and the clinical belief that abrupt changes in the serum urate level may prolong the attack. Our approach to the patient with a gout flare in the perioperative period is to treat with oral NSAIDs (i.e., indomethacin 50 mg orally three times daily, naproxen 500 twice daily, or celecoxib 200 to 300 twice daily, which does not interfere with platelet function) if the patient is able to tolerate oral medications and is without relative contraindications to NSAID therapy (gastrointestinal risk, renal risk, bleeding risk). The NSAID dose is not reduced until after complete improvement is documented. We attempt to taper the NSAID within 10 to 14 days. Parenteral NSAIDs have no safety advantage over oral therapy. For the patient who has a history of tolerating colchicine, low-dose therapy (0.6 mg once to twice daily) can be added for several weeks to prevent another attack. Corticosteroids are a valid alternative to NSAID therapy. We generally prescribe 40 mg prednisone or its equivalent daily; after complete response is documented, the steroid is tapered to discontinuation over approximately 10 days. Using too low a dose or too short a course frequently results in inadequate resolution or a rebound flare. Intra-articular corticosteroid injections can be used if the attack is limited to one or a few joints if infection can be excluded.

MYOSITIS (POLYMYOSITIS, DERMATOMYOSITIS, MYOSITIS ASSOCIATED WITH OTHER DISEASES)

Disease Characteristics

Polymyositis and dermatomyositis are associated with cardiomyopathy, cardiac conduction disease, interstitial lung disease, and respiratory muscle dysfunction. Consideration should be given to the preoperative need to assess these parameters on an individual basis. Patients, particularly those with active disease, should be assessed in advance for potential difficulty in weaning from a ventilator.

The transaminases, the myocardial band enzymes of creatine phosphokinase (CPK-MB), and rarely troponin may be elevated in patients with peripheral myositis (without cardiac involvement). Baseline measurements may be of value in patients at risk for myocardial events.

Initiation of swallowing may be compromised in patients with acute or severe disease. The ability to swallow pills should be inquired about in advance. Adult patients with dermatomyositis, particularly those more than 40 years old, are at increased risk of malignant disease. The preoperative consultation should take this into consideration, especially in the setting of (1) high-risk elective surgery in patients with recently diagnosed dermatomyositis if a malignant disease has not been excluded or (2) recently diagnosed dermatomyositis and "exploratory surgery" (e.g., an abdominal surgical procedure for unexplained obstruction).

Medications

Treatment of myositis usually requires a prolonged course of high-dose corticosteroids. Methotrexate, calcineurin antagonists, and azathioprine are also frequently utilized in relatively high doses to maintain remission and to permit tapering of steroids. The myositis is not likely to flare with short-term holding of these latter medications; thus, it is reasonable not to give these drugs within a few days of the surgical procedure, given the theoretical risk of infection and the adverse effects of the calcineurin antagonists on renal blood flow. No data exist to support this suggestion. If held, medications should be resumed postoperatively as soon as the patient is stable. Steroid myopathy does not increase CPK levels and usually does not affect respiratory muscle function.

Hydroxychloroquine

Hydroxychloroquine is often used to suppress the rash of dermatomyositis, and it is also used in systemic lupus erythematosus (SLE) and RA. It has a prolonged tissue half-life. Long-term use has been associated with the rare occurrence of vacuolar cardiomyopathy. Hydroxychloroquine has a weak antithrombotic effect but seems unlikely to cause bleeding. It can be continued in the perioperative period.

Intravenous Immune Globulin

Some patients with myositis receive intravenous immune globulin (IVIg; γ-globulin) in high doses on a monthly basis to induce or maintain remission. If possible, IVIg should not be given in temporal proximity to any potential renal insult, because administration can cause acute intrarenal hypoperfusion and renal failure.

Postoperative Complications

Weaning from the ventilator may be difficult in patients with respiratory muscle involvement, and having the patient in a seated position may provide significant advantage. There is also an increased risk for aspiration because of dysphagia as well as ineffective cough resulting from muscle weakness. The diagnosis of myocardial infarction may be difficult as a result of inflammatory muscle disease that causes an elevation in serum enzymes traditionally linked to acute myocardial infarction. Although CPK-MB is classically a marker of myocardial injury or infarction, elevated levels may be detected in the patient with inflammatory skeletal muscle disease as a result of skeletal muscle injury and regeneration. Cardiac troponin T may also be elevated in patients with polymyositis or dermatomyositis. Troponin I is much less likely to be elevated as a direct result of skeletal muscle inflammation, although it has been reported in rare instances. It is the cardiac biomarker of choice in patients with inflammatory skeletal muscle disease in whom myocardial infarction is suspected.

SYSTEMIC LUPUS ERYTHEMATOSUS

Disease Characteristics

Patients with SLE, like those with RA, are at an increased risk for coronary artery disease unexplained by traditional risk factors. Pulmonary hypertension may be present yet unrecognized. Interstitial lung disease occurs less frequently. Cytopenias are common. A baseline complete blood count should be obtained. Thrombocytopenia should prompt questioning regarding features that could suggest antiphospholipid antibody syndrome (APLAS), such as miscarriage or thrombosis, because there is an association of thrombocytopenia with this syndrome. It is our practice to test for lupus anticoagulant and antiphospholipid antibodies (APLAs) when thrombocytopenia is noted in the patient with SLE. APLAs or lupus anticoagulant may be present in more than 30% of patients with SLE. This situation predisposes at least some of these patients to thrombosis. Other than by a history of prior thrombosis, this subset of patients cannot be readily recognized. A prolonged partial thromboplastin time must not be assumed to reflect a lupus anticoagulant without completing a full coagulation laboratory evaluation. Factor deficiency and antifactor antibodies must be excluded because these are associated with significant hemorrhage.

Glomerulonephritis is usually asymptomatic and may be accompanied by a normal serum creatinine concentration. If the urine dipstick detects leukocytes or blood, microscopic evaluation of a fresh urine sample, not one that has required time to be transported to the laboratory, is mandatory in the evaluation of possible glomerulonephritis. Pyuria may be present as a result of glomerulonephritis, not infection.

Medications

Drugs, other than corticosteroids, used to maintain remission may be held during the immediate perioperative period as noted earlier and in Table 19-2. Corticosteroids taken on a long-term basis should be continued during the perioperative period, given intravenously until enteral absorption is ensured. Some clinicians recommend a slight elevation in corticosteroid dose to prevent a flare induced by the stress of surgery. Data are inadequate to support or refute this practice. The need for aggressive antithrombotic prophylaxis should be considered at the time of preoperative assessment in patients who have APLAs and especially lupus anticoagulant.

Postoperative Complications

Flares in disease may occur in the perioperative setting and may be difficult to distinguish from infection, corticosteroid withdrawal syndromes, drug reactions, or a surgical complication. Fever may be a manifestation of disease activity, thrombosis, infection, or drug reaction. Acute leukopenia or thrombocytopenia favors the diagnosis of lupus flare instead of infection. The presence of rigors favors infection. Acute-phase reactants may be elevated in the postoperative period in the absence of an SLE flare. They are of minimal clinical utility during that period.

SCLERODERMA

Disease Characteristics

Severe disease may produce facial tightening with decreased ability to open the mouth wide enough to permit easy intubation. Dental health may be poor. Vascular and soft tissue

TABLE 19-2	Immunosuppressive and Rheumatic Disease Medications in the Perioperative Period	
Drug	**Preoperative Recommendations**	**Comments**
NSAID (nonselective)	Stop four to five half-lives before surgical procedure	Reversibly inhibits platelet function, demonstrated increased postoperative bleeding; risk of gastric ulceration; can decrease renal function, decrease drug excretion
Aspirin	Unless used as antithrombotic drug, stop ~10 days preoperatively	Irreversible platelet inhibition; increased postoperative bleeding
COX-2 selective NSAIDs	Can continue through surgery unless renal concerns	No antiplatelet effects; may be prothrombotic; can decrease renal function; effective as analgesic: narcotic sparing
Prednisone	Continue; consider SHORT-TERM hydrocortisone, 25–100 IV q8h	Concern with wound healing and infection with long-term use; cause leukocytosis, hyperglycemia; NO NEED for protracted tapering if stress doses are prescribed; study shows baseline dosing is sufficient to avoid hypotension; pick dose based on hemodynamic stress of specific procedure
Hydroxychloroquine	Can continue	Some antithrombotic effect (has been used as prophylactic antithrombotic in orthopedic surgery)
Methotrexate	Can continue	Avoid administration within 24–48 hours of possible acute renal insufficiency; preoperative discontinuation associated with flares in rheumatoid arthritis
Azathioprine	Can continue	
Leflunomide	Can continue or hold few days preoperatively	Limited data
Cyclophosphamide	Can continue	Acute renal failure could cause buildup of metabolites
Sulfasalazine	Can continue	
IV immune globulin	Can continue	Avoid within few days of potential acute renal injury (i.e., hypoperfusion)

Table continued on following page

TABLE 19-2	Immunosuppressive and Rheumatic Disease Medications in the Perioperative Period (Continued)	
Drug	**Preoperative Recommendations**	**Comments**
Anti-TNF agents	Stop four to five half-lives preoperatively	Limited but growing amount of data
Colchicine	Can continue in baseline chronic dose; adjust if renal failure occurs	IV bioavailability higher than oral; use IV route only with extreme care, if at all; renal insufficiency or administration of some medications (macrolides) can increase drug levels
Allopurinol	Can continue	Resume as soon as possible postoperatively; do not initiate therapy in acute perioperative period

COX, cyclooxygenase; IV, intravenous; NSAID, nonsteroidal anti-inflammatory drug; q, every; TNF, tumor necrosis factor.

involvement may make vascular access extremely difficult, and the need for central venous access should be considered in advance. The requirement for placement of arterial lines should be carefully considered because ulnar artery occlusion is common and digital circulation is often tenuous. Radial artery line placement can occasionally produce severe tissue damage. Brachial artery lines should be avoided. Digital ischemia resulting from Raynaud's phenomenon may make digital oximetry unreliable.

Pulmonary hypertension may be severe, yet clinically unrecognized. The symptoms may be incorrectly attributed to pulmonary fibrosis. Pulmonary hypertension may make the patient significantly dependent on preload, and modest hypovolemia, with associated preload reduction, can elicit severe hypotension in the presence of pulmonary hypertension. Patients receiving continuous epoprostenol (Flolan) infusion for pulmonary artery hypertension must *not* have their infusion interrupted. The baseline electrocardiogram may reveal conduction disease or a pseudoinfarction pattern. Interstitial lung disease is common.

Bowel pseudo-obstruction occurs and may result in surgical procedures for what is believed to be true structural obstruction. Hematologic abnormalities are not typical of uncomplicated, even severe, scleroderma. Fever is not characteristically part of the disease.

Medications

Medications that the patient takes on a long-term basis for Raynaud's phenomenon, pulmonary hypertension, and gastroesophageal reflux should be continued in the perioperative period.

Postoperative Complications

Fever is not expected from a disease flare, so alternative causes of fever must be sought. Scleroderma involvement of the gut may make oral drug absorption slow and unreliable. Bacterial overgrowth is common. Postoperative ileus may be particularly problematic. Reflux and esophageal dysmotility are often severe and place patients at high risk for aspiration when they are supine. The patient should be positioned in bed to limit the likelihood of aspiration.

Even mild hypothermia or vasoconstrictive medications may cause peripheral, renal, or central vasoconstriction. Severe vasospastic peripheral ischemia may necessitate acute vasodilator therapy.

ANTIPHOSPHOLIPID ANTIBODY SYNDROME

Disease Characteristics and Postoperative Complications

APLAS includes both venous and arterial thrombosis. Patients with a history of thrombotic events and persistent APLAS or the lupus anticoagulant are at extremely high risk for perioperative thrombosis. **Patients with a history of thrombosis are likely at particularly high risk for thrombosis at the time of warfarin withdrawal accompanied by** the additional thrombotic risk of surgery [⊙ *Erkan et al, 2002*]. We typically continue the patient's long-term warfarin therapy as close to the time of the surgical procedure as possible and use bridge anticoagulation therapy with either full-dose continuous unfractionated heparin or low-molecular-weight heparin. Heparin anticoagulation is withheld preoperatively to allow for appropriate hemostasis and is then restarted along with the patient's warfarin as soon as hemostasis is stable in the postoperative period.

Patients with APLAS are statistically predisposed to cardiac valve disease, particularly thickening of the mitral or aortic valve leaflets, nonbacterial valve leaflet vegetations, and in some cases valve regurgitation. Routine echocardiography is not necessary, but careful examination is warranted. At present, data are insufficient to implicate APLAS with an increased risk of postoperative thrombosis in the absence of prior thrombosis. Cardiovascular findings of the APLAS include peripheral vascular disease and premature stenosis of coronary artery bypass grafts. Patients with APLAS, even without a history of thrombosis, who undergo valve replacement surgery present many difficult management problems. These include increased surgical complications, difficulty in the choice of valve type, and potential problems in monitoring anticoagulation therapy.

The presence of thrombocytopenia is not protective against thrombosis in the setting of APLAS. Severe thrombocytopenia may increase the risk for anticoagulant-associated bleeding. In this setting, corticosteroid or IVIg therapy may be used (in conjunction with anticoagulation) to increase the platelet count while protecting the patient from thrombosis.

Immunosuppressive therapy is unlikely to be of benefit in preventing thrombosis. Women with a history of otherwise unexplained miscarriages and APLAS may also be at high risk for thrombosis.

In the presence of a lupus anticoagulant, routine monitoring of the partial thromboplastin time may be unreliable

[Bartholomew and Kottke-Marchant, 1998]. Low-molecular-weight heparin can be dosed by weight. Alternatively, factor Xa activity or thrombin time may be monitored. Monitoring of heparin effect during bypass may be unreliable if the activated coagulation time is used. Monitoring of heparin levels should be considered.

In addition to the increased risk of thrombosis, these patients may be at higher risk for development of heparin-associated thrombocytopenia. The medicine consultant should have special vigilance for the development of the HELLP (hemolysis, elevated liver enzymes, low platelets) syndrome in the third trimester of pregnancy, fat embolism syndrome (after arthroplasty), and heparin-induced thrombocytopenia with thrombosis in patients with APLAS because these distinctive diagnoses may be extremely difficult to make in this setting.

OSTEOARTHRITIS

Disease Characteristics and Postoperative Complications

OA is the most common underlying disease warranting arthroplasty. Although frequently a multifocal process involving cartilage and periarticular bone, OA has no systemic manifestations affecting the perioperative course. OA is not characterized by inflammatory joint flares. Patients with acute joint swelling, particularly with swelling or warmth, should be evaluated by arthrocentesis for crystal disease or infection. Because the joint pain is not primarily the result of inflammation in the usual sense, postoperative joint pain can generally be managed with pure analgesics. Fever immediately following hip or knee arthroplasty (done for any indication) is common and is usually not related to infection. However, persistent fever for several days or fever developing a few days postoperatively warrants detailed evaluation for infection, thrombosis, drug allergy, or crystalline arthritis.

Selected Readings

Aberra FN, Lewis JD, Hass D, et al: Corticosteroids and immunomodulators: Postoperative infectious complication risk in inflammatory bowel disease patients. Gastroenterology 125:320-327, 2003.

Bartholomew JR, Kottke-Marchant K: Monitoring anticoagulation therapy in patients with the lupus anticoagulant. J Clin Rheumatol 4:307-311, 1998.

Caples SM, Utz JP, Allen MS, Ryu JH: Thoracic surgical procedures in patients with rheumatoid arthritis. J Rheumatol 31:2136-41, 2004.

Collins DN, Barnes CL, Fitzrandolph RL: Cervical spine instability in rheumatoid patients having total hip or knee arthroplasty. Clin Orthop Relat Res 272:127-35, 1991.

Craig MH, Poole GV, Hower CJ: Postsurgical gout. Am Surg 61:56-59, 1995.

Erkan D, Leibowitz E, Berman J, Lockshin MD: Perioperative medical management of antiphospholipid syndrome: Hospital for special surgery experience, review of literature, and recommendations. J Rheumatol 29:843-849, 2002. ©

Giles JT, Bartlett SJ, Gelbert AC, et al: Tumor necrosis factor inhibitor therapy and risk of serious postoperative orthopedic infection in rheumatoid arthritis. Arthritis Rheum 55:333-337, 2006.

Grauer JN, Tingstad EM, Rand N, et al: Predictors of paralysis in the rheumatoid cervical spine in patients undergoing total joint arthroplasty. J Bone Joint Surg Am 86:1420-1424, 2004.

Grennan DM, Gray J, Loudon J, Fear S: Methotrexate and early postoperative complications in patients with rheumatoid arthritis undergoing elective orthopaedic surgery. Ann Rheum Dis 60:214-217, 2001.

Hogan WJ, McBane RD, Santrach PJ, et al: Antiphospholipid syndrome and perioperative hemostatic management of cardiac valvular surgery. Mayo Clin Proc 75:971-976, 2000.

Kolman J, Morris I: Cricoarytenoid arthritis: A cause of acute upper airway obstruction in rheumatoid arthritis. Can J Anaesth 49:729-732, 2002. ©

Maradit-Kremers H, Crowson CS, Nicola PJ, et al: Increased unrecognized coronary heart disease and sudden deaths in rheumatoid arthritis. Arthritis Rheum 52:402-411, 2005. ©

Neal B, Gray H, MacMahon S, Dunn L: Incidence of heterotopic bone formation after major hip surgery. Aust N Z J Surg 72:808-21, 2002.

Nguyen HV, Ludwig SC, Silber J, et al: Rheumatoid arthritis of the cervical spine. Spine J 4:329-334, 2004. ©

Pioro M, Mandell BF: Septic arthritis. In Mandell BF (ed): Life-threatening complications of autoimmune disease. Rheum Dis Clin North Am 23:239-258, 1997.

Reynolds LW, Hoo RK, Brill RJ, et al: The COX-2 specific inhibitor, valde-coxib, is an effective, opioid-sparing analgesic in patients undergoing total knee arthroplasty. J Pain Symptom Manage 25:133-41, 2003.

Robinson CM, Christi J, Malcom-Smith N: Nonsteroidal anti-inflammatory drugs, perioperative blood loss, and transfusion requirements in elective hip arthroplasty. J Arthroplasty 8:607, 1993.

Romano CL, Duci D, Romano D, et al: Celecoxib versus indomethacin in the prevention of heterotopic ossification after total hip arthroplasty. J Arthroplasty 19:14-18, 2004.

Salem M, Tainsh RE, Bromberg J, et al: Perioperative glucocorticoid cover-age: A reassessment 42 years after emergence of a problem. Ann Surg 219:416-425, 1994. ©

Shaw JA, Chung R: Febrile response after knee and hip arthroplasty. Clin Orthop Relat Res 367:181-189, 1999.

Shaw M, Mandell BF: Perioperative management of selected problems in patients with rheumatic diseases. Rheum Dis Clin North Am 25: 623-637, 1999.

Slappendel R, Weber EWG, Benraad B, et al: Does ibuprofen increase perioperative blood loss during hip arthroplasty? Eur J Anaesthesiol 19:829-831, 2002.

20 | Perioperative Care of the Patient with Psychiatric Illness

JENNY Y. WANG, MD
DANIEL K. HOLLERAN, MD
BARRY S. ZIRING, MD

This chapter covers the various psychiatric medications, their side effects, and general recommendations for these agents in the perioperative period. It also discusses the evaluation of patients undergoing electroconvulsive therapy (ECT) and reviews the risks of cardiac and cerebrovascular complications associated with ECT. The neuroleptic malignant syndrome (NMS) and its possible relation to malignant hyperthermia are also discussed.

PSYCHIATRIC MEDICATIONS

The major classes of psychiatric medications include benzodiazepines, tricyclic antidepressants, selective serotonin reuptake inhibitors (SSRIs), neuroleptic agents, monoamine oxidase (MAO) inhibitors, and lithium. The only agents that are contraindicated during the perioperative period are the MAO inhibitors; however, knowledge of the side effect profiles, drug interactions, and withdrawal syndromes may be helpful in interpreting clinical problems of patients undergoing surgery. Perioperative recommendations for different psychiatric medication classes are summarized in Table 20-1.

Levels of Evidence:

A—Randomized controlled trials (RCTs), meta-analyses, well-designed systematic reviews of RCTs. **B**—Case-control or cohort studies, nonrandomized controlled trials, systematic reviews of studies other than RCTs, cross-sectional studies, retrospective studies. **C**—Consensus statements, expert guidelines, usual practice, opinion.

TABLE 20-1	Psychiatric Drugs and Perioperative Management	
Drug Category	**Perioperative Concerns**	**Recommendations for Management**
Benzodiazepines	Abrupt discontinuation can lead to withdrawal symptoms Mild: insomnia, dysphoria Moderate: agitation, delirium, tremors, abdominal cramps, diaphoresis, seizures Concurrent narcotics may lead to excessive sedation, confusion, hypotension, or respiratory depression	Continue perioperatively to avoid withdrawal, using intravenous forms if NPO Postoperatively, reduce benzodiazepine doses gradually if concurrent narcotics lead to increased side effects
Tricyclic Antidepressants	Hypotension may be more prevalent with other drugs that also cause hypotension, including some anesthetics (atropine, pancuronium) Interactions with sympathomimetics can cause hypertension Interactions with some volatile anesthetics can increase potential for arrhythmias Can lead to slowed cardiac conduction	Consider holding TCA a few days preoperatively and restarting them a few days postoperatively, particularly in patients who are at higher risk for falls, hypotension, confusion or arrhythmias or in patients who are taking lower doses of TCAs who have less risk of withdrawal symptoms Watch for mild withdrawal symptoms (gastrointestinal symptoms, dizziness) No IV form available Watch for slowed cardiac conduction including P-R and Q-T prolongation and bundle branch block, especially with concurrent atrioventricular node blockers, such as β-blockers and calcium channel blockers
Selective Serotonin Reuptake Inhibitors	May interact with warfarin, digoxin, phenytoin Stopping SSRIs suddenly may exacerbate mood disorders Concurrent use with MAO inhibitors can lead to serotonin syndrome	Continue SSRI perioperatively; no IV form available In patients on warfarin and SSRI, monitor INR closely Monitor for phenytoin toxicity in patients on SSRI

MAO Inhibitors	Hypertensive crisis with sympathomimetics, caffeine Interaction with meperidine, dextromethorphan, leading to autonomic instability, agitation, cyanosis (potentially fatal) Interaction with SSRIs, leading to autonomic instability, rigidity, myoclonus, confusion, coma	Stop MAO inhibitors at least 2 wk before elective surgery to allow complete elimination For emergency surgery, or if psychiatrist believes it unsafe to stop the MAO inhibitor, anesthesiologist should be notified to avoid sympathomimetics and to monitor blood pressure closely If MAO inhibitor is continued perioperatively, avoid foods containing higher amounts of tyramine Avoid meperidine (Demerol) and dextromethorphan within 2 wk of using an MAO inhibitor Avoid SSRIs within 2 wk of using an MAO inhibitor (5 wk with fluoxetine)
Neuroleptics	At high doses, some antipsychotics can prolong the Q-T interval, leading to risk of torsades de points	Continue therapy perioperatively; IV haloperidol available for patients who are NPO Follow ECG in patients on other agents that can prolong the Q-T interval and for patients on high doses of antipsychotics
Lithium	Narrow safety margin Possible perioperative side effects: nausa, nephrogenic diabetes insipidus, delirium, coma, ventricular arrhythmias May prolong the effects of neuromuscular blocking agents and anesthetics May cause T-wave flattening or inversion	Stop lithium 1–2 days preoperatively and restart when taking oral medications; no parenteral form available If continued, follow lithium levels and check baseline ECG preoperatively

ECG, electrocardiogram; INR, international normalized ratio; IV, intravenous; MAO, monoamine oxidase; NPO, nothing by mouth; SSRI, selective serotonin reuptake inhibitor; TCA, tricyclic antidepressant.

Benzodiazepines

Benzodiazepines are used as antianxiety agents and for insomnia. They are generally divided into long-acting agents with a half-life of more than 24 hours (diazepam, chlordiazepoxide, and flurazepam), intermediate-acting agents with a half-life of 6 to 24 hours (lorazepam, temazepam, and oxazepam), and short-acting agents with a half-life less than 6 hours (estazolam and triazolam). These half-lives are determined not only by the parent compound, but also by the presence and half-life of any active metabolites. Side effects of benzodiazepines at therapeutic doses may include sedation, dizziness, and confusion.

Perioperatively, the major adverse effect of these agents is the potential for acute withdrawal if they are discontinued abruptly. Mild withdrawal symptoms can present as insomnia and dysphoria. More severe symptoms include tremors, abdominal cramps, diaphoresis, agitation, delirium, and seizures. If a patient taking benzodiazepines requires a surgical procedure, the drugs should be continued postoperatively to prevent withdrawal. If the patient is receiving nothing by mouth (NPO) and is taking a benzodiazepine without a parenteral formulation, lorazepam, diazepam, and chlordiazepoxide can be used intravenously. Postoperatively, benzodiazepine doses may need to be reduced if concurrently administered narcotics lead to excessive sedation, confusion, or hypotension.

Tricyclic and Related Antidepressants

The tricyclic antidepressants are used for a variety of problems, including depression, panic disorder, anxiety, and neuropathic pain (Table 20-2). These drugs have a 70% response rate for depression when therapeutic blood levels are achieved. Their mechanism of action is by potentiating the effects of both serotonin and norepinephrine. Unfortunately, they have many side effects, especially cardiovascular.

Side effects of the tricyclic antidepressants include orthostasis, anticholinergic effects (dry eyes, blurry vision, dry mouth, urinary hesitancy, constipation), conduction delays, and

TABLE 20-2	Tricyclic Antidepressants					
Medication	**Orthostasis**	**Anticholinergic Effect**	**Conduction Delay**	**Sedation**	**Major Drug Interaction**
First-Generation Agents					
Amitriptyline (Elavil)	High	Very high	High	High	Volatile anesthetics: tachycardia and hypotension
Nortriptyline (Pamelor)	Moderate	Moderate	High	Moderate	Antiarrhythmic agents: arrhythmia
Desipramine (Norpramin)	High	Moderate	High	Mild	Warfarin: prolonged INR
Doxepin (Sinequan)	High	High	High	High	Sympathomimetics: hypertension
Imipramine (Tofranil)	High	High	High	High	Thyroid hormones: arrhythmia
Protriptyline (Vivactil)	Moderate	High	High	Mild	Atropine: increased anticholinergic effect
Trimipramine (Surmontil)	High	High	High	High	β-Blockers: bradyarrhythmias, hypotension
Newer Agents					
Amoxapine (Asendin)	Moderate	Moderate	High	High	Same as first-generation tricyclics
Maprotiline (Ludiomil)	Moderate	Moderate	High	High	Same as first-generation tricyclics
Trazodone (Desyrel)	Moderate	Low	Moderate	High	Phenytoin, digoxin: increased levels of toxicity

INR, international normalized ratio.

sedation. Orthostasis occurs in up to 24% of patients receiving tricyclic drugs. In addition, tricyclic antidepressants have multiple interactions with other drugs. Specific comparisons of side effects and drug interactions for the various tricyclic antidepressants are listed in Table 20-2. In general, second-generation tricyclic antidepressants cause less orthostasis, anticholinergic effect, and sedation, but they tend to be very sedating.

Clinicians have long known that tricyclic agents can result in significant ventricular arrhythmia when they are taken in overdose. As a result, tricyclic antidepressants were believed to be arrhythmogenic. More recent studies have not substantiated this belief. Tricyclic drugs at therapeutic levels have been shown to suppress ventricular premature contractions. Electrophysiologic studies have supported this finding by demonstrating that tricyclic agents have properties similar to those of the class 1A antiarrhythmic agents.

Tricyclic agents were also believed initially to depress left ventricular function. Several studies using radionucleotide angiography, however, demonstrated that several tricyclic drugs have no adverse effect on left ventricular function.

The observation that atrioventricular block was a frequent complication of tricyclic antidepressant overdose led to concern regarding the use of these medications in patients with preexisting cardiac conduction disease. Patients with preexisting bundle branch block are at increased risk for the development of significant conduction complications when they are treated with a tricyclic drug. For patients with preexisting bundle branch block, tricyclic agents should probably be avoided unless a pacemaker is in place. If tricyclic medications are used, the patient should be followed with serial electrocardiograms (ECGs) as therapeutic levels are achieved. The optimal frequency for obtaining these ECGs is unknown and probably depends on the kinetics of the drug and how fast it achieves therapeutic levels. Twice weekly seems reasonable. For patients with other conduction abnormalities, care should be taken when initiating therapy with tricyclic agents, and a follow-up ECG should be obtained to look for widening of the QRS complexes or increased P-R or Q-T intervals.

Perioperatively, these side effects, particularly the potential for impairment of cardiac conduction, hypotension, and sedation, should be considered before starting tricyclic antidepressants. This concern is especially important for the patient at risk for falls. Potential drug interactions can also be problematic during the perioperative period. Tricyclic medications have varying degrees of anticholinergic properties. In the perioperative period, the anticholinergic and α-adrenergic blocking properties of tricyclic drugs may potentiate similar effects caused by anesthetic agents, including atropine and pancuronium. Additional drug interactions result from the concomitant use of tricyclic agents with sympathomimetic agents, which can cause either hypertension or paradoxical hypotension with epinephrine. The mechanism is the additive vasodilatory effect of β_2-adrenergic stimulation by epinephrine in addition to α-blockade by the tricyclic drug. The tricyclic agents may interact with warfarin and increase the prothrombin time and cause bleeding. Cimetidine has been shown to alter steady-state concentrations of tricyclic agents significantly and to result in side effects from overdose. As a result of the high potential for drug interaction, it may be preferable to withhold tricyclic medications for several days preoperatively and resume them several days postoperatively, particularly in patients at risk for falls, hypotension, confusion, and arrhythmias. This approach rarely causes a depressive episode. The medical consultant should be aware that withdrawal of tricyclic antidepressants can cause mild symptoms, including nausea, abdominal pain, diarrhea, and dizziness. Patients taking lower doses of tricyclic antidepressants may be at less risk for withdrawal symptoms.

Selective Serotonin Reuptake Inhibitors and Related Agents

SSRIs are the fastest growing class of antidepressant medications. They are used in depression, premenstrual dysphoric disorder, panic disorder, obsessive-compulsive disorder, anxiety, phobias, and eating disorders. At this time, they include fluoxetine (Prozac), paroxetine (Paxil), sertraline (Zoloft), fluvoxamine (Luvox), venlafaxine (Effexor), citalopram (Celexa), and escitalopram (Lexapro). These drugs have the same clinical efficacy (70%) as conventional antidepressants. Unlike the tricyclic antidepressants, they cause no associated orthostatic hypotension or anticholinergic effects. SSRIs are associated only rarely with conduction abnormalities and tend to be stimulating rather than sedating. They may cause nausea and insomnia. The foregoing SSRIs are listed in the order of those with the most to the least cytochrome P-450 2D6–inhibiting properties. Those with more cytochrome P-450 activity are more likely to interact with warfarin, thus leading to an increased bleeding risk. These also may increase phenytoin levels and, consequently, the risk of toxicity. Venlafaxine inhibits the reuptake of both norepinephrine (like a tricyclic agent) and serotonin. Its side effects are more similar to those of other SSRIs, with transient nausea and vomiting. Cardiac conduction is not affected. Venlafaxine may also cause an increase in systolic blood pressure.

Other agents with some effects on the serotonin pathway are bupropion (Wellbutrin), buspirone (BuSpar), nefazodone, and mirtazapine (Remeron). Bupropion works primarily on the dopamine system and is used in depression with excessive somnolence and psychomotor slowing. It is also used in smoking cessation. Although the drug it is generally well tolerated, there is a risk of seizures with bupropion, particularly in the patient with a history of seizures or epileptogenic focus, in those patients taking large doses of bupropion (>450 mg/day), or in patients withdrawing from alcohol or sedative-hypnotics. Bupropion should be used with caution with other dopaminergic agents. Buspirone has effects on serotonin, dopamine, and α_2- receptors. It is used primarily for generalized anxiety disorder. This drug tends to cause a moderate degree of sedation, unlike the other SSRIs. Nefazodone works on the serotonin and norepinephrine pathways and blocks

α_1-receptors. It is used to treat depression. Unlike most other antidepressants, it does not tend to affect sleep patterns. Nefazodone is structurally similar to trazodone and can be accompanied by anticholinergic effects, orthostasis, agitation, bradycardia, and idiosyncratic liver toxicity. It increases levels of benzodiazepines, digoxin, haloperidol, and carbamazepine. Mirtazapine works by blocking α_2-receptors, with effects on serotonin and norepinephrine levels. It is used in depression and is associated with sedation but is less likely to cause sexual side effects than other antidepressants. It may reduce the effectiveness of clonidine.

Monoamine Oxidase Inhibitors

The MAO antidepressants include phenelzine (Nardil) and tranylcypromine (Parnate). These drugs are infrequently used because of the potential for severe reactions with many classes of drugs, both psychiatric and nonpsychiatric. MAO inhibitors can interact with sympathomimetic agents such as epinephrine, amphetamines, decongestants, and even excessive amounts of caffeine and can result in hypertensive crisis. MAO inhibitors should be stopped at least 2 weeks before elective surgical procedures to allow complete elimination. If emergency surgery is necessary, the anesthesiologist should be notified so that sympathomimetic agents can be avoided and careful monitoring can be performed. A poorly understood and potentially fatal interaction can occur between MAO inhibitors and meperidine (Demerol). Patients become agitated, disoriented, cyanotic, hyperthermic, hypertensive, and tachycardic. The MAO inhibitors may also interact with the SSRIs, leading to autonomic instability, hyperthermia, rigidity, myoclonus, confusion, and coma. There should be at least a 2-week interval between using MAO inhibitors and agents of these classes. Because long-term use of fluoxetine (Prozac) can saturate the tissues, the interval between long-term fluoxetine and MAO inhibitors should be 5 weeks.

Neuroleptic Agents (Antipsychotics)

This class of agents can be divided into first-generation antipsychotics and second-generation, or atypical, antipsychotics (Table 20-3). First-generation antipsychotics generally are less expensive than second-generation agents, but they have more side effects, including anticholinergic effects, sedation, and orthostasis. The neuroleptic agents can also cause extrapyramidal syndromes of parkinsonism, tardive dyskinesia, akathisia, and dystonia. At high doses, they may cause repolarization changes with Q-T prolongation and T-wave changes. Thioridazine (Mellaril), in particular, may produce a dose-related prolongation of the Q-T interval and may lead to torsades de pointes.

Second-generation neuroleptics are generally much better tolerated and have fewer side effects. Clozapine (Clozaril) has minimal extrapyramidal symptoms but has a 1% to 2% risk of agranulocytosis. Fatalities have been reported even with close monitoring of the complete blood count. For this reason, this drug is primarily used in patients who are not responding to other treatments. Risperidone (Risperdal) and olanzapine

TABLE 20-3	Neuroleptic Agents
First-Generation Agents	
Chlorpromazine (Thorazine)	
Thioridazine (Mellaril)	
Fluphenazine (Prolixin)	
Mesoridazine (Serentil)	
Perphenazine (Trilafon)	
Trifluoperazine (Stelazine)	
Loxapine (Loxitane)	
Haloperidol (Haldol)	
Second-Generation Agents	
Clozapine (Clozaril)	
Olanzapine (Zyprexa, Zyprexa Zydis)	
Risperidone (Risperdal, Risperdal M-Tab, Risperdal Consta)	
Quetiapine (Seroquel)	
Ziprasidone (Geodon)	
Aripiprazole (Abilify)	

(Zyprexa) are other second-generation neuroleptics, with minimal extrapyramidal side effects but without agranulocytosis. They both come in formulations that are orally disintegrating (Zyprexa Zydis, Risperdal M-tab). Risperidone also comes as a depot form given intramuscularly every 2 weeks. Olanzapine is more likely to cause weight gain and to affect diabetes and lipids. Risperidone may have more dopaminergic side effects. Quetiapine (Seroquel), ziprasidone (Geodon), and aripiprazole (Abilify) are newer agents that are well tolerated.

In general, it is not necessary to discontinue neuroleptics perioperatively. While a patient is NPO, intravenous haloperidol, orally disintegrating tablets of either risperidone or olanzapine, or intramuscular injections of haloperidol, fluphenazine, or risperidone can be used. If high doses of neuroleptics are used, serial ECGs should be monitored to watch for Q-T prolongation.

Lithium

Lithium is used to treat mania. It has a narrow margin of safety and is dangerous when overdosed. Minor side effects occur even at therapeutic levels (0.8 to 1.5 mEq/L). These side effects include nausea, anorexia, and nephrogenic diabetes insipidus with polyuria and polydipsia. These last two symptoms occur in 50% of new patients but in only 5% of patients taking lithium on a long-term basis. Lithium can also affect thyroid function. Many drugs can raise lithium levels, including thiazides, NSAIDs, and metronidazole (Flagyl). Major side effects may occur at blood levels greater than 2 mEq/L. They consist of progressive delirium, coma, seizures, and ventricular arrhythmias. Unlike many other psychiatric drugs, lithium does not cause sedation at therapeutic levels. Lithium may also prolong the effects of neuromuscular blocking and anesthetic agents. Therefore, these agents should be used with caution in patients receiving lithium. In addition, lithium may cause changes on the ECG, including T-wave flattening or inversion, which may provoke confusion in the perioperative period with ischemic changes. A baseline ECG may be helpful. Except in unusual circumstances, lithium should be stopped 1 to 2 days preoperatively and restarted when the patient resumes full oral intake. Lithium is not available in a parenteral formulation.

ELECTROCONVULSIVE THERAPY

ECT is one of the most successful methods of treating depression, with up to an 80% response rate. It is also effective in mania and in some psychoses. In general, ECT is often used when rapid antidepressant response is necessary or in refractory psychiatric conditions. The procedure consists of electrical stimulation lasting approximately 5 seconds, followed by a convulsion lasting approximately 30 seconds. ECT is performed using general anesthesia with cardiac and blood pressure monitoring. Patients receive mask ventilation and are given a bite block.

ECT is capable of causing profound changes in hemodynamics. These include acute hypertension, hypotension, and arrhythmias, with resultant alterations in cardiac output. These disturbances result from changes in parasympathetic and sympathetic tone. Initially, these alterations are manifested by a decrease in blood pressure and heart rate. The blood pressure may decrease by 10% with the induction of anesthesia and then increase by up to 80% during the convulsion. These hemodynamic changes increase myocardial oxygen consumption and cause ischemia. As a result, hypertension should be well controlled before ECT. The noncardiac surgery guideline of the American College of Cardiology/American Heart Association classifies ECT as a low-risk procedure. Because ECT is generally an elective procedure, patients with recent myocardial infarction (≤30 days) should probably not undergo ECT. **The American Psychiatric Association has suggested that patients with unstable or severe cardiac disease are at increased risk for morbidity** with ECT [● *American Psychiatric Association, 2001*]. In the pre-ECT medical evaluation, cardiac history, including risks for arrhythmia, ischemia, and congestive heart failure, should be reviewed. In patients with a higher risk for arrhythmias, electrolytes should be checked and optimized. In patients with a higher ischemic risk, cardiology consultation should be obtained, and β-blockers should be considered, although these drugs may increase the risk of asystole during ECT. Patients at higher risk for congestive heart failure either from cardiomyopathy or from severe valvular disease should also have cardiac consultation before ECT.

ECT also causes fluctuations in cerebrovascular blood flow. Initial cerebrovascular constriction is followed by a significant increase in blood flow of up to seven times baseline. This change results in increased intracranial pressure. Intraocular pressure also increases. Glaucoma should be controlled before ECT. The American Psychiatric Association has suggested that patients with space-occupying intracranial lesions with evidence of elevated intracranial pressure, recent stroke or cerebral hemorrhage, or unstable aneurysms are at increased risk for morbidity with ECT. These patients should receive neurologic or neurosurgical consultation before considering ECT.

Current anesthetic practices to control blood pressure and heart rate and to minimize skeletal muscle contraction have certainly improved the safety of ECT. Even high-risk patients with one of the absolute contraindications have undergone ECT successfully. In addition, considering that ECT can lower the mortality rate of depressed patients back to normal levels, one author has suggested that ECT should be considered potentially lifesaving and has no absolute contraindications.

NEUROLEPTIC MALIGNANT SYNDROME

NMS occurs in approximately 1.5% of all patients taking neuroleptic drugs and has a 20% morality rate. NMS is an idiosyncratic reaction to neuroleptic agents that consists of fever, mental status changes, muscle rigidity, autonomic dysfunction, respiratory distress, and rhabdomyolysis. The syndrome is treated with the dopamine agonist bromocriptine and supportive measures such as a cooling blanket and intravenous fluids, as well as with discontinuation of the neuroleptic agent. Dantrolene sodium has also been used.

The issue of NMS in the perioperative period relates to its similarity to malignant hyperthermia. The latter is a rare state triggered by anesthetic agents and the muscle relaxant succinylcholine. NMS is inherited in an autosomal dominant mode, and it has been suggested that patients with a history of NMS may be at greater risk for the development of malignant hyperthermia during procedures requiring anesthesia. This would include ECT.

Selected Readings

American Psychiatric Association: Practice guideline for the treatment of patients with major depressive disorder (revision). Am J Psychiatry 157:1-45, 2000.

American Psychiatric Association: The Practice of Electroconvulsive Therapy: Recommendations for Treatment, Training, and Privileging, 2nd ed. Washington, DC, 2001. ●

Boehnert MT, Lovejoy FH Jr: Value of the QRS duration versus the serum drug level in predicting seizures and ventricular arrhythmias after an acute overdose of tricyclic antidepressants. N Engl J Med 313:474-479, 1985.

Burke WJ, Rubin EH, Zerumski CF, Wetzel RD: The safety of ECT in geriatric psychiatry. J Am Geriatr Soc 35:516-521, 1987.

Cohen BM, Baldessarini RJ, Pope MG, et al: Neuroleptic malignant syndrome. N Engl J Med 313:1293, 1985.

Fink M: Contraindications to electroconvulsive therapy. Anesth Analg 66:913-922, 1987.

Gerry JP, Shields HM: The identification and management of patients with a high risk for cardiac arrhythmias during modified ECT. J Clin Psychiatry 42:1403-1406, 1982.

Moore DP, Jefferson JW: Handbook of Medical Psychiatry, 2nd ed. St. Louis, MO, Mosby, 2004.

Paroxetine. Med Lett 35:24-25, 1993.

Richelson E: Treatment of acute depression. Psychiatr Clin North Am 16:461-478, 1993.

Roose SP, Glassman AH, Dalack GW: Depression, heart disease and tricyclic antidepressants. J Clin Psychiatry 50(Suppl):12-16, 1989.

Roose SP, Glassman AH, Giardiner EG, et al: Tricyclic antidepressants in depressed patients with conductive disease. Arch Gen Psychiatry 44:273-275, 1987.

Wells DG, Davies GG: Hemodynamic changes associated with electroconvulsive therapy. Anesth Analg 66:1193-1195, 1987.

Williams RB Jr, Sherter C: Cardiac complications of tricyclic antidepressant therapy. Ann Intern Med 74:395-398, 1971.

Yacoub OF, Morrow DM: Malignant hyperthermia and ECT. Am J Psychiatry 143:1027-1029, 1986.

21 Managing Medication in the Perioperative Period

WALTER K. KRAFT, MD, MS
GRETCHEN DIEMER, MD

ROLE OF THE MEDICAL CONSULTANT IN MANAGING MEDICATIONS

The medical consultant plays a critical role in preventing drug-related adverse events, in managing disease-specific complications associated with surgery, and in providing guidance for control of concomitant medical conditions. The risk of medication-related adverse events is elevated in the perioperative period as a result of physiologic changes related to surgery and the cessation of oral medications. Patients taking medications on a regular basis have a higher incidence of postoperative complications than those not taking daily medications. When one is caring for surgical patients seen initially in the inpatient setting, all attempts should be made to ascertain the patient's outpatient drug regimen, as well as the level of adherence to this regimen. Existing medications should be examined to ensure that no interaction with drugs added for surgical purposes will occur. The preoperative evaluation should include a detailed plan regarding administration of the patient's long-term medications in the perioperative period. This is especially important for patients administered multiple medications, because polypharmacy itself is a risk for adverse drug reactions. Specific attention should be given to dose and

---

Levels of Evidence:

Ⓐ—Randomized controlled trials (RCTs), meta-analyses, well-designed systematic reviews of RCTs. Ⓑ—Case-control or cohort studies, nonrandomized controlled trials, systematic reviews of studies other than RCTs, cross-sectional studies, retrospective studies. Ⓒ—Consensus statements, expert guidelines, usual practice, opinion.

route of administration, with contingencies provided for patients who will be unable to resume oral medications immediately after the surgical procedure. As part of continuing inpatient care through the perioperative period, the medical consultant can optimize therapeutics by daily review of medication lists.

Specific recommendations could include the following: (1) removal of unnecessary or potentially harmful medications, (2) switch from parenteral to oral forms of medication as tolerated by the patient, (3) dosage adjustment for changes in renal or hepatic function, (4) management strategies for unrecognized withdrawal syndromes or drug interactions, (5) identification and management of delirium, (6) postdischarge medication regimen review and reconciliation, and (7) communication with primary care physician for treatment-related changes in existing care.

DRUG ABSORPTION CHANGES ASSOCIATED WITH SURGERY

The stomach is primarily an organ of maceration and acid production and not one of absorption. In the postsurgical state, as under normal conditions, a key determinant of the rate of drug absorption is the rate of gastric emptying. Manipulation of abdominal organs, anesthesia, pain, opioid analgesics, anticholinergic drugs, and electrolyte disturbances all contribute to gastric stasis associated with postoperative ileus. Additionally, decreased splanchnic flow, edema, and villous atrophy contribute to decreases in rate and extent of drug absorption in the postoperative period. Common management of patients with ileus is the use a nasogastric (NG) tube to decompress the stomach. If there is delay in the resumption of enteral function, intravenous administration of important or essential medications is preferred.

Essential medications that are not available in intravenous form are often administered through an NG tube, followed by clamping for 30 minutes and subsequent resumption of intermittent suction. However, **the oral bioavailability of medications administered in this manner in the postoperative period is decreased relative the presurgical state [⊕** *Elfant et al, 1995*]. The degree to which absorption is impaired is unpredictable, owing to variability of interpatient and intrapatient gut motility with incomplete evacuation of drug to the duodenum and dissolution and absorptive kinetics specific to individual drugs. Although it is difficult to predict the extent of drug absorption through the NG route, absorption can be expected to be less than in the normal physiologic state. A general principle is to use parenteral forms of critical medications until gastric motility and absorption are established by the toleration of enteral nutrition. Additionally, although the efficacy of a multimodality approach to shortening the duration of postoperative ileus has not been established, the dose of opioids should be minimized as much as possible while maintaining control of pain. Uncomplicated surgery is not associated with significant changes in volume of distribution or elimination of drugs, and oral drug doses generally do not need to be altered.

DRUGS ASSOCIATED WITH ADVERSE EVENTS ON SUDDEN CESSATION

Numerous medications that are administered on a long-term basis are associated with withdrawal syndromes (Table 21-1). These syndromes are typically class specific and not drug specific, although members of the class with a longer half-life are associated with milder withdrawal syndromes. For procedures with a limited period of discontinued oral intake (nothing by mouth [NPO] status), withdrawal syndromes are uncommon, because oral administration can quickly be resumed. Onset of withdrawal, if it occurs, is usually within the first 24 hours of missing a dose. Symptoms, such as irritability, hypertension, tachycardia, and even delirium, are often nonspecific. Because many of these symptoms could have multiple causes unrelated to drugs in the postsurgical period, patients are often not recognized as suffering from a withdrawal syndrome. The best

TABLE 21-1	Drugs and Substances Associated with Withdrawal Syndrome on Sudden Cessation	
Drugs and Substances	**Symptoms**	**Potential Severity**
β-Blockers	Hypertension, tachycardia	Increased risk of cardiovascular mortality and morbidity
Clonidine	Hypertension, tachycardia	Increased risk of cardiovascular mortality and morbidity
Benzodiazepines	Agitation, tachycardia, hallucinosis	Potentially severe and life-threatening
Alcohol	Agitation, tachycardia, hallucinosis	Potentially severe and life-threatening
Opioids	Gastrointestinal distress, diaphoresis, irritability, sleep disturbance, rhinorrhea	Unpleasant but not life-threatening
Antipsychotics	Insomnia, nausea, vomiting, anxiety, agitation	Generally self-limited
Selective serotonin reuptake inhibitors	Dizziness, light-headedness, vertigo or feeling faint, paresthesia, anxiety, diarrhea, fatigue, gait instability, headache, insomnia, irritability, nausea or emesis, tremor, visual disturbance	Generally self-limited
Tricyclic antidepressants	Agitation, irritability, insomnia	Generally self-limited
Caffeine	Irritability, sleepiness, dysphoria, delirium, nausea, vomiting, rhinorrhea, nervousness, restlessness, anxiety, muscle tension, muscle pains, flushed face	Self-limited

management strategy is to plan for potential withdrawal syndromes preoperatively. This approach includes use of parenteral forms where available or the tapering of a medication in the immediate preoperative period. Table 21-2 gives general recommendations for the preoperative management of commonly prescribed medications.

The medical consultant must also recognize withdrawal in the postoperative period. The importance of an accurate, first-person account of outpatient medications and of ongoing substance abuse cannot be overemphasized. The treatment of withdrawal generally depends on the specific drug identified or suspected. Replacement of the responsible drug is generally the first goal.

β-Adrenergic Receptor Blockers

Initiation of β-Blockers to Decrease the Perioperative Risk of Cardiac Complications

Data from small clinical trials suggest that β-blockers decrease the risk of cardiac complications (e.g., myocardial infarction) in the perioperative period. An observational study found that perioperative β-blockers have their greatest benefit in patients at increased risk of cardiac complications, that is, patients with three or more of the following clinical features: (1) ischemic heart disease, (2) cerebrovascular disease, (3) renal insufficiency, (4) diabetes mellitus, or (5) high-risk surgical procedure.

The American College of Cardiology/American Heart Association 2006 Update on Perioperative Beta Blocker Therapy recommended that β-blockers be continued in patients already receiving β-blockers and initiated in patients undergoing vascular surgery who are estimated to be at high cardiac risk as determined by the presence of ischemia on preoperative testing [◐ *Fleisher et al, 2006*]. This guideline states that β-blockers are probably recommended for patients undergoing vascular surgery who have a history of coronary artery disease or who have multiple coronary artery disease risk factors and for patients with multiple cardiac risk factors who undergo intermediate-risk or high-risk surgical procedures. β-Blockers may be considered for patients who undergo intermediate-risk or high-risk surgical procedures who have a single clinical cardiac risk factor and may also be considered for patients who undergo vascular surgery who have no cardiac risk factors. Ideally, β-blocker therapy should be initiated 2 weeks preoperatively, but in practice that is not always achievable. Not uncommonly, the clinician is faced with settings in which β-blocker therapy is initiated the day before or even the day of surgery. In all cases, a key point is that β-blocker therapy should be titrated to achieve a heart rate of

TABLE 21-2   Management of Commonly Prescribed Medications

Medication	Preoperative Management
β-Blockers	Continue through procedure with parenteral dosage
ACE inhibitors	Hold day of surgery
Angiotensin II receptor blockers	Hold day of surgery
Calcium channel blockers	Hold day of surgery
α$_2$-Agonists	Continue through procedure with parenteral dosage
Antiarrhythmics	Administer the morning of surgery
Nitrates	Hold oral nitrates the day of surgery
Diuretics	Hold day of surgery
HMG-CoA reductase inhibitors (statins)	Administer through the perioperative period
Nonstatin lipid-lowering agents	Discontinue preoperatively
Low-molecular-weight heparin	Hold 12 hr before procedure
Unfractionated heparin drip	Hold 6 hr before procedure
Warfarin	Hold 4-5 days before surgery with or without heparin bridge, depending on indication for anticoagulation
Aspirin	Hold 5-7 days before procedures with high bleeding risk
Clopidogrel	Hold 5-7 days before procedures with high bleeding risk
NSAIDs	Hold 1-2 days before procedure
β$_2$-Agonists	Continue the morning of surgery through postoperative period
Inhaled anticholinergics	Continue the morning of surgery through postoperative period
Leukotriene modifiers	Administer the morning of surgery through postoperative period
Hormone replacement therapy	Discontinue 4-6 wk before procedures with high risk of venous thromboembolism
Selective estrogen receptor modifiers	Discontinue 4-6 wk before procedures with high risk of venous thromboembolism
Oral contraceptives	Administer the morning of surgery through postoperative period
Antiretroviral agents	Continue if anticipate patient will be able to take PO; if NPO status anticipated, stop all simultaneously, except: hold efavirenz 4 days and nevirapine 2 days before stopping other antiretrovirals

arenteral Equivalents	Comments
metoprolol, labetalol, esmolol	
enalaprilat	Has been associated with intraoperative hypotension with ACE inhibitors responsive only to vasopressin; could administer day of surgery for minor procedures or with anticipated hypertension or dysrhythmia
	Similar profile as ACE inhibitors; IV enalaprilat reasonable parenteral substitution for PO ARB; could administer day of surgery for minor procedures or with anticipated hypertension or dysrhythmia
diltiazem, verapamil, nicardipine	Could administer day of surgery for minor procedures or with anticipated hypertension or dysrhythmia
Clonidine transdermal patch	Use in high-cardiovascular risk patients who have contraindications to β-blockers
amiodarone	Amiodarone generally not required during NPO period owing to long half-life of drug
nitroglycerin	Benefit established only in patients with active ischemia
furosemide, bumetanide	Avoid preoperative overdiuresis
	Restart as soon enteral function returns
	Restart when renal and gastrointestinal function stability ensured
	For once-daily administration, hold 24 hr before procedure
	On restarting postoperatively, use the previous therapeutic dose without a loading bolus
unfractionated heparin drip or low-molecular-weight heparin subcutaneously	Patients restarting warfarin after an extended period of NPO status may be more sensitive to warfarin
	Aspirin should be continued during vascular and cardiac surgery, and possibly in for those at high cardiovascular risk, depending on bleeding risk of planned surgery
	Clopidogrel should not be discontinued within the first 6 wk following cardiac stent placement
torolac	COX-2 inhibitors do not inhibit platelet aggregation but do influence renal hemodynamics and are associated with poorer outcomes in cardiac surgical patients
	Avoid oral preparations
	For lower-risk procedures, continue through surgery using DVT prophylaxis
	For lower-risk procedures, continue through surgery using DVT prophylaxis
	If patient is NPO and misses any doses, counsel for the need for alternate contraception through the next cycle
	All agents should be restarted simultaneously

Table continued on following page

TABLE 21-2	Management of Commonly Prescribed Medications *(Continued)*
Medication	**Preoperative Management**
Transplantation antirejection medications	Continue through surgery
Selective serotonin reuptake inhibitors	Administer half dose for 3 days preoperatively if NPO period is anticipated postoperatively
Tricyclic antidepressants	Continue through surgery with precautions
Monoamine oxidase inhibitors	Consult with anesthesiologist regarding use of MAO inhibitor–safe anesthesia
Lithium	Administer the morning of surgery through postoperative period
Antipsychotics	Administer the morning of surgery through postoperative period

ACE, angiotensin-converting enzyme; ARB, angiotensin II receptor blocker; COX, cyclooxygenase; DVT, deep venous thrombosis; HMG-CoA, hepatic 3-methylglutaryl–coenzyme A; IM, intramuscular; IV, intravenous; MAO, monoamine oxidase; NPO, nothing by mouth; NSAID, nonsteroidal anti-inflammatory drug; PO, oral.

60 to 70 beats/ minute in the perioperative period. For the patient who requires perioperative β-blocker therapy but does not have indications for the long-term use of β-blockers, we typically continue the β-blocker for 30 days postoperatively and then rapidly taper it.

Adverse Events with Perioperative Initiation of β-Blockers

In the perioperative period, risks specifically associated with initiation of β-blockers include worsening of severe obstructive lung disease or congestive heart failure and bradycardia.

Adverse Events with Cessation of Long-Term β-Blocker Use

For patients who take β-blockers on a long-term basis, sudden cessation of these agents may be associated with adverse cardiovascular events. The most dramatic manifestation is the

arenteral Equivalents	Comments
eroids, tacrolimus, cyclo-sporine, mycophenolate	Monitor drug levels
	Watch for serotonin syndrome induced by meperidine and antiemetics in patients with long-term fluoxetine preoperatively
	Monitor drug levels
ultiple IV/IM forms available	Long-acting decanoate forms can be administered if a long period of NPO status is anticipated

well-known *hyperadrenergic withdrawal syndrome*, characterized by increased blood pressure and heart rate. However, even in the absence of symptomatic or overt signs of increased sympathetic drive, postoperative withdrawal of β-blockers increases the rate of subsequent myocardial infarctions in vascular surgical patients [Hoeks et al, 2007]. Withdrawal syndromes are less severe with longer-acting agents such as atenolol. For patients unable to take oral medications postoperatively, adverse events related to withdrawal can be prevented through the use of intravenous preparations, with transition back to oral administration when oral medications are tolerated.

Angiotensin-Converting Enzyme Inhibitors

Only modest amounts of research have specifically examined the use of angiotensin-converting enzyme (ACE) inhibitors in the perioperative period. What is established is that ACE inhibitors are not associated with increased perioperative mortality and do not potentiate or attenuate the level of anesthesia, although long-term treatment with ACE inhibitors may increase the frequency of hypotension during induction of anesthesia. This effect does not appear to be present during spinal anesthesia. ACE inhibitor-associated intraoperative hypotension can be made worse by hypovolemia and is sometimes refractory to vasopressors. Although long-term ACE inhibitor use has been linked to postoperative renal dysfunction, other investigators have postulated renoprotective effects in patients undergoing coronary artery bypass grafting surgery.

No hypertensive withdrawal syndrome or immediate decompensation of otherwise stable congestive heart failure has been reported following cessation of ACE inhibitors. Therefore, in an effort to avoid ACE inhibitor-related perioperative hypotension or renal dysfunction, we recommend that ACE inhibitors be withheld the day of surgery and resumed as soon as possible in the postoperative period. For minor surgical procedures, particularly in patients with blood pressure that is difficult to control, administration of a usual dose of an ACE inhibitor with a sip of water on the morning of surgery may be warranted. Postoperatively, patients who are receiving ACE inhibitors on a long-term basis and who have left ventricular dysfunction or postoperative hypertension with indications for ACE inhibition (i.e., diabetes) should be administered an intravenous ACE inhibitor (enalaprilat) if they are unable to resume oral intake. Anesthesiologists should be made aware of the patients' long-term use of inhibitors of the renin-angiotensin-aldosterone system, because intraoperative hypotension may be refractory to standard pressors and may require the use of vasopressin.

Angiotensin II Receptor Blockers

Like the ACE inhibitors, the angiotensin II receptor blockers (ARBs) derive their efficacy from inhibition of signals downstream from the angiotensinogen II receptor. In contrast to the ACE inhibitors, the ARBs do not potentiate the effects of the vasodilatory bradykinin system. The clinical implication of this differential inhibition remains unclear. ACE inhibitors and ARBs have comparable efficacy and safety in the treatment of chronic heart failure and high-risk myocardial infarction, although ARBs have a modestly decreased frequency and severity of side effects. Although some investigators have suggested that candesartan may protect against mesenteric ischemia in the setting of hypovolemia, the hemodynamic influences of the ARBs in the perioperative period are probably similar to those seen with the ACE inhibitors. Similarly, although ARBs theoretically cause less intraoperative hypotension than ACE inhibitors, treatment-resistant intraoperative hypotension has been noted with the ARBs. Given a lack of convincing data suggesting an advantage of the use of ARBs over ACE inhibitors in the perioperative period, the management of these two classes of medications should be similar. In the absence of known hypersensitivity to ACE inhibitors, intravenous enalaprilat should be used as an intravenous alternative to an ARB.

Calcium Channel Antagonists

Common practice has been to continue calcium channel blockers on the day of surgery and postoperatively, for hemodynamic stability and control. Most observational studies have not demonstrated a cardiac protective effect of calcium channel antagonists when these drugs are administered in the perioperative period. Calcium channel blockers do not appear to increase perioperative mortality, interact with anesthesia, or cause a significant withdrawal syndrome. Therefore, they may be continued through the perioperative period. For patients dependent on the rate-control properties of diltiazem or verapamil, these agents should be administered the morning of surgery. Use of these drugs on the morning of surgery is also warranted in patients who have a history of poorly controlled hypertension or in those undergoing minor procedures. Intravenous preparations are available for patients with extended periods of NPO status.

α_2-Adrenergic Agonists

Clonidine is the most commonly used agent of this class. The hypotensive effect of clonidine is mediated primarily by agonism of central nervous system α_2-receptors, which leads to increased parasympathetic tone and decreased circulating catecholamines. This global reduction in sympathetic output has made the drug a useful adjunct in the treatment of opiate withdrawal. Similarly, in a mechanism likely analogous to that seen with perioperative β-adrenergic blockade, clonidine use is associated with decreased mortality following vascular surgery and decreased ischemia and likely decreased mortality following cardiac surgery. This appears to be a class effect, because mivazerol (not available in the United States) has been shown to improve hemodynamic stability intraoperatively, to reduce cardiac ischemia during emergence from anesthesia, and to decrease late postoperative tachycardia and hypertension in patients at risk for or with coronary artery disease. On the basis of these findings, the American College of Cardiology suggested that some evidence (level IIB) indicates that α_2-adrenergic agonists may be cardioprotective in the perioperative period. Clonidine should be used for cardioprotective prophylaxis in patients with a contraindication to β-blockers.

Aside from cardiovascular indications, α_2-agonists are occasionally used de novo perioperatively, because they are known to have sedative, analgesic, and anxiolytic properties. Intrathecal clonidine has been used as part of an anesthesia regimen for postoperative pain control, whereas preoperative oral clonidine has been associated with decreased postoperative pain. Anesthesia induction with clonidine helps to prevent postoperative nausea and vomiting.

Particular care must be exercised for patients who take clonidine on a regular basis in the perioperative period. Cessation of clonidine can be associated with a *hyperadrenergic withdrawal syndrome* characterized by hypertension, tremor, and agitation. Given the benefits of sympatholysis in the surgical period and the risks associated with clonidine withdrawal, patients who have been taking this drug should have it administered orally the day surgery and resumed as soon as possible postoperatively. If a delay in the resumption of oral intake is anticipated, the patient should be transitioned to the clonidine transdermal patch preoperatively until enteral status allows oral administration of the medication. Although other α_2-agonists such as methyldopa have less of a propensity to cause a withdrawal syndrome, it is prudent to continue these agents during the perioperative period or transition to a clonidine patch.

The most effective treatment of postoperative clonidine withdrawal is resumption of clonidine. If this cannot be accomplished, labetalol (combined α- and β-blocker) may be used. Standard β-blockers should not be used to treat the patient with clonidine withdrawal syndrome because they block the peripheral β-receptors that facilitate peripheral vasodilation. Therefore, β-blockers could exacerbate clonidine withdrawal-related hypertension by preventing peripheral vasodilation in the setting of excessive α-stimulation.

Antiarrhythmics

Given the proarrhythmic effects of many traditional agents, the most commonly encountered antiarrhythmic drugs aside from the β-blockers and calcium channel blockers are amiodarone and sotalol. Amiodarone appears safe in operative patients, and the drug should be continued until the day before surgery. The drug has a half-life of 40 to 55 days, with pharmacodynamic effects lasting up to 50 days after the last dose. In light of this pharmacokinetic profile, pharmacologic efficacy is minimally influenced by missed doses. Unless there are extended periods of NPO status or serious arrhythmia, use of the intravenous formulation of amiodarone is not indicated. Intravenous formulations of flecainide, propafenone, or sotalol are not available. Patients who take these agents on a long-term basis should take them with a sip of water on the day of surgery. Patients who develop recurrent atrial fibrillation in the postoperative period should have their atrial rate controlled with intravenous diltiazem or a β-blocker, and oral agents can be resumed with the return of enteral motility.

Nitrates

For the treatment of intraoperative myocardial ischemia, vasospasm, or hypertension, intravenous nitroglycerin is preferable to transdermal preparations because of more reliable drug delivery. Unfortunately, nitrates can be associated with intraoperative hypotension, especially when these drugs are used in conjunction with anesthesia in a hypovolemic patient. **The use of prophylactic intravenous nitroglycerin is not associated with a reduction in ischemia in patients undergoing noncardiac surgical procedures** [❶ *Dodds et al, 1993*].

On the basis of available evidence, the American College of Cardiology and American Heart Association guidelines endorsed the use of intravenous intraoperative nitroglycerin in patients with clear signs of myocardial ischemia (level A). In contrast, even for high-risk patients, the use of intraoperative nitroglycerin as a prophylactic against ischemia is not well supported by the evidence (level IIB) and should be reserved for carefully screened patients. In all cases, nitroglycerin should be avoided in hypovolemic or hypotense patients.

In long-term users of these agents, a nitrate withdrawal syndrome of increased angina and myocardial ischemia has been suggested, but clinical studies of this possible effect yielded divergent results. Given inconsistent clinical observations, when nitrate withdrawal does cause an increase in arterial reactivity, the effect is likely modest. Because of the lack of demonstrated benefit in most patients, the risk of intraoperative hypotension, and the lack of well-characterized withdrawal syndrome, oral and transdermal nitrates should be held on the morning of surgery for patients without active ischemia. These preparations should be restarted in the postoperative period only when the patient has demonstrated hemodynamic stability.

Diuretics

Little evidence exists to guide the management of diuretic therapy in the perioperative period. Decompensated congestive heart failure is associated with poor surgical outcomes, so in patients with clinical volume overload, diuretics should be used until euvolemia is reached. In the more common case of a stable patient receiving diuretic maintenance therapy, management is ideally guided by clinical volume status. Hypovolemia places patients at risk for intraoperative hypotension and associated cardiovascular and cerebrovascular complications. Additionally, hypovolemia and associated hypotension are risk factors for postoperative renal failure, with diabetic and elderly patients at particularly high risk. **Unfortunately, clinical estimation of volume status and of the risk of postoperative hypovolemic hypotension in hospitalized and preoperative patients is often difficult** [● *McGee et al, 1999*]. For near-euvolemic patients, diuretics should be discontinued the day before the surgical procedure. Although diuretic-associated hypokalemia is well tolerated by patients in the perioperative period, attention should be paid to this phenomenon in patients taking digoxin or requiring large doses of β_2-agonists.

Hepatic 3-Methylglutaryl–Coenzyme A Reductase Inhibitors and Other Lipid-Lowering Agents

Hepatic 3-Methylglutaryl–Coenzyme A Reductase Inhibitors

The hepatic 3-methylglutaryl–coenzyme A (HMG-CoA) reductase inhibitors ("statins") have demonstrated efficacy in primary and secondary reduction of cardiovascular mortality and morbidity. Several lines of evidence support the continued use of statins in the perioperative period, especially in patients with established cardiovascular disease. Retrospective studies in noncardiac vascular surgical patients suggest an independent survival benefit associated with statin use in the perioperative period. The use of these drugs in thoracic surgical patients has been associated with preservation of renal function, decreased incidence of postoperative atrial fibrillation, and improved overall mortality. A mechanistic basis for beneficial effects of the statins is not explained entirely by reductions in low-density lipoprotein cholesterol and may be related to alterations of the release of endothelial nitric oxide. Evidence indicates that, in patients with acute coronary syndrome, withdrawal of statins may lead to worse outcome. Although no prospective randomized studies have been conducted to guide the use of statins in the perioperative period, the lack of interaction with anesthesia, coupled with the possibility of harm associated with withdrawal, lead us to recommend that statins be continued through the perioperative period. A rule of thumb is that if there are good clinical indications for statin use, they should be started for patients not previously administered these agents.

Fibrates, Ezetimibe, and Bile Acid Sequestrants

No evidence exists to indicate a rebound in cardiovascular events associated with the cessation of nonstatin lipid medications. The risk reduction in cardiovascular events is the result of long-term control of lipids with these agents, with generally little effect of short-term cessation. Because niacin and gemfibrozil have the potential to interact with statins to cause myopathy and rhabdomyolysis, these agents should not be restarted with statins until stable postoperative renal function is established. Fenofibrate appears less likely to have this interaction. Ezetimibe can cause diarrhea, whereas the bile acid sequestrants (cholestyramine, colestipol) can cause constipation and interfere with drug absorption. These agents can be resumed when the patient has documented stability of enteral function.

Anticoagulants

Decisions regarding the management of anticoagulants are based primarily on the risk of hemorrhage if anticoagulation is continued in the perioperative period as opposed to the risk and consequences of thrombosis if anticoagulation is withdrawn preoperatively. No prospective RCTs exist to offer definitive guidance to this problem. Our clinical approach has been to attempt to weigh the risks and benefits of discontinuing versus continuing anticoagulants on a case-by-case basis.

For patients receiving long-term warfarin therapy, most ophthalmologic procedures, dental extractions, joint injections, and many dermatologic procedures can be safely performed without interruption of anticoagulation or with an international normalized ratio (INR) at or slightly lower than the therapeutic range. Bleeding with dental procedures can be managed with tranexamic acid or ε-aminocaproic acid mouthwash. **Gastrointestinal procedures not requiring cessation of long-term anticoagulation include endoscopy or colonoscopy with or without biopsy, endoscopic retrograde cholangiopancreatography, enteroscopy, and biliary stent placement** [◉ Eisen et al, 2002]. Whether to perform a biopsy during esophagogastroduodenoscopy or colonoscopy while a patient is receiving anticoagulant or antithrombotic therapy is controversial and should be decided on a case-by-case basis.

For the patient with atrial fibrillation who is receiving long-term warfarin anticoagulation, we attempt to estimate the risk of systemic embolic phenomena without anticoagulation. If that risk is high, we use bridging anticoagulant therapy to minimize the amount of time the patient is not systemically anticoagulated. **The CHADS2 score is helpful in estimating thromboembolic risk** [◉ Gage et al, 2001]. In this scoring system, the patient with atrial fibrillation is assigned 1 risk point for the presence of each factor (C, congestive heart failure; H, history of hypertension; A, age >75 years; and D, diabetes mellitus) and 2 points if he or she has had a stroke or transient ischemic attack (S2). The patient with 0 points is at low risk for systemic thromboembolic phenomena, the patient with 1 to 2 points is at intermediate risk, and the patient with 3 or more points is at high risk. For the patient who is estimated to be at low risk of thromboembolic phenomena and who is to undergo a surgical procedure, we typically discontinue warfarin 4 days preoperatively and then restart it as soon as possible following surgery. For the patient at high risk, we discontinue the warfarin 4 days preoperatively and then initiate either a continuous infusion of unfractionated heparin (UFH) or low-molecular-weight heparin (LMWH) once the INR decreases to less than 2.0. Heparin is discontinued approximately 12 hours preoperatively and is then resumed as soon as possible following the surgical procedure. Warfarin is restarted when oral intake resumes. Heparin is discontinued when the INR is therapeutic. For the patient at intermediate risk of thromboembolic phenomena, we decide on a case-by-case basis whether to use the low-risk or the high-risk approach to treatment.

For the patient who is receiving warfarin anticoagulation for treatment of deep venous thrombosis (DVT), we consider the duration of their DVT treatment as well as ongoing DVT risk factors in determining perioperative anticoagulation management. For most patients with a cause of DVT that has been resolved and no ongoing DVT risk factors, the duration of anticoagulation is usually 3 months. For the patient with idiopathic DVT or DVT, the duration of therapy is 6 to 12 months. For the patient with DVT and antiphospholipid antibody syndrome or the presence of two thrombophilic conditions (e.g., factor V Leiden, prothrombin 20210 gene mutation), indefinite anticoagulation therapy is recommended. It has been estimated that stopping anticoagulation in the first month after the onset of acute DVT is associated with a 1% per day absolute increase in risk of recurrent venous thromboembolism. Stopping anticoagulation during the second or third month after an acute episode of DVT may be associated with a 0.2% per day increase in the absolute risk of recurrent thromboembolism. After 3 months of anticoagulant therapy, this risk decreases markedly. If the patient is nearing completion of the anticoagulation therapy, we often recommend that surgery be delayed until the completion of anticoagulant therapy. If that cannot be done or if the patient is receiving anticoagulant therapy indefinitely, we use a bridging anticoagulation strategy in a manner similar to the high-risk patient with atrial fibrillation.

Patients with prosthetic heart valves and atrial fibrillation and mechanical heart valves in the mitral position are at high risk of systemic thromboembolism if not anticoagulated. Our approach to their perioperative anticoagulation management has been to use a bridging approach similar to the high-risk patient with atrial fibrillation. An exception is the pregnant patient who has a mechanical heart valve. **We advise particular caution in the case of the pregnant patient who has a mechanical heart valve that requires long-term anticoagulation** [● Bates et al, 2004]. Currently available studies are inadequate to make definitive recommendations regarding anticoagulation management. The difficulties relate to the risk of fetal embryopathy resulting from warfarin and the inadequacy of efficacy data of LMWH and subcutaneous heparin in preventing mechanical valve thrombosis. The American College of Chest Physicians recommended one of the following approaches to anticoagulant management for the pregnant patient with a mechanical heart valve:

1. Adjusted dose twice-daily LMWH throughout pregnancy, either to keep a 4-hour postinjection anti–factor Xa level at 1.0 to 1.2 U/mL or according to weight.
2. Aggressive adjusted-dose UFH throughout pregnancy (generally 17,500 to 20,000 U subcutaneously) every 12 hours, to keep a midinterval partial thromboplastin time at least twice control or to attain an anti–factor Xa heparin level at 0.35 to 0.50 U/mL.
3. LMWH or UFH as per options 1 or 2 until the 13th week of pregnancy, then change to warfarin until the middle of the third trimester, and finally return to LMWH or UFH.

Small case series have shown that LMWH is not effective in minimizing thromboembolic risk in patients with mechanical heart valves. Until more robust data are available, we use continuous UFH to bridge anticoagulation during the period of warfarin withdrawal. The patient who has an aortic valve mechanical prosthesis and is in sinus rhythm is at a lower short-term risk of valve thrombosis or thromboembolic phenomena. If it is anticipated that anticoagulation will be resumed promptly following the surgical procedure, we typically discontinue warfarin 4 days preoperatively and then restart warfarin as soon as possible postoperatively. If anticoagulation is not expected to resume promptly after the surgical procedure, we not infrequently initiate therapy with UFH heparin or LMWH once the INR falls to less than 2.0 following the cessation of warfarin preoperatively. The heparin preparation is discontinued 12 to 24 hours before the surgical procedure and is then restarted as soon as possible postoperatively. We believe that this approach minimizes the time during which anticoagulation is discontinued in this group.

Anticoagulation Use in Neuraxial Anesthesia (Spinal Anesthesia and Epidural Anesthesia)

Bleeding associated with an epidural catheter has been linked to potentially devastating hematomas as a result of mass effect within the closed space of the spinal cord. If an epidural catheter is already in place, initiation of UFH for DVT prophylaxis (5000 U subcutaneously every 12 hours) is considered safe. Similarly, intravenous UFH is considered safe as long as it is started more than 1 hour following epidural needle placement. The epidural catheter should not be removed until 2 to 4 hours after cessation of heparin. Postoperatively, if LMWH is to be administered at prophylactic doses, the first dose should be held until 6 to 8 hours postoperatively, and the catheter should be removed at least 10 to 12 hours after the previous dose. Full-dose LMWH anticoagulation should not be used while an epidural catheter is in place. In all cases, LMWH should not be administered within 2 hours after removal of an epidural catheter. Fondaparinux should not be used in patients receiving neuraxial anesthesia.

For patients receiving postoperative warfarin, an epidural catheter should be removed before the INR is greater than 1.5. Nonsteroidal anti-inflammatory drugs (NSAIDs) do not appear to increase the risk of epidural hematoma formation.

Aspirin, Other Nonsteroidal Anti-inflammatory Drugs, and Antiplatelet Agents

Aspirin

Aspirin's antiplatelet effect preferentially protects against high shear conditions seen in the arterial vascular bed. This effect accounts for the key role of aspirin in the prevention of arterial thrombosis in patients undergoing coronary artery bypass grafting or vascular surgical procedures and, to a much lesser degree, in the reduction in postoperative venous thrombosis. Aspirin is routinely administered in the perioperative period to patients who undergo coronary artery bypass grafting. Similarly, patients undergoing infrainguinal vascular bypass or carotid endarterectomy should have aspirin therapy initiated in, or continued through, the preoperative period.

The incidence of surgical bleeding complications in aspirin users is increased by a factor of 1.5, although with the exception of neurosurgery, the severity of the complications is not increased. Withdrawal of aspirin is associated with an increase in cardiovascular events. For patients undergoing nonvascular surgical procedures, the decision to discontinue long-term preoperative aspirin administration should be driven primarily by bleeding risk and the indication for which aspirin was prescribed (primary or secondary cardiac prevention). Ocular surgery is associated with low risks of bleeding, and aspirin should not be discontinued. Patients undergoing higher-risk procedures such as neurosurgery or spinal surgery should have aspirin held 5 to 7 days preoperatively. It is not unreasonable to hold aspirin 3 to 5 days preoperatively with an intermediate risk of bleeding and then restart aspirin therapy 24 hours postoperatively in patients taking the drug for secondary prevention.

Thienopyridines and Dipyridamole

Clopidogrel has supplanted ticlopidine as the preferred adenosine diphosphate-mediated inhibitor of platelet function. Clopidogrel irreversibly inhibits platelets and has the same rate of hemorrhagic events as aspirin. Thus, patients who are receiving these agents on a long-term basis as an adjunct to antianginal therapy and are at low risk of acute cardiovascular events should have this medication held for 5 to 7 days before surgical procedures with higher risks of bleeding and then restarted 24 hours postoperatively if hemostasis is ensured. One of the most frequent uses of clopidogrel is in conjunction with aspirin to prevent acute and subacute stent thrombosis following implantation of a drug-eluting stent. For the patient who undergoes implantation of a sirolimus-coated coronary stent or **a paclitaxel-coated stent, the minimum course of postimplant aspirin and clopidogrel is 6 months. The time course of this mandatory antiplatelet regimen must be considered when planning noncardiac surgery** [● *Grines et al, 2007*]. For the patient who requires urgent or emergency surgery before completion of the mandatory aspirin-clopidogrel therapeutic regimen, we typically continue aspirin and clopidogrel in the perioperative period and use platelet transfusions if life-threatening hemorrhage occurs. One exception is the patient who requires neurosurgery. Because even a small amount of bleeding can be catastrophic in these patients, we review the management of antithrombotic therapy with a focus on the risks versus the benefits of antithrombotic discontinuation on a case-by-case basis.

Nonsteroidal Anti-inflammatory Drugs

Like aspirin, the non–cyclooxygenase-2 (non–COX-2)–selective NSAIDs exert an antiplatelet effect mediated by inhibition of the thromboxane pathway. In contrast to aspirin, this inhibition is reversible and will abate if the drug is eliminated. Platelet function returns to baseline 24 hours after cessation of long-term ibuprofen use, so NSAIDs should be held 1 to 2 days preoperatively. The propensity of NSAIDs to increase bleeding when they are administered postoperatively is unclear. In addition to their effects on platelets, the actions of NSAIDs on prostaglandins place the postoperative patient at a higher risk of gastrointestinal hemorrhage and renal failure. NSAIDs should therefore be used sparingly in patients at risk for these conditions, especially if pain can be managed by other modalities. NSAIDS have limited ability to cause postoperative renal dysfunction in patients without underlying kidney disease.

COX-2–specific agents do not inhibit platelet aggregation and may provide modest protection from gastric bleeding relative to nonselective agents. However, these agents have effects on renal hemodynamics that are similar to the effects of nonspecific agents. COX-2–specific drugs are additionally associated with an increase in postoperative cardiovascular events when they are used in cardiac surgical patients and thus should be avoided in favor of alternate means of pain control, such as opiates or acetaminophen.

Pulmonary Medications and Antihistamines

Most pulmonary medications administered on a long-term basis are those used in the treatment of the obstructive lung diseases. The inhaled anticholinergics have minimal systemic absorption or cardiovascular effects and should be continued through the perioperative period. Similarly, continuing the administration of regularly used inhaled β_2-specific agonists has been associated with a decrease in perioperative complications in patients with an obstructive lung process. Patients taking oral β_2-agonists are more at risk for dose-dependent side effects and should have these replaced with inhaled preparations, especially patients with concomitant cardiovascular disease. Similarly, no evidence indicates that parenteral β_2-agonists are more effective than inhaled formulations, although the parenteral agents carry increased cardiovascular risks of arrhythmias and myocardial ischemia. Inhaled bronchodilators are best delivered in mechanically ventilated patients by way of an in-line, spacer-equipped metered dose inhaler with actuation during the inhalation phase.

Stable patients who are managed with inhaled corticosteroids are not at higher risk of postoperative infection or adrenal insufficiency, and these medications should be administered throughout the perioperative period. Nebulized budesonide is available for patients with severe disease who are unable to use a metered dose inhaler. The few patients who require systemic corticosteroids should have these continued in the perioperative period, with potential use of stress doses, depending on the patient's standing dose and the extent of the surgical procedure.

The leukotriene modifiers are generally adjuncts to inhaled corticosteroids. They have excellent safety profiles, although no intravenous preparations are commercially available. These agents should be administered the morning of surgery and then resumed following the recovery of enteral function. Theophylline provides modest efficacy in chronic obstructive pulmonary disease, although it is associated with significant side effects, even within the therapeutic range. Given the narrow therapeutic index of theophylline, oral forms can be given until 1 or 2 days before the surgical procedure, and intravenous preparations should not be used.

First-generation antihistamines such as diphenhydramine, promethazine, and meclizine are effective in reducing postoperative nausea and vomiting. Antihistamines have been demonstrated to reduce intraoperative histamine-mediated adverse reactions. Thus, patients who take these agents on a long-term basis should continue taking them until the day before the surgical procedure. Routine use of intravenous postoperative antihistamines for allergic indications is not recommended, owing to the potential for sedation or urinary retention. Second-generation antihistamines such as fexofenadine, desloratadine, and cetirizine are very well tolerated and can be resumed in the immediate postoperative period. If first-generation agents are used, clinicians should be aware of the potential anticholinergic effects of urinary retention and decreased gastric motility.

Oral Contraceptives and Hormone Replacement Therapy

Both combination oral contraceptive pills and postmenopausal hormone replacement therapy have been associated with an increased risk of venous thromboembolic disease. Some concern exists that the higher risk associated with surgery can cause additional events in patients who continue these medications through the operative and postoperative periods. In one prospective study, the risk of postoperative thromboembolism in oral contraceptive users was found to be 0.96% versus 0.5% in nonusers. Simply stopping oral contraceptives just before a surgical procedure does not lower the risk of thromboembolism. The hypercoagulable state associated with combination oral contraceptive pills does not resolve until 4 to 6 weeks after discontinuation. Unplanned pregnancy also carries health risks. **Given these concerns and the small absolute increase in risk of venous thromboembolism, oral contraceptives should not be discontinued before elective surgery**. Instead, patients should be managed with aggressive DVT and pulmonary embolism prophylaxis. This approach is supported by the evidence-based clinical management guidelines of the American College of Obstetricians and Gynecologists. Oral contraceptives should be administered on the day of surgery. Particular attention should be paid to alternate forms of contraception in the subsequent month if the patient misses a contraceptive dose in the perioperative period.

As with oral contraceptive preparations, oral estrogen hormone replacement is associated with an increased risk of venous thromboembolism. Although older patients who take these medications are at higher risk of venous thromboembolism than are patients taking oral contraceptives, no good studies have evaluated the preoperative discontinuance of hormone replacement therapy. The guidelines of the American College of Obstetricians and Gynecologists suggest that these medications be continued during the perioperative period, with the use of appropriate DVT prophylaxis. For the patient who will undergo a procedure associated with a high risk of thrombosis, such as orthopedic surgery, hormone replacement should be discontinued 4 to 6 weeks preoperatively. A similar approach is indicated for the selective estrogen receptor modifiers, because they are also associated with an increased risk of venous thrombosis. If a selective estrogen receptor modifier is used for breast cancer treatment, consultation regarding optimal management should be made with the patient's medical oncologist.

Antiretroviral Medications

Special attention is required for the patient receiving antiretroviral medications whose surgical procedure necessitates cessation of oral intake in the perioperative period. Zidovudine is the only antiretroviral medication that is available in intravenous formulation. Because even short periods of monotherapy can generate resistance to antiretrovirals, all antiretroviral drugs should be stopped and resumed at the same time. Exceptions to this rule are the non-nucleoside reverse transcriptase inhibitors nevirapine and efavirenz, because of their extended half lives (20 to 30 hours and 40 to 55 hours, respectively) and the rapidity with which human immunodeficiency virus develops resistance to this class of medications. Nevirapine should be held 2 days and efavirenz 4 days before the cessation of other antiretrovirals. Patients who receive maintenance therapy with the subcutaneously administered fusion inhibitor enfuvirtide should have this medication held with other antiretrovirals. Administration of antiretrovirals sensitive to food effects should be resumed when oral intake has been firmly established. For minor procedures and those with no anticipated interruption in oral intake, antiretrovirals can be taken with a sip of water on the morning of surgery. Orally administered antibiotics taken for prophylaxis of opportunistic infections can be taken until the day of surgery and can generally be restarted when the patient has resumed enteral feeding.

Immunosuppressants Used in Organ Transplantation

Patients with transplanted organs are generally treated with numerous immunosuppressant mediations. Most antirejection medications have parenteral forms that are continued through the perioperative period. Sirolimus is available only as an oral form, but it has an extended half-life and can be administered through the NG route. Although no clear consensus guidelines exist for perioperative patients, most of these patients can safely miss a few doses of antirejection drugs, especially patients with a lower rejection risk (e.g., no prior rejection, >1 year from transplant, white race). Judicious use of therapeutic drug monitoring will aid in dosage adjustments. Patients with active infectious processes or difficulty healing may benefit from medication adjustment to decrease the degree of immunosuppression. Decisions about stopping and starting immunosuppressive medications in the perioperative period should be made in advance of surgery in collaboration with the patient's transplant physician or, if that is not possible, in consultation with a physician skilled in the use of immunosuppressives and the care of patients who have undergone organ transplantation.

Antidepressants

Selective Serotonin Reuptake Inhibitors
Serotonin amplifies platelet aggregation in the presence of agonists such as collagen and epinephrine. The selective serotonin reuptake (SSRIs) inhibitors decrease intraplatelet serotonin levels by 80%, and this leads to a decreased thrombogenic potential to normal or pathologic stimuli.

Mild attenuation of platelet activity by this and other mechanisms may be partly responsible for both the improved cardiovascular outcomes in patients taking SSRIs who have concomitant coronary arthrosclerotic disease, as well as the increased risks of gastrointestinal bleeding. A retrospective study noted a 3.7-fold increase in the need for transfusion in orthopedic surgery in patients who took SSRIs, but not in patients taking other classes of antidepressants. Although a relationship between dose and risk of bleeding has not been established, the degree of platelet inhibition is considerably less than that produced by aspirin or clopidogrel.

The bleeding risk from SSRIs in the preoperative period must be balanced with the risk of a withdrawal syndrome associated with sudden cessation of SSRIs. Dizziness, lethargy, paresthesia, nausea, vivid dreams, irritability, and lowered mood are the most common manifestations of discontinuation of these drugs. As with all discontinuation syndromes, symptoms are more common and severe with shorter-acting agents, such as paroxetine. Symptoms are not life-threatening and resolve within 24 hours of resumption of treatment. The return of depressive symptoms following discontinuation of SSRIs is much more gradual and only of concern after a week of cessation. Little good evidence is available to guide an approach to management of this drug class in the perioperative period. One approach that balances risks of bleeding with discontinuation symptoms is to administer half the dose of shorter-acting agents 3 days preoperatively and hold the day of surgery if NPO status is anticipated postoperatively. These medications should be resumed as soon as possible following surgery. Fluoxetine has a prolonged half-life and, if held, should be stopped 1 week preoperatively. For patients undergoing neurosurgical or other procedures with a high risk of operative bleeding and who have a lower risk of severe mood disorders, consideration should be given to earlier ($\approx$1 week preoperatively) discontinuation of SSRIs. This duration would need to be approximately 1 month in the case of fluoxetine.

Physicians caring for postoperative patients taking SSRIs, and especially fluoxetine, should also be aware of the potential for drug interactions causing the *serotonin syndrome.* This syndrome is characterized by agitation, hyperreflexia, hyperactive bowel sounds, and increased neuromuscular tone, often with hyperthermia. It can occur even if the patient is no longer taking fluoxetine because of the prolonged half-life of this particular SSRI. Drugs that could cause this interaction include other SSRIs or other antidepressants, tramadol, meperidine, fentanyl, and antiemetics. Treatment of the serotonin syndrome is with a benzodiazepine and the serotonin agonist cyproheptadine.

Tricyclic Antidepressants

The clinician should be aware of several risks if patients continue taking tricyclic antidepressants (TCAs) into the perioperative period. These drugs inhibit the reuptake of biogenic amines in the central and peripheral nervous system. This action can predispose patients to cardiac arrhythmias, and the effect may be increased with the use of pancuronium and volatile anesthetics such as enflurane. There have also been case reports of decreased seizure threshold in patients taking TCAs on a long-term basis who undergo anesthesia with enflurane. Agents with sympathomimetic properties may have exaggerated effects in the presence of TCA, and the dose of these medications may need to be reduced.

Discontinuation syndromes have been described that include agitation, irritability, and insomnia. When TCAs are used to treat depression, these agents should be tapered, when possible, over a week and held the day before surgery. For patients taking TCAs for pain, a prudent course is to allow preoperative withdrawal for a period of three to four drug half-lives, with control of pain provided by other, non-TCA agents.

Monoamine Oxidase Inhibitors

With the advent of SSRIs, the use of monoamine oxidase (MAO) inhibitors became less common. MAO inhibitors have been shown to have adverse drug interactions with meperidine and dextromethorphan and have the potential to cause hypertensive crisis if indirectly acting sympathomimetics are used concurrently. Although many clinicians recommend holding these agents 2 weeks preoperatively if possible, this approach raises the possibility of aggravating the patient's depression and the complications that could arise thereafter. It is best in these cases to work closely with an anesthesiologist who can follow MAO inhibitor-safe anesthetic protocols, with the avoidance of offending agents and the use regional nerve blocks for pain control when possible.

Lithium

Lithium is used in the treatment of bipolar disorder. It is likely that lithium can potentiate the duration of neuromuscular blocking agents (e.g., succinylcholine and decamethonium) that are used during induction of anesthesia and may prolong the effects of muscle relaxants, but lithium may safely be continued through the perioperative period with attention paid to monitoring levels. There is no intravenous preparation of lithium. Lithium is eliminated entirely by the kidneys, so we monitor postoperative renal function before restarting this drug. Additionally, because long-term lithium use can cause nephrogenic diabetes insipidus resulting in hypernatremia, the medical consultant should be aware of sodium and free water balance, especially when patients are not taking oral hydration.

Antipsychotics

The typical antipsychotics such as haloperidol and chlorpromazine are generally considered safe for use in surgery, and some of these agents have been used as anesthetic adjuncts for the treatment of emesis. Aside from the potential for Q-T prolongation and some mild anticholinergic effects, the newer atypical agents such as olanzapine and quetiapine are also considered safe in the perioperative period. A mild withdrawal syndrome of insomnia and agitation has been noted. This would be expected to be more common with the short-acting agents quetiapine and ziprasidone. Patients unable to take oral agents who require treatment for psychosis or agitation can be given parenteral forms of these drugs (e.g., haloperidol). Patients undergoing procedures with extended anticipated periods of NPO status can be administered long-acting decanoate forms (e.g., risperidone or haloperidol).

Herbal Medications

The use of herbal remedies and supplements is common and has been reported in up to 22% of preoperative patients. Most patients do not consider these substances "medications" and do not list them with their medications unless they are specifically asked about them. Management of patients taking these products is difficult for a variety of reasons. Preparations often vary in amount of herbal product present, as well as other ingredients. Neither a mechanism of purported action nor a dose response has been identified for most products, and very few have efficacy demonstrated by well-performed clinical trials. Adverse reactions to some products have been identified, such as induction of cytochrome P-450 3A4 by St. John's wort and adverse cardiovascular events from ephedra (ma huang). A proposed management approach is outlined in Table 21-3.

TABLE 21-3	Herbal Medicines in the Perioperative Period			
Herb	Purported Indications	Potential Drug Interactions	Possible Side Effects	Recommended Discontinuation
Ephedra (ma huang)	Increase energy, weight loss, asthma/bronchitis	Antidepressants, CNS stimulants, halothane	Increases in blood pressure, heart rate, arrhythmias	≥24 hr preoperatively
Garlic	Hypercholesterolemia, atherosclerotic disorders, hypertension	Aspirin, antiplatelet agents, and anticoagulants	Bleeding	≥7 days preoperatively
Ginkgo	Cognitive disorders, peripheral vascular disease, macular degeneration, erectile dysfunction	Aspirin, antiplatelet agents, anticoagulants, anticonvulsants, TCAs	Bleeding, decreased seizure threshold	≥36 hr preoperatively
Ginseng	Protection of the body against stress	Corticosteroids, MAO inhibitors, warfarin	Hypoglycemia, decreased INR	≥7 days preoperatively
St. John's wort	Depression and dysthymia	Antidepressants, piroxicam, tetracyclines, CNS stimulants, theophylline, cyclosporine, indinavir, ethinyl estradiol, midazolam, lidocaine, calcium channel blockers, warfarin	Increased photosensitivity, serotonin syndrome, induction of cytochrome P-450 3A4 (reduced INR, cyclosporine levels), possible withdrawal syndrome similar to SSRIs	≥5 days preoperatively

CNS, central nervous system; INR, international normalized ratio; SSRI, selective serotonin reuptake inhibitor; MAO, monoamine oxidase; TCA, tricyclic antidepressant.

Selected Readings

Ang-Lee M, Moss J, Yuan C: Herbal medicines and perioperative care. JAMA 286:208-216, 2001.

Bates S, Greer I, Hirsh J, Ginsberg J: Use of antithrombotic agents during pregnancy: Seventh ACCP Conference on Antithrombotic and Thrombolytic Therapy. Chest 126:627-644, 2004. **C**

Bertrand M, Godet G, Meersschaert K, et al: Should the angiotensin II antagonists be discontinued before surgery? Anesth Analg 92:26-30, 2001.

Burger W, Chemnitius JM, Kneissl GD, Rucker G: Low-dose aspirin for secondary cardiovascular prevention—cardiovascular risks after its perioperative withdrawal versus bleeding risks with its continuation: Review and meta-analysis. J Intern Med 257:399-414, 2005.

Comfere T, Sprung J, Kumar MM, et al: Angiotensin system inhibitors in a general surgical population. Anesth Analg 100:636-644, 2005.

Coriat P, Richner C, Douraki T, et al: Influence of chronic angiotensin converting enzyme inhibition on anesthetic induction. Anesthesiology 81:299-307, 1994.

Dodds TM, Stone JG, Coromilas J: Prophylactic nitroglycerine infusion during noncardiac surgery does not reduce perioperative ischemia. Anesth Analg 76:705-713, 1993. **B**

Eisen GM, Baron TH, Dominitz JA, et al: Guideline on the management of anticoagulation and antiplatelet therapy for endoscopic procedures. Gastrointest Endosc 55:775-779, 2002. **C**

Elfant AB, Levine SM, Peikin SR, et al: Bioavailability of medication delivered via nasogastric tube is decreased in the immediate postoperative period. Am J Surg 169:430-432, 1995. **B**

Fleisher LA, Beckman JA, Brown KA, et al: ACC/AHA 2006 guideline update on perioperative cardiovascular evaluation for noncardiac surgery: Focused update on perioperative beta-blocker therapy. A report of the American College of Cardiology/American Heart Association Task Force on Practice Guidelines. J Am Coll Cardiol 47:2343-2355, 2006. **C**

Gage BF, Waterman AD, Shannon W, et al: Validation of clinical classification schemes for predicting stroke: Results from the National Registry of Atrial Fibrillation. JAMA 285:2864-2870, 2001. **B**

Grines CL, Bonow RO, Casey DE Jr, et al: Prevention of premature discontinuation of dual antiplatelet therapy in patients with coronary artery stents: A science advisory from the American Heart Association, American College of Cardiology, Society for Cardiovascular Angiography and Interventions, American College of Surgeons, and American Dental Association, with representation from the American College of Physicians. Catheter Cardiovascular Interv 69:334-340, 2007. **C**

Hoeks SE, Scholte OP, Reimer WJ, et al: Increase of 1-year mortality after perioperative beta-blocker withdrawal in endovascular and vascular surgery patients. Eur J Vasc Endovasc Surg 33:13-19, 2007.

Horlocker TT, Wedel DJ, Benzon H, et al: Regional anesthesia in the anticoagulated patient: Defining the risks. The second ASRA Consensus Conference on Neuraxial Anesthesia and Anticoagulation. Reg Anesth Pain Med 28:172-197, 2003. ⓒ

Kearon C, Hirsh J: Management of anticoagulation before and after elective surgery. N Engl J Med 336:1506-1511, 1997.

Lindenauer PK, Pekow P, Wang K, et al: Lipid-lowering therapy and in-hospital mortality following major noncardiac surgery. JAMA 291: 2092-2099, 2004.

McGee S, Abernethy WB, Simel DL: The rational clinical examination: Is this patient hypovolemic? JAMA 281:1022-1029, 1999. ⓒ

Wijeysundera DN, Naik JS, Beattie WS: Alpha-2 adrenergic agonists to prevent perioperative cardiovascular complications: A meta-analysis. Am J Med 114:742-752, 2003.

Appendix A
THORACOSCOPY AND VIDEO-ASSISTED THORASCOPIC SURGERY

MARK G. GRAHAM, MD
GREGORY MOKRYNSKI, MD

The indications for video-assisted thoracic surgery (VATS) are rapidly increasing, obviating the need for open thoracotomies. This appendix is limited to laparoscopic surgical procedures of the thorax.

I. Diagnostic Pleural Biopsy

A. Definition: fiberoptic scope–guided biopsy of pleural tissue through intercostal approach
B. Indications
   1. Pleural effusion of unknown origin (20% nondiagnostic rate after thoracentesis, 70% of these diagnosed with thoracoscopic biopsy)
   2. Primary pleural disease (mesothelioma, asbestosis-related changes, rheumatoid disease, pleural tuberculosis)
   3. Lung cancer (to identify the small percentage of patients with effusions who would benefit from lobectomy)
C. Duration of surgery: less than 1 hour
D. Anesthesia: conscious sedation
E. Transfusion requirements: none
F. Mortality: less than 1%
G. Postoperative complications
   1. Pneumothorax
   2. Hemothorax

H. Deep venous thrombosis prophylaxis
   1. Aggressive early mobilization
   2. For patients with additional thromboembolic risk factors (see Chapter 5, Table 5-1, on risk factors for deep venous thrombosis and pulmonary embolism), choose one of the following:
      a. Unfractionated heparin, 5000 U subcutaneously every 12 hours
      b. Low-molecular-weight heparin
         i. Enoxaparin, 40 mg subcutaneously every 24 hours
         ii. Dalteparin, 5000 U subcutaneously every 24 hours
      c. Intermittent pneumatic compression sleeves

II. Diagnostic Lung Biopsy

A. Definition: fiberoptic scope–guided biopsy of lung tissue through intercostal approach
B. Indications: failure of less invasive techniques to yield diagnosis of
   1. Peripheral lung lesions
   2. Diffuse pulmonary disease (e.g., infection, pneumoconiosis)
C. Duration of surgery: less than 1 hour
D. Anesthesia: conscious sedation or general anesthesia
E. Transfusion requirements: rare
F. Surgical mortality: less than 1%
G. Postoperative complications
   1. Pneumothorax
   2. Hemothorax
H. Deep venous thrombosis prophylaxis
   1. Aggressive early mobilization
   2. For patients with additional thromboembolic risk factors (see Chapter 5, Table 5-1, on risk factors for deep venous thrombosis and pulmonary embolism), choose one of the following:

   a. Unfractionated heparin, 5000 U subcutaneously
      every 12 hours
   b. Low-molecular-weight heparin
      i. Enoxaparin, 40 mg subcutaneously every
         24 hours
      ii. Dalteparin, 5000 U subcutaneously every
         24 hours
      iii. Intermittent pneumatic compression sleeves

III. Diagnostic Mediastinal Biopsy

A. Definition: fiberoptic scope–guided biopsy of mediastinal
   structures
B. Indication: to obtain tissue diagnosis of anterosuperior
   mediastinal masses, thus obviating the need for open
   mediastinotomy
C. Duration of surgery: less than 1 hour
D. Anesthesia: conscious sedation or general anesthesia
E. Transfusion requirements: rare
F. Surgical mortality: less than 1%
G. Postoperative complications
   1. Pneumothorax
   2. Hemothorax
H. Deep venous thrombosis prophylaxis
   1. Aggressive early mobilization
   2. For patients with additional thromboembolic risk fac-
      tors (see Chapter 5, Table 5-1, on risk factors for deep
      venous thrombosis and pulmonary embolism), choose
      one of the following:
      a. Unfractionated heparin, 5000 U subcutaneously
         every 12 hours
      b. Low-molecular-weight heparin
         i. Enoxaparin, 40 mg subcutaneously every
            24 hours
         ii. Dalteparin, 5000 U subcutaneously every
            24 hours
      c. Intermittent pneumatic compression sleeves

IV. Therapeutic Evacuation of Pleural Space

A. Definition: fiberoptic scope–guided procedure to remove loculated fluid or adhesions from the pleural space and fiberoptic scope–guided application of sclerosing agents into the pleural space

B. Indications
   1. Multiple adhesions preventing drainage of pleural space (e.g., empyema, malignant effusions)
   2. Need to prevent reaccumulation of pleural effusions (malignant effusions)
   3. Prevention of recurrent spontaneous pneumothorax

C. Duration of surgery: less than 1 hour

D. Anesthesia: conscious sedation or general anesthesia

E. Transfusion requirements: rare

F. Surgical mortality: less than 1%

G. Postoperative complications
   1. Persistent loculations with fluid
   2. Pneumothorax
   3. Hemothorax
   4. Inflammatory reaction to sclerosing agent
   5. Respiratory failure due to talc poudrage

H. Deep venous thrombosis prophylaxis
   1. Aggressive early mobilization
   2. For patients with additional thromboembolic risk factors (see Chapter 5, Table 5-1, on risk factors for deep venous thrombosis and pulmonary embolism), choose one of the following:
      a. Unfractionated heparin, 5000 U subcutaneously every 12 hours
      b. Low-molecular-weight heparin
         i. Enoxaparin, 40 mg subcutaneously every 24 hours
         ii. Dalteparin, 5000 U subcutaneously every 24 hours
      c. Intermittent pneumatic compression sleeves

V. Video-Assisted Thorascopic Surgery (VATS)

A. Definition: introduction of fiberoptic scope into the pleural space to assist the surgeon with thoracic surgical procedures (as listed here)

B. Indications
  1. Stapled lung biopsy
  2. Lobectomy/pneumonectomy
  3. Peripheral lung nodule resection
  4. Transthoracic vagotomy
  5. Creation of pericardial window
  6. Sympathetic trunk ablation
  7. Bronchopleural fistuloplasty

C. Duration of surgery: 1 hour

D. Anesthesia: general anesthesia

E. Transfusion requirements: rare

F. Surgical mortality: less than 1%

G. Postoperative complications
  1. Pneumothorax
  2. Hemothorax
  3. Infection
  4. Horner's syndrome

H. Deep venous thrombosis prophylaxis
  1. Aggressive early mobilization
  2. For patients with additional thromboembolic risk factors (see Chapter 5, Table 5-1, on risk factors for deep venous thrombosis and pulmonary embolism), choose one of the following:
     a. Unfractionated heparin, 5000 U subcutaneously every 12 hours
     b. Low-molecular-weight heparin
        i. Enoxaparin, 40 mg subcutaneously every 24 hours
        ii. Dalteparin, 5000 U subcutaneously every 24 hours
     c. Intermittent pneumatic compression sleeves

Selected Readings

Ballanleyne GH, Leahy PF, Modlin IM: Laparoscopic Surgery. Philadelphia, WB Saunders, 1994.

Boutin C, Viallat PR, Cargnino P, Farisse P: Thoracoscopy in malignant pleural effusions. Am Rev Respir Dis 124:588-592, 1981.

Davis RD, Oldham HN Jr, Sabiston DC Jr: Primary cysts and neoplasms of the mediastinum: Recent changes in clinical presentation, methods of diagnosis, management and results. Ann Thorac Surg 44:229-237, 1987.

Frantzider CT: Laparoscopic and Thoracoscopic Surgery. St. Louis, Mosby-Yearbook, 1994.

Hamed H, Fentiman IS, Chaudary MA, Rubens RD: Comparison of intracavitary bleomycin and talc for control of pleural effusion secondary to carcinoma of the breast. Br J Surg 78:12661267, 1989.

Lewis RJ: Thoracoscopy. In Grillo HG, Austin GW, Wilkins EW, et al (eds): Current Therapy in Cardiothoracic Surgery. Philadelphia, BC Decker, 1989, p 31.

Light RW: Pleural Diseases. Philadelphia, Lea & Febiger, 1990.

Loddenkemper R: Thoracoscopy: Result in cancerous and idiopathic pleural effusion. Poumon Coeur 37:261-264, 1981.

Menzies R, Charbonneau M: Thoracoscopy for the diagnosis of pleural disease. Ann Intern Med 114:271-276, 1991.

Pepper JR: Thoracoscopy in the diagnosis of pleural effusions and tumors. Br J Dis Chest 72:74-75, 1978.

Appendix B
LAPAROSCOPIC SURGERIES

MARK G. GRAHAM, MD
JEFFREY M. RIGGIO, MD

I. Laparoscopic Cholecystectomy

A. Definition: endoscopic removal of the gallbladder
B. Indications: cholelithiasis or cholecystitis, or both, without common duct stenosis
C. Duration of surgery: less than 1 hour
D. Anesthesia: general endotracheal anesthesia
E. Transfusion requirements: rare
F. Mortality: less than 1%
G. Complications
  1. Major bleeding: less than 2%
  2. Wound infection: less than 1%
  3. Biliary injury: less than 1%
  4. Bowel injury: less than 1%
  5. Need to convert to open procedure: 5% to 10%
H. Specific recommendations
  1. Deep venous thrombosis prophylaxis
    a. Aggressive early mobilization
    b. For patients with additional thromboembolic risk factors (see Chapter 5, Table 5-1, on risk factors for deep venous thrombosis and pulmonary embolism), choose one of the following:
      i. Unfractionated heparin, 5000 U subcutaneously every 12 hours
      ii. Low-molecular-weight heparin
        (a) Enoxaparin, 40 mg subcutaneously every 24 hours
        (d) Dalteparin, 5000 U subcutaneously every 24 hours
      iii. Intermittent pneumatic compression sleeves

2. Prophylactic antibiotics
    a. High risk: ampicillin, 2 g intravenously, and gentamicin, 1.5 mg/kg, 30 minutes before the procedure, followed by amoxicillin, 1 g orally, intramuscularly or intravenously, 8 hours after the procedure; for penicillin-allergic patients, delete ampicillin and amoxicillin and add vancomycin, 1 g intravenously, 1 to 2 hours before the procedure
    b. Moderate risk: amoxicillin, 2 g orally, or ampicillin, 2 g intravenously, 30 minutes before the procedure; for penicillin-allergic patients, substitute with vancomycin, 1 g intravenously, 1 to 2 hours before the procedure
    c. Low risk: none suggested
I. Advantages over open procedure
    1. Less morbidity
    2. Preoperative diagnosis unclear (gallbladder versus appendix versus gynecologic problem)

II. Laparoscopic Appendectomy

A. Definition: removal of appendix by laparoscope
B. Indications: acute or chronic appendicitis
C. Duration of surgery: less than 1 hour
D. Anesthesia: general anesthesia
E. Transfusion requirements: rare
F. Surgical mortality: less than 1%
G. Postoperative complications
    1. Hemorrhage
    2. Local infection
    3. Peritonitis
    4. Sepsis
H. Specific recommendations
    1. Deep venous thrombosis prophylaxis
        a. Aggressive early mobilization
        b. For patients with additional thromboembolic risk factors (see Chapter 5, Table 5-1, on risk factors for

deep venous thrombosis and pulmonary embolism), choose one of the following:

   i. Unfractionated heparin, 5000 U subcutaneously every 12 hours

   ii. Low-molecular-weight heparin

      (a) Enoxaparin, 40 mg subcutaneously every 24 hours

      (b) Dalteparin, 5000 U subcutaneously every 24 hours

   iii. Intermittent pneumatic compression sleeves

   2. Prophylactic antibiotics: same as earlier

I. Advantages over open procedure

   1. Less morbidity

   2. Preoperative diagnosis unclear

III. Laparoscopic Fundoplasty/Fundoplication

A. Definitions

   1. Fundoplasty: repair of lax lower esophageal sphincter for gastroesophageal reflux

   2. Fundoplication: reduction of gastric volume by placation of gastric fundus (a form of bariatric surgery)

B. Indications

   1. Fundoplasty: intractable gastroesophageal reflux disorder

   2. Fundoplication: morbid obesity

C. Duration of surgery: 1 to 3 hours

D. Anesthesia: general anesthesia

E. Transfusion requirements: rare

F. Surgical mortality: 0.5% to 1%

G. Postoperative complications

   1. Bowel perforation

   2. Surgical failure

   3. Herniation at trochar site

H. Specific recommendations

   1. Deep venous thrombosis prophylaxis

      a. Aggressive early mobilization

    b. For patients with additional thromboembolic risk factors (see Chapter 5, Table 5-1, on risk factors for deep venous thrombosis and pulmonary embolism), choose one of the following:

       i. Unfractionated heparin, 5000 U subcutaneously every 12 hours

      ii. Low-molecular-weight heparin

        (a) Enoxaparin, 40 mg subcutaneously every 24 hours

        (b) Dalteparin, 5000 U subcutaneously every 24 hours

      iii. Intermittent pneumatic compression sleeves

  2. Antibiotic prophylaxis unnecessary

IV. Laparoscopic Highly Selective Vagotomy

A. Definition: interruption of selective vagus nerve fibers

B. Indication: duodenal ulcer disease refractory to medical therapy

C. Duration of surgery: 3 hours

D. Anesthesia: general anesthesia

E. Transfusion requirements: usually none

F. Surgical mortality: less than 1%

G. Postoperative complications

  1. Dumping syndrome

  2. Diarrhea

  3. Recurrent ulcer disease

H. Specific recommendations

  1. Deep venous thrombosis prophylaxis

    a. Aggressive early mobilization

    b. For patients with additional thromboembolic risk factors (see Chapter 5, Table 5-1, on risk factors for deep venous thrombosis and pulmonary embolism), choose one of the following:

       i. Unfractionated heparin, 5000 U subcutaneously every 12 hours

      ii. Low-molecular-weight heparin

  (a) Enoxaparin, 40 mg subcutaneously every 24 hours
  (b) Dalteparin, 5000 U subcutaneously every 24 hours
   iii. Intermittent pneumatic compression sleeves
  2. Antibiotic prophylaxis unnecessary

V. Laparoscopic Nephrectomy

A. Definition: removal of a kidney by laparoscopy
B. Indication: diseased kidney
C. Duration of surgery: 1 to 2 hours
D. Anesthesia: general anesthesia
E. Transfusion requirements: usually none
F. Surgical mortality: less than 1%
G. Postoperative complications
  1. Vascular injury: 7%
  2. Other (e.g., small bowel obstruction): 17%
  3. Two to three times more complications when compared with open nephrectomy
H. Specific recommendations
  1. Deep venous thrombosis prophylaxis
   a. Aggressive early mobilization
   b. For patients with additional thromboembolic risk factors (see Chapter 5, Table 5-1, on risk factors for deep venous thrombosis and pulmonary embolism), choose one of the following:
    i. Unfractionated heparin, 5000 U subcutaneously every 12 hours
    ii. Low-molecular-weight heparin
     (a) Enoxaparin, 40 mg subcutaneously every 24 hours
     (b) Dalteparin, 5000 U subcutaneously every 24 hours
    iii. Intermittent pneumatic compression sleeves
  2. Antibiotic prophylaxis: unnecessary

Selected Readings

Ballanleyne GH, Leahy PF, Modlin IM: Laparoscopic Surgery. Philadelphia, WB Saunders, 1994.

Buchwald H, Avidor Y, Braunwald E, et al: Bariatric surgery: A systematic review and meta-analysis. JAMA 292:1724-1737, 2004.

Dajani AS, Taubert KA, Wilson W, et al: Prevention of bacterial endocarditis: Recommendations by the American Heart Association. JAMA 277:1794-1801, 1997.

Geerts WH, Pineo GF, Heit JA, et al: Prevention of venous thromboembolism: The Seventh ACCP Conference of Antithrombotic and Thrombolytic Therapy. Chest 126:338S-400S, 2004.

Jacobs SC, Cho E, Foster C, Liao P: Laparoscopic donor nephrectomy: The University of Maryland 6-year experience. J Urol 171:47-51, 2004.

Matas AJ, Bartlett ST, Leichtman AB, Delmonico FL: Morbidity and mortality after living kidney donation, 1999-2001: Survey of United States transplant centers. Am J Transplant 3:830-834, 2003.

Strasberg SM, Soper NJ: An analysis of the problem of biliary injury during laparoscopic cholecystectomy. J Am Coll Surg 180:101-125, 1995.

Appendix C
OBSTETRIC AND GYNECOLOGIC SURGERY

SUSAN E. WEST, MD
JOSEPH M. MONTELLA, MD

I. Vaginal Hysterectomy

A. Definition: removal of the uterus through the vaginal approach

B. Indications
   1. Uterine prolapse
   2. Carcinoma in situ of the cervix
   3. Obesity with pelvic relaxation
   4. Small leiomyomata with some relaxation

C. Duration of surgery: approximately1 hour, longer if laparoscopically assisted

D. Anesthesia: general (usually), spinal, or epidural anesthesia

E. Transfusion requirements: infrequent

F. Overall surgical mortality: less than 1%

G. Postoperative complications
   1. Ureteral injury (rare for vaginal approach) may occur during clamping or ligation of the uterine artery, with resulting flank pain with fever and ileus.
   2. Sciatic and peroneal injury (1 in 500) is more common than in abdominal hysterectomy.
   3. Vaginal cuff or adnexal infections are more common than in abdominal hysterectomy.
   4. Postoperative hemorrhage is more common than in abdominal hysterectomy.
   5. Deep venous thrombosis
   6. Vesicovaginal fistula

H. Specific recommendations
  1. Antibiotic prophylaxis for wound infection
    a. Cefazolin, 1 to 2 g intravenously, cefoxitin, 2 g, or metronidazole, 1 g as a single dose 30 minutes before the incision
    b. Bacterial vaginosis is a known risk factor for vaginal cuff infection. Metronidazole, 500 mg twice daily, should be given for 1 week, ideally starting at least 4 days preoperatively.
  2. Deep venous thrombosis prophylaxis
    a. Heparin, 5000 U subcutaneously given 2 hours before surgery and every 8 to 12 hours until the patient is ambulatory or discharged.

II. Abdominal Hysterectomy

A. Definition: removal of the uterus and cervix through an abdominal incision
B. Indications
  1. Malignant disease of cervix, endometrium, fallopian tubes, or ovaries
  2. Benign diseases: leiomyoma, endometriosis, or pelvic inflammatory disease
  3. Menorrhagia refractory to other medical or surgical therapies
C. Duration of surgery: approximately 1 to 2 hours
D. Anesthesia: general (usually), epidural, or spinal anesthesia
E. Transfusion requirements: usually not necessary, dependent on degree of dissection performed or size of uterus
F. Overall surgical mortality: less than 1%
G. Postoperative complications
  1. Ureteral injury during clamping or ligating the vascular bundle occurs in less than 1%. This may result in decreased urine output, flank pain, ileus, or unexplained fever.

2. Bladder injury occurs in 1.8%.
3. Sciatic and peroneal nerve damage is less common than in vaginal hysterectomies. Femoral neuropathy secondary to use of self-retaining retractors is a rare complication.
4. Ileus may last 3 to 4 days postoperatively.
5. Wound infections may manifest on postoperative days 4 to 5.
6. Deep venous thrombosis occurs in 12% to 15% of surgical procedures for benign disease but in 12% to 35% of hysterectomies performed for malignancy if patients are not given prophylaxis.
7. Septic pelvic thrombophlebitis may occur with unexplained high spiking fevers.

H. Specific recommendations
1. Antibiotic prophylaxis for wound infection: same as for vaginal hysterectomy
2. Deep venous thrombosis prophylaxis: same as for vaginal hysterectomy

III. Radical Hysterectomy

A. Definition: extended abdominal hysterectomy with bilateral deep pelvic lymphadenectomy, removal of parametrial tissue lateral to cervix and vagina, and removal of upper third of vagina with mobilization of ureters
B. Indications: stage IB and IIA carcinoma of the cervix
C. Duration of surgery: longer than 3 hours
D. Anesthesia: general (usually) or spinal anesthesia
E. Transfusion requirements: usually necessary, approximately 2 U of packed red blood cells
F. Overall surgical mortality: less than 1%
G. Postoperative complications: same as those in abdominal hysterectomy plus the following:
1. Deep venous thrombosis occurs in up to 40%.
2. Urinary fistulas may occur secondary to ureteral dissection and hypogastric artery ligation.

  3. Atonic bladder may result from interruption of para-sympathetic innervation in up to 30%.
  4. Ureteral injury from mobilization occurs in 2%.
H. Specific recommendations: same as those for abdominal hysterectomy

IV. Uterine Dilatation and Curettage

A. Definition: evacuation of endometrial tissue with curette following cervical dilatation
B. Indications: incomplete abortion; dysfunctional uterine bleeding, and postmenopausal bleeding if office endometrial biopsy is inadequate or difficult
C. Duration of surgery: less than 15 minutes
D. Anesthesia: usually general but also regional anesthesia
E. Transfusion requirements: rare
F. Overall surgical mortality rate: rare, less than 1%
G. Postoperative complications
  1. Uterine perforation occurs in 0.6% and is usually initially asymptomatic. Occult retroperitoneal or intra-abdominal hemorrhage may present with postoperative hypotension.
  2. Uterine artery damage can produce hemorrhage.
H. Specific recommendations
  1. Prophylactic antibiotics are not recommended for uncomplicated dilatation and curettage.
  2. Deep venous thrombosis prophylaxis is usually not necessary if the patient will be ambulatory on the day of surgery.

V. Abortion

A. Definition: removal of products of conception during the first trimester, usually accomplished by dilatation and suction curettage, rarely sharp curettage; during the second trimester, by suction, amniotomy, instillation, or curettage

B. Indications: termination of pregnancy
C. Duration of surgery: less than 1 hour
D. Anesthesia: general or regional anesthesia
E. Transfusion requirements: rare
F. Overall surgical mortality: rare, less than 1 in 50,000 by one account
G. Postoperative complications
   1. Uterine perforation
   2. Endometritis and parametritis with pain, fever, and vaginal discharge
   3. Amniotic fluid embolism rarely, with resultant disseminated intravascular coagulation
   4. Hypernatremia rarely if instilled hyperosmolar solution reaches the intravascular space
   5. Hyponatremia rarely with high-dose oxytocin infusions

H. Specific recommendations
   1. Antibiotic prophylaxis
      a. Doxycycline, 100 mg orally 1 hour before the procedure, then 200 mg orally after the procedure
   2. Endometritis should be treated with clindamycin, 600 mg intravenously every 8 hours, and gentamicin or tobramycin, dosed according to weight and renal function.

VI. Cesarean Section
A. Definition: delivery of fetus transabdominally
B. Indications: dystocia, breech or other abnormal presentations, placenta previa, abruptio placentae, failure of labor to progress or nonreassuring fetal heart rate tracing, maternal medical indications (cardiac, pulmonary)
C. Duration: less than 1 hour
D. Anesthesia: general or epidural anesthesia
E. Transfusion requirements: required in only 1% to 2%
F. Overall surgical mortality: less than 1%

G. Postoperative complications
   1. Postoperative ileus
   2. Hemorrhage from injury to uterine arteries or veins, uterine atony, or placenta accreta
   3. Injury to bladder or bowel occur in less than 1%
   4. Risk of endomyometritis is increased with increased length of labor and duration of ruptured membranes. It may present with fever, uterine tenderness, and foul lochia. Endometritis may progress to pelvic cellulitis and septic pelvic thrombophlebitis.
   5. Wound infections as per previous abdominal surgical procedures
H. Specific recommendations
   1. Antibiotic prophylaxis can decrease the incidence of endomyometritis, wound infection, and urinary tract infections. Ampicillin, 2 g intravenously, or cefazolin 1 g intravenously, is administered immediately after cord clamping. Penicillin-allergic patients may receive metronidazole, 500 mg intravenously, after the cord is clamped.
   2. Deep venous thrombosis prophylaxis is indicated for women at high risk.
      a. Heparin, 5000 U subcutaneously 12 hours before surgery and then 5000 U every 8 to 12 hours until patient is ambulatory or discharged.
      b. Pneumatic compression sleeves should be worn during surgery and then postoperatively until patient is ambulatory. They may be removed for out-of-bed activities or bathroom use.

VII. Laparoscopy

A. Definition: insertion of a fiberoptic scope into the abdominal cavity following needle insertion through abdominal wall into the peritoneal cavity with carbon dioxide insufflation
B. Indications: surgery for tubal occlusion, biopsy, aspiration of fluid, myomectomy, oophorectomy, ovarian

cystectomy, lysis of pelvic adhesions, pelvic pain, and recovery of ova for in vitro fertilization

C. Duration of surgery: dependent on indication but generally less than 1 hour

D. Anesthesia: general or local anesthesia

E. Transfusion requirements: none

F. Overall surgical mortality: rare, less than 8 in 100,000

G. Postoperative complications
   1. Uncontrolled hemorrhage may occur if the epigastric or mesenteric vessels are perforated.
   2. Abdominal wall injuries occur in 0.6%.
   3. Perforated viscus may occur.

H. Specific recommendations
   1. No indication for antibiotic prophylaxis
   2. Deep venous thrombosis prophylaxis only if the patient is not ambulatory

VIII. Pelvic Exenteration

A. Definition: radical hysterectomy, vaginectomy, total cystectomy, resection of rectosigmoid with formation of a colostomy and urinary conduit

B. Indications: locally recurrent or persistent cervical cancer after radiation therapy

C. Duration of surgery: 4 to 8 hours

D. Anesthesia: general anesthesia or combined general and epidural anesthesia

E. Transfusion requirements: often needed, may require 2 to 6 U of packed red blood cells

F. Overall surgical mortality: 3% to 5%

G. Postoperative complications
   1. Severe persistent ileus with third spacing of fluid is common. Extensive fluid shifts in volume similar to those in burn victims may occur.
   2. Hemorrhage
   3. Ureteral injury or obstruction may produce oliguria, acute renal failure, and fistulas.

4. Wound infections become apparent on postoperative day 3 or 4.

5. Deep venous thrombosis occurs in up to 45%.

H. Specific recommendations: same as for abdominal hysterectomy

IX. Correction of Female Urinary Incontinence

A. Definition: procedures in the form of retropubic suspensions or suburethral (midurethral) slings to address pelvic support or urethral sphincter deficiency

   1. Retropubic urethropexies: suspension of urethrovesical angle by suturing endopelvic fascia to the pectineal ligaments on the posterior surface of the pubic ramus

   2. Sling procedures: attachment of strips of rectus fascia, fascia lata, or cadaveric, allograft, xenograft, or synthetic material through an abdominal or combined vaginal-abdominal approach; newer categories of midurethral slings made of synthetic material done through a vaginal approach

B. Indications: stress incontinence from loss of support of the urethrovesical junction or urethral sphincter deficiency

C. Duration of surgery: approximately 1 hour

D. Anesthesia: general, spinal, or epidural anesthesia

E. Transfusion requirements: infrequently required

F. Overall surgical mortality: less than 1%

G. Postoperative complications

   1. Urethral occlusion from overaggressive surgery or edema may produce postoperative urinary retention.

   2. Ureteral kinking or ligation may occur with any procedure. Obstruction of the urethra causing urinary retention occurs in 13% to 20% of traditional slings and in less than 2% of midurethral slings and retropubic suspensions.

   3. Urinary tract infections may occur with urinary retention.

4. Bladder or ureteral injury may occur.

5. Hemorrhage is rarely a serious postoperative complication.

6. De novo detrusor overactivity occurs in 15% to 20%.

H. Specific recommendations

1. Antibiotic prophylaxis for wound infection: same as for vaginal hysterectomy

2. Deep venous thrombosis prophylaxis: same as for vaginal hysterectomy

Selected Readings

ACOG Committee on Practice Bulletins: ACOG Practice Bulletin 74: Antibiotic prophylaxis for gynecologic procedures. Obstet Gynecol 108:225-234, 2006.

Capeless E, Damron DP: Caesarian delivery. Available at http://www.Uptodate.com

Dajani AS, Taubert KA, Wilson W, et al: Prevention of bacterial endocarditis: Recommendations by the American Heart Association. Circulation 96:358-366, 1997.

Geerts WH, Pineo GF, Heit JA, et al: Prevention of venous thromboembolism: The Seventh ACCP Conference on Antithrombotic and Thrombolytic Therapy. Chest 126(Suppl):338S-400S, 2004.

Mann WJ Jr: Preoperative evaluation and preparation of women for gynaecologic surgery. Available at http://www.Uptodate.com

Appendix D
UROLOGIC SURGERY
SUSAN E. WEST, MD
DEBORAH T. GLASSMAN, MD

I. Transurethral Prostate Resection (TURP)

A. Definition: circumferential excision of prostatic tissue by resectoscope to the depth of the pseudocapsule
B. Indications: enlargement of prostatic tissue causing severe obstruction to urination
C. Duration of surgery: less than 1.5 hours
D. Anesthesia: general, spinal, or epidural anesthesia
E. Transfusion requirements: rarely needed; transfusions possibly required for large adenoma
F. Overall surgical mortality: less than 1% (2% if patient older than 80 years or with azotemia)
G. Postoperative complications
   1. Transurethral resection syndrome occurs from absorption of hyposmolar, nonelectrolyte irrigating fluid through the periprostatic veins with dilutional hyponatremia and hypervolemia. Clinical signs include hypertension, restlessness, confusion, tachycardia or bradycardia, muscle twitches, seizures, and eventually vascular collapse.
   2. Hemorrhage from arterial or venous sinus sources may be severe.
   3. Fibrinolysis may occur if excessive amounts of fibrinolysin are liberated into the blood from prostatic tissues, thus producing a fall in fibrinogen levels and bleeding diathesis.
   4. Postobstructive diuresis may occur.
   5. Disseminated intravascular coagulation may occur in patients with prostate cancer from release of thromboplastin from prostate cells.

6. If distilled water is used as an irrigating solution, hemolysis may occur.

7. Large fluid shifts may occur from absorption of irrigating solution, thus producing a transient expansion of circulating volume with hypertension, after which hypotension may occur from the shift into the extravascular space.

8. Deep venous thrombosis occurs rarely.

9. Septic shock may occur if infected urine is not treated preoperatively.

H. Specific recommendations

1. Limit resection time to less than 1.5 hours.

2. Transurethral resection syndrome requires supportive measures, and mild cases correct themselves within the first day. Hypertonic saline and furosemide may be necessary for sodium levels less than 110 mmol/L or for seizures.

3. Deep venous thrombosis prophylaxis is not recommended.

4. No prophylactic antibiotics are recommended if the urine is sterile. Infected urine should be sterilized with appropriate antibiotics preoperatively. Prophylaxis for subacute bacterial endocarditis should be given for patients with enterococcal urinary tract infections.

5. Preoperative coagulation studies should be checked in a patient with suspected or known prostate cancer or with symptoms of bleeding diathesis.

II. Open Prostatectomy

A. Definition: Simple prostatectomy is the enucleation of the prostate from within the prostatic pseudocapsule. Radical prostatectomy involves removal of the prostate, its capsule, and the seminal vesicles.

B. Indications
   1. Radical prostatectomies are performed for prostate cancer.
   2. Open simple prostatectomies are performed for urinary outlet obstruction and are preferred over transurethral prostate resection if the prostate is larger than 50 to 60 g or there is a concomitant bladder pathologic condition.
C. Duration of surgery: 2 to 3 hours
D. Anesthesia: general anesthesia is preferred; epidural and spinal anesthesia are alternatives.
E. Transfusion requirements: often less than 2 U of packed red blood cells
F. Overall surgical mortality: less than 1%
G. Postoperative complications
   1. Simple: Hemorrhage from the prostatic arteries and venous sinuses may be profuse. Radical: Dorsal venous plexus bleeding may be profuse.
   2. Postobstructive diuresis may result, producing hypovolemia and hyponatremia if fluid and electrolytes are not replaced. This is a rare complication and must be kept in mind.
   3. Deep venous thrombosis occurs in 30% to 50% of patients with open prostatectomies if no prophylaxis is used.
   4. Epididymitis occurs in 3% to 6% of patients.
   5. Urosepsis is common if infected urine is not sterilized before surgery.
   6. Urethrocutaneous fistula, persistent leakage of urine through the anastomosis, may occur. Prolonged drainage almost universally treats this condition.
H. Specific recommendations
   1. Antibiotics: No prophylactic antibiotics are required unless the urine is infected. Infected urine should be sterilized 24 to 48 hours before surgery. Prophylaxis for subacute bacterial endocarditis is given to patients with enterococcal UTIs.

2. Deep venous thrombosis prophylaxis (see Chapter 5)

III. Cystectomy and Urinary Diversion

A. Definition: removal of the bladder and lymph nodes. In men, the prostate and seminal vesicles are removed. In women, the uterus, cervix, and one third of the vagina are removed.

1. Ileal loop incontinent diversion: short segment of ileum interposed between the ureters and skin with creation of an external stoma to the loop of intestine

2. Continent urinary diversions: ureters anastomosed to reconstructed bowel, typically ileum, and right colon, with continent stoma allowing intermittent catheterization

3. Ureterosigmoidostomy: ureters ligated at ureterovesical junction and anastomosed to the sigmoid colon

B. Indications: malignancy or malfunction of lower urinary tract or other malignant diseases (e.g., cervical or rectal) requiring cystectomy

C. Duration of surgery: 4 hours or more; if performed with continent diversion, 6 hours or more

D. Anesthesia: general anesthesia preferred but also epidural or spinal anesthesia

E. Transfusion requirements: 2 U or more of packed red blood cells often required.

F. Overall surgical mortality: up to 4%

G. Postoperative complications

1. Prolonged postoperative paralytic ileus is expected.

2. Postoperative oliguria or anuria is often related to edema at the ureterointestinal anastomosis. This usually resolves in 12 to 24 hours as the edema subsides. Ureteral catheters are placed to prevent this complication.

3. Deep venous thrombosis occurs in 5% to 10% of patients not given prophylaxis.

4. Pyelonephritis occurs in 6% (>50% in ureterosigmoidostomies).

    5. Fecal or urinary leakage may occur immediately post-operatively or may be delayed because of necrosis at the bowel or ureteral anastomotic sites.

    6. Electrolyte disturbances may follow ureterosigmoid-ostomy in 50% of patients, with hypokalemia, hyper-chloremia, and acidosis.

    7. Obturator nerve injury, manifested as diminished ad-duction of the leg, may occur.

H. Specific recommendations

    1. Infected urine should be treated before surgery.

    2. Deep venous thrombosis prophylaxis is the same as for prostatectomy.

IV. Cystoscopy

A. Definition: insertion of fiberoptic scope into the bladder through the urethra

B. Indications: evaluation of hematuria; abnormalities of the urethra, bladder, or prostate; and difficult micturition

C. Duration of surgery: less than 1 hour. Simple diagnostic cystoscopy may only take 10 minutes.

D. Anesthesia: topical anesthesia if flexible cystoscope is used; otherwise, general or local anesthesia

E. Transfusion requirements: very rare

F. Overall surgical mortality: very rare, less than 0.01%

G. Postoperative complications

    1. Urethral or bladder perforation may occur.

    2. Mild hematuria is common.

    3. Urinary retention may occur.

    4. If urethral dilatation is performed, bacteremia may occur.

H. Specific recommendations: No prophylactic antibiotics are necessary, except for prophylaxis against subacute bacterial endocarditis, in patients with enterococcal UTIs. Infected urine should be sterilized before the procedure.

V. Nephrectomy

A. Definition

1. Simple nephrectomy: removal of kidney, usually through incision or laparoscopy

2. Radical nephrectomy: removal of kidney, Gerota fascia, ipsilateral adrenal gland, and retroperitoneal lymph nodes, usually by a transabdominal, flank, or thoracoabdominal approach or by laparoscope for tumors up to 10 cm in size

B. Indications: neoplasm (radical nephrectomy), severe trauma, chronic infection, renovascular hypertension, or renal donation (simple nephrectomy)

C. Duration of surgery: 2 hours for uncomplicated simple nephrectomy, 3 hours or more for difficult radical nephrectomy or laparoscopic procedures

D. Anesthesia: general anesthesia

E. Transfusion requirements: uncommon for straightforward cases; 2 to 3 U for radical nephrectomies or nephrectomies complicated by adhesions or abscesses. Transfusion for laparoscopic nephrectomy is infrequent.

F. Overall surgical mortality: 2% for radical nephrectomy; 1% for simple nephrectomy

G. Postoperative complications

1. Hemorrhage requiring multiple units of packed red blood cells may occur, especially with radical nephrectomies.

2. Pneumothorax may occur if the pleural cavity is entered.

3. Postoperative atelectasis is common, even if the pleural cavity is not entered. The intraoperative flank position decreases vital capacity by 15%.

4. Pancreatic injury may occur intraoperatively with typical postoperative signs and symptoms of pancreatitis.

5. Tumor thrombus extends into the inferior vena cava in 4% to 10% of renal cell carcinomas, thereby increasing the risk of pulmonary embolism. Deep venous thrombosis is a complication of simple or radical nephrectomies.

H. Specific recommendations

1. Prophylactic antibiotics are not necessary unless the kidney is infected. Pyelonephritis should be adequately treated preoperatively.

2. Deep venous thrombosis prophylaxis is the same as for prostatectomy.

3. Incentive spirometry should be taught preoperatively and continued postoperatively every waking hour.

VI. Renal Vascular Surgery and Percutaneous Transluminal Angioplasty

A. Definition: correction of renal artery lesions surgically or through intra-arterial balloon catheter

B. Indications: renovascular hypertension, renal failure from vascular disease, or structural lesions of renal artery (e.g., aneurysm)

C. Duration of surgery: less than 1 hour for percutaneous transluminal angioplasty (PTA); 1 to 2 hours for renal vascular surgery

D. Anesthesia: local anesthesia for PTA; general (usually), epidural, or spinal anesthesia for surgery

E. Transfusion requirements: rare in PTA, usually none with vascular surgery

F. Overall surgical mortality: less than 1%, up to 2% with severe atherosclerosis

G. Postoperative complications

1. Renovascular surgery

a. Postoperative hypertension may be severe and may be caused by intraoperative renal ischemia, pain, or hypervolemia.

    b. Hemorrhage may occur, especially with hypertension or unrecognized coagulopathy.

    c. Renal artery thrombosis occurs in less than 5%, usually within the first few days postoperatively. Embolism of atheroma from aorta may also produce occlusion of the renal artery. Symptoms include sudden hypertension and elevated creatinine levels. Nuclear medicine scans or arteriography may be necessary.

    d. Acute renal failure induced by ischemia may occur if the renal artery is occluded for more than 30 minutes intraoperatively.

  2. Percutaneous transluminal angioplasty

    a. Thrombosis or intramural dissection of the renal artery and perforation of the renal artery with retroperitoneal hemorrhage are possible.

    b. Acute renal failure from ischemia or contrast dye may occur.

    c. Cholesterol emboli from the aorta or renal artery may cause renal infarction or failure, or embolism from the aorta to the mesentery or lower extremities may occur.

H. Specific recommendations

  1. The patient should be well hydrated to minimize the risk of postoperative acute renal failure.

  2. Severe hypertension immediately postoperatively should be managed in a monitored setting, by maintaining diastolic pressure at 90 to 100 mm Hg to ensure renal perfusion.

  3. Deep venous thrombosis prophylaxis is the same as for prostatectomy

  4. Prophylactic antibiotics are not necessary. Infected urine should be sterilized preoperatively.

VII. Extracorporeal Shock Wave Lithotripsy (ESWL)

A. Definition: High-energy shock waves are used to break upper urinary tract stones into fragments small enough for spontaneous discharge.

B. Indications: upper urinary tract stones causing infection, obstruction, refractory pain, or significant bleeding

C. Duration of surgery: 1 hour

D. Anesthesia: general, spinal, or epidural anesthesia

E. Transfusion requirements: very rare

F. Overall surgical mortality: 0.01%

G. Postoperative complications
   1. Gross hematuria occurs in most patients.
   2. Sepsis can occur if the urine is infected at the time of the procedure.

H. Specific recommendations
   1. Patients with pacemakers may receive ESWL, but precautions should be undertaken to minimize the likelihood of inhibition of the pacemaker by the ESWL shock. Those precautions include programming the pacemaker to the VVI or VOO mode, synchronizing the ESWL shock wave to the electrocardiogram R wave, and monitoring the patient's electrocardiogram during the procedure. The pacemaker should be interrogated and reprogrammed following ESWL.
   2. Incentive spirometry should be taught before the procedure and continued thereafter.
   3. Urine output and serum electrolytes should be monitored and replaced as necessary.
   4. Prophylactic antibiotics are not needed unless the urine is infected. If the urine or kidney is infected, appropriate intravenous antibiotics should be started 24 to 48 hours before the procedure.

5. Deep venous thrombosis prophylaxis is not needed if the patient is discharged the same day. Otherwise, pneumatic compression sleeves should be worn on call to the operating room and continuously until the patient is ambulatory.

VIII. Percutaneous Stone Removal

A. Definition: nephrostomy tube insertion under fluoroscopy, urinary tract dilatation, and removal of upper urinary tract stone

B. Indications: upper urinary tract stones causing infection, obstruction, pain, or bleeding; favored over ESWL for large (>2 cm) or complex calculi, cystine stones, anatomic abnormalities, and stones within caliceal diverticula

C. Duration of surgery: less than 1 hour

D. Anesthesia: usually general anesthesia

E. Transfusion requirements: rare

F. Overall surgical mortality: less than 1%

G. Postoperative complications
   1. Hemorrhage with hematoma occurs in 5% to 13% but is usually self-limited. Macroscopic hematuria is common for the first 1 to 2 days.
   2. Arteriovenous fistula or pseudoaneurysm formation occurs in 0.5%, manifesting with brisk bleeding from the nephrostomy tube.
   3. Sepsis may occur with infected stones or urine.
   4. Rarely, guidewire perforation of the kidney, liver, pleura, spleen, duodenum, or colon may occur.

H. Specific recommendations
   1. Prophylactic antibiotics are not required. Infected stones or urine should be treated with appropriate intravenous antibiotics 24 to 48 hours preoperatively.
   2. Deep venous thrombosis prophylaxis is usually not required. Pneumatic compression sleeves may be used if the patient remains hospitalized.

IX. Retroperitoneal Lymph Node Dissection

A. Definition: dissection of lymph nodes from renal vessels to iliac vessels by an extensive midline approach

B. Indications: testicular cancer as well as renal, adrenal, prostate, and bladder cancer

C. Duration of surgery: more than 3 hours for extensive retroperitoneal dissection

D. Anesthesia: general anesthesia

E. Transfusion requirements: unusual unless a major vessel is injured

F. Overall surgical mortality: less than 1%.

G. Postoperative complications

    1. Sequestration of fluid into the retroperitoneum can produce hypotension. Rarely, damage to the cisterna chyli can produce chylous ascites.

    2. Vascular injury may produce hemorrhage and hypotension.

    3. Ureteral, splenic, pancreatic, and diaphragmatic injuries are possible.

    4. The risk of deep venous thrombosis is increased with the length of surgery.

    5. Sympathetic trunk injury may result in an ejaculation.

    6. Postoperative ileus is expected.

H. Specific recommendations

    1. Deep venous thrombosis prophylaxis is the same as for prostatectomy.

    2. Prophylactic antibiotics are advocated by some authors, such as cefazolin, 1 g intramuscularly or intravenously 1 hour preoperatively and then every 8 hours postoperatively for 3 days.

Selected Readings

Geerts WH, Heit JA, Clagett GP, et al: Prevention of venous thromboembolism: The Seventh ACCP Conference on Antithrombotic and Thrombolytic Therapy. Chest 126(3 suppl):338S-400S, 2004.

Taneja SS, et al: Complications of Urologic Surgery: Prevention and Management. Philadelphia, WB Saunders, 2001.

Wilson W, Taubert KA, Gewitz M, et al: Prevention of infective endocarditis: Guidelines from the American Heart Association: A guideline from the American Heart Association Rheumatic Fever, Endocarditis, and Kawasaki Disease Committee, Council on Cardiovascular Disease in the Young, and the Council on Clinical Cardiology, Council on Cardiovascular Surgery and Anesthesia, and the Quality of Care and Outcomes Research Interdisciplinary Working Group. Circulation 116:1736-1754, 2007. Epub 2007 Apr 19.

Appendix E
OTOLARYNGOLOGIC SURGERY

MARK G. GRAHAM, MD
JANINE V. KYRILLOS, MD

Note 1: Prophylactic antibiotics are indicated for some oto-rhinolaryngologic procedures that produce bacteremia in patients at high risk for infective endocarditis. Where indicated, the American Heart Association recommendations are as follows: (1) standard: amoxicillin, 2 g orally 1 hour before procedure; and (2) alternative: substitute amoxicillin with clindamycin, 600 mg, or cephalexin, 2 g, or cefadroxil, 2 g, or azithromycin 500 mg.

Note 2: Recommendations for VTE prohylaxis are based on the Seventh ACCP Conference on Antithrobotic and Thrombolytic Therapy, section on General Surgery recommendations. Evidence for VTE prophylaxis for minor procedures in VTE risk-free patients suggests the recommendation of early mobilization alone (Grade $1C^+$); evidence for those undergoing moderate-risk surgeries or patients with VTE risk factors undergoing minor surgeries suggests the use of either unfractionated heparin, 5000 bid, or LMWH, up to 3400 units/day (Grade 1A); evidence for those undergoing high-risk surgeries or patients with multiple VTE risk factors suggests the recommendation of either unfractionated heparin, 5000 tid, or LMWH of at least 3400 units/day (Grade $1C^+$). Grade 1A refers to randomized control trials (RCTs) without significant limitations; Grade $1C^+$ refers to no RCTs, but strong results can be unequivocally extrapolated, or overwhelming evidence from observational studies.

I. Otoplasty/Pinnaplasty

A. Definition: Plastic surgery of the auricle
B. Indications: correction of structural abnormalities of the auricle
C. Duration of surgery: variable, approximately 1 hour
D. Anesthesia: local anesthesia in adults, general anesthesia in children
E. Transfusion requirements: none
F. Surgical mortality: less than 1%
G. Postoperative complications
   1. Hematoma
   2. Perichondritis
H. Deep venous thrombosis prophylaxis
   1. Early mobilization

II. Foreign Body Removal from the External Ear

A. Definition: foreign body removal from the external ear
B. Indications: foreign body in ear
C. Duration of surgery: less than 1 hour
D. Anesthesia: local or general anesthesia
E. Transfusion requirements: none
F. Surgical mortality: less than 1%
G. Postoperative complications
   1. Local infection
   2. Hematoma
H. Deep venous thrombosis prophylaxis
   1. Early mobilization

III. Myringotomy

A. Definition: puncture of the tympanic membrane
B. Indications: serous otitis media
C. Duration of surgery: less than 1 hour
D. Anesthesia: general anesthesia
E. Transfusion requirements: none
F. Surgical mortality: less than 1%

G. Postoperative complications
  1. Persistent perforation
  2. Scarring of tympanic membrane
  3. Disruption of ossicular chain
  4. Perforation of jugular bulb with bleeding
H. Deep venous thrombosis prophylaxis
  1. Early mobilization

IV. Exploratory Tympanotomy

A. Definition: exposure of the tympanic cavity for diagnostic inspection
B. Indications: to clarify diagnosis of middle ear disorder
C. Duration of surgery: less than 1 hour
D. Anesthesia: general anesthesia
E. Transfusion requirements: none
F. Surgical mortality: less than 1%
G. Postoperative complications
  1. Disruption of ossicular chain
  2. Perforation of tympanic membrane
  3. Injury to chorda tympani nerve
H. Deep venous thrombosis prophylaxis
  1. Early mobilization

V. Stapes Surgery

A. Definition: removal of stapes, replacement with prosthesis
B. Indications: otosclerosis
C. Duration of surgery: 1 to 2 hours
D. Anesthesia: local or general anesthesia
E. Transfusion requirements: none
F. Surgical mortality: less than 1%
G. Postoperative complications
  1. Vertigo
  2. Nausea
  3. Vomiting
  4. Acute otitis media

5. Facial nerve paralysis
6. Sensorineural deafness
H. Specific recommendations
1. Vertigo prophylaxis with meclizine, 25 mg orally twice daily
2. Deep venous thrombosis prophylaxis: early mobilization

VI. Facial Nerve Decompression

A. Definition: decompression of facial nerve in or near the bony canal
B. Indications: facial nerve paralysis resulting from temporal bone fracture
C. Duration of surgery: 4 to 5 hours
D. Anesthesia: general anesthesia
E. Transfusion requirements: none
F. Surgical mortality: less than 1%
G. Postoperative complications: none
H. Deep venous thrombosis prophylaxis
1. Early mobilization

VII. Acoustic Neuroma Surgery

A. Definition: resection of the neuroma through craniotomy or the translabyrinthine route
B. Indications: symptomatic neuroma of the eighth cranial nerve
C. Duration of surgery
1. First stage: 5 to 7 hours
2. Second stage, 1 to 2 weeks later: 6 to 8 hours
D. Anesthesia: general anesthesia
E. Transfusion requirements: variable
F. Surgical mortality: less than 1%
G. Postoperative complications
1. Anteroinferior cerebellar artery thrombosis
2. Local bleeding/hematoma

3. Edema
4. Cerebrospinal fluid leak
H. Deep venous thrombosis prophylaxis
    1. Intermittent pneumatic compression

VIII. Glomus Jugulare Tumor Excision

A. Definition: resection of a glomus jugulare tumor
B. Indications: presence of a glomus jugulare tumor
C. Duration of surgery: 4 to 5 hours
D. Anesthesia: general anesthesia
E. Transfusion requirements: variable
F. Surgical mortality: less than 1%
G. Postoperative complications
    1. Bleeding
    2. Air embolism
H. Deep venous thrombosis prophylaxis
    1. Intermittent pneumatic compression

IX. Tympanoplasty

A. Definition: repair of injured tympanic membrane
B. Indications: tympanic membrane injury
C. Duration of surgery: 3 to 5 hours
D. Anesthesia: local or general anesthesia
E. Transfusion requirements: none
F. Surgical mortality: less than 1%
G. Postoperative complications: bleeding
H. Deep venous thrombosis prophylaxis
    1. Intermittent pneumatic compression

X. Nasal Fracture Reduction

A. Definition: reduction of nasal bone fractures
B. Indications: nasal bone fracture with disfigurement or airway obstruction
C. Duration of surgery: approximately 1 hour
D. Anesthesia: local or general anesthesia

E. Transfusion requirements: none
F. Surgical mortality: less than 1%
G. Postoperative complications: none
H. Deep venous thrombosis prophylaxis
   1. Early mobilization

XI. Nasal Polypectomy

A. Definition: removal of a nasal polyp
B. Indications: nasal polyp
C. Duration of surgery: approximately 1 hour
D. Anesthesia: local or general anesthesia
E. Transfusion requirements: none
F. Surgical mortality: less than 1%
G. Postoperative complications: none
H. Deep venous thrombosis prophylaxis
   1. Early mobilization

XII. Rhinoplasty

A. Definition: plastic surgery on the nose
B. Indications: cosmetic
C. Duration of surgery: approximately 1 hour
D. Anesthesia: local or general anesthesia
E. Transfusion requirements: none
F. Surgical mortality: less than 1%
G. Postoperative complications: none
H. Deep venous thrombosis prophylaxis
   1. Early mobilization

XIII. Caldwell-Luc Sinusotomy

A. Definition: access to the maxillary sinus by creating a window through the canine fossa
B. Indications
   1. Sinusitis refractory to medial or endoscopic surgery
   2. Sinus tumors
C. Duration of surgery: 1 to 2 hours
D. Anesthesia: general anesthesia

E. Transfusion requirements: none
F. Surgical mortality: less than 1%
G. Postoperative complications: bleeding
H. Deep venous thrombosis prophylaxis
1. Early mobilization

XIV. Ethmoidectomy

A. Definition: conversion of multichannel ethmoid labyrinth into a single large cell, thus providing effective drainage
B. Indications: chronic ethmoid sinusitis
C. Duration of surgery: approximately 1 hour
D. Anesthesia: local or general anesthesia
E. Transfusion requirements: none
F. Surgical mortality: less than 1%
G. Postoperative complications
1. Bleeding
2. Cerebrospinal fluid leak
H. Deep venous thrombosis prophylaxis
1. Early mobilization

XV. Frontal Sinus Trephination

A. Definition: external incision to expose the floor of sinus with creation of a conduit for drainage
B. Indication: chronic frontal sinusitis
C. Duration of surgery: 1 to 2 hours
D. Anesthesia: local or general anesthesia
E. Transfusion requirements: none
F. Surgical mortality: less than 1%
G. Postoperative complications: bleeding
H. Deep venous thrombosis prophylaxis
1. Early mobilization

XVI. Sphenoid Sinus Surgery

A. Definition: enlargement of sphenoid sinus ostium, providing effective drainage
B. Indications: sphenoidal sinusitis

C. Duration of surgery: approximately 1 hour
D. Anesthesia: local anesthesia in adults, general anesthesia in children
E. Transfusion requirements: none
F. Surgical mortality: less than 1%
G. Postoperative complications: bleeding
H. Deep venous thrombosis prophylaxis
   1. Early mobilization

XVII. Laryngectomy

A. Definition: removal of larynx
B. Indication: malignant laryngeal tumors
C. Duration of surgery: 6 to 7 hours
D. Anesthesia: general anesthesia
E. Transfusion requirements: 0.5 to 1.5 U
F. Surgical mortality: less than 1%
G. Postoperative complications
   1. Pneumothorax
   2. Pneumomediastinum
   3. Hypotension, bradycardia, apnea resulting from carotid sinus reflex
   4. Laryngospasm
   5. Bronchospasm
   6. Venous air embolism
   7. Pharyngeal fistula
   8. Hematoma
   9. Chylofistula
H. Deep venous thrombosis prophylaxis (one of the following)
   1. Unfractionated heparin, 5000 U subcutaneously every 8 hours
   2. Low-molecular-weight heparin
      a. Enoxaparin, 40 mg subcutaneously every 24 hours
      b. Dalteparin, 5000 U subcutaneously every 24 hours
   3. Intermittent pneumatic compression

XVIII. Tracheostomy

A. Definition: creation of a tracheocutaneous fistula
B. Indications
   1. Tracheal stenosis
   2. Need for prolonged mechanical ventilation
C. Duration of surgery: approximately 1 hour
D. Anesthesia: local anesthesia
E. Transfusion requirements: none
F. Surgical mortality: none
G. Postoperative complications
   1. Early: bleeding, tube displacement, aspiration pneumonia, recurrent laryngeal nerve paralysis, subcutaneous emphysema, mediastinal emphysema, esophageal injury
   2. Late: ostomy site infection, cannula occlusion, tracheal stenosis, tracheoesophageal fistula
H. Specific recommendations: none

XIX. Hemimandibulectomy/Radical Neck Dissection

A. Definition: excision of part of the floor of the tongue, mouth, palate, lip, and cheek
B. Indications: malignant oropharyngeal disease
C. Duration of surgery: 3 to 5 hours
D. Anesthesia: general anesthesia
E. Transfusion requirements: variable
F. Surgical mortality: less than 1%
G. Postoperative complications
   1. Loss of airway
   2. Bleeding
H. Specific recommendations: deep venous thrombosis prophylaxis (see Note 2)

XX. Mandibular Fracture Repair

A. Definition: mandibular fracture repair
B. Indications: fracture of mandible

C. Duration of surgery: 1 to 2 hours
D. Anesthesia: general anesthesia
E. Transfusion requirements: none
F. Surgical mortality: less than 1%
G. Postoperative complications: none
H. Specific recommendations: deep venous thrombosis prophylaxis (see Note 2)

XXI. LeFort Maxillary Fracture Repair

A. Definition: repair of fractures of maxilla
B. Indications: fractures of maxilla
C. Duration of surgery: 1 to 2 hours
D. Anesthesia: general anesthesia
E. Transfusion requirements: none
F. Surgical mortality: less than 1%
G. Postoperative complications: none
H. Specific recommendations: deep venous thrombosis prophylaxis (see Note 2)

Selected Readings

Ballenger J, Snow J: Otorhinolaryngology: Head and Neck Surgery, 15th ed. Baltimore, Williams & Wilkins, 1996.

Cummings CW: Otolaryngology: Head and Neck Surgery, 3rd ed. St Louis, Mosby–Year Book, 1998.

Dajani AS, Taubert KA Wilson W, et al: Prevention of bacterial endocarditis: Recommendations of the American Heart Association. JAMA 277: 1794-1801, 1997.

Dickens JR: Comparative study of otologic surgery in outpatient and hospital settings. Laryngoscope 96:774-785, 1986.

Gates GA: Current Therapy in Otolaryngology: Head and Neck, 5th ed. St. Louis, MO, Mosby, 1994.

Lee K: Essential Otolaryngology: Head and Neck Surgery, 6th ed. Norwalk, CT, Appleton & Lange, 1995.

Levine SB, Kimmelman CP, Zwillenberg S, Silberstein L: Blood transfusions in surgery of the larynx and neck. Laryngoscope 96:1095-1098, 1986.

I. Extracapsular Cataract Extraction

A. Definition: procedure to remove cataractous lens that leaves the posterior capsule of the lens intact; this allows an intraocular lens to be placed in the posterior chamber. In patients with severe glaucoma, this procedure may be combined with trabeculectomy.
B. Indications
   1. Decreased visual acuity interfering with activities of daily living
   2. Enlarged cataractous lens causing shift of the lens-iris diaphragm and secondary glaucoma
   3. Morgagnian cataract: an advanced cataract in which the lens protein liquefies and produces uveitis
C. Duration of surgery: less than 1 hour
D. Anesthesia: local or general anesthesia
E. Specific recommendations
   1. Early ambulation is encouraged.
   2. Resumption of preoperative medications is encouraged.

II. Intracapsular Cataract Extraction

A. Definition: cataract extraction that removes the entire lens, including the posterior capsule
B. Indications
   1. Marfan's syndrome or homocystinuria (both syndromes produce subluxation of the lens)
   2. Traumatic subluxation of the lens
C. Duration of surgery: less than 1 hour
D. Anesthesia: local or general anesthesia

E. Specific recommendations
   1. Early ambulation is encouraged.
   2. Resumption of preoperative medications is encouraged.

III. Trabeculectomy

A. Definition: a partial-thickness scleral flap is created so that a portion of the sclera and trabecular meshwork can be removed to create an alternative pathway for the egress of aqueous humor from the anterior chamber of the eye. In patients with visually significant cataracts, this procedure may be combined with cataract extraction.
B. Indications: primary open-angle glaucoma not responsive to medical therapy
C. Duration of surgery: less than 2 hours
D. Anesthesia: local or general anesthesia
E. Specific recommendations
   1. Patient may require 1 to 2 days postoperatively in the hospital.
   2. Patients' carbonic anhydrase inhibitors are typically stopped postoperatively to encourage the production and flow of aqueous humor through the surgically created fistula.
   3. Patients often need frequent atropine and phenylephrine drops, which may produce central nervous side effects.

IV. Cyclocryotherapy

A. Definition: A freezing probe is applied to the bulbar conjunctiva above the ciliary body to destroy the ciliary body and thereby to decrease the amount of aqueous humor produced.
B. Indications: treatment of glaucoma that has not responded to medical therapy
C. Duration of surgery: less than half an hour
D. Anesthesia: local anesthesia
E. Specific recommendations: none

V. Peripheral Iridectomy

A. Definition: an intraocular procedure to create an opening in the iris (as compared with peripheral iridotomy [see later], which is a closed procedure using a laser)

B. Indications
   1. Angle-closure glaucoma refractory to medical management in which the cornea is too clouded to perform laser iridotomy
   2. Peripheral iridectomy is also often performed as a part of other intraocular procedures (e.g., cataract extraction), when there is a concern about a possible element of angle closure or pupillary block glaucoma.

C. Duration of surgery: less than half an hour

D. Anesthesia: local or general anesthesia

E. Specific recommendations: none

VI. Laser Trabeculoplasty (Argon Laser Trabeculoplasty)

A. Definition: production of argon laser burns in the trabecular meshwork of the eye to improve aqueous humor outflow from the anterior chamber

B. Indications: primary open-angle glaucoma refractory to medical management

C. Duration of surgery: less than 15 minutes

D. Anesthesia: topical anesthesia

E. Specific recommendations: Patients typically need to have their intraocular pressures checked 1 hour after this procedure because there can be a significant elevation of intraocular pressure after laser treatment; the pressure elevation can be marked enough to necessitate an emergency trabeculectomy.

VII. Temporal Artery Biopsy

A. Definition: removal of a small portion of the temporal artery for histopathologic examination

B. Indications: suspected cases of temporal arteritis

C. Duration of surgery: less than 15 minutes

D. Anesthesia: local or general anesthesia

E. Specific recommendations: If the clinical suspicion of arteritis is extremely high, the patient is often given steroids before biopsy to avoid any delay in treatment. If the biopsy result is abnormal, the corticosteroids are continued.

VIII. Extraocular Muscle Surgery

A. Definition: reattachment of the extraocular muscles to the globe either to increase (resection) or to reduce (recession) their mechanical effect on eye movements

B. Indications: ocular misalignment producing either diplopia or a cosmetically unacceptable appearance to the patient

C. Duration of surgery: less than 1 hour

D. Anesthesia: local or general anesthesia

E. Specific recommendations: none

IX. Scleral Buckle

A. Definition: An encircling silicon ring is placed around the globe to indent the sclera and "buckle" it so that a retinal detachment will lie flat against the choroid.

B. Indications: retinal detachment

C. Duration of surgery: 2 hours

D. Anesthesia: local or general anesthesia

E. Specific recommendations
   1. Patients typically require 1 postoperative day in the hospital.
   2. Patients may be required to remain at bed rest if an intraocular gas bubble was used to help tamponade a retinal break.

X. Pars Plana Vitrectomy

A. Definition: removal of the vitreous humor from the eye by placing special suction, cutting, and irrigation instruments through the pars plana

B. Indications
   1. Vitreous hemorrhages that do not clear
   2. Often must be performed in cases of neovascularization or proliferative vitreoretinopathy with retinal tears and detachments associated with vitreal hemorrhages
C. Duration of surgery: 1 hour
D. Anesthesia: local or general anesthesia
E. Specific recommendations: same as those for scleral buckle

XI. Enucleation

A. Definition and indications: removal of an eye; performed for either a blind, painful eye or an eye with an intraocular malignant tumor
B. Duration of surgery: 1 hour
C. Anesthesia: local or general anesthesia
D. Specific recommendations: Patients typically spend a postoperative day in the hospital. Note: Vasovagal response to ocular pressure may result in bradycardia.

XII. Evisceration

A. Definition and indications: removal of the intraocular contents, leaving the sclera and extraocular muscles intact. It is performed when inflammation has destroyed the eye irreversibly or when severe panophthalmitis has created an abscess within the eye; its advantage over enucleation (see earlier) is that the prosthesis will have some mobility; it has the disadvantage that because the uveal tract is violated, there is a risk of sympathetic ophthalmia.

XIII. Orbitotomy

A. Definition: an exploratory procedure of the orbit behind the globe
B. Indications
   1. Mass lesions within the orbit

2. Infectious processes within the orbit
3. To decompress the enlarged extraocular muscles in thyroid eye disease

C. Duration of surgery: less than 3 hours
D. Anesthesia: general anesthesia
E. Specific recommendations: Patients typically spend 1 to 2 postoperative days in the hospital.

Selected Readings

Fraunfelder F, Roy F, Randall J: Current Ocular Therapy, 5th ed. Philadelphia, WB Saunders, 2000.

Kanski J: Clinical Ophthalmology: A Systematic Approach, 6th ed. London, Butterworth-Heinemann, 2007.

Riordan-Eva P, Whitcher J: Vaughan and Asbury: General Ophthalmology, 16th ed. New York, McGraw-Hill, 2004.

Appendix G
ORTHOPEDIC SURGERY
GENO J. MERLI, MD
JAVAD PARVIZI, MD

I. Cervical Fusion

A. Definition: immobilization of a joint to create a bony continuity between two or more adjacent vertebrae (may be performed by anterior or posterior approach)

B. Indications: intractable pain, instability, or neurologic deficit (from fracture or dislocation, degenerative disease, inflammatory lesion, neoplasm, subluxation or impaction, destabilizing procedure) that is not responsive to nonoperative treatment

C. Duration of surgery: 3 to 4 hours

D. Anesthesia: general anesthesia with nasotracheal or endotracheal intubation

E. Transfusion requirements
   1. Usually not required
   2. Approximate blood loss commonly 200 to 300 mL

F. Overall surgical mortality: less than 1%

G. Postoperative complications
   1. Bleeding
      a. The amount depends on the anatomic level, the number of segments to be fused, and the surgical approach.
      b. Arterial or venous bleeding is most common.
      c. Vertebral artery laceration is uncommon and is usually related to fusions near C1.
      d. Hematoma after anterior approach must be evacuated immediately because of the risk of airway obstruction.

2. Wound infection
   a. Infection usually occurs after the third postoperative day.
   b. Presentation may include wound erythema, induration, drainage, pain, and elevated white blood cell count.
   c. Incidence is correlated with the type of surgery, the use of antibiotics, and the length of the procedure.
   d. Treatment is determined by culture, early wound débridement, and pulsed irrigation.
3. Extension of fusion mass (very common)
4. Damage to laryngeal nerve from laceration, edema, or contusion (may result in temporary or even permanent hoarseness)
5. Paresthesias may be associated with passage of wires into the spinal canal.
6. Damage to or perforation of the esophagus or trachea
7. Graft extrusion with collapse and nonunion of fusion
8. Dural laceration
9. Damage to sympathetic chain (Horner's syndrome)
10. Pain, bleeding, or infection at the bone graft site
11. Air embolism
    a. This can occur intraoperatively during the posterior approach owing to the development of a gravitational gradient between an open vessel and the dependent right atrium.
    d. Presentation may include sudden hypotension, alterations in respiratory patterns, electrocardiographic changes, and cardiac arrest.
    c. Air embolism can be detected by end-expiratory carbon dioxide concentration monitoring.
12. Deep venous thrombosis and pulmonary embolism (see Chapter 5)

H. Specific recommendations
   1. Antibiotic prophylaxis
      a. Cefazolin, 1 g intravenously within 60 minutes preoperatively and every 8 hours for 24 hours, or

cefuroxime, 1.5 g intravenously within 60 minutes preoperatively and every 12 hours for 24 hours

b. β-Lactam allergy: vancomycin, 1 g 120 minutes before surgery and then every 12 hours for 24 hours, or clindamycin, 600 mg intravenously 60 minutes before surgery and then every 6 hours for 24 hours

II. Surgery for Hip Fracture

A. Definition: repair of fracture of the proximal femur by reduction and then fixation using one of a variety of metallic devices

B. Indications
   1. Relief of pain from fracture
   2. To increase ambulation to return the patient to previous functional status

C. Anesthesia: general or regional anesthesia

D. Duration of surgery: 1 to 2 1/2 hours

E. Transfusion requirements
   1. Blood loss of 50 to 500 mL may occur from the fracture itself before surgery.
   2. Operative blood loss may vary from 250 mL to more than 1 L depending on the extent of surgery.

F. Overall surgical mortality
   1. Operative: less than 1%
   2. Postoperative in hospital: 10% to 20%
   3. Within 6 months: 20% to 30%

G. Postoperative complications
   1. Deep vein thrombosis and pulmonary embolism (see Chapter 5)
   2. Infection
      a. Wound infection
         i. Superficial drainage (incidence of 5%)
         ii. Deep infection: Incidence is increased in elderly patients, in patients with decubitus ulcers, in bladder infections, when the wound is in close proximity to the perineum, and

with prolonged operative time. Symptoms include fever, hip pain, and decreased range of motion.

b. Urinary tract infection
   i. Incidence: up to 30%
   ii. Increased incidence with bladder catheterization

3. Osteonecrosis of the femoral head
   a. Occasional complication of femoral neck fractures that can occur after intracapsular, and especially displaced, fractures. Disruption of the major blood supply to the femoral head is believed to result in ischemia.
   b. Osteonecrosis may be followed by late segmental collapse (collapse of the subchondral bone and articular cartilage that overlies the infarcted area).
   c. Osteonecrosis of the femoral head may be an indication for total hip replacement.

4. Nonunion
   a. This is diagnosed by lack of radiographic evidence of healing 6 months after fracture.
   b. Incidence is related to fracture type, vascularity, and type of fixation.

5. Fat embolism
   a. This may occur 6 to 24 hours after surgery.
   b. Signs include tachycardia, dyspnea, confusion, petechial hemorrhage (of axillae, chest, and conjunctivae), and acute respiratory distress syndrome.
   c. Hypoxia is uniformly present.
   d. Anemia and thrombocytopenia may be present.
   e. Diagnosis is by exclusion of other causes.
   f. It may be self-limited if adequate ventilatory support and oxygenation are provided.

6. Post-traumatic osteoarthritis
7. Heterotopic ossification
8. Acute cholecystitis

H. Specific recommendations
  1. Antibiotic prophylaxis
    a. Cefazolin, 1 g intravenously 60 minutes preoperatively and every 8 hours for 24 hours, or cefuroxime, 1.5 g intravenously 60 minutes preoperatively and every 12 hours for 24 hours.
    b. β-Lactam allergy: vancomycin, 1 g 120 minutes before surgery and then every 12 hours for 24 hours, or clindamycin, 600 mg intravenously, 60 minutes before surgery and then every 6 hours for 24 hours
  2. Deep venous thrombosis and pulmonary embolism prophylaxis (see Chapter 5)

III. Total Knee Replacement

A. Definition: replacement of the three components of the knee joint (femoral, tibial, and patellar) with prosthetic components
B. Indications
  1. Severe pain, instability, or functional limitations not responsive to conservative management
    a. Osteoarthritis (primary or secondary to trauma)
    b. Inflammatory polyarthritis (rheumatoid arthritis, systemic lupus erythematosus, psoriatic arthritis)
  2. Failed previous knee surgery
C. Duration of surgery: 2 to 3 hours
D. Anesthesia: general or regional anesthesia
E. Transfusion requirements: usually not required
F. Overall surgical mortality: less than 0.1%
G. Postoperative complications
  1. Infection
    a. Infection may be caused by hematogenous spread or by spread from a contiguous site such as infected hematoma, cellulitis, or a suture abscess.
    b. Approximately 50% of infections are caused by *Staphylococcus aureus* or *S. epidermidis;* 25% are

caused by streptococci; and 25% are caused by gram-negative bacilli.
   c. The most frequent symptom of infection is pain. Other symptoms, including fever, erythema, swelling, and drainage, are variable. Wound drainage that persists for more than 10 days should be investigated
   d. Diagnosis of infection is made by serology, knee aspiration, blood culture, or open arthrotomy.
   e. Treatment consists of incision and drainage, débridement or removal of prosthetic components, and antibiotic administration.
2. Bleeding: Oozing from the wound may account for blood loss of 200 to 300 mL.
3. Deep vein thrombosis and pulmonary embolism
4. Component loosening
   a. Loosening may be septic or aseptic
   b. Aseptic loosening is a major long-term complication of total knee replacement.
5. Periprosthetic fracture
   a. The incidence approximates 0.5%.
   b. Fracture may be associated with rheumatoid arthritis, steroid use, osteopenia, neurologic disorders, and poor surgical technique.
   c. Signs and symptoms include pain, swelling, and inability to bear weight.
6. Dislocation or subluxation of components
7. Local wound complications
   a. May be secondary to beginning motion or physical therapy too early
   b. Delayed wound healing (wound separation, skin necrosis) or wound drainage, or both, may be seen.
8. Nerve injury
   a. Peroneal nerve injury occurs in up to 0.8% of patients.
   b. Symptoms occur from a few hours to 5 to 6 days postoperatively.

      c. Injury may be related to traction, local trauma, pressure from a dressing, splint, or cast, or disturbance of the vascular supply.

      d. Recovery may be incomplete in up to 50% of patients.

   9. Vascular injury

  10. Urinary retention and urinary tract infection occur in up to 20% of patients.

H. Specific recommendations

   1. Antibiotic prophylaxis

      a. Cefazolin, 1 g intravenously within 60 minutes preoperatively and every 8 hours for 24 hours, or cefuroxime, 1.5 g intravenously 60 minutes preoperatively and every 12 hours for 24 hours.

      b. β-Lactam allergy: vancomycin, 1 g 120 minutes before surgery and then every 12 hours for 24 hours, or clindamycin, 600 mg intravenously, 60 minutes before antibiotic prophylaxis with either cefazolin, 1 g, or vancomycin, 1 g intravenously preoperatively

   2. Deep venous thrombosis and pulmonary embolism prophylaxis (see Chapter 5)

IV. Total Hip Replacement

A. Definition: replacement of both sides of the hip joint by excision of the native femoral head and part of the neck and enlargement of the native acetabulum, followed by insertion of a femoral prosthesis into the femoral medullary canal and an acetabular component into the enlarged acetabular space. The components may be fixed either with cement or inserted press fit.

B. Indications

   1. Disabling pain or severe functional limitation, or both, not responsive to nonsurgical management

      a. Osteoarthritis (primary or secondary to trauma)

      b. Inflammatory polyarticular arthritis (rheumatoid arthritis, ankylosing spondylitis)

c. Other conditions such as developmental dysplasia, Paget's disease, benign neoplasm, and avascular necrosis

2. Reconstruction of previously unsuccessful hip surgery (osteotomy, prosthesis, cup arthroplasty)
3. Fracture, dislocation

C. Duration of surgery: 1 1/2 to 2 hours
D. Anesthesia: general, spinal, or epidural anesthesia
E. Transfusion requirements: 2 U of packed red blood cells
F. Overall surgical mortality: less than 1%
G. Postoperative complications
   1. Infection
      a. Sterile drainage (incidence: ≈8%)
         i. Clear serous drainage in benign-appearing wound without fever, pain, or change in appearance of wound margins
         ii. Not infected, but rather delayed wound healing
         iii. More common in obesity as a result of trauma of subcutaneous tissues
      b. Suprafascial
         i. Usually about suture or drain site
         ii. Localized swelling and redness with or without purulent drainage
         iii. No pain or temperature elevation
         iv. No progression to late deep infection
         v. Treatment with local care and intravenous antibiotics
      c. Deep (subfascial)
         i. Single most serious complication
         ii. Incidence: less than 1% (early postoperative period, 40%; 2 to 24 months, 45%; 2 to 5 years after surgery, 15%)
         iii. Cause: contamination during surgery, draining hematoma, or hematogenous spread from distant focus (dental infection, pneumonia, or urinary infection)

    iv. Causative agents: 55% staphylococci, 20% streptococci, 25% gram-negative species (*Pseudomonas, Escherichia coli*)

    v. Diagnosis: persistent and increasing pain, elevated sedimentation rate, positive aspiration, and culture results. Fever, drainage, wound inflammation, and swelling may not be present

    vi. Treatment: early aggressive débridement and intravenous antibiotics

  d. Urinary retention and infection occur with an incidence of 15% to 30%.

2. Bleeding
  a. Occurs in approximately 1%
  b. Develops on the 5th to the 12th postoperative day
  c. Presents with sudden onset of pain and fullness in the wound area
  d. May be implicated as a cause of late deep infection or sepsis, or both
  e. Nonoperative management: cessation of anticoagulants with reversal of anticoagulation if necessary, cold packs, and bed rest
  f. May drain in 24 to 48 hours
  g. Indications for surgery: impending necrosis of skin margins, uncontrollable pain, continued expansion of hematoma, neurologic signs, or symptoms

3. Deep venous thrombosis and pulmonary embolism (see Chapter 5)

4. Mechanical complications
  a. Occur after initial good result
  b. May present as abrupt onset of pain made worse with activity
  c. Periprosthetic loosening
    i. Process may be septic or aseptic (incidence of aseptic loosening: 1.2% to 2.4%)
    ii. Can often be demonstrated by plain radiographs

    d. Periprosthetic fracture
       i. Rare after primary total hip arthroplasty (0.1%) but may be higher in revision arthroplasty (4.2%)
      ii. May be secondary to trauma or to abnormal stresses placed on the native bone by the prosthesis
5. Hip dislocation
    a. Most common in first few months after surgery but can occur several years later
    b. Incidence: 0.8% to 2.4%
    c. Presents as acute pain in hip with extreme position as well as inability to stand on hip or return hip to functional position
6. Heterotopic ossification
    a. May occur to some extent in 20% to 50% of patients undergoing total hip replacement but causes symptoms in less than 4%
    b. Patients at risk include those with previous heterotopic ossification, diffuse idiopathic skeletal hyperostosis, Paget's disease, or ankylosing spondylitis.
7. Neuropathy
    a. Incidence: less than 1%
    b. Prognosis for recovery is good.
    c. May involve sciatic, femoral, obturator, or gluteal nerve
    d. May be caused by bleeding, surgical trauma, dislocation, stretching of nerve secondary to leg lengthening, entrapment by wire, or damage from cement
8. Fat embolism
    a. This occurs 12 to 72 hours postoperatively.
    b. It manifests with sudden tachycardia, respiratory distress, petechial rash on upper body, fat in retinal vessels, delirium, and coma
    c. Diagnosis is by exclusion of other causes.

    d. Treatment with corticosteroids, heparin, or ethanol has been proposed, but none has proved effective. Treatment remains supportive.

    e. The mortality rate is high.

  9. Cholecystitis

H. Specific recommendations

  1. Antibiotic prophylaxis

    a. Cefazolin, 1 g intravenously 60 minutes preoperatively and every 8 hours for 24 hours, or cefuroxime, 1.5 g intravenously 60 minutes preoperatively and every 12 hours for 24 hours

    b. β-Lactam allergy: vancomycin, 1 g 120 minutes before surgery and then every 12 hours for 24 hours, or clindamycin, 600 mg intravenously, 60 minutes before

  2. Deep venous thrombosis and pulmonary embolism prophylaxis (see Chapter 5).

Selected Readings

Bratzler D, Houck P: Antimicrobial prophylaxis for surgery: An advisory statement from the National Surgical Infection Prevention Project. Am J Surg 189:394-404, 2005.

Greenfield LJ (ed): Complications in Surgery and Trauma. Philadelphia, JB Lippincott, 1990.

Lawrence VA, Hilsenbeck SG, Noveck H, et al: Medical complications and outcomes after hip fracture repair. Arch Intern Med 162:2053-2057, 2002.

Quinlet RJ, Winters EG: Total joint replacement of the hip and knee. Med Clin North Am 76:1235-1251, 1992.

Appendix H
NEUROSURGERY
GENO J. MERLI, MD
KENNETH LIEBMAN, MD

I. Craniotomy

A. Definition: opening of a portion of the skull to obtain access for surgical intervention

B. Indications
   1. Establishment of histologic diagnosis for optimal adjuvant treatment and estimation of prognosis
   2. Provision of immediate palliation of increased intracranial pressure

C. Duration of surgery: variable, depending on the reason for procedure

D. Anesthesia
   1. General anesthesia
   2. Sedation with local anesthesia (to monitor patient's language function)

E. Transfusion requirement: minimal

F. Overall surgical mortality: less than 3%

G. Postoperative complications
   1. Postoperative intracranial hemorrhage is most frequently seen in the first 24 to 48 hours postoperatively. The cardinal sign is a change in mental status.
   2. Cerebral edema
      a. Most frequently seen in the first 48 to 72 hours postoperatively and manifested by a change in mental status
      b. Most frequently seen in central nervous system neoplastic disease
   3. Infection: In clean craniotomies, 2% to 5% will experience postoperative infections. This rate is decreased

by the use of antibiotics. Reoperation increases the incidence to 3% to 5% for each reexploration.

4. Seizures
   a. They occur in fewer than 5% of patients.
   b. Other systemic causes should always be considered.
5. Fluid and electrolytes
   a. Syndrome of inappropriate antidiuretic hormone
      i. Hypo-osmolality of serum
      ii. Hyperosmolality of urine: increased urinary sodium
   b. Diabetes insipidus
      i. Urine output 16 to 24 L/day
      ii. Urine specific gravity less than 1.01
      iii. Urine osmolality less than 290 mOsm/kg
6. Cardiac disorders
   a. Supraventricular tachycardia is the most common arrhythmia.
   b. Ventricular and atrial premature contractions can be seen but are not treated unless the patient is hemodynamically compromised.
7. Deep venous thrombosis and pulmonary embolism: incidence of 18% to 43% in patients not receiving prophylaxis
H. Specific recommendations
   1. Wound prophylaxis: cefazolin, 2 g intravenously
   2. Steroid prophylaxis depends on the reason for performing the craniotomy. Dexamethasone is begun before surgery and is continued postoperatively in the following manner:
      a. Administer a 20-mg intravenous loading dose followed by 4 mg intravenously every 6 hours.
      b. Taper over 7 to 10 days postoperatively.
      c. Maintain for patients receiving radiation therapy.
   3. Seizure prophylaxis with phenytoin
      a. Loading dose of 15 to 18 mg/kg intravenously, then a maintenance dose of 4 to 8 mg/kg intravenously (divided dose)

b. Loading 300 mg, 300 mg, 400 mg orally every 2 hours, then 300 mg every 12 hours

4. Fluid and electrolytes
   a. Syndrome of inappropriate antidiuretic hormone
      i. Restrict fluids to 500 to 800 mL/day
      ii. Intravenous hypertonic saline if serum sodium level less than 115 mEq/L
      iii. Demeclocycline, 300 to 600 mg orally twice a day
   b. Cerebral salt wasting
      i. Avoid fluid restriction
      ii. Salt replacement
   c. Diabetes insipidus
      i. Vasopressin, 5 to 10 U (0.25 to 0.5 mL) subcutaneously or intramuscularly; repeat two or three times daily as needed.
      ii. Desmopressin, 10 to 40 μg/day (0.1 to 0.4 mL) intranasally either as a single dose or two to three divided doses.

5. Deep venous thrombosis and pulmonary embolism prophylaxis: External pneumatic compression sleeves should be used intraoperatively and postoperatively until the patient is ambulatory.

II. Intracranial Pressure Monitoring

A. Definition: direct monitoring of intracranial pressure by intraventricular cannulation, intracerebral bolt, intraparenchymal probe, or epidural transducer
B. Indications: severe central nervous system trauma and postoperative intracranial tumor resections (postoperatively when intracranial pressures are a concern)
C. Duration of surgery: 30 minutes
D. Anesthesia: monitoring system is placed intraoperatively or under local anesthesia
E. Transfusion requirements: none

F. Overall surgical mortality: none
G. Postoperative complications: 4% to 5% risk of infection, with increased risk for wound infection
H. Specific recommendations: infection prophylaxis (variable) with vancomycin, 1 g intravenously every 12 hours while the catheter is in place

III. Lumbar Disk Surgery

A. Definition: disk herniation or rupture resulting in nerve root or spinal cord compression
B. Indications
   1. Neurologic signs (weakness, atrophy, sensory deficit, absent or asymmetric reflex, bowel or bladder dysfunction)
   2. Mechanical signs not responsive to conservative management
   3. Intolerable or increasing pain
C. Duration of surgery: 2 to 2 1/2 hours
D. Anesthesia: general or epidural anesthesia
E. Blood loss: 100 to 1000 mL, depending on procedure
F. Overall surgical mortality: 0.2% to 0.4%
G. Postoperative complications
   1. Infection
      a. Incidence: overall 4% to 5% risk of infection, with increased risk of local wound infection
      b. May include local wound infection, osteomyelitis, diskitis, meningitis, empyema, or abscess
   2. Hemorrhage (risk is small)
   3. Persistent pain may occur in 10% to 15% of cases.
   4. Dural tear with possible cerebrospinal fluid leak, which may result from excessive manipulation of the dura and must be repaired before closure
   5. Colonic ileus is seen 24 to 72 hours postoperatively.
   6. Deep venous thrombosis and pulmonary embolism incidence: 40% to 50%

H. Specific recommendations: Antibiotic prophylaxis with vancomycin, 1 g intravenously every 12 hours while the catheter is in place, is controversial.
   1. Wound infection prophylaxis
      a. Cefazolin, 1 g intravenously 60 minutes preoperatively and every 8 hours for 24 hours, or cefuroxime, 1.5 g intravenously 60 minutes preoperatively and every 12 hours for 24 hours
      b. β-Lactam or penicillin allergy: vancomycin, 1 g 120 minutes before surgery and then every 12 hours for 24 hours, or clindamycin, 600 mg intravenously 60 minutes before surgery and then every 6 hours for 24 hours
   2. Prophylaxis for deep venous thrombosis and pulmonary embolism (see Chapter 5)

IV. Transsphenoidal Surgery

A. Definition: an approach to the sella turcica through the sphenoid sinus with or without the assistance of an endoscope
B. Indications: ablative hypophysectomy; management of tumors of the area of the pituitary, such as pituitary adenoma, craniopharyngiomas, chordomas, and cholesteatomas; diseases of the sphenoid sinuses such as mucoceles, carcinomas, or cysts
C. Duration of surgery: 1 to 3 hours
D. Anesthesia: general anesthesia
E. Transfusion requirements: none
F. Overall surgical mortality: less than 1%
G. Postoperative complications
   1. Diabetes insipidus
      a. Usually does not appear before 12 to 24 hours postoperatively
      b. Criteria for diagnosis
         i. Urine output 16 to 24 L/day
         ii. Urine specific gravity less than 1.01
         iii. Urine osmolality less than 290 mOsm/kg

2. Cerebrospinal fluid rhinorrhea
   a. Cerebrospinal fluid assessment
      i. Cerebrospinal glucose concentration is 50% of the serum concentration.
      ii. Nasal glucose concentration is 10 mg/100 mL or less.
      iii. A spinal drain may need to be placed to treat the leak.
      iv. If the leak does not resolve in 10 days, a second surgical procedure will be necessary.
3. Sinusitis
4. Hypopituitarism requiring hormone replacement
H. Specific recommendations
   1. Wound prophylaxis
      a. Cefazolin, 1 g intravenously 60 minutes preoperatively and every 8 hours for 24 hours, or cefuroxime, 1.5 g intravenously 60 minutes preoperatively and every 12 hours for 24 hours
      b. β-Lactam allergy: vancomycin, 1 g 120 minutes before surgery and then every 12 hours for 24 hours, or clindamycin, 600 mg intravenously 60 minutes before surgery then every 6 hours for 24 hours
   2. Hypopituitarism treatment with hydrocortisone
      a. 100 mg intravenously every 6 hours before surgery and then tapered postoperatively
      b. Patients are discharged on physiologic maintenance doses, and their pituitary-adrenal axis is assessed on an outpatient basis.
   3. Diabetes insipidus
      a. Aqueous vasopressin, 5 to 10 U (0.25 to 0.5 mL) subcutaneously, two to three times daily
      b. Desmopressin, 10 to 40 μg/day (0.1 to 0.4 mL) intranasally as a single dose or two to three divided doses or 2 to 4 μg/day intravenously or subcutaneously in two divided doses

4. Deep venous thrombosis and pulmonary embolism prophylaxis (see Chapter 5)

V. Carpal Tunnel Release

A. Definition: complete division of the transverse carpal ligament to free the median nerve and its branches; can be accomplished through a traditional longitudinal palmar incision, "mini-incision," or endoscopically through single-portal or two-portal techniques

B. Indications: signs or symptoms (pain, paresthesias, muscle atrophy) of median nerve compression that do not respond to conservative measures (nonsteroidal anti-inflammatory drugs, splinting, local steroid injection)

C. Duration of surgery: 20 to 40 minutes

D. Anesthesia: local anesthesia under pneumatic tourniquet control or general anesthesia or regional anesthesia by axillary or brachial block

E. Transfusion requirements: none

F. Overall surgical mortality: negligible

G. Postoperative complications

1. Persistence or recurrence of symptoms for the following reasons:
   a. Incorrect initial diagnosis
   b. Incomplete section of transverse carpal ligament
   c. Injury to or laceration of the median nerve or its branches
   d. Flexor tenosynovitis
   e. Scar tissue, fibrosis, or adhesions
   f. Neuroma (of the median palmar sensory branch)

2. Temporary nerve dysfunction resulting from tourniquet use

3. Grip weakness from "bowstringing" of the flexor tendons (may result from inadequate immobilization)

4. Damage to or laceration of the superficial palmar arch

5. Postoperative wound infection (incidence ≈0.5%; may be increased risk with prolonged operative time or use of a surgical chain)
6. Hematoma
7. Hypertrophic scar
8. Reflex sympathetic dystrophy

Selected Readings

Berger RA: Endoscopic tunnel release: A current perspective. Hand Clin 10:625-636, 1994.

Lang EW, Chestnut RM: Intracranial pressure: Monitoring and management. Neurosurg Clin North Am 5:573-605, 1994.

Rosner M: Complications of craniotomy and trauma. *In* Greenfield L (ed): Complications of Craniotomy and Trauma. Philadelphia, JB Lippincott, 1990, pp 677-713.

Young H: Complications of spine surgery and trauma. *In* Greenfield L (ed): Complications of Surgery and Trauma. Philadelphia, JB Lippincott, 1990, pp 713-746.

Index

Note: Page numbers followed by the letter b refer to boxes, those followed by the letter f refer to figures, and those followed by the letter t refer to tables.

A